Handbook of CLINICAL ANAESTHESIA

This book is dedicated to my mother in gratitude for her never-ending support and encouragement over more than half a century

Commissioning Editor: Paul Fam/Alison Ashmore
Project Development Manager: Belinda Henry
Project Manager: Jess Thompson
Design Manager: Jayne Jones
Illustration Manager: Mick Ruddy
Illustrator: Robin Dean

Handbook of CLINICAL ANAESTHESIA

SECOND EDITION

Edited by

Brian J Pollard B Pharm MB ChB MD FRCA

Professor of Anaesthesia
University Department of Anaesthesia
Manchester Royal Infirmary
Manchester
UK

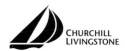

CHURCHILL
LIVINGSTONE

Edinburgh London New York Oxford Philadelphia St Louis Sydney Toronto 2004

CHURCHILL LIVINGSTONE
An imprint of Elsevier Ltd

First edition 1996

ISBN 0443072590

British Library Cataloguing in Publication Data
A catalogue record for this book is available from the British Library

Library of Congress Cataloging in Publication Data
A catalog record for this book is available from the Library of Congress

Notice
Medical knowledge is constantly changing. Standard safety precautions must be followed, but as new research and clinical experience
broaden our knowledge, changes in treatment and drug therapy may
become necessary or appropriate. Readers are advised to check the
most current product information provided by the manufacturer of
each drug to be administered to verify the recommended dose, the
method and duration of administration, and contraindications. It is
the responsibility of the practitioner, relying on experience and knowledge of the patient, to determine dosages and the best treatment for
each individual patient. Neither the Publisher nor the editor assume
any liability for any injury and/or damage to persons or property arising from this publication.

The Publisher

Printed in China

The
publisher's
policy is to use
**paper manufactured
from sustainable forests**

Contents

Contributors

O. Abdelatti MBBS DEAA FFARCS
Consultant Anaesthetist
Rochdale Infirmary
Rochdale
Lancashire
UK

A. Addei MB ChB FRCA
Specialist Registrar
Department of Anaesthesia
Bart's and London NHS Trust
London
UK

M. Y. Aglan MBBCH MSc FFARCSI FRCA DEAF
Consultant in Pain Management and Anaesthesia
Chronic Pain Service
Burnley General Hospital
Manchester
UK

T. Ainley FRCA
Consultant Anaesthetist
Department of Anaesthesia
Charing Cross Hospital
London
UK

U. Akhigbe FRCA
Staff Grade Anaesthetist
Department of Anaesthesia
William Harvey Hospital
Ashford, Kent
UK

R. Alcock MBBS FRCA
Consultant Anaesthetist
Robert Jones and Agnes Hunt Orthopaedic and District Hospital,
Owestry
Shropshire
UK

M. Alveraz FRCA
Specialist Registrar
Department of Anaesthesia
Royal Manchester Infirmary
Manchester
UK

B. Al-Shaikh MBChB FFARCSI
Consultant in Anaesthesia,
Honorary Senior
Lecturer (GKT Medical School) and Clinical Tutor
William Harvey Hospital
Ashford
Kent
UK

I. Appleby MBBS FRCA
Consultant Anaesthetist
Department of Anaesthesia
The National Hospital for Neurology and Neurosurgery
London
UK

K. Ashpole MBBS FRCA
Specialist Registrar in Anaesthesia
Chiswick
London
UK

W. Aveling MA MB BChir FRCA
Consultant Anaesthetist
Department of Anaesthesia
University College London Hospitals
London
UK

R. Balon MBBS FRCA
Consultant Anaesthetist
Department of Anaesthesia
St Mary's Hospital
London
UK

I. Banks MBBS FRCA
Consultant Anaesthetist
Hull Royal Infirmary
Yorkshire
UK

M. Barnard
Cardiothoracic Anaesthetist
The Middlesex Hospital
London
UK

J. Barrie FRCA
Consultant Anaesthetist
Department of Anaesthesia
The Royal Oldham Hospital
Oldham
UK

A. Batchelor MBChB FRCA
Consultant Anaesthesia and Intensive Care Medicine
Royal Victoria Infirmary
Newcastle
UK

J. Beattie MB ChB
Consultant Anaesthetist
Anaesthetic Department
Royal Liverpool University Hospital
Liverpool
UK

M. C. Bellamy BA MBBS MA FRCA
Consultant in Anaesthesia
The Intensive Care Unit
St James's University Hospital
Leeds
UK

S. Berg BSc FRCA
Consultant Paediatric Anaesthetist
Department of Anaesthesia
John Radcliff Hospital
Oxford
UK

P. J. Bickford-Smith FRCA
Consultant Anaesthetist
Anaesthetic Department
Bradford Royal Infirmary
Bradford
West Yorkshire
UK

R. Bingham BS
Consultant Paediatric
    Anaesthetist
Department of Anaesthesia
Great Ormond Street Hospital
London
UK

M. J. Boscoe MBBS FRCA
Consultant Anaesthetist
Department of Anaesthetics
Royal Brompton and Harefield
    NHS Trust
Middlesex
UK

J. Broadfield
Chairman and Consultant
    Anaesthetist,
Department of Anaesthesia
Kings College Hospital
London
UK

**L. Bromley BSc MBBS FRLA
    MHM**
Senior Lecturer in Anaesthesia
Centre for Anaesthesia
Middlesex Hospital
London
UK

K. A. Bruce MSc BSc Hons RGN
Resuscitation Officer
Resuscitation Department
Department of Anaesthesia
Manchester Royal Infirmary
Manchester
UK

H. Buglass MB ChB FRCA
Specialist Registrar
    Anaesthetics
Department of Anaesthesia
St James's University Hospital
Leeds
UK

I. Calder FRCA
Consultant Neuroanaesthetist
National Hospitals for
    Neurology and Neurosurgery
London
UK

A. Campbell MB ChB FRCA
Clinical Fellow in Cardiothoracic
    Anaesthesia and
Intensive Care
The Heart Hospital
University College London
    Hospitals
London
UK

I. T. Campbell MD FRCA
Consultant Anaesthetist
Department of Anaesthesia
Wythenshawe Hospital
Manchester
UK

**C. A. Carr MA(OXON) MBBS
    FRCA**
Consultant Anaesthetist
Moorfields Eye Hospital NHS
    Trust
London
UK

A. J. Charlton MB ChB FRCA
Consultant Paediatric
    Anaesthetist, Honorary
Lecturer, University of
    Manchester
Department of Anaesthesia
Manchester Royal Infirmary
Manchester
UK

P. Charters MD FRCA MRCP
Senior Lecturer in Anaesthesia
Department of Anaesthesia
University Hospital Aintree
Liverpool
UK

S. Christian
Specialist Registrar
Department of Anaesthesia
Good Hope Hospital NHS Trust
Sutton Coldfield
UK

S. Cottam MB CHB FRLA
Consultant Anaesthetist
Department of Anaesthesia
King's College Hospital
London
UK

N. Curry
Specialist Registrar
Department of
    Neuroanaesthesia
The National Hospital for
    Neurology and
Neurosurgery
London
UK

N. Curzen BM (Hons) MRCP
Consultant Anaesthetist
Manchester Royal Infirmary
Manchester
UK

**W. Davies MB ChB DRCOG DCH
    FRCA**
Consultant Anaesthetist
London
UK

M. W. Davies BSc FRCA
Consultant Anaesthetist
Department of Anaesthesia
Royal Liverpool University
    Hospital
Liverpool
UK

K. Demaine MB ChB FRCA
Specialist Registrar in
    Anaesthesia
Department of Anaesthesia
Hope Hospital
Salford
UK

N. Denny FRCA
Consultant Anaesthetist
Department of Anaesthesia
Kings Lynn
Norfolk
UK

J. Desborough MD FRCA
Consultant Anaesthetist
Department of Anaesthetics
Epsom General Hospital
Epsom
Surrey
UK

J. Dinsmore MBBS FRCA
Consultant Anaesthetist
 Department of Anaesthesia
Grosvenor Wing
London
UK

M. Dresner MBBS FRCA
Consultant Obstetric
 Anaesthetist
Department of Anaesthesia
Leeds General Infirmary
Leeds
UK

O. Duff MB
Specialist Registrar in
 Anaesthesia
William Harvey Hospital
Ashford
Kent
UK

R. Edwards MBBS FRCA
Consultant in Anaesthesia and
 Intensive Care Medicine
Anaesthetics Department
Eastbourne District General
 Hospital
East Sussex
UK

W. J. Fawcett MBBS FRCA
Consultant Anaesthetist
Department of Anaesthetics
Royal Surrey County Hospital
Guildford
Surrey
UK

R. Fox
Consultant in Anaesthesia and
 Intensive Care
Royal National Orthopaedic
 Hospital
Stanmore
UK

J. Frossard FRCA
Consultant Anaesthetist
University College School of
 Medicine
The Middlesex Hospital
London
UK

S. Galton
Specialist Registrar
Department of
 Neuroanaesthesia
The National Hospital for
 Neurology and
Neurosurgery
London
UK

J. C. Goldstone MD FRCA
Consultant Department of
 Anaesthesia
and Intensive Care Medicine
UCL Medical School
London
UK

**J. W. W. Gothard MBBS Dip
 (obst) RCOG FRCA**
Consultant Anaesthetist
Department of Anaesthesia
Royal Brompton Hospital
London
UK

**H. Gray MB ChB DA(UK)
 FANZCA**
Clinical Fellow
Department of
 Neuroanaesthesia
The National Hospital for
 Neurology and
Neurosurgery
London
UK

**S. J. Greenhough MB ChB
 FRCA**
Consultant Paediatric
 Anaesthetist
Department of Anaesthesia
Manchester Royal Infirmary
Manchester
Greater Manchester
UK

**E. M. Grundy RD BSc MRCP
 FRCA**
Consultant Anaesthetist
Department of Anaesthetics
University College London
 Hospitals
London
UK

C. Gomersall FRCA
Assistant Professor
Department of Anaesthesia and
 Intensive Care
The Chinese University of Hong
 Kong
Prince of Wales Hospital
Shatin
Hong Kong

C. Gwinnutt MBBS FRCA
Consultant Anaestheist
Hope Hospital
Salford
UK

**G. Hall MBBS MRCS LRCP PhD
 DSc(Med) CBiol FIBiol FRCA**
Chairman & Professor of
 Anaesthesia
Department of Anaesthesia and
 Intensive Care Medicine
St George's Hospital Medical
 School
London
UK

**C. Hamilton-Davies MD MBBS
 FRCA**
Consultant Cardiothoracic
 Anaesthetist
Department of Anaesthetics
University College London
 Hospitals
London
UK

J. Hammond MBBS FRCA
Senior Registrar in Anaesthesia
Department of Anaesthesia
Withington Hospital
Manchester
UK

J. Handy BSc MBBS FRCA
Specialist Registrar in
 Anaesthesia and Intensive
 Care Medicine
Imperial College School of
 Medicine
London
UK

**R. J. Harding MBBS BMedSci
    FRCA**
Specialist Registrar in
    Anaesthesia
Department of Anaesthesia
St James's University Hospital
Leeds
UK

**W. Harrop-Griffiths MA MBBS
    FRCA**
Consultant Anaesthetist
Department of Anaesthetics
St. Mary's NHS Trust
London
UK

N.P Hirsch MBBS FRCA
Consultant in Neuroanaesthesia
The National Hospital for
    Neurology and
Neurosurgery
London
UK

C. A. Hodgson BSc MBBS FRCA
Consultant Anaesthetist
Department of Anaesthesia
University Hospital Aintree
Liverpool
UK

P. M. Hopkins MBBS MF FRCA
Professor of Anaesthesia
Academic Unit of Anaesthesia
St. James's University Hospital
Leeds
UK

J. M. Hopkinson MB ChB FRCA
Consultant Anaesthetist
Bolton Hospitals NHS Trust
UK

E. L. Horsman FRCA
Consultant Anaesthetist
Department of Anaesthesia
Manchester Royal Infirmary
Manchester
UK

J. M. Hull FRCA
Consultant Anaesthetist
Department of Anaesthesia
Good Hope Hospital NHS Trust
Sutton Coldfield
UK

K. Hunt FRCA
Consultant Anaesthetist
Department of
    Neuroanaesthesia
The National Hospital for
    Neurology and
Neurosurgery
London
UK

M. J. Jones FRCA
Consultant Anaesthetist
Department of Anaesthesia
Glenfield Hospital
Leicester
UK

J. Jones BA BsC FRCP FFARCS
Consultant Anaesthetist
Department of Anaesthesia
St Mary's Hospital
London
UK

**M. J. Jordan MA MB BChir
    FRCA**
Consultant Anaesthetist
Ashford St Peter's Hospital
Chertsy
Surrey
UK

R. Kandasamy MBBS FRCA
Consultant Anaesthetist
Department of Anaesthesia
University Hospital Aintree
Liverpool
UK

B. Keogh MBBS FRCA
Consultant Anaesthetist
Department of Anaesthesia
Royal Brompton Hospital
London
UK

S. K. Kodakat MBBS MD FRCA
Consultant in Anaesthesia and
    Intensive Care
Manchester Royal Infirmary
Manchester
UK

R. Langford
Consultant in Anaesthesia
Intensive Care Unit
St Bartholemew's Hospital
London
UK

A. Leonard
Acute Pain Sister
Department of Anaesthesia
Manchester Royal Infirmary
Manchester
UK

A. Loach MA MB BChir FRCA
Department of Anaesthesia
The John Radcliffe Hospital
Headley Way
Oxford,
UK

A. T. Lovell
Consultant Anaesthetist
Department of Anaesthesia
Bristol Royal Infirmary
Bristol
UK

D. T. Moloney
Consultant in Anaesthesia
University Hospital Aintree
Liverpool
UK

I. McConachie FRCA
Consultant Anaesthetist
Blackpool Victoria Hospital
Blackpool
UK

P. McKenzie MD FRCA
Consultant Anaesthetist
John Radcliffe Hospital
Headington
UK

P. McQuillan FRCA FFICANZCA
Consultant in Anaesthesia and
    Intensive Care
Department of Intensive Care
    Medicine
Queen Alexandra Hospital
Portsmouth
UK

A. MacKillop
Specialist Registrar
Consultant Anaesthetist
Bury General Hospital
Bury
UK

S. Mallet
Consultant Anaesthetist
Department of Anaesthesia
Royal Free Hospital
London
UK

G. H. Meakin MB ChB MD FRCA
Senior Lecturer in Paediatric
  Anaesthesia, Honorary
Consultant in Paediatric
  Anaesthesia
University Department of
  Anaesthesia
Royal Manchester Children's
  Hospital
Manchester
UK

R. Milaszkiewicz MBBS FRCA
Consultant Anaesthetist
Department of Anaesthesia
Barnet General Hospital
UK

**D. M. Miller MB ChB FFA(SA)
  PhD**
Consultant Anaesthetist
GKT Department of Anaesthesia
New Guy's House
London
UK

L. Milligan BSc MB ChB FRCA
Specialist Registrar in
  Anaesthesia
Intensive Care Unit
St James's University Hospital
Leeds
UK

C. Morgan BM FRCA
Consultant Anaesthetist
Department of Anaesthetics
Royal Brompton Hospital
London
UK

**A. J. Mortimer BSc (Hons) MD
  FRCA**
Consultant in Anaesthesia and
  Intensive Care
Department of Anaesthesia
Wythenshawe Hospital
Manchester
UK

S. M. Mostafa MD FRCA
Consultant in Anaesthesia and
  Intensive Care Medicine
Royal Liverpool Hospital
Liverpool
UK

I. Munday FRCA
Consultant Anaesthetist
Department of Anaesthesia
Cambridge
UK

P. Newman FRCA
Anaesthetics Department
St Georges Hospital
London
UK

**N. I. Newton MA BM BcH DA
  FRCA**
Consultant Anaesthetist
Department of Anaesthetics
Guy's and St Thomas' Hospital
  Trust
London
UK

M. Newton FRCA MBBS
Consultant Neuroanaesthetist
Department of
  Neuroanaesthesia
The National Hospital for
  Neurology and
Neurosurgery
London
UK

**P. Nightingale MBBS FRCA
  FRCP**
Consultant Anaesthetist
Intensive Care Unit
Acute Block
Withenshawe Hospital
Manchester
UK

D. M. Nolan MB ChB FRCA
Consultant Anaesthetist
Department of Anaesthesia
Withenshawe Hospital
Manchester
UK

D. O'Connor FRCA
Consultant Anaesthetist
Department of Anaesthesia
Royal Perth Hospital
Perth
Australia

D. O'Malley RGN
Department of Anaesthesia
Manchester Royal Infirmary
Manchester
UK

D. Østergaard MD
Department of Anaesthesiology
University of Copenhagen
Herlev Hospital
Herlev
Denmark

H. Owen Reece BSc FRCA
Consultant in Anaesthesia
Department of Anaesthesia
The Middlesex Hospital
London
UK

**C. Parker MA MB Bchir MD
  FRCA**
Consultant Anaesthetist
Royal Liverpool University
  Hospital
Liverpool
UK

D. Patel MBChB FRCA
Consultant Paediatric
  Anaesthetist
Department of Anaesthesia
Royal Manchester Children's
  Hospital
Manchester
Greater Manchester
UK

A. C. Pearce MB BChir FRCA
Consultant Anaesthetist
Department of Anaesthesia
Guy's Hospital (2nd Floor)
London
UK

D. Phillips MB ChB FRCA
Consultant Anaesthetist
Lincoln County Hospital
Lincoln
UK

S. Piggott FRCA
Consultant Anaesthetist
Department of Anaesthesia
Derby City Hospital
Derby
UK

S. Polhill MB
Specialist Registrar in
  Anaesthesia
William Harvey Hospital
Ashford
Kent
UK

B. J. Pollard B Pharm MB ChB MD FRCA
Professor of Anaesthesia
University Department of
   Anaesthesia
Manchester Royal Infirmary
Manchester
UK

C. J. D Pomfrett BSc PhD
Lecturer in Neurophysiology
   Applied to Anaesthesia
University Department of
   Anaesthesia
University of Manchester
Manchester
UK

J. S. Porter
Department of Anaesthesia
The National Hospital for
   Neurology and Neurosurgery
Queens Square
London
UK

M. Price BSc MBBS FRCA
Consultant Anaesthetist
Department of Anaesthesia
St Mary's Hospital
London
UK

A. Quinn MBChB FFARCSI
Consultant Neuroanaesthetist
Anaesthetics Department
Leeds General Infirmary
Leeds
UK

J. J. Radcliffe FRCA
Consultant Neuroanaesthetist
National Hospital for Neurology
   and Neurosurgery
London
UK

N. P. C. Randall BM FRCA
Consultant in Anaesthesia
Department of Anaesthesia
Victoria Hospital
Blackpool
UK

P. R. Saunders MBBS FRCA
Consultant Anaesthetist
Department of Anaesthesia
Royal Surrey County Hospital
Surrey
UK

M. Scallan MB ChB FRCA
Consultant Anaesthetist
Department of Anaesthesia
Royal Brompton Hospital
London
UK

S. M. Scuplak MBBS
Consultant Anaesthetist
Great Ormond Street Hospital
   for Children
London
UK

J. R. Shelgaonkar FRCA
Specialist Registrar in
   Anaesthesia
William Harvey Hospital
Ashford
Kent
UK

A. M. Severn MA FRCA
Consultant Anaesthetist
Department of Anaesthesia
Royal Lancaster Infirmary
Lancaster
UK

M. Simpson
Consultant Anaesthetist
Department of Anaesthetics
Manchester Royal Infirmary
Manchester
UK

M. Sivaloganathan FRCA
Research Fellow in Anaesthesia
Department of Anaesthesia
Institute of Child Health
London
UK

R. M. Slater FRCA
Consultant Anaesthetist
Queen's Medical Centre
Nottingham
UK

G. B. Smith BM ICTM FRCA FRCP
Consultant in Intensive Care
   Medicine
Honorary Senior Lecturer in
   Critical Care
Portsmouth Hospitals NHS
   Trust
Portsmouth
UK

M. Smith MBBS FRCA
Consultant Neuroanaesthetist
Department for
   Neuroanaesthesia and
   Critical Care
The National Hospital For
   Neurology &
Neurosurgery
London
UK

N. Soni MB ChB FRCA FANZCA MD FFICANZCA
Consultant in Anaesthesia and
   Intensive Care
Chelsea and Westminster
   Hospital
London
UK

S. Stacey FRCA
Consultant Anaesthetist
Bart's and London NHS Trust
London
UK

R. Stephens BA MBBS FRCA
Academy of Medical Sciences
   Research Training
Fellow
Protex Unit
London
UK

T. Strang MB ChB DCH FRCA
Consultant Anaesthetist
CICU
South Manchester University
   Hospital
Manchester
UK

B. L. Taylor BSc FRCA DCH
Consultant in Anaesthesia and
   Intensive Care Medicine
Department of Anaesthesia
Portsmouth Hospitals NHS
   Trust
Portsmouth
UK

V. Taylor MB ChB FRCA
Consultant Anaesthetist
Royal National Orthopaedic
   Hospital
Middlesex
UK

G. Thomas
Specialist Registrar
Department of
    Neuroanaesthesia
The National Hospital for
    Neurology and
Neurosurgery
London
UK

**N. M. Tierney BSc MB ChB
    FRCA**
Consultant Anaesthetist
Department of Anaesthesia
Fairfield General Hospital
Bury
UK

R. Vanner FRCA
Consultant Anaesthestist
Department of Anaesthesia
Gloucestershire Royal NHS
    Trust Hospital
Gloucester
UK

S. Varley MBBS FRCA
Consultant Anaesthetist
Manchester Royal Infirmary
Manchester
UK

G. Venkatesan FRCA
Specialist Registrar Anaesthesia
Department of Anaesthesia
Blackpool Victoria Hospital
Blackpool
UK

M. Venning
Consultant Anaesthetist
Department of Anaesthesia
Manchester Royal Infirmary
Manchester
UK

J. Viby-Mogenson MD DMSc
Professor and Chairman
Department of Anaesthesia and
    Intensive Care
The National University Hospital
Rigshospitalet
Blegdamsvej
Denmark

A. Vohra MB ChB DA FRCA
Consultant in Cardiothoracic
    Anaesthesia and Critical
Care
Department of Anaesthesia,
Manchester Royal Infirmary
Manchester
UK

U. Waheed FRCA
Specialist Registrar in
    Anaesthesia and Intensive
    Care
National Hospital for Neurology
    and Neurosurgery
London
UK

R. Walker MBChB DCH FRCA
Consultant in Paediatric
    Anaesthesia
University Department of
    Anaesthesia
Royal Manchester Childrens
    Hospital
Manchester
UK

N. Watson MBBS FRCA
Consultant Anaesthetist &
    director of Critical Care
Department of Anaesthesia
Eastbourne District General
    Hospital
East Sussex
UK

M. Weisz MB ChB FRCA
Consultant Anaesthetist
Department of Anaesthesia
Peterborough Hospital NHS
    Trust
Cambridgeshire
UK

R. Wenstone MBChB, FRCA
Consultant in Intensive Care
    and Anaesthesia
Royal Liverpool University
    Hospital
Liverpool
UK

S. Wilmshurst MB ChB FRCA
Specialist Registrar in
    Anaesthesia
Department of Anaesthesia
Wythenshawe Hospital
Manchester

S. R. Wilson FRCA
Consultant Neuroanaesthetist
Department of
    Neuroanaesthesia
The National Hospital for
    Neurology and
Neurosurgery
London
UK

Preface

Preparing the second edition of a book is a very important step. It is an indication that the first edition was popular and that there is a need for a new version. It is also an appropriate time to critically evaluate the contents. I hope that this second edition lives up to its expectations.

The overall philosophy of this second edition of the *Handbook* is identical to that of the first, namely to approach individual problems and to address them in a concise and readable form, readily assimilated by busy clinicians. Each article tries to maintain as consistent a format as possible beginning with the pathophysiology and continuing through the anaesthetic sequence ending with postoperative management. This sort of structured approach is one favoured by many examiners in postgraduate examinations. The monographs are written by individuals almost all of whom are practising clinicians and who have experience in the field and an appreciation of the important issues.

The articles have been collected together in a problem orientated way and an attempt has been made to arrange the problems in a similar fashion to their appearance in the clinical situation. Thus a surgical referral is usually the starting point. Issues with respect to the surgery as well as co-existing medical problems become apparent at the preoperative visit. The particular anaesthetic technique is planned and consideration given to various related matters. Finally, variations in technique, complications and potential solutions to these are presented. There are inevitable areas of overlap between some sections and topics but these are necessary in a work such as this.

The book has been divided up into three principal parts, namely Patient Conditions, Surgical Procedures and Anaesthetic Factors. Each of these is subdivided systematically. An overall index is supplied to guide the reader rapidly to specific facts, and cross references are supplied at the end of most of the monographs to guide the reader in appropriate onward directions. Not every eventuality has been covered of course – that would be impossible in a book of this size. It is not a replacement for major texts or review articles but in it the reader should find guidance to cover most everyday problems. There will be many ways to use this book and individuals will develop their own method, probably annotating the margins with additional points relevant to their own particular practice.

I must thank each and every contributor who has written for the book. They were presented with near-impossible deadlines and still delivered! Some of the contributors who wrote for the first edition have retired, disappeared without trace, or for other reasons were unable to work on the revision. I should like to thank them also for their original contribution to the first edition because in a few cases the monographs for this second edition have been built onto their original text.

Finally I must sincerely thank my friend and colleague Dr John Goldstone who was my co-editor in the first edition. We both began to pull together this second edition as a two-man team at the start. Owing to other pressures on his time, however, John had to unfortunately withdraw during the early phases of the project. I am grateful to him for helping to start the project in the first place and I hope that he approves of the way it has turned out.

BJP
Manchester
2003

PART 1

PATIENT CONDITIONS

1

CENTRAL NERVOUS SYSTEM
J. J. Radcliffe
M. Smith

Autonomic dysfunction

N. P. Hirsch

Autonomic dysfunction (dysautonomia) may be either a result of a central nervous disorder (congenital, idiopathic, degenerative) or, commonly, a disorder of the peripheral nervous system (Box 1.1).

BOX 1.1

Classification of clinically important autonomic neuropathies

- Central nervous system disorders
- Pure autonomic failure
- Autonomic failure with multisystem atrophy (Shy–Drager syndrome)
- Autonomic failure with Parkinson's disease
- Peripheral nervous system disorders
- Diabetes
- Primary amyloidosis
- Porphyria
- Guillain–Barré syndrome
- Familial dysautonomia (Riley–Day syndrome)

PATHOPHYSIOLOGY

Although the pathophysiological mechanisms causing the autonomic dysfunction vary depending on the aetiology, the symptoms that result are remarkably similar.

CARDIOVASCULAR
In normal individuals, assumption of the erect position from the supine position results in a transient fall in arterial blood pressure due to a decrease in the venous return to the heart. Compensatory mechanisms involving aortic and carotid baroreceptors and the vasomotor and cardioinhibitory centres result in an increase in vasomotor tone and heart rate. Arterial blood pressure is rapidly returned to normal levels. In patients with autonomic dysfunction the compensatory mechanisms are impaired and, on standing, a sustained period of hypotension follows (orthostatic hypotension). Similarly, the response to the Valsalva manoeuvre is abnormal.

RESPIRATORY SYSTEM
Heart rate normally increases during inspiration (sinus arrhythmia) due to inhibition of the cardioinhibitory vasomotor centres by the central inspiratory drive centres. This response is lost in some forms of autonomic dysfunction.

In the Shy–Drager syndrome, abductor vocal cord paralysis may result in problems with phonation and in inspiratory stridor. Poor central respiratory control, weakness of respiratory muscles and recurrent aspiration pneumonia are common features of familial dysautonomia.

GUT
Disorders of oesophageal and gastric motility may occur, as may poor sphincter control. Gastric emptying may be delayed, resulting in greater than normal resting gastric volume. Constipation may be a feature.

GENITOURINARY SYSTEM
Urinary retention is common, as is impotence.

OTHER
The normal sweating response may be impaired.

PREOPERATIVE ASSESSMENT AND TREATMENT

HISTORY:
- Of the underlying disorder if present (e.g. diabetes mellitus) and any coexisting disorder (e.g. ischaemic heart disease)
- Of postural hypotension, syncope, intestinal stasis and disorders of sweating
- In the case of the Shy–Drager syndrome, look for history of problems with phonation associated with vocal cord paralysis.

INVESTIGATIONS:
- Assessment of the underlying medical disorder
- Response of heart rate (using R-R interval of ECG) to altered posture and to the Valsalva manoeuvre
- More specialised investigations, including sympathetic skin response testing, sweat tests and plasma catecholamine levels.

PREOPERATIVE TREATMENT
In most cases, autonomic disturbances are not of sufficient severity to warrant specific preoperative therapy. If postural hypotension is causing symptoms, treatment is directed to increasing blood volume by increasing dietary intake of salt, and by the use of fludrocortisone. Simple measures such as the wearing of graded elastic stockings may help.

In the period leading up to surgery, attention should be directed towards ensuring adequate hydration, using intravenous crystalloid if necessary.

PERIOPERATIVE MANAGEMENT

PREMEDICATION
Drugs that have major effects on the autonomic system (e.g. anticholinergic drugs, the phenothiazines and butyrophenones) should be avoided. If sedative premedication is necessary, a benzodiazepine should be given.

H_2-receptor antagonists should be given to patients with delayed gastric emptying.

MONITORING
Prior to anaesthetic induction:
- ECG (lead CM5)
- Blood pressure measurement (via indwelling arterial cannula if autonomic dysfunction is severe)
- SpO_2
- Central venous pressure (CVP) or pulmonary capillary wedge pressure (PCWP) measurement, if indicated
- Temperature measurement (poor temperature homeostasis may result in hypothermia if procedure is prolonged).

INDUCTION AND MAINTENANCE OF ANAESTHESIA
Induction of anaesthesia and the maintenance of anaesthesia with volatile anaesthetic agents may cause precipitous falls in arterial blood pressure in this group of patients. Such agents must therefore be used with great care and in the lowest doses possible. Similarly, the introduction of intermittent positive-pressure ventilation (IPPV) may cause hypotension.

A rapid sequence induction may be indicated in patients with delayed gastric emptying and those with a history of recurrent aspiration.

If hypotension occurs, treat initially with a fluid challenge. If this proves unsuccessful, give a small dose of an α-receptor agonist (e.g. methoxamine). Be aware that this may result in a large rise in arterial blood pressure; sensitivity to direct-acting sympathomimetics and an unpredictable response to indirect agents is a feature. If bradycardia is present, this is readily treated with an anticholinergic drug.

REGIONAL ANAESTHESIA
The hypotensive effect of extradural and spinal anaesthesia may be exaggerated in these patients, perhaps due to a combination of intravascular volume depletion and impaired compensatory vasoconstriction.

POSTOPERATIVE CARE

- Maintain adequate hydration.
- Adequate postoperative pain relief is essential. Apnoea following narcotic administration is common.
- Stridor may occur in the postoperative period in the Shy–Drager syndrome.

BIBLIOGRAPHY

Axelrod FB, Donenfield RF, Danzier F, Turndorf H. Anaesthesia in familial dysautonomia. Anesthesiology 1988; 68:631–635

Drury PME, Williams EGN. Vocal cord paralysis in the Shy–Drager syndrome. Anaesthesia 1991; 46:466–468

Hutchinson RC, Sugden JC. Anaesthesia for Shy–Drager syndrome. Anaesthesia 1984; 39:1229–1231

CROSS-REFERENCES

Diabetes mellitus (IDDM)
    Patient Conditions 2: 56
Intraoperative hypotension
    Anaesthetic Factors 31: 758

Brain stem death

U. Waheed and S. R. Wilson

1

The brain stem determines the ability to breathe independently and is a conduit for nerve fibres between the periphery and the central nervous system. Because the reticular activating system passes through the brain stem, the capacity for consciousness is lost when the brain stem dies. The brain stem also influences cardiovascular function (asystole follows brain stem death).

Brain stem death is defined as the irreversible loss of the capacity for consciousness, combined with the irreversible loss of the capacity to breathe. It is important to differentiate between the diagnoses of brain stem death and persistent vegetative state for the purposes of management, the latter being associated with massive cortical damage and intact brain stem reflexes.

The criteria governing the diagnosis were first highlighted in the USA at Harvard in 1968 and then in Minnesota in 1976. In the UK in 1976, the Conference of Medical Royal Colleges and Faculties described what is now accepted as the criteria for testing brain stem death. This has remained essentially unchanged except for modifications by 'The Working Party' in 1998. The important difference between the UK and USA is that the tests in the UK are purely clinical.

PHYSIOLOGICAL CHANGES AFTER BRAIN STEM DEATH

CARDIOVASCULAR
Sympathetic storm (increases in heart rate, blood pressure, cardiac output, systemic vascular resistance (SVR) – Cushing's reflex), followed by:
- Myocardial impairment
- Pulmonary oedema
- Hypotension
- Arrhythmias.

ENDOCRINE:
- Pituitary failure, resulting in:
  —reduced levels of T3 and T4 (undetectable after 16 h)
  —diabetes insipidus (antidiuretic hormone (ADH) undetectable after 6 h) leading to inappropriate diuresis, hypovolaemia, hyperosmolality, hypernatraemia
  —reduced cortisol levels (up to 50%)
  —hyperglycaemia secondary to reduced insulin secretion (20% of normal after 13 h) or iatrogenic treatment of hypernatraemia with 5% dextrose and increased levels of catecholamines.
- Coagulopathy:
  —tissue thromboplastin release leading to disseminated intravascular coagulation.
- Hypothermia:
  —loss of hypothalamic control
  —fall in metabolic rate and muscle activity
  —peripheral vasodilatation.

METABOLIC:
- Reduced myocardial energy stores
- Increased anaerobic metabolism
- Increased lactate and free fatty acids
- Metabolic acidosis.

BRAIN STEM TESTS

The declaration of brain stem death requires not only a series of careful neurological tests but also the fulfilment of set preconditions and exclusions.

PRECONDITIONS:
1. Apnoeic coma – the patient is unresponsive and dependent on a ventilator
2. Proven irremediable structural brain damage – may be obvious when associated with a primary intracranial event. However, when associated with hypoxia secondary to cardiac arrest or cerebral air or fat embolism, it may take longer to establish the diagnosis and to be confident of the prognosis.

Major causes include:
- Severe head injury (50%)
- Intracranial haemorrhage (30%)

- Cerebral malignancy, abscess, meningitis, encephalitis (19%)
- Cerebral oedema secondary to hypoxia (1%).

EXCLUSIONS:

- Drug intoxication; sedatives, neuromuscular blocking agents, narcotics, etc.
- Allow greater than three times half-life of drug before testing.
- Benzodiazepine and barbiturates are cumulative in their actions and it may be necessary to measure drug concentrations to ensure that the levels are subhypnotic.
- Hypothermia – temperature must be higher than 35°C.
- Severe hypotension – adequate mean arterial pressure needs to be maintained
- Primary metabolic or endocrine disturbance, such as:
  —diabetic coma
  —uraemia
  —hepatic encephalopathy.

Hypernatraemia is a symptom rather than a cause. If hypernatraemia is secondary to brain stem death, it can be ignored and does not need to be corrected before the tests are performed.

Two physicians are required independently or together to perform the tests, although no data have suggested that a second assessment by a different physician reduces error or the possibility of negligence. The tests may be carried out separately or together. Both physicians (one a consultant) should be experienced (registered with the General Medical Council for more than 5 years) and not part of any transplant team.

Examination of the brain stem reflexes involves measurement of the pathways in the mesencephalon, pons and medulla oblongata. Patients often lose their reflexes in a rostral to caudal direction, with the medulla being the last part of the brain to cease to function.

CLINICAL DETERMINATION OF BRAIN STEM DEATH

The following reflexes must be absent:
- *Pupillary reflex* – pupils remain fixed and dilated to an external light stimulus (cranial nerves II and III).
- *Corneal reflex* – elicited by touching the edge of the cornea (nerves V and VII). Care must be taken not to damage the cornea, as this may be required for donation.
- *Vestibulo-ocular reflex* – no tonic deviation towards the side of the cold stimulus provided by ice-cold water in the external

ear. The eardrums must be viewed first. If they are not visible, for example if there is clotted blood or wax present, they must be cleared. The doll's eye reflex – the absence of oculocephalic movements on rapid turning of the head (VIII, III, VI) – is occasionally used.
- *Gag or cough reflex* – the cough reflex is elicited by introducing a suction catheter deep in the trachea. Moving the tracheal tube back and forth may not be an adequate stimulus and is not recommended. The gag reflex is tested by bilateral pharyngeal stimulation (IX, X).
- *Cranial motor response to pain* – determined by the absence of grimacing or eye opening following pressure on either (or both) condyles at the level of the temporomandibular joint, on the supraorbital ridge or on the nail bed of the fingers. Body movements may be seen that are manifestations of primal spinal reflexes and are therefore ignored in this context. It is important to note that in the presence of proven spinal injury the test may be concentrated solely on the cranial nerves (V, VII).

APNOEA TEST:

- Preoxygenation with 100% oxygen for 10 min. This eliminates the stores of respiratory nitrogen and accelerates the transport of oxygen.
- Perform an arterial blood gas analysis.
- Ideally disconnect the ventilator when normocapnoea is present. A catheter is then passed via the tracheal tube (the tip should be placed at the carina) to deliver oxygen at about 6 l min^{-1}. The patient must be observed for 10 min. Signs of chest and/or abdominal wall movements must be noted together with any changes in vital signs. The test should be abandoned if cardiovascular complications arise (e.g. hypotension or cardiac arrhythmias). These two complications are often due to failure to provide an adequate source of oxygen or inadequate preoxygenation.
- A repeat arterial blood gas is obtained after 10 min and the patient is deemed apnoeic when the PCO$_2$ is greater than 6.65 kPa.

The legal time of death is after the first set of tests, although death is usually pronounced after the second set. Legally, the relatives' permission is not required to discontinue ventilation, but in practice this is desirable. Organ donation should be considered in all brain-dead patients, and the

1

relatives should be approached after the first set of tests.

CONFIRMATORY TESTS

In many European, Asian and South American countries additional testing is required by law to support the diagnosis of brain death. Physicians in Sweden require cerebral angiography, and in the USA the choice is left to the discretion of the examining doctors, although bedside tests seem to be the preference. These additional tests may include the following.

Cerebral angiography

This is performed with an injection in the aortic arch to visualise both the anterior and posterior circulation. No blood flow on a four-vessel angiogram establishes the irreversibility of coma. Arrest of flow in the posterior circulation is found at the foramen magnum and at the petrosal portion in the anterior circulation.

Magnetic resonance angiography may produce similar views.

Electroencephalography

The most popular and validated of the confirmatory tests. Recordings are obtained for 30 min. Electrical activity is absent at levels higher than 2 μV in patients who are found to be brain dead. However, it has been shown that over-sedated patients who subsequently recover also show an absence of activity at this level.

Transcranial Doppler ultrasonography

This method shows there is absent diastolic or reverberating flow of the middle cerebral and vertebral arteries caused by the contractive force of the vessels.

Nuclear imaging

This method detects the uptake of technetium by cerebral tissue, although this technique is not as sensitive as the other tests.

Brain stem evoked potentials

The absence of brain stem evoked potentials establishes the irreversibility of coma.

BIBLIOGRAPHY

The Working Party. A code of practice for the diagnosis of brain stem death. London: Department of Health; 1998

Van Norman GA. A matter of life and death: what every anesthesiologist should know about the medical, legal, and ethical aspects of declaring brain death. Anesthesiology 1999; 91:275–287

Wijdicks Eelco FM. The diagnosis of brain death. New England Journal of Medicine 2001; 344:1215–1221

CROSS-REFERENCES

Management of the organ donor
Surgical Procedures 21: 528

1

Epilepsy

M. Smith

Epilepsy is a common disorder occurring in approximately 1 in 200 of the general population. It is a chronic illness resulting from an underlying disorder of neuronal activity, and characterised by recurrent seizure activity. Despite considerable progress in the medical management of epilepsy and the development of new anticonvulsant drugs, some patients remain refractory to therapy or develop intolerable side-effects. Surgery is an alternative and increasingly favourable option for patients with a discrete seizure focus that may be resected without producing neurological deficits.

PATHOPHYSIOLOGY

Epilepsy may be long-standing or develop *de novo* secondary to another pathology (e.g. brain tumour). Electrical activity in the brain is normally well controlled, but in epileptogenic disorders normal brain regulatory functions are altered. Sudden and disordered neuronal activity is responsible for the clinical manifestations of epilepsy. In epilepsy there is:

- Loss of postsynaptic inhibition
- Introduction of significant excitatory synaptic connections
- The appearance of pacemaker neurones.

Pacemaker neurones appear to be the centre of the epileptic focus and have the capacity to produce spontaneous burst discharges, which are recognised as interictal spikes on the EEG. Increased cellular activity and loss of normal inhibitory tone allow spread of these discharges to surrounding areas, resulting in uncontrolled neuronal firing and seizure activity. Changes in membrane flux, impaired γ-aminobutyric acid (GABA)-mediated synaptic inhibition and alterations in local neurotransmitter levels are implicated in this process.

CLASSIFICATION

Epilepsy may be generalised or partial (Box 1.2). Generalised epilepsies occur in 20% of

patients with epilepsy, involve both hemispheres, and are associated with an initial impairment of consciousness. Simple partial seizures are caused by a localised discharge and there is no impairment of consciousness. In complex partial seizures the initial focal discharge spreads widely and secondary loss of consciousness occurs. This is the most common seizure disorder and includes temporal lobe epilepsy (TLE). The typical EEG finding is the interictal spike and, in a high proportion of patients, high-quality magnetic resonance imaging (MRI) demonstrates hippocampal sclerosis. Under such circumstances, extended temporal lobectomy may offer a reduction of seizure frequency and severity.

BOX 1.2

Classification of the epilepsies

- Generalised epilepsy:
  - —generalised absence – petit mal
  - —generalised tonic–clonic – grand mal
  - —myoclonic
  - —tonic–atonic – drop attacks
- Partial epilepsy:
  - —complex partial – temporal lobe epilepsy
  - —simple partial

ANTICONVULSANT THERAPY

The aim of medical treatment in epilepsy is a seizure-free patient with minimal side-effects. Correct choice of anticonvulsant agent involves consideration of seizure type, seizure history, patient age and side-effects (Table 1.1). Therapy is initiated with a single agent given in a dose sufficient to produce adequate plasma levels. If seizures continue, or if unacceptable side-effects develop, a second agent is substituted for the first. Monotherapy is sufficient to control seizures in many patients, but some require addition of second- or third-line agents.

1

TABLE 1.1

Anticonvulsants: first-line indications and side-effects

Drug	First-line indication	Side-effects
Phenytoin	Grand mal Complex partial Tonic-clonic	Rash, gingival hypertrophy, ataxia, megaloblastic anaemia, Stevens–Johnson syndrome, neuropathy, encephalopathy
Sodium valproate	Grand mal Tonic-clonic	Tremor, weight gain, alopecia, thrombocytopaenia raised hepatic transaminase, hepatic failure
Carbamazepine	Complex	Rash, sedation, thrombocytopaenia, diplopia, leukopaenia, cholestasis, hyponatraemia
Phenobarbital	Complex	Rash, hypersensitivity, sedation, megaloblastic anaemia, osteomalacia, folate deficiency
Ethosuximide	Petit mal	Nausea, sedation, ataxia, confusion, photophobia, thrombocytopaenia
Primidone	Complex	Ataxia, nystagmus, sedation, thrombocytopaenia, leukopaenia
Vigabatrin	Second line	Sedation, irritability, aggression, psychosis, weight gain, mild anaemia
Lamotrigine	Second line	Rash, diplopia, dizziness, sedation, headache, ataxia, irritability, gastrointestinal disturbance, Stevens–Johnson syndrome

PREOPERATIVE ASSESSMENT

The patient's history should be evaluated in relation to the epilepsy and other coexisting medical problems. Particular attention should be paid to:
• Seizure frequency
• Seizure type and pattern
• Current anticonvulsant therapy (including plasma levels)
• Complications of anticonvulsant therapy (Table 1.1)
• IQ (poorly controlled chronic epilepsy may be associated with low IQ).
Anticonvulsant therapy must be continued up to and including the day of operation. Plasma anticonvulsant levels must be checked and doses adjusted as appropriate. Premedication may be prescribed as required, and benzo-diazepines are appropriate.

ANAESTHETIC AGENTS AND THE EEG

The action of anaesthetic agents on the EEG is complex. Paradoxically, many agents have been reported to cause clinical seizure activity whilst also possessing anticonvulsant actions. This effect is dose related. Low doses generally have proconvulsant actions and higher doses anticonvulsant activity.

BARBITURATES
Most barbiturates are anticonvulsants at normal clinical doses, and thiopental may be used to control seizures. Thiopental infusion has also been used in the treatment of status epilepticus. Methohexitone, however, activates the EEG and should be avoided in epileptic patients.

PROPOFOL
Propofol has been shown to activate the EEG in temporal lobe epilepsy, and to produce seizures and opisthotonos in non-epileptic patients. Conversely, anticonvulsant effects have also been reported, and propofol is widely used in the treatment of status epilepticus resistant to other therapies. It is now clear that propofol has a profound dose-dependent effect on the EEG and produces activation at small doses and burst suppression (anticonvulsant action) at higher (clinical) doses.

BENZODIAZEPINES
Diazepam and other benzodiazepines have anticonvulsant EEG effects and are widely used in the treatment of seizures.

INHALATIONAL AGENTS AND NITROUS OXIDE

The EEG effects of inhalational anaesthetic agents are dose dependent. EEG activity is maintained with isoflurane concentrations of less than 1 minimum alveolar concentration (MAC), although background epileptiform activity may be suppressed. Low-dose isoflurane has been used in the treatment of resistant status epilepticus. Higher inspired concentrations of isoflurane have profound effects on the EEG and at levels greater than 2 MAC the EEG becomes isoelectric. Sevoflurane and desflurane have isoflurane-like effects on the EEG. The effects of halothane are also similar to those of isoflurane, with background epileptic activity being suppressed at clinically useful concentrations. High-dose enflurane, on the other hand has convulsant activity, which is exaggerated in the presence of increased $PaCO_2$. Dose-dependent EEG changes occur with nitrous oxide, with anticonvulsant effects predominating at higher inspired concentrations.

OPIOIDS

Opioids have minimal effect on the EEG at usual clinical doses, although marked EEG slowing occurs at high doses. Fentanyl at moderate doses ($25 \mu g\ kg^{-1}$) causes modest activation of the EEG, whereas high-dose opioid techniques result in EEG slowing. Alfentanil increases epileptiform activity and should be avoided in patients with epilepsy. Remifentanil, however, appears to be safe in epileptic patients and may be used during epilepsy surgery with minimal impact on intraoperative EEG recording.

LOCAL ANAESTHETICS

Lidocaine (lignocaine) has a biphasic effect on the EEG. At low plasma levels it has anticonvulsant-like actions, whereas at high levels it causes excitation of the central nervous system, including the provocation of seizures.

ANAESTHETIC TECHNIQUE

Patients with epilepsy may present for surgery for incidental conditions, following injury during a seizure, or for neurosurgery for medically intractable epilepsy. General or local anaesthesia may be provided using standard techniques that avoid factors known to precipitate seizures (Box 1.3). Anaesthetic agents that are proconvulsant at usual clinical doses should be avoided.

BOX 1.3

Causes of seizures in the perioperative period

- Pre-existing epilepsy
- Subtherapeutic anticonvulsant levels
- Hypoxia
- Hypercarbia
- Proconvulsant drugs and anaesthetic agents
- Electrolyte disturbances:
  —hyponatraemia
  —hypoglycaemia
  —uraemia
- Related disorders:
  —head injury
  —eclampsia

Specific requirements for the management of a patient undergoing epilepsy surgery include the recording of intraoperative cerebral electrical activity (the electrocorticogram or ECoG) and/or activation of the epileptic focus. Knowledge of the effects of anaesthetic agents on the EEG allows a rational choice of technique to be made (see above). Careful titration of the end-tidal concentration of a volatile agent in combination with moderate doses of a short-acting opioid allow a depth of anaesthesia to be maintained that does not interfere with ECoG recording whilst minimising the risk of awareness. Alternatively, anaesthesia may be maintained by propofol infusion, although the effect on the ECoG is not yet fully characterised. Neuromuscular blockade should be maintained during the lighter stages of anaesthesia necessary for ECoG recording, and monitoring of neuromuscular function is essential because of interactions between muscle relaxant drugs and anticonvulsants.

Intraoperative seizures during general anaesthesia are rare but may be masked by neuromuscular blockade. Unexpected tachycardia, hypertension or increases in end-tidal carbon dioxide are suspicious warning signs. An intravenous bolus of propofol or thiopental, followed by deepening of anaesthesia, is usually sufficient to bring seizures under control.

POSTOPERATIVE CARE

Postoperative care is directed towards the nature of the operation. It is essential to continue anticonvulsant therapy into the postoperative period, and anticonvulsant levels must be checked after surgery.

Recurrent seizures leading to status epilepticus are more common in the postoperative period and may be precipitated by use of pro-convulsant drugs or anaesthetic agents, hypoxia or electrolyte disturbances, or subtherapeutic levels of long-acting anticonvulsant drugs (Box 1.3). Treatment of seizures in the postoperative period must be rapid and aggressive, and precipitating factors should be corrected. Seizures should be terminated rapidly with a short-acting anticonvulsant such as thiopental or a benzodiazepine. A top-up dose of the long-acting anticonvulsant should be added if plasma levels are low.

BIBLIOGRAPHY

Chapman MG, Smith M, Hirsch NP. Status epilepticus. Anaesthesia 2001; 56:648–659

Herrick IA, Gelb AW. Anesthesia for temporal lobe epilepsy surgery. Canadian Journal of Neurological Sciences 2000; 27:S64–S67

Kofke WA, Tempelhoff R, Dasheiff RM. Anesthesia for epileptic patients and for epilepsy surgery. In: Cottrell JE, Smith DS, eds. Anesthesia and neurosurgery. St Louis: Mosby; 2001

Modica PA, Tempelhoff R, White PF. Pro- and anti-convulsant effects of anaesthetics (part 1). Anesthesia and Analgesia 1990; 70:303–315

Modica PA, Tempelhoff R, White PF. Pro- and anti-convulsant effects of anaesthetics (part 2). Anesthesia and Analgesia 1990; 70:433–443

Smith M. Anaesthesia in epilepsy surgery. In: Shorvon S, Dreifus F, Fish D, Thomas D, eds. The treatment of epilepsy. Oxford: Blackwell Scientific; 1995

CROSS-REFERENCES

Raised ICP/CBF control
    Anaesthetic Factors 31: 781

1

Guillain–Barré syndrome

N. P. Hirsch

Guillain–Barré syndrome (GBS) is an acute infective neuropathy characterised by progressive neuropathic weakness of more than one limb and areflexia. Criteria necessary for diagnosis may be divided into essential and supportive criteria (Box 1.4).

BOX 1.4

Diagnostic criteria for Guillain–Barré syndrome

Essential criteria

- Progressive weakness of more than one limb due to neuropathy
- Areflexia
- Duration of progression less than 4 weeks

Supportive criteria
Clinical features:

- Weakness is usually symmetrical
- Sensory signs are mild
- Cranial nerve involvement is common
- Autonomic dysfunction is common

Laboratory features:

- CSF — after first week, total protein content is increased (in 80%); white cell count is near normal (in 90%)
- EMG — nerve conduction slowed, suggesting demyelination

PATHOPHYSIOLOGY

The incidence is 1–2 per 100 000 population. In 60% of cases of GBS the condition is preceded (usually 1–2 weeks beforehand) by a viral infection, often affecting the respiratory or gastrointestinal tract. Commonly implicated organisms include cytomegalovirus, Epstein–Barr and human immunodeficiency viruses as well as the bacteria *Mycoplasma pneumoniae* and *Campylobacter jejuni*. Antibody-mediated demyelination following infection has been proposed as the pathogenesis of GBS.

CLINICAL FEATURES

NEUROLOGICAL
GBS starts with pain, mild sensory symptoms and weakness. Weakness is usually symmetrical and is more pronounced proximally. Cranial nerves, especially facial and bulbar nerves, are commonly affected. Areflexia occurs early and urinary retention is common. The Miller–Fisher variant of GBS is characterised by external ophthalmoplegia, diminished pupillary reflexes, ataxia and areflexia.

RESPIRATORY SYSTEM
Respiratory muscle weakness requiring positive-pressure ventilation occurs in 25–30% of patients. Bulbar dysfunction occurs in a similar proportion and may require tracheal intubation for airway protection.

AUTONOMIC DYSFUNCTION
Approximately 70% of patients show a persistent tachycardia with or without accompanying paroxysmal hypertension. Postural hypotension occurs in 20% of patients. Cardiac arrhythmias may include bradycardia and asystole. ECG changes include T-wave inversion. Excessive sweating occurs in 30% of patients.

METABOLIC DERANGEMENTS
Hyponatraemia occurs commonly and may be related to excessive ADH secretion.

TREATMENT

The mortality rate is in the range 2–13%, depending on severity, where nursed, etc.

GENERAL CARE
- Good general medical and nursing care (including monitoring) are essential.
- Early tracheal intubation is indicated if respiratory muscle weakness occurs (i.e. if vital capacity falls) or bulbar function is compromised.

1

- Tracheostomy should be performed early if it is obvious that a prolonged period of artificial ventilation is necessary.
- Measures to prevent deep venous thrombosis and pulmonary embolus (e.g. subcutaneous heparin therapy, graded elastic stocking, etc.) are mandatory.

IMMUNOGLOBULIN

High-dose intravenous immunoglobulin therapy appears to be effective in accelerating recovery in patients with GBS. The relative efficacy of plasma exchange and intravenous immunoglobulin (or a combination of the two) has yet to be fully defined. There appears to be a similar course of improved recovery, but immunoglobulin therapy is less hazardous although still associated with morbidity.

PLASMA EXCHANGE

Plasma exchange accelerates recovery if performed within 2 weeks of onset of the disease. Patients likely to benefit most are those exchanged within 1 week of onset of symptoms and those with rapid deterioration of limb power.

STEROIDS

A number of series have failed to show any benefit of steroid therapy.

ANAESTHETIC CONSIDERATIONS

Patients usually present for elective tracheostomy and are already intubated.

PREOPERATIVE ASSESSMENT:

- If unintubated, assess airway, mouth, dentition, neck. Special examination of bulbar function to assess risk of pulmonary aspiration at induction.
- Assess respiratory muscle function – vital capacity, mouth occlusion pressures, cough.
- Assess autonomic function – ECG, postural hypotension, excessive sweating.

INVESTIGATIONS

Electrolyte determination for signs of dehydration or hyponatraemia.

PERIOPERATIVE MANAGEMENT:

- Monitoring should include ECG, non-invasive or invasive blood pressure monitoring, and oxygen saturation.
- If bulbar function is poor or a full stomach is suspected, a rapid sequence induction is indicated.
- Suxamethonium should be avoided in the chronic stages of the condition, as widespread denervation may result in hyperkalaemia.
- If respiratory muscle weakness is present, the patient's lungs should be ventilated during surgery.
- Non-depolarising muscle relaxants should be used sparingly and neuromuscular monitoring undertaken.

POSTOPERATIVE MANAGEMENT:

- Adequate pain relief must be administered, even if this means a period of postoperative ventilation is necessary.
- Monitoring of postoperative respiratory function should ideally be carried out in an intensive care setting.

BIBLIOGRAPHY

Guillain–Barré Syndrome Study Group. Plasmapheresis for acute Guillain–Barré syndrome. Neurology 1985; 35:1096–1104

Hughes RAC. Guillain–Barré syndrome. London: Springer; 1990

Slater R, Rostami A. Treatment of Guillain–Barré syndrome with intravenous immunoglobulin. Neurology 1998; 51:S9–S15

CROSS-REFERENCES

Autonomic dysfunction
    Patient Conditions 1: 4
Weaning from mechanical ventilation
    Anaesthetic Factors 31: 803

Head injury

I. Appleby and M. Smith

Between 700 000 and 1 000 000 people attend accident and emergency (A&E) departments in the UK each year with a history of head injury, but the majority present with minor or mild head injury (Glasgow Coma Score (GCS) > 12). Fewer than 20% of those attending A&E are admitted to hospital and the majority of those with a poor outcome are in the moderate (GCS 9–12) or severe (GCS < 8) head injury groups, which account for only 10% of total A&E attenders. Some 72% of patients with head injury are male and 30% are children under 15 years of age. Although the incidence of head injury is high, the mortality rate is low, accounting for 6–10 deaths per 100 000 population. This represents 1% of overall deaths but 15% of deaths in the 15–45-years age group. Fewer than 0.2% of people attending A&E with head injury will suffer a fatal outcome, but the incidence of significant morbidity is higher than has previously been appreciated. Head injury is therefore a huge clinical problem because it affects mainly children and young adults, and contributes massively to the prevalence of long-term disability.

The anaesthetist plays a key role in the management of head-injured patients during initial resuscitation, imaging and interhospital transfer, and also by providing anaesthesia for neurosurgical and non-neurosurgical trauma.

PATHOPHYSIOLOGY

This is divided into primary and secondary brain injury. Primary brain injury occurs at the time of the initial impact and encompasses diffuse axonal injury and focal contusions. It is not amenable to treatment and can only be prevented. Secondary brain injury is essentially ischaemic in nature and occurs at any time after the primary injury. It may occur due to intracranial or extracranial factors and is preventable or treatable (Box 1.5). Potential mechanisms contributing to secondary cerebral ischaemia include cerebral vasoconstriction (especially in the first few hours after head injury) and impaired pressure autoregulation. Acute intracranial injury also initiates a cascade of ionic and metabolic changes that render the brain susceptible to secondary insults.

BOX 1.5

Causes of secondary brain injury

Intracranial factors

- Expanding haematoma
- Cerebral oedema
- Seizures

Extracranial factors

- Hypotension
- Hypoxaemia
- Hypercapnia
- Hypocapnia

Because autoregulation may be lost or impaired following head injury, cerebral perfusion pressure (CPP) becomes dependent on mean arterial pressure (MAP):

$$CPP = MAP - ICP$$

It is therefore necessary to maintain MAP at supranormal levels in the presence of increased intracranial pressure (ICP).

PRIMARY TREATMENT AND RESUSCITATION

The primary goal of acute management is the prevention, recognition and treatment of conditions known to cause secondary brain injury, including the identification and evacuation of surgically remedial compressive lesions. The importance of securing the airway and of maintaining adequate oxygenation and blood pressure in all patients with severe head injury cannot be overemphasised because secondary brain injury begins and continues from the moment of impact.

AIRWAY

Severely head-injured patients are unlikely to be able to protect their airway and often have impaired gas exchange, with hypoxaemia occurring in up to 65% of cases. Therefore the airway must be cleared of blood, teeth and foreign bodies, and protected if necessary. Early intubation and ventilation is necessary to maintain adequate oxygenation and normal arterial carbon dioxide tension (Box 1.6). To facilitate endotracheal intubation, a sleep dose of thiopental or propofol should be used to attenuate the rise in ICP associated with laryngoscopy. Hypotension should, however, be avoided. A full stomach must be assumed and suxamethonium used as part of a rapid sequence induction technique. The small rise in ICP following administration of suxamethonium is of little concern compared with the risks of hypoxaemia and hypercapnia during prolonged intubation attempts with inadequate relaxation. The neck must be immobilised by in-line cervical stabilisation or a rigid collar, as there is a high association between head injury and cervical spine fracture. Nasotracheal intubation should be avoided because of the risk of a skull base fracture. Following intubation an orogastric tube should be inserted to prevent acute gastric dilatation.

BOX 1.6

Indications for intubating the head-injured patient

Airway protection

Loss of protective laryngeal reflexes
Unconscious patient (GCS < 8)
Copious bleeding into the mouth
Facial injuries compromising the airway

Hypoventilation

Hypoxaemia (PaO_2 < 10 kPa on air)
Hypercapnia ($PaCO_2$ > 6 kPa)
Spontaneous hyperventilation ($PaCO_2$ < 4.0 kPa)
Associated chest injury

In preparation for transfer

Unconscious patient (GCS < 8)
When neurological deterioration is likely in transit
When seizures have occurred

BREATHING

Inadequate ventilation, or abnormal ventilatory patterns, may be central or peripheral in origin. Central causes result from cerebral damage or cervical cord injury, whereas peripheral causes include airway obstruction, aspiration and chest injuries such as pneumothorax. Rapid correction of hypoventilation is essential to prevent secondary brain injury due to hypoxaemia and a rise in ICP secondary to hypercapnia. Following intubation, the lungs should be mechanically ventilated to maintain PaO_2 > 13.5 kPa and $PaCO_2$ between 4.5 and 5.0 kPa. Judicious moderate hyperventilation ($PaCO_2$ 4.0–4.5 kPa) may be a useful means of emergency control of ICP pending definitive treatment. However, prolonged empirical hyperventilation may precipitate cerebral ischaemia.

CIRCULATION

Hypotension results in reduced cerebral perfusion, and maintenance of systemic blood pressure at normal or supranormal levels is a prerequisite for good neurological outcome after head injury. Closed head injury is never a cause of hypotension in adults, and blood loss from other injuries should be sought. Volume replacement may be achieved with 0.9% saline or colloid, and blood loss should be replaced with blood products as usual. Dextrose solutions are best avoided, as the glucose is metabolised to lactate in the ischaemic brain and the free water may worsen cerebral oedema, both of which may adversely affect outcome.

DYSFUNCTION (NEUROLOGICAL)

Initial conscious level is assessed using the GCS (Table 1.2). In addition, localising signs and pupillary reaction are noted.

EXAMINATION

About 40% of head-injured patients have associated injuries that may affect outcome. These should be excluded by a full trauma survey and appropriate investigations. Extracranial injuries must always be dealt with prior to definitive management of the head injury. Active bleeding and other life-threatening chest and abdominal injuries must be treated, but it is sufficient to stabilise non-life-threatening injuries.

SECONDARY MANAGEMENT

- Mannitol 20% (0.5 g kg^{-1}) may be used as a temporary means of reducing ICP following consultation with the neurosurgical centre.

TABLE 1.2

Glasgow Coma Score

	Score
Best motor response (observed in the upper limb)	
Obeys commands	6
Withdraws from painful stimuli	5
Localises to painful stimuli	4
Flexes to painful stimuli	3
Extends to painful stimuli	2
No response	1
Best verbal response	
Oriented	5
Confused speech	4
Inappropriate words	3
Incomprehensible sounds	2
None	1
Eye-opening response	
Spontaneously	4
To speech	3
To pain	2
None	1

- Anticonvulsants are used following post-traumatic seizures.
- There has been recent interest in the use of moderate hypothermia for cerebral protection, but the evidence to date suggests that active cooling of patients is not effective in improving outcome after head injury. However, the active warming of patients with severe head injuries who present with spontaneous hypothermia (a practice commonly adopted with trauma patients in the A&E department) may be detrimental. Pyrexia should be avoided because increased core temperature is associated with worsened outcome.

TRANSFER

Many head-injured patients require intrahospital transfer for computed tomography (CT) and other imaging, and/or interhospital transfer for neurosurgical management. Transfer time itself contributes little to morbidity and mortality rates, but interhospital transfer can be a hazardous procedure because it is often poorly managed.

The key to successful and safe transfer includes:

- Adequate resuscitation and stabilisation prior to transfer
- Adequate monitoring during transfer with the availability of appropriate equipment and drugs
- A doctor and assistant with suitable skills and experience of transfer of patients with head injury
- Good communication between referring and receiving centres, including the development of joint protocols and collaboration between senior medical staff. See also Box 1.7.

BOX 1.7

Guidelines for transfer of head-injured patients

- The patient must be stabilised prior to transfer
- The doctor escorting the patient should be of appropriate seniority and have sufficient skill to recognise and treat deteriorations that may occur during transfer
- All equipment and drugs, including oxygen, should be checked before departure.
- All intubated patients require:
  —sedation (propofol), to prevent increases in ICP
  —paralysis (vecuronium or atracurium), to prevent coughing and to facilitate mechanical ventilation
  —analgesia (fentanyl), if indicated
- Monitoring should be of the same standard as in the operating theatre:
  —ECG, invasive blood pressure, SpO_2 and temperature are the minimum acceptable
  —$EtcO_2$ should be considered
  —urinary catheter

ANAESTHETIC CONSIDERATIONS

PREOPERATIVE:

- Treatment of an expanding intracranial haematoma may require urgent surgical intervention and should ideally be available within 4 h. Some 20–30% of extradural haematomas present as rapid neurological deterioration following a lucid interval after the initial injury (the 'talk and die' patient). Delay in surgical treatment is a major preventable cause of morbidity and the key point is that deterioration in conscious level is an urgent clinical sign that requires immediate attention.

1

- The timing of surgery for non-neurological injuries should ideally allow time for a period of stable neurological observation.

INTRAOPERATIVE:

- In addition to minimum monitoring, $EtCO_2$, direct blood pressure, CVP and temperature measurement are necessary. Urinary catheterisation is also recommended.
- The patient should be positioned on the table with 15° head-up tilt and unobstructed venous drainage from the head.
- Use IPPV with neuromuscular paralysis.
- Sevoflurane at < 1.5 minimum alveolar concentration (MAC) (in an air : oxygen mix) is a suitable maintenance agent because it is not associated with a significant increase in cerebral blood flow.
- Total intravenous anaesthesia (TIVA) with propofol and remifentanil is an increasingly used option.

POSTOPERATIVE:

- Neurological observation should be continued into the postoperative period.
- Meticulous fluid balance is required.
- Admission to ITU for postoperative ventilation or observation may be necessary; ICP monitoring is desirable if the patient requires sedation.
- Any deterioration in neurological status warrants early rescanning.

OUTCOME

This depends on the patient's age, GCS on admission, and the pupillary state. Mortality and long-term outcome can be significantly improved by aggressive treatment in the first few hours after injury, although morbidity after head injury remains high. Almost 50% of surviving head-injured patients have some form of disability at 1 year. This ranges from significant neurological disability to problems such as memory loss and difficulty with concentration. Early rehabilitation plays a crucial part in the management of the head-injured patient.

BIBLIOGRAPHY

Association of Anaesthetists of Great Britain and Ireland. Recommendations on transfer of the severely head injured patient. London: AAGBI; 1996

Brain Trauma Foundation. Guidelines for the management of severe head injury. Journal of Neurotrauma 1996; 13:639–734

Chesnut RM. Avoidance of hypotension: conditio sine qua non of successful severe head-injury management. Journal of Trauma 1997; 42:S4–S9

Gentleman D, Dearden M, Midgley S, Maclean D. Guidelines for resuscitation and transfer of patients with serious head injury. British Medical Journal 1993; 307:547–552

Lam AM, Winn HR, Cullen BF et al. Hyperglycaemia and neurological outcome in patients with head injury. Journal of Neurosurgery 1991; 75:545–551

Maas AI, Dearden M, Teasdale GM et al. EBIC-guidelines for management of severe head injury in adults. Acta Neurochirurgica (Wien) 1997; 139:286–294

Muizelaar JP, Marmarou A, Ward JD et al. Adverse effects of prolonged hyperventilation in patients with severe head injury. A randomized clinical trial. Journal of Neurosurgery 1991; 75:731–739

CROSS-REFERENCES

Transport of the critically ill patient
    Anaesthetic Factors 31: 795
Raised ICP/CBF control
    Anaesthetic Factors 31: 787

1

Motor neurone disease

N. P. Hirsch

This condition is characterised by degeneration of motor neurones within the motor cortex, the brain stem motor nuclei of the cranial nerves, and the anterior horn cells of the spinal cord. It therefore produces:

- Amyotrophic lateral sclerosis – due to an upper motor neurone lesion with pyramidal tract damage resulting in neuronal loss in the motor cortex. This results in spastic limb weakness. Bulbar motor neurone lesions cause a pseudobulbar palsy.
- Progressive bulbar palsy – due to lower motor neurone lesions of the brain stem motor nuclei of the cranial nerves.
- Progressive muscular atrophy – due to a lower motor neurone lesion of the anterior horn cells.

The majority of patients exhibit a combination of these defects.

The prevalence is 5 per 100 000 population, with men more commonly affected than women. The peak age of onset is 50–70 years. In 5–10% of cases there is an autosomal dominant inheritance, these patients presenting at an earlier age.

The spinal muscular atrophies are a group of rare inherited conditions (including Werdnig–Hoffman and Wohlfart–Kugelberg–Welander diseases) that are characterised by degeneration of motor neurones. They occur in infancy, childhood or adolescence.

CLINICAL FEATURES

NERVOUS SYSTEM

Presentation is variable, depending on which part of the nervous system is predominantly affected. If the picture is one of a lower motor neurone deficit, patients may present with weakness and wasting of the small muscles of the hand or with wasting of the distal leg muscles and foot drop. Fasciculation is a characteristic feature. Other patients may present with an upper motor neurone picture with spastic weakness of the limbs. Reflexes are characteristically brisk. In a high proportion of patients, bulbar symptoms may be present with difficulty in phonation, chewing and swallowing. As bulbar dysfunction becomes more impaired, pulmonary aspiration may occur during swallowing. These patients characteristically have poor tongue and palatal movements with accompanying fasciculation and atrophy of the tongue.

Distressingly, there is no impairment of intellect. The sensory system is unaffected.

RESPIRATORY SYSTEM

The respiratory muscles are usually affected late in the disease process. Progressive respiratory muscle failure leads to breathlessness (especially when lying flat), poor cough, recurrent pneumonia and respiratory failure. Nocturnal hypoventilation may lead to characteristic symptoms, such as morning headaches and daytime hypersomnolence. The poor bulbar function results in recurrent pulmonary aspiration, which further compromises respiratory function. Most patients die from associated pulmonary problems within 3 years of diagnosis.

PREOPERATIVE ASSESSMENT

HISTORY AND EXAMINATION:

- General details of disease and any associated conditions.
- Bulbar function – ask whether patient has problem with phonation, chewing and swallowing. Does food or liquid 'go the wrong way'? Examine palatal movement while testing the gag reflex. Look for pooling of saliva in the pyriform fossae.
- Respiratory function – ask about recurrent chest infections. Measure vital capacity both standing and lying. A drop of more than 30% on lying suggests significant diaphragmatic weakness. Breathlessness on lying flat, especially when associated with paradoxical abdominal movement on inspiration, will confirm the suspicion. Ask

1

about symptoms of nocturnal hypoventilation.

INVESTIGATIONS:

- To confirm diagnosis (e.g. EMG and nerve conduction studies)
- Routine haematological and biochemical investigations
- Chest radiography, pulmonary function tests, arterial blood gases, tests of diaphragmatic function (e.g. mouth occlusion pressures)
- Videofluoroscopy to investigate the swallowing mechanism may be indicated.

PERIOPERATIVE MANAGEMENT

PREMEDICATION

Opioid premedication should be avoided because of its respiratory depressant action. If premedication is required, a small dose of a benzodiazepine is appropriate.

If bulbar function is poor, prophylaxis against pulmonary aspiration (i.e. an H_2-receptor antagonist) should be administered.

MONITORING:

- Should start in the anaesthetic room
- ECG (CM5)
- Blood pressure measurement
- SpO_2
- $EtCO_2$ (maintain patient at normocarbia as defined by preoperative arterial blood gases)
- Neuromuscular function monitoring.

INDUCTION AND MAINTENANCE OF ANAESTHESIA

Patients are very sensitive to the respiratory depressant effects of anaesthetic induction agents, which should be titrated carefully against response.

Poor bulbar function dictates that the patient is intubated in order to protect the airway. Although a rapid sequence induction may be indicated, suxamethonium is contraindicated in motor neurone disease, and therefore tracheal intubation must be effected without this agent.

The administration of suxamethonium may result in dangerous hyperkalaemia in the pre-

sence of the widespread denervation found in motor neurone disease.

Because of increased sensitivity to non-depolarising neuromuscular blocking drugs, these agents should be used in the lowest possible doses and neuromuscular blockade should be monitored continuously.

During anaesthesia controlled ventilation is recommended.

Tracheal extubation should be performed with the patient fully awake to ensure maximal function of the laryngeal reflexes.

REGIONAL ANAESTHESIA

If appropriate, this would appear to have distinct advantages over general anaesthesia. However, if extradural or spinal anaesthesia is planned, care must be taken to ensure that the level of block does not compromise an already weak respiratory musculature.

POSTOPERATIVE MANAGEMENT

Effective postoperative pain relief must be administered without the use of agents that depress respiratory function. The use of regional analgesia should be considered.

Postoperative ventilation may be required and weaning may be prolonged.

BIBLIOGRAPHY

Gregory S, Siderowf A, Golaszewski A, McCluskey L. Gastrostomy insertion in ALS patients with low vital capacity: respiratory support and survival. Neurology 2002; 58:485–487

Gronert GA, Lambert EM, Theye RA. The response of denervated skeletal muscle to succinylcholine. Anesthesiology 1973; 39:13–22

Rosenbaum KJ, Neigh JT, Strobel GE. Sensitivity to non-depolarizing muscle relaxants in amylotrophic lateral sclerosis: report of two cases. Anesthesiology 1971; 35:638–641

CROSS-REFERENCES

Restrictive lung disease
    Patient Conditions 3: 101

1

Movement disorders

R. Stephens and J. J. Radcliffe

The commonest movement disorder is parkinsonism, a syndrome characterised by tremor, rigidity, bradykinesia and autonomic instability. Anaesthestists may be called on to see patients with rarer conditions that include movement and degenerative disorders such as Huntington's disease, Sydenham's chorea, Wilson's disease, Shy–Drager syndrome and Alzheimer's disease.

Parkinson's disease affects 0.3% of the general population, increasing to 3% in those aged over 65 years. It is a worldwide disease, affecting all ethnic groups.

AETIOLOGY

IDIOPATHIC
Parkinson's disease is the commonest cause of parkinsonism.

SECONDARY:
- Drugs (e.g. phenothiazines, metoclopramide)
- Toxins (e.g. carbon monoxide)
- Encephalitis
- Cerebrovascular disease
- Heavy metal poisoning (manganese and copper)
- Other degenerative CNS diseases (e.g. Alzheimer's disease)
- Anoxic brain damage (e.g. postcardiac arrest).

PATHOLOGY

Parkinsonism is due to an imbalance of the antagonistic basal ganglion cholinergic and dopaminergic systems. In Parkinson's disease, pigmented cells in the substantia nigra are lost along with associated dopaminergic activity, so that there is more than twice the normal degree of ageing. As there is no loss of cholinergic activity, there is a functional deficit of dopamine, which treatment is aimed to correct.

CLINICAL FEATURES

There is a classical 'triad' of features, which is usually asymmetrical:
- Tremor ('pill rolling' – improved by voluntary movement)
- Rigidity (with tremor – 'cogwheel rigidity')
- Bradykinesia (paucity of movement).

OTHER RELEVANT FEATURES:
- Autonomic:
  —postural hypotension
  —seborrhoea (excess sweating)
  —difficulty with micturition, impotence.
- Respiratory:
  —upper airway dysfunction
  —excess bronchial secretions
  —speech impairment.
- Gastrointestinal:
  —excessive salivation (sialorrhoea)
  —gastro-oesophageal reflux.
- Cardiovascular:
  —postural hypotension
  —dysrhythmias.
- Neurological
  —dementia
  —depression
  —sleep disturbance.

MANAGEMENT

GENERAL
Education, physiotherapy, laxatives, support stockings.

DOPAMINERGIC DRUGS
L-Dopa, an inactive form of dopamine (which itself does not cross the blood–brain barrier) is converted to dopamine by decarboxylases in the CNS. Peripheral decarboxylase inhibitors (e.g. benserazide, carbidopa), themselves unable to cross the blood–brain barrier, reduce peripheral conversion resulting in fewer side-effects and reducing the dosage needed. Intravenous dopamine is ineffective.

1

Selegiline, a monoamine oxidase (MAO) type B inhibitor, reduces the central breakdown of dopamine. It does not produce the tyramine 'cheese' reaction seen with MAO type A inhibitors.

Ergot derivatives (e.g. bromocriptine, pergolide, lisuride, cabergoline, ropinirole, pramipexole) are dopamine receptor agonists; nausea, hypotension and psychiatric disturbance may occur. They are mostly reserved as adjuvant therapy or for those with L-dopa side-effects.

Catechol-O-methyl transferase inhibitors (e.g. entacapone) improve the dopamine concentration profile, resulting in fewer on–off symptom fluctuations.

Apomorphine is the only available parenteral dopaminergic drug and should be given with the antiemetic domperidone.

ANTICHOLINERGIC DRUGS

Examples are procyclidine, benzatropine, biperiden, trihexyphenidyl (benzhexol) and orphenadrine. These have limited efficacy and several side-effects (confusion, urinary retention, glaucoma). Procyclidine and benzatropine can be used intravenously for drug-induced dystonias.

SURGICAL THERAPY

Stereotactic unilateral and even bilateral pallidotomy, thalamotomy and deep brain stimulation are increasingly used in the awake patient. Fetal cell transplantation currently remains experimental.

ANAESTHESIA

PREOPERATIVE ASSESSMENT:
- Cardiovascular – postural hypotension and dysrhythmias
- Respiratory – poor cough and retained secretions
- Gastrointestinal – dysphagia, excess salivation, risk of reflux
- Neurological – cause of parkinsonism, mental state, severity of symptoms, cooperation with a regional technique
- Co-morbid illness
- Drug – interactions are frequent, normal timing of antiparkinsonian medication is often disrupted by hospital admission. The balance of on–off periods may be crucial to the return to activity.

PREOPERATIVE PREPARATION:
- Cardiovascular – ensure adequate hydration, ECG

- Respiratory – consider baseline chest radiography, spirometry (restrictive pattern)
- Gastrointestinal – dysphagia, excess salivation, reflux
- Urological – consideration for a urinary catheter
- Neurological – clear explanation of procedure
- Drugs – check antiparkinsonian medication has been continued as usual, or modified when subcutaneous apomorphine infusion is required for longer operations.

CONDUCT OF ANAESTHESIA

L-Dopa therapy must be continued, by nasogastric tube if necessary. Regional anaesthesia may avoid some of the complications of general anaesthesia, but tremor, confusion and exaggerated hypotension may cause difficulty for the operator. Potential drug interactions should be considered.

Intravenous induction agents
Thiopental, etomidate and ketamine have been used in patients with Parkinson's disease without harm, although there may be concern regarding a hypertensive reaction to ketamine. There are reports of propofol causing exacerbation of dyskinesia and reduction of tremor, and for this reason it is generally not used in patients undergoing surgery for Parkinson's disease.

Volatile agents
Halothane, in particular, may potentiate the hypotension and dysrhythmias seen in treated parkinsonism.

Analgesics
Non-steroidal anti-inflammatory drugs (NSAIDs) and simple analgesics may be used as normal. Fentanyl, alfentanil and morphine have all caused rigidity in individual cases; the use of local and regional anaesthetic techniques should minimise potent opioid requirements.

Neuromuscular blockade and reversal
Non-depolarising neuromuscular agents have been used, as has neostigmine–glycopyrronium. One report of suxamethonium causing hyperkalaemia has not been confirmed in a subsequent case series.

Antihypertensives
Direct-acting vasodilators may be preferred and employed with caution.

Antiemetics and antipsychotics
These agents, including chlorpromazine, droperidol and metoclopramide, may exacerbate

parkinsonian symptoms. Ondansetron is an appropriate antiemetic, being a specific inhibitor of serotonin type 3 receptors and devoid of extrapyramidal actions.

POSTOPERATIVE CARE:
- Mobilising may be delayed; attention to pressure areas and thromboprophylaxis is necessary.
- Drug interactions – many are unexpected (Tables 1.3 & 1.4).

- Ensure L-dopa therapy is continued. Confusion may need to be treated by a benzodiazepine or an 'atypical' antipsychotic while the cause is sought.
- Patient-controlled analgesia may be awkward for the patient; regional techniques should be continued.
- Physiotherapy for the chest (impaired cough, laryngeal function and increased secretions) and mobility.

TABLE 1.3

Interactions of commonly used drugs in patients taking treatment for Parkinson's disease

Drugs	Effects	Comments
Antiemetics Metoclopramide Droperidol Prochlorperazine	Extrapyramidal side-effects or parkinsonian symptoms	Use domperidone, 5-HT$_3$ antagonist (e.g. ondansetron) or antihistamine (e.g. cyclizine)
Analgesics Pethidine	↑ BP and rigidity with selegiline	? Resembles malignant hyperpyrexia
Synthetic opiates	↑ Rigidity	Dose related
Volatile agents	↑ L-Dopa-induced dysrhythmias	Avoid halothane if ECG abnormal
Antihypertensives	Exaggerated drug effects ↑ BP with indirect antihypertensives and selegiline	
Antipsychotics	Extrapyramidal side-effects or parkinsonian symptoms	Use 'atypical' antipsychotics (e.g. clozapine or olanzapine)
Antidepressants Tricyclics SSRIs	↑ L-Dopa-induced dysrhythmias ↑ Blood pressure and cerebral excitation with selegiline	

BP, blood pressure; SSRI, selective serotonin-reuptake inhibitor.

1

TABLE 1.4

Interaction of drugs taken for Parkinson's disease with other drug therapy

Drug	Interactions
Amantadine	Anticholinergics, levodopa, CNS depressants and stimulants, diuretics
Biperiden	Antihistamines, CNS depressants, quinidine, metoclopramide
Levodopa–benserazide	MAOIs, potent opioids, antihypertensives, sympathomimetics, ferrous sulfate
Trihexyphenidyl (benzhexol)	MAOIs, phenothiazines, antihistamines, antidepressants, disopyramide, amantadine
Benzatropine	MAOIs, phenothiazines, antihistamines, antidepressants, disopyramide, amantadine
Bromocriptine	Erythromycin, metoclopramide, alcohol
Cabergoline	Neuroleptics, ergot alkaloids, dopamine antagonists, macrolides, hypotensive agents
Entacapone	MAOIs, rimiterol, sympathomimetics, methyldopa, antidepressants, iron, bromocriptine
Levodopa–carbidopa	MAOIs, antihypertensives, sympathomimetics
Orphenadrine	Phenothiazines, antihistamines, antidepressants, amantadine, disopyramide
Pergolide	Dopamine antagonists, antihypertensives, anticoagulants, competition for protein binding
Pramipexole	Amantadine, cimetidine, ranitidine, diltiazem, quinidine, quinine, verapamil, digoxin, procainamide, triamterene, sedatives, alcohol
Procyclidine	Phenothiazines, antihistamines, antidepressants, amantadine, disopyramide, ketoconazole, quinidine, MAOIs
Ropinirole	Antihypertensives, antiarrhythmics, neuroleptics, oestrogens, alcohol, drugs affecting cytochrome P450
Selegiline	Fluoxetine, sertraline, paroxetine, pethidine, non-selective MAOIs, tricyclic antidepressants, anticoagulants, digitalis

MAOI, monoamine oxidase inhibitor.

BIBLIOGRAPHY

Lang AE, Lozano AM. Parkinson's disease: first of two parts. New England Journal of Medicine 1998; 339 (15):1130–1143

Lang AE, Lozano AM. Parkinson's disease: second of two parts. New England Journal of Medicine 1998; 339(16):1044–1052

Nagele P, Hammerle AF. Sevoflurane and mivacurium in a patient with Huntington's chorea. British Journal of Anaesthesia 2002; 85(2):320–321

Nicholson G, Pereira AC, Hall GM. Parkinson's disease and anaesthesia. British Journal of Anaesthesia 2002; 89(6):904–916

Severn AM. Parkinsonism and the anaesthetist. British Journal of Anaesthesia 1988; 61:761–770

CROSS-REFERENCES

The elderley
    Anaesthetic Factors 27: 606
N Malignant Syndrome
    Anaesthetic Factors 31: 769

Multiple sclerosis

M. Sivaloganathan

Multiple sclerosis (MS) is a chronic inflammatory disease of the CNS white matter. It is the commonest cause of chronic neurological disability in young adults, with an acute onset followed by slow progression.

AETIOLOGY

Epidemiological evidence suggests two factors involved with causation: exposure to an environmental agent (assumed to be infective, probably viral) and genetic susceptibility (multiple genes being involved, including HLA-DR2).

INCIDENCE

This varies from 5 to more than 30 per 100 000 population, being highest in northern Europe, southern Australia and mid North America, and lowest in the equatorial regions. The reason for the variance is not understood, and both genetic and environmental factors probably play a role.

PATHOGENESIS

MS is believed to have autoimmune aetiology in which myelin proteins serve as autoantigens, leading to the destruction of the myelin sheaths of nerve fibres. There are characteristic multifocal inflammatory and demyelinating plaques disseminated in space and time throughout the CNS. They have a predilection for the periventricular, optic nerve, brain stem, cerebellum and spinal cord white matter, and are easily imaged with magnetic resonance imaging (MRI).

Demyelination produces a conduction block and plays a part in the resulting signs and symptoms of MS.

CLINICAL COURSE

MS appears to include distinct clinical subtypes. The main forms are:

- Relapsing remitting (RR) MS, which often proceeds to a secondary progressive (SP) form; and
- Primary progressive (PP) MS.

Around 80% patients with MS have the RR form. This has a female : male preponderance of 2 : 1, and affects young adults in the second and third decades of life. Symptoms and signs typically evolve over a period of several days before stabilising either spontaneously or in response to corticosteroid therapy. RR MS typically starts with sensory disturbances, optic neuritis, diplopia, Lhermitte's sign (trunk and limb paraesthesias evoked by neck flexion), limb weakness, gait ataxia, and neurogenic bladder and bowel symptoms. Cortical and extrapyramidal signs are more rare. Eventually there is cognitive impairment, depression, emotional lability, dysarthria, dysphagia, progressive quadraparesis, spasticity and other CNS disability.

PP MS often presents with a slowly progressive upper motor neurone weakness of the legs, which worsens gradually resulting in quadraparesis. There is also cognitive decline, visual loss, brain stem syndromes, and the whole gamut of signs and symptoms typical of RR MS.

Overall, 10% of patients do well for more than 20 years and are considered to have benign multiple sclerosis. Approximately 70% will have secondary progression.

DIAGNOSIS

Based on clinical, laboratory and MRI criteria.

CLINICAL:
- History of exacerbations and remissions
- Clinical manifestations suggesting multiple lesions in different regions of the CNS
- Abnormal visual, auditory or somatosensory evoked potentials.

LABORATORY

Abnormal cerebrospinal fluid:
- Increased white cell count
- Increased total protein count
- Oligoclonal bands on electrophoresis.

MRI:
- Multifocal lesions of varying ages, especially involving the peri-ventricular white matter, brain stem, cerebellum and spinal cord white matter
- Gadolinium-enhancing lesions indicate sites of active lesions.

TREATMENT

- Exposure to viral illness needs to be limited as infection can trigger relapse.
- Transient worsening of symptoms occurs with increased temperature or fatigue.
- Multidisciplinary approach to therapy and psychological support. Depression and suicide is common; patients face enormous prognostic uncertainty.

THERAPIES
No treatment predictably slows the course of MS. Commonly used agents are corticosteroids, immunomodulatory agents such as β-interferon 1b, 1a and glatiramer acetate.

Corticosteroids
Often used to treat relapses to hasten recovery. Usually methylprednisolone for 5 days followed by prednisolone.

β-Interferon
Trials show that early treatment with the 1a subtype can delay the development of a second clinically significant episode of MS.

β-Interferon 1b reduces the frequency of relapse in RR MS by approximately 30%.

Glatiramer acetate
A synthetic polymer with immunological similarities to myelin basic protein. Treatment resulted in a 29% reduction in annual relapse rate in a 2-year trial.

New development
These are all based on new technologies used to manipulate the immune system; they vary from administration of monoclonal antibodies to bone marrow transplantation.

ANAESTHETIC MANAGEMENT

The stress of anaesthesia and surgery alone has been implicated in the exacerbation of symptoms in MS; involvement of the patient in planning of the anaesthetic technique may reduce anxiety.

PREOPERATIVE ASSESSMENT

- Disease progress in the patient should be noted, as well as evidence of relapse so that postoperative complications may be interpreted.
- Evidence of infection – a rise in temperature of 0.5–1.0°C exacerbates conduction block in demyelinated neurones.
- Respiratory reserve can be poor – respiratory function tests and arterial blood gas analysis may be indicated.
- Signs of impairment of bulbar function and recurrent pulmonary aspiration should be sought.
- Autonomic dysreflexia has been reported in patients with extensive spinal cord demyelination from 3 weeks to 12 years after initial demyelination. This is characterised by a massive disordered autonomic response to certain stimuli below the level of the demyelinating lesion, causing hypertension, flushing or pallor, and reflex bradycardia.
- Steroid medication.
- Mental state.
- The presence of pressure sores and contractures.

PREMEDICATION

- Sedative premedication to reduce anxiety
- Continuation of antispasmodic medication
- H_2-receptor antagonists if there is any suggestion of recurrent aspiration
- Avoid agents with anticholinergic properties as they may increase body temperature
- Deep vein thrombosis prophylaxis (there is an increased tendency for platelet aggregation in patients with MS)
- Steroid supplementation as indicated.

GENERAL VERSUS REGIONAL ANAESTHESIA

There is no absolute contraindication to regional blockade in patients with MS. It has been suggested that the demyelination predisposes to local anaesthetic toxicity at the site of injection. Epidural and subarachnoid blockade has been employed successfully in obstetric anaesthesia practice and in most other disciplines. Many still believe that regional techniques lead to symptomatic exacerbation, although without evidence to support this the decision to proceed with a general or regional technique must therefore be based on careful discussion with the patient, bearing in mind the nature of the operation and other risk factors.

GENERAL ANAESTHESIA:

- Suxamethonium should be avoided as it may produce profound increases in serum potassium concentration in patients with extensive demyelination. Response to non-depolarising neuromuscular blockade is normal, but monitoring is advisable. It has been suggested that nitrous oxide should be avoided in longer cases in view of its time-weighted effect on vitamin B_{12} metabolism.
- Deep general anaesthesia usually ensures control of autonomic dysreflexia. Labetalol or hydralazine may be indicated in hypertensive crises.
- Central temperature should be monitored and normothermia maintained.
- If there is poor bulbar function, tracheal intubation is often preferred.
- Careful positioning of patients with contractures and pressure sores.

POSTOPERATIVE CARE

The mode of postoperative analgesia chosen should take into account the patient's pre-operative respiratory function. Maintenance of normothermia is advisable. Intensive physiotherapy to remove pulmonary secretions and prevent worsening contractures may be required. A postoperative neurological examination will allow interpretation of the exacerbation or the development of new symptoms.

BIBLIOGRAPHY

Hambly PR, Martin B. Anaesthesia for chronic spinal cord lesions. Anaesthesia 1998; 53:273–289

Jones RM, Healy TEJ. Anaesthesia and demyelinating disease. Anaesthesia 1980; 35:879–884

Noseworthy JH, Lucchinetti C, Rodriguez M, Weinshenker BG. Medical progress: multiple sclerosis. New England Journal of Medicine 2000; 343(13):938–952

Polman CH, Uitedhaag BMJ. Drug treatment of multiple sclerosis. British Medical Journal 2000; 321:490–494

CROSS-REFERENCES

Autonomic Dysfunction
    Patient Conditions 1: 4
Preoperation Assessment of pulmonary risk
    Anaesthetic Factors 27: 638

1

Neurofibromatosis

S. M. Scuplak and J. J. Radcliffe

Neurofibromatosis is a heterogeneous group of disorders characterised by cutaneous pigmentation and tumour formation. Von Recklinghausen or type 1 neurofibromatosis is the most common form in clinical practice (Box 1.8). It is inherited as an autosomal dominant trait with a prevalence of 1 in 5000 population; half of the cases represent new mutations.

PATHOPHYSIOLOGY

The severity of disease and the occurrence of complications cannot be predicted owing to variable gene expression. Neurofibromas virtu-

---

BOX 1.8

Clinical features of von Recklinghausen neurofibromatosis

Major defining features (diagnostic if two or more)

- Café-au-lait spots – usually more than six greater than 1.5 cm in diameter
- Peripheral neurofibromas
- Iris hamartomas (Lisch nodules)
- Axillary or groin freckling
- Optic glioma
- Distinctive bony lesion – dysplastic sphenoid or long bone
- First-degree relative with neurofibromatosis type 1

Minor features

- Short stature
- Macrocephaly

Disease complications

- Intellectual handicap
- Epilepsy
- CNS tumours
- Bone dysplasias, scoliosis
- Hypertension
- Pulmonary fibrosis

---

ally always involve the patient's skin, but can also affect any peripheral nerve or visceral tissue innervated by the autonomic nervous system. Involvement of the pharynx, larynx, trachea, spinal canal and cardiac ventricular outflow has been reported.

CARDIOVASCULAR

Neurofibromas developing in blood vessel walls can produce vascular obstruction or aneurysmal dilatation. Renal artery stenosis occurs in approximately 2% of patients, giving rise to hypertension, most commonly in children. Hypertension occurring in adults is not generally due to phaeochromocytoma, although there is a strong association.

RESPIRATORY

Restrictive lung disorders are common. Diffuse pulmonary fibrosis associated with bullous emphysema can result in arterial hypoxaemia and cor pulmonale; it may also present as pneumothorax. Lung volumes are further reduced by chest wall abnormalities such as scoliosis and intrathoracic neurofibromas. Obstructive disorders may be produced by neurofibromas within the airway.

ENDOCRINE

Phaeochromocytoma develops in approximately 1% of patients and may be part of the multiple endocrine neoplasia syndrome, which includes medullary carcinoma of the thyroid.

CENTRAL NERVOUS SYSTEM

Epilepsy occurs in at least 4% of patients, although no underlying abnormality is usually found. Occasionally it may signal the presence of an intracranial tumour, especially glioma.

PREOPERATIVE ASSESSMENT

HISTORY:

- Review of cardiovascular and respiratory systems.

- Symptoms of airway obstruction:
  —dyspnoea
  —dysphagia
  —dysphonia.
- Phaeochromocytoma:
  —paroxysmal tachycardia
  —sweating.

EXAMINATION:
- Assess distribution of neurofibromas – some patients with new mutations may present as mosaics
- Posture and presence of scoliosis
- CNS deficits indicative of intracranial or spinal neurofibromas.

INVESTIGATIONS:
- Chest radiography to detect intrathoracic abnormalities and assess thoracic spine
- Lung function tests for obstructive and restrictive disease
- Arterial blood gases
- CT/MRI imaging of the airway in the presence of obstructive symptoms
- The investigation of hypertension should include plasma catecholamine or urinary metabolite levels.

PERIOPERATIVE MANAGEMENT

PREMEDICATION
Respiratory depressant drugs are contraindicated only in the presence of severe respiratory insufficiency. Anticholinergic agents should be given if difficulty in intubation is anticipated.

MONITORING
This should commence in the anaesthetic room.
- ECG
- SpO_2
- Arterial cannula, if hypertensive
- Peripheral nerve stimulator
- Airway pressure monitor.

GENERAL ANAESTHESIA
No particular anaesthetic technique or drug has advantages over another. Evidence of airway obstruction may be an indication for awake fibreoptic intubation. If muscle atrophy is present, succinylcholine should be avoided. Succinylcholine, pancuronium and D-tubocurarine have been reported to produce prolonged neuromuscular blockade, and monitoring of blockade and the use of shorter-acting drugs is recommended; however, it is unlikely that this is a common feature of the condition in the absence of hepatic or renal impairment. Positioning of the unconscious patient must be carried out with care to avoid undue pressure on large cutaneous neurofibromas. Severe kyphoscoliosis may also hinder positioning. High airway pressures can be achieved in patients with severe restrictive lung disease, and the possibility of pneumothorax must be considered.

REGIONAL ANAESTHESIA
Regional anaesthesia has been used successfully. The presence of cutaneous neurofibromas overlying the site of injection may hinder successful placement of the needle, and this can be further complicated by bony abnormalities such as scoliosis.

POSTOPERATIVE CARE

- Position with adequate padding; cutaneous neurofibromas can be tender
- Continuous oxygen therapy
- Chest physiotherapy.

BIBLIOGRAPHY

Fisher MMcD. Anaesthetic difficulties in neurofibromatosis. Anaesthesia 1975; 30:648–650

Hirsch NP, Murphy A, Radcliffe JJ. Neurofibromatosis: clinical presentations and anaesthetic implications. British Journal of Anaesthesia 2001; 86:555–564

Van Aken H, Scherer R, Lawin P. A rare intra-operative complication in a child with Von Recklinghausen's neurofibromatosis. Anaesthesia 1982; 37:827–829

CROSS-REFERENCES

Epilepsy
    Patient Conditions 1: 9
Restrictive lung disease
    Patient Conditions 3: 101
Hypertension
    Patient Conditions 4: 151

1

Spinal cord injury (acute)

J. S. Porter and M. Smith

AETIOLOGY

The incidence of spinal trauma is about 50 per million population per year. The cervical spine is the most susceptible to injury as it is the least supported, C5–C6 being the level most commonly affected. In the thoracolumbar spine T12–L1 is the commonest level affected by trauma. Injuries may involve fracture of bony elements, disruption of intervertebral discs, or ligamentous and soft tissue injury. Other injuries occur in 60% of cases, with head injury being a common association. Road traffic accidents account for about 70% of all cervical spine injuries.

PATHOPHYSIOLOGY

The primary injury is caused by stretching or direct trauma to the spinal cord and is characterised by vasodilatation and disruption of the microvasculature and marked oedema in the grey matter. Local hypoxia sets up a chain of events culminating in neuronal death. Rises in intracellular calcium levels, synthesis of vasoactive peptides, free radical production and lipid peroxidation are all implicated in this process. Secondary ischaemic injury may follow because of hypotension, hypoxaemia and progressive cord oedema. Treatment is directed at respiratory and cardiovascular support to minimise secondary injury.

NERVOUS SYSTEM

'Spinal shock' occurs due to interruption of visceral and somatic sensation with flaccid paralysis and absent autonomic and somatic reflexes following spinal cord injury. It may last for up to 6 weeks, followed by progressive spasticity of the affected levels (see Chronic spinal cord injury, p. 33). Interruption of the spinal cord outflow has major effects on other physiological systems.

CARDIOVASCULAR SYSTEM:

- Hypertension occurs at the time of the injury
- Hypotension follows within minutes as a result of loss of sympathetic (autonomic) tone, with marked cutaneous vasodilatation
- Hypotension may be exacerbated by bleeding from other injuries
- Loss of compensatory reflexes for changes in cardiac output and blood pressure if lesion is above T1
- Severe bradycardia may occur due to unopposed vagal activity.

RESPIRATORY SYSTEM:

- Respiratory insufficiency is common, although the degree depends on the level of cord damage. Respiratory impairment may also result from associated injuries.
- *Lesion above C4* – diaphragmatic paralysis, loss of intercostal function and paralysis of all four limbs occurs. Such patients require ventilatory support. If the lesion extends to the upper cervical levels and lower cranial nerves, accessory muscle function is also lost.
- *Lesion at C4–C5* – voluntary control of breathing is maintained under cervical control at 20–25% of normal vital capacity. Such patients often require ventilatory assistance, especially in the early stages.
- *Lesion below C5* – diaphragmatic sparing occurs but the intercostal muscles are affected to varying degrees. There is a decrease in alveolar ventilation and paradoxical respiration. A decreased cough occurs due to loss of intercostal function and paralysed abdominal musculature.
- In the early stages of injury, during the phase of spinal cord oedema, the level of the lesion may ascend and a patient requiring minimal respiratory support may become entirely ventilator dependent.
- Pulmonary oedema is common after spinal cord injury and is a common cause of death

– it may be neurogenic in origin or due to the inability to cope with fluid overload.

GASTROINTESTINAL TRACT:
- Acute gastric dilatation and paralytic ileus
- Increased risk of regurgitation and pulmonary aspiration.

TEMPERATURE
Temperature regulation is impaired due to the inability to sweat combined with cutaneous vasodilatation.

GENITOURINARY TRACT
Bladder atony and urinary retention occur.

ACUTE MANAGEMENT

The resuscitation of patients with spinal cord injuries should follow routine guidelines for any patient with major trauma.

AIRWAY
The airway should be secured and supplemental oxygen delivered to prevent hypoxaemia. Tracheal intubation may be necessary (Box 1.9). Airway control is considered below.

BOX 1.9

Indications for tracheal intubation after acute spinal cord injury

- $Pao_2 < 10.0$ kPa
- $Paco_2 > 6.5$ kPa
- Vital capacity < 20 ml kg^{-1}
- Pulmonary aspiration
- Pulmonary oedema
- Associated chest and lung injuries

BREATHING
Artificial ventilation may be necessary to maintain oxygenation and normocapnia (see above).

CIRCULATION
Bradycardia should be treated with atropine. Hypovolaemia due to vasodilatation or venodilatation requires aggressive intravascular filling to ensure adequate cardiac output and blood pressure. Central venous pressure (CVP) monitoring is mandatory and, because of the inability to deal with fluid overload, monitoring of pulmonary artery capillary wedge pressure (PCWP) may be required. Vasoconstrictors or inotropes are necessary when perfusion is in-

adequate and fails to improve with adequate filling.

DRUGS
Steroids and naloxone have been used in an attempt to block the cascade of neuronal damage after spinal cord injury. Steroids should be given in high dosage and within 8 h of the injury.

OTHER
A nasogastric tube and urinary catheter should be inserted.

SURGICAL MANAGEMENT
Open reduction and stabilisation of unstable spinal fractures with decompression may prevent further spinal cord damage and allow earlier mobilisation.

CONSERVATIVE MANAGEMENT
The spine can be immobilised with traction to the cervical spine applied using skull tongs. This entails prolonged bed rest with an increased incidence of decubitus ulcers and thromboembolic episodes. A halo body jacket device allows mobilisation.

ANAESTHESIA FOR ACUTE SPINAL CORD INJURY

PREOPERATIVE ASSESSMENT:
- Careful attention must be paid to the respiratory and cardiovascular systems (see above).
- Other injuries should be dealt with as appropriate.
- Respiratory depressant drugs should be avoided in patients who are self-ventilating.
- An antisialagogue may be useful in those in whom fibreoptic nasal intubation is required.
- Atropine should be given prior to intubation if the patient is bradycardic.

AIRWAY CONTROL
There is much debate over the safest method of tracheal intubation in patients with an unstable cervical spine. Secondary damage to the spinal cord is common if precautions are not taken. No difference in neurological outcome has been shown between the different intubation methods.
- Awake fibreoptic nasal intubation using topical anaesthesia. In skilled hands this may be the method of choice.
- Oral or nasal intubation under direct laryngoscopy. The neck should be

1

immobilised by either a hard collar, external fixation device or manual in-line stabilisation by an assistant.
- Tracheostomy under local anaesthesia.
Problems associated with tracheal intubation in patients with spinal cord injury include:
- Inability to extend the neck
- Cervical spine fixation devices
- Associated facial injuries
- Full stomach or gastric dilatation
- Cricoid pressure difficult – may exacerbate cervical spine subluxation.

MONITORING:
- ECG, pulse oximeter, invasive blood pressure, CVP, temperature and urine output, as a minimum
- PCWP and cardiac output may guide fluid therapy
- Somatosensory evoked potentials during procedures involving spinal cord manipulation.

ANAESTHETIC TECHNIQUE:
- No one specific technique is better than another.
- Falls in blood pressure should be avoided by cautious use of intravenous induction agents, minimum airway pressures, maintenance of normovolaemia and careful positioning.
- Suxamethonium should be avoided beyond day 3 after the injury.

POSTOPERATIVE CONSIDERATIONS:
- Continuation of respiratory support may require full ventilation or assisted ventilation with CPAP
- Maintenance of adequate circulating volume and urinary output
- Skilled physiotherapy is essential
- Adequate analgesia
- Careful positioning to avoid decubitus ulcers

- Deep vein thrombosis prophylaxis – thromboembolism-deterrent (TED) stockings, intermittent calf compression and subcutaneous heparin should all be considered
- Gastric ulcer prophylaxis – adequate nutrition should be maintained; enteral feeding is usually possible.

BIBLIOGRAPHY

Durret JM. The early management of spinal injuries. Current Anaesthesia and Critical Care 1994; 5:17–22

Johnston RA. The management of acute spinal cord compression (review). Journal of Neurology, Neurosurgery and Psychiatry 1993; 56:1046–1054

MacKenzie CF, Shin B, Krishnaprasad D, McCormack F, Illingworth W. Assessment of cardiac and respiratory function during surgery on patients with acute quadriplegia. Journal of Neurosurgery 1985; 62:843–849

Mansel JK, Norman JR. Respiratory complications and management of spinal cord injuries. Chest 1990; 97:1446–1451

Mendoza ND, Bradford R, Middleton F. Spinal injury. In: Greenwood R, Barnes M, Macmillan T, Ward C, eds. Neurological rehabilitation. Edinburgh: Churchill Livingstone; 0000:545–560

CROSS-REFERENCES

The failing heart
    Patient Conditions 4: 146
Intraoperative hypotension
    Anaesthetic Factors 31: 758
Spinal cord injury
    Patient Conditions 1: 30

1

Spinal cord injury (chronic)

K. Hunt and R. Fox

Characteristics of chronic spinal cord injury typically appear 6–8 weeks after the initial insult, the hallmark being the return of reflex activity in the cord causing hyperreflexia and hypertonia. Good anaesthetic management relies on understanding the complex pathophysiology of these patients, including changes in the cardiovascular, respiratory and neuromuscular systems.

BOX 1.10

Clinical features of autonomic dysreflexia

- Hypertension
- Cardiac arrhythmias
- Flushing and sweating above level of lesion
- Headache
- Myocardial ischaemia
- Cerebral haemorrhage
- Triggers include blocked urinary catheter, bowel distension, uterine contractions

CENTRAL NERVOUS AND NEUROMUSCULAR SYSTEMS

The body below the cord injury is initially flaccid and areflexic. After a period of between 6 days and 6 weeks disinhibited cord function returns, leading to spasticity and augmented reflexes. In addition to spasticity, patients with chronic spinal cord injury may suffer from sensory deprivation, phantom limb and body pain, and psychological conditions including depression and frank psychosis. Violent muscle spasms may be caused by seemingly minor cutaneous or proprioceptive stimuli.

CARDIOVASCULAR SYSTEM

AUTONOMIC DYSREFLEXIA (BOX 1.10)

Stimulus below the level of injury produces massive autonomic discharge from the sympathetic chain below the cord lesion. This leads to intense peripheral and central vasoconstriction, which may cause rapid and profound hypertension. Depending on the level of cord injury, and the amount of remaining functioning cord, compensatory reflex vasodilatation may occur; this minimises the degree of hypertension and is at the same time responsible for 'flushing' noted above the level of injury.

Autonomic dysreflexia occurs in approximately 60% of patients with cervical lesions and in 20% of those with thoracic lesions. It may be triggered by multiple stimuli, including bladder and bowel distension, uterine contrac-

tion, urinary tract infections, and cutaneous and proprioceptive stimuli. The condition is associated with significant morbidity, with side-effects including myocardial ischaemia, pulmonary oedema and intracranial haemorrhage – all of which may lead to death.

Treatment:
- Rapid-onset, short-acting vasodilators such as sublingual or intravenous glyceryl trinitrate or nifedipine
- Identify and treat stimulus – a blocked urinary catheter is the commonest cause
- Long-term prophylaxis with agents including glyceryl trinitrate, guanethidine or prazosin may be considered.

OTHER CARDIOVASCULAR PROBLEMS:
- Orthostatic hypotension – may be evident in the first few weeks after spinal cord injury. It improves as time progresses due to adaptation mechanisms, including an increase in renin activity and autoregulation of cerebral blood flow.
- Cardiac arrhythmias, including vagally mediated bradycardias, may occur.

RESPIRATORY SYSTEM

Patients with chronic spinal cord injury have a globally reduced respiratory function including

1

reduced inspiratory flow, tidal volume, forced vital capacity (FVC) and inspiratory capacity. FVC may be affected by posture, being most markedly reduced in the supine position, particularly in tetraplegic patients.

Patients with high thoracic injuries lose innervation to the abdominal and intercostal muscles, leading to an inability to cough and loss of expiratory reserve volume. These patients, however, are able to breathe independently using their diaphragmatic and accessory muscles.

Partial or complete loss of respiratory muscle function may lead to retention of secretions, atelectasis, recurrent chest infections and chronic respiratory failure requiring night-time or continuous ventilatory support.

GASTROINTESTINAL SYSTEM

Patients with chronic spinal cord injury may have delayed gastric emptying, constipation and bowel distension. Characteristic signs of an acute abdomen are often unreliable in these patients, and they are more likely to exhibit symptoms including autonomic dysreflexia, referred shoulder-tip pain and increased spasticity with this condition.

GENITOURINARY SYSTEM

Many spinal cord injured patients require permanent or intermittent catheterisation to evacuate the bladder, although some may develop the ability to initiate and control voiding using spinal reflexes. Recurrent problems of the genitourinary system in patients with spinal injury include urinary tract infection, ureteric reflux, urethral trauma, development of renal calculi and, less commonly, renal failure.

SKIN AND TEMPERATURE CONTROL

Sensory deprivation coupled with immobility and poor nutrition renders patients with spinal injury extremely susceptible to the rapid development of pressure sores. Patients with high cord lesions lack the ability to regulate temperature via normal thermostatic mechanisms such as shivering, sweating and vasodilatation. This may lead to large swings in temperature during the perioperative period.

OTHER SYSTEMS

Chronic spinal cord injured patients frequently develop hypoalbuminaemia and a normochromic, normocytic anaemia. Osteoporosis, leading to an increased incidence of bone fracture, and thromboembolic disease are also common in this population.

ANAESTHETIC CONSIDERATIONS

PREOPERATIVE ASSESSMENT:
- Liable to have frequent surgical procedures, particularly urological and orthopaedic. Latex allergy must be considered.
- Identify cause, nature and timing of injury. Sensory and motor level of patient should be ascertained. Vagally mediated visceral sensation may be intact.
- Assessment of frequency and severity of muscle spasms and autonomic dysreflexia.
- Respiratory assessment – lung function tests and arterial blood gas analysis may be necessary.
- Drug history – avoid cessation of antispasmodics (e.g. baclofen, dantrolene, tizanidine) if possible. Oxybutynin, frequently used to treat bladder spasticity, may enhance the sedative effects of general anaesthesia. Patients may be taking large doses of opiates for the treatment of chronic pain.

Table 1.5 indicates the common findings with preoperative investigations.

ANAESTHESIA
No anaesthesia
In compliant patients, who suffer only infrequently from muscle spasm and autonomic dysreflexia, anaesthesia may not be necessary. If this option is to be used, it must be remembered that pain may be produced with surgery carried out on vagally mediated viscera, and should be treated appropriately.

Regional anaesthesia
Spinal anaesthesia reliably eradicates both autonomic dysreflexia and muscle spasms. Epidural anaesthesia also performs this function but to a lesser degree. Many patients with spinal injuries have undergone posterior surgery and have metalwork in place that can make performing a spinal or epidural anaesthetic technically challenging.

TABLE 1.5

Common findings with preoperative investigations

Investigation	Finding
Full blood count	Anaemia, raised white cell count
Biochemistry	Electrolyte disturbances, low albumin level, chronic or cute renal impairment
ECG	Bradycardia, other arrhythmias
Chest radiography	Infection, kyphoscoliosis
Microbiology	Infected sputum or urine
Arterial blood gases	Hypoxaemia or hypercarbia
Pulmonary function tests	Reduced vital capacity, expiratory reserve volume (ERV) and functional residual capacity (FRC)

General anaesthesia

Deep general anaesthesia also abolishes muscular spasm and diminishes autonomic dysreflexia. Fluid challenges before induction of anaesthesia help to prevent hypotension, which is common to this group of patients. Spontaneous ventilation is possible, although respiratory function and risk of aspiration should be assessed when considering this technique. Some patients with high spinal cord lesions may require postoperative ventilation and intensive physiotherapy to prevent chest infection. Suxamethonium should be avoided between 72 h and 9 months after injury because of the risk of hyperkalaemia.

Obstetric anaesthesia

Women in labour, with chronic spinal cord injury, are highly susceptible to autonomic dysreflexia. Episodes may be induced by uterine contractions alone, instrumental delivery, oxytocin and perineal distension. There is a significant risk of these life-threatening episodes continuing for 24–48 h after delivery. Epidurals, containing a standard low-dose mixture (0.125% bupivacaine with fentanyl 2–4 μg ml^{-1}) are recommended for these women and should be continued for 48 h after delivery. If it is technically impossible to site an epidural, hypertension from autonomic dysreflexia should be controlled using hydralazine or nifedipine.

MONITORING AND OTHER CONSIDERATIONS

As well as standard anaesthetic monitoring, invasive blood pressure and central venous monitoring should be considered, particularly in patients prone to frequent episodes of cardiovascular instability, or in those with lesions above T10. Urinary catheterisation, if not already in place, should be considered. Temperature control and careful positioning and padding must be implemented in all patients with chronic spinal injury undergoing surgery.

BIBLIOGRAPHY

Fox R, Watling G. Anaesthesia for patients with chronic spinal cord injury. Current Anaesthesia and Critical Care 2001; 12:154–158

CROSS-REFERENCES

Spinal cord injury-acute
    Patient Conditions 1: 30
Autonomic dysfunction
    Patient Conditions 1: 4

Subarachnoid haemorrhage

H. Gray and S. R. Wilson

Subarachnoid haemorrhage (SAH) refers to the presence of blood in the subarachnoid space. SAH may occur as a result of a head injury (traumatic SAH) or be non-traumatic, most commonly resulting from the rupture of an intracerebral aneurysm or arteriovenous malformation. Other less common causes are listed in Box 1.11. SAH is a devastating neurological disease with multisystem sequelae.

BOX 1.11

Causes of non-traumatic SAH

- Intracerebral saccular aneurysm
- Arteriovenous malformation
- Bleeding diathesis
- Cocaine use
- Bleeding into meningeal tumour
- Amyloid angiopathy

1

TRAUMATIC SAH

The incidence of traumatic SAH is estimated to be 100 per 100 000 population per year. Up to 40% of patients with moderate to severe head injury have evidence of subarachnoid blood on CT, accumulated following rupture of bridging veins or arteries. Traumatic SAH is associated with an increased incidence of hypoxia, hypotension, skull fractures, cerebral contusions, raised intracranial pressure (ICP) and consequently a high rate of morbidity and death.

The effects of traumatic SAH are thought to be similar to those of non-traumatic SAH. There is associated vasospasm demonstrated by transcranial Doppler ultrasonography and angiography.

When the history preceding the head injury is unclear, cerebral angiography should be performed to exclude non-traumatic SAH. The main priority in treating those with traumatic SAH is to prevent secondary insults.

NON-TRAUMATIC SAH

- The incidence of non-traumatic SAH is 6–16 per 100 000 population per year, with the highest rates in Finnish and Japanese populations. Women have a higher incidence than men.
- Some 1–2% of patients who present to A&E departments with headache have SAH; 25% of those who present with 'the worst headache of their lives' and abnormal neurology have SAH.
- SAH is a notable cause of maternal mortality, contributing to a number of deaths in the Confidential Enquiry into Maternal Deaths triennial reports.
- The commonest causes of non-traumatic SAH are ruptured intracranial aneurysm (80%) and arteriovenous malformations (10%).

INTRACRANIAL ANEURYSMS

The natural history of intracranial aneurysms is incompletely understood, but the annual rupture rate is thought to be 0.5–2%. Aneurysms greater than 10 mm in diameter are at particular risk of haemorrhage.

As the pressure within the aneurysm or the radius of the aneurysm increases and the wall thickness reduces, the tension within the aneurysm and therefore its propensity to rupture increases (Laplace's law). With rupture, blood is released under arterial pressure into the subarachnoid space, causing a massive and sudden rise in ICP. Blood then spreads through the cerebrospinal fluid in the subarachnoid space around the brain and spinal cord. This is often associated with intracerebral and subdural haematoma.

ARTERIOVENOUS MALFORMATIONS

These may rupture, causing SAH – usually with associated intracerebral haemorrhage. The mortality rate from the first bleed is 10%, and the rebleed rate and incidence of vasospasm is low. Patients who do rebleed have a high rate of ongoing rebleeding and death.

PRESENTATION

The typical presentation of SAH is sudden onset of a severe headache. There may be associated nausea, vomiting and photophobia. Loss of consciousness can be caused by the sudden increase in ICP. Drowsiness, agitation and restlessness are common.

Some 15–30% of patients die at aneurysm rupture secondary to sustained rises in ICP.

The SAH may be preceded by days or weeks by a prodromal headache. This is caused by a 'sentinel bleed' and probably represents extravasation of blood into the aneurysmal wall or subarachnoid space.

The breakdown products of blood in the subarachnoid space cause meningeal irritation with neck stiffness. Back pain and bilateral radicular leg pain may also occur.

Following SAH, patients are graded, for example using the World Federation of Neurological Surgeons' scale (WFNS) (Table 1.6), to correlate operative risk and prognosis.

OTHER SIGNS AND SYMPTOMS OF SAH
Hydrocephalus:
- Acute obstructive hydrocephalus (within 72 h) is common, particularly in patients with a poor grade. It is caused by a subarachnoid clot in the basal cisterns and is managed with external ventricular drainage. Any signs of a falling GCS is an indication for immediate CT.
- Late communicating hydrocephalus (after 30 days) occurs in 25% of patients and may require a permanent ventricular shunt.

TABLE 1.6

WFNS classification of SAH and associated morbidity and mortality

Grade	GCS	Motor deficit	Morbidity [%]	Mortality [%]
I	15	Absent	< 5	< 5
II	14–13	Absent	10	5–10
III	14–13	Present	25	5–10
IV	12–7	Absent or present	25	25–30
V	6–3	Absent or present	40	40

Hyponatraemia:
- This complicates up to 35% of SAHs. It is caused by cerebral salt wasting with excessive natruresis, leading to hypovolaemia. The treatment is intravascular volume expansion.
- Other electrolyte disturbances, particularly hypokalaemia and hypocalcaemia, are common.

Seizures:
- Occur in up to 25% of patients with SAH
- Prophylactic treatment is not usually recommended after aneurysm control.

Cardiac:
- Transient myocardial dysfunction (as evidenced by ECG changes) is common and correlates with the WFNS grade and amount of intracranial blood.
- A neurogenic stunned myocardium is a rare complication of SAH associated with refractory hypotension, lactic acidosis and regional wall motion abnormalities.
- ECG changes are seen in 50–100% of patients with SAH, and may mimic myocardial infarction with a T-wave inversion, ST elevation and rhythm disturbances. The changes are thought to be the result of hyperactivity of the sympathetic system – particularly noradrenaline (norepinephrine) release – and sensitisation of the myocardium to catecholamines by raised corticosteroid levels.
- Such ECG changes do not correlate with postoperative myocardial morbidity, and therefore isolated ECG changes are not an indication to postpone definitive surgical or interventional radiological treatment.
- If other symptoms or signs suggest myocardial injury, cardiac enzyme analysis (troponins), echocardiography and thallium scanning should be undertaken.

Respiratory
These cause 23% of non-neurological causes of death and consist of:
- Pneumonia
- Cardiogenic pulmonary oedema
- Neurogenic pulmonary oedema
- Pulmonary embolus.

DIAGNOSIS

COMPUTED TOMOGRAPHY:
- Thin-slice (3 mm) non-contrast CT is highly sensitive (> 95%) for blood in the

subarachnoid space within 24 h of acute haemorrhage.
- Blood is cleared rapidly from the subarachnoid space, and sensitivity decreases to 30% at 2 weeks.
- The increased density of blood on CT is a function of haemoglobin concentration and SAH may not be apparent in anaemic patients.
- CT detects associated intracranial haemorrhage and hydrocephalus.
- The distribution of the blood may suggest the site of bleeding.

LUMBAR PUNCTURE:
- Any patient whose clinical presentation suggests SAH, but whose scan is negative or equivocal, must have a lumbar puncture as soon as possible.
- Blood-stained 'traumatic taps' occur in 20% of lumbar punctures, and must be distinguished from true SAH.
- Following SAH the released haemoglobin is metabolised within 2 h to oxyhaemoglobin and by 12 h to bilirubin, resulting in xanthochromia.
- When clear CSF is obtained, this excludes SAH. If the CSF is bloody, the lumbar puncture should be repeated at 12 h and examined for the presence of xanthochromia.

ANGIOGRAPHY:
- Conventional four-vessel intra-arterial angiography remains the 'gold standard' for confirming the presence of an aneurysm or arteriovenous malformation.
- This can then be used to plan further treatment.
- Magnetic resonance angiography and helical (spiral) CT angiography are used in some centres.

MEDICAL MANAGEMENT OF SAH

The main aims of treatment are to:
- Optimise cerebral perfusion in the area of the bleed
- Reduce the risk of rebleeding prior to definitive treatment (surgical clipping or Guglielmi coil embolisation)
- Reduce the risk of vasospasm, which may cause delayed ischaemic deficit and subsequent cerebral infarction
- At all times in the course of a SAH a high index of suspicion must be

maintained for the development of hydrocephalus.

REBLEEDING

The rate of rebleeding following the initial SAH is 4% for the first 24 h and then 1–2% per day for the next 2 weeks. Without definitive treatment, 50% of patients will rebleed within 6 months. The mortality rate from a rebleed is 50–60%, mainly due to vasospasm.

Rebleeding is related to variations and changes, rather than the absolute level of blood pressure. Bed rest, analgesia and stabilisation of blood pressure are recommended. Aggressive blood pressure reduction should not be attempted as there may be raised ICP following the SAH, and an adequate cerebral perfusion pressure must be maintained.

VASOSPASM

Up to 67% of patients who initially survive a SAH develop vasospasm (narrowing of cerebral vessels when demonstrated by angiography) and this remains an important cause of morbidity and death. Half of these patients will be symptomatic with delayed ischaemic deficit manifesting as an alteration in conscious level, disorientation or focal neurological deficits.

Vasospasm is most likely to occur in patients with poor initial grades and in those with larger clots in the basal cisterns. It typically occurs between 3 and 10 days after the SAH, with a peak incidence at day 7. Without treatment the mortality rate is 30–50%.

DIAGNOSIS:
- Angiography
- Transcranial Doppler (TCD)
- Both methods have limitations and so a diagnosis is usually made on clinical grounds (i.e. altered neurology).

PATHOPHYSIOLOGY
This remains unclear, but it is thought that vasoactive substances in the subarachnoid blood cause severe vasoconstriction. Oxyhaemoglobin is thought to have a major role by producing superoxide free radicals that inactivate nitric oxide. Intracellular calcium stores are released, and produce prolonged smooth muscle contraction. There may also be a calcium-mediated imbalance between prostaglandins.

TREATMENT OF VASOSPASM

Triple H therapy

The rationale for triple H therapy (haemodilution, hypertension, hypervolaemia) is based on the presumption that cerebral blood flow in affected areas of the brain is pressure dependent (hence hypertension) and the observation that flow in ischaemic brain varies with cardiac output (hence hypervolaemia). Triple H therapy has been shown to reduce the incidence of delayed ischaemic deficit by 50%.

Volume loading with a colloid is most important and is done prophylactically to a CVP of 12–15 mmHg. Caution is needed to avoid vasogenic cerebral oedema or cardiac overload and pulmonary oedema. Many patients with SAH are volume depleted and the haemodynamic goals are to improve cerebral oxygenation.

A vasopressor – usually noradrenaline (norepinephrine) – is used to create a supranormal blood pressure. This is done most safely following definitive treatment when the risk of rebleeding is low. Invasive monitoring of arterial blood pressure is needed and a non-invasive measure of cardiac output may be useful.

Haemodilution to a haematocrit of 32% produces optimal cerebral microvascular rheology and occurs with volume loading.

Calcium channel antagonists

Nimodipine administered orally (60-mg, 4-hourly) decreases the incidence of cerebral infarction following SAH by 34% and the incidence of poor outcomes by 40%, with minimal side effects. Nimodipine is thought to provide benefit by inhibiting calcium entry into smooth muscle cells and vasoactive substance release from platelets and endothelial cells. It does not reduce the incidence of angiographic vasospasm.

Angioplasty

- Balloon angioplasty for discrete lesions in proximal arteries if instituted within 2 h of onset of delayed ischaemic deficit
- Chemical angioplasty using papaverine directly instilled into the cerebral circulation for diffuse, distal vasospasm or catheter-induced vasospasm during coil embolisation.

BIBLIOGRAPHY

Edlow JA, Caplan LR. Avoiding pitfalls in the diagnosis of subarachnoid haemorrhage. New England Journal of Medicine 2000; 342:29–36

Lam AM. Cerebral aneurysms: anesthetic considerations. In: Cottrell JE, Smith DS, eds. Anesthesia and neurosurgery. 4th edn. St Louis: Mosby; 2001:367–397

Mayberg MR. AHA medical/scientific statement: guidelines for the management of aneurysmal subarachnoid haemorrhage. Stroke 1994; 25(11):2315–2328

Schievink WI. Intracranial aneurysms. New England Journal of Medicine 1997; 336:28–39

Treggiari-Venzi MM, Suter PM, Romand J-A. Review of medical prevention of vasospasm after aneurysmal subarachnoid haemorrhage: a problem of neurointensive care. Neurosurgery 2001; 48(2):249–262

Vermeulen M. Subarachnoid haemorrhage: diagnosis and treatment. Journal of Neurology 1996; 243:496–501

CROSS-REFERENCES

Raised ICP/CBF control
Anaesthetic Factors 31: 787

1

Tetanus

S. K. Kodakat and J. J. Radcliffe

Tetanus is a preventable endemic disease of the developing world, frequently requiring expensive modern critical care for effective management. The disease is rare in the developed world. It is caused by *Clostridium tetani*, an obligate, anaerobic, spore-forming bacillus, ubiquitous in soil and animal gut. The bacilli are heat susceptible, but the spores are very resistant to heat and thorough autoclaving (at least 15 min at 1 atmosphere, 120°C) is needed to ensure decontamination.

EPIDEMIOLOGY

Although the incidence is declining, there are an estimated one million cases worldwide annually. Neonatal tetanus may account for half of these. Approximately 15 cases each year are reported in the UK. In the developed world tetanus is more often diagnosed in older people (with no or incomplete primary vaccination or declining immunity). Tetanus may follow elective surgery, injected drug abuse (especially heroin), burns, otitis media, dental infection, abortion, childbirth, animal bites, diabetic foot, deep puncture wounds or crush wounds. The injury may be trivial in up to 50% of cases.

PATHOPHYSIOLOGY

Under anaerobic conditions in necrotic or infected tissue spores germinate and the vegetative organism secretes the two exotoxins tetanospasmin (mol. wt. 56 000), which causes clinical tetanus, and tetanolysin, which produces local tissue injury. Toxins are disseminated locally and via the bloodstream, subsequently entering motor nerve endings and travelling intra-axonally to the cell body. Motor endplates, spinal cord and sympathetic nervous system are usually affected. The most significant clinical effects are through a presynaptic blockade of inhibitory interneurones, leading to overactivity of α-motor neurones.

There can be an incubation period of 1–60 days (usually 7–10 days). Onset may be quicker if the injury is nearer to the cranium.

CLINICAL FEATURES

Tetanus is characterised by a clinical triad of trismus (lockjaw), local or generalised muscle rigidity, and autonomic dysfunction (Box 1.12). Neck stiffness, dysphagia and difficulty in opening the jaw are usually the earliest signs. Severe muscle spasm, laryngospasm, convulsion, coma and arrhythmias are seen in severe cases. Diagnosis is made on clinical grounds. A history of injury or other mode of transmission may not be obtained in all cases.

BOX 1.12

Clinical features of tetanus

Early manifestations

- Muscle stiffness
- Spasm of masseter muscle (trismus or lockjaw)

Later manifestations

- Tetanospasms occur, causing:
  —clenching of the jaw (risus sardonicus)
  —arching of the back (opisthotonos)
  —flexion of arms, extension of legs
- Autonomic involvement – hypotension or hypertension, arrhythmias
- Respiratory failure, aspiration pneumonia
- Fractures, especially of thoracic vertebrae

COMPLICATIONS

Aspiration pneumonia (50–70% of autopsies), respiratory failure due to sustained muscle spasms, convulsions, fracture of spines or long bones, autonomic nervous system instability leading to hypertension, paroxysmal tachycardia or other arrhythmia, and profuse salivary and bronchial hypersecretion may all occur. A prolonged hospital stay can be associated with nosocomial infections, pulmonary embolism, decubitus ulcers and gastrointestinal bleeding.

PROGNOSIS

The reported overall mortality rate varies from 12% to 50%. A poor prognosis is associated with a shorter incubation period, rapid progression from local spasm to generalised spasm and the extremes of age. Residual effects relate principally to complications of the acute illness and prolonged intensive care.

PREVENTION

Active immunity is provided with tetanus toxoid. Passive immunity can be secured with tetanus immune globulin administered after the injury if the patient has not had a full course of tetanus toxoid. Early debridement of contaminated wounds should be performed (under 6 h).

TREATMENT

- Secondary debridement of even small or hidden wounds in established tetanus.
- Tetanus immune globulin (3000–6000 units i.m.) will neutralise unbound toxins.
- Benzylpenicillin has been used most frequently; tetracyclines are an alternative in allergic patients. Intravenous metronidazole may be the antibiotic of choice where seizures are present.
- Admission to HDU or ICU is indicated except for those with only local symptoms. Avoid unnecessary stimulation; monitor closely in a quiet room.
- Control of spasms may need sedation (diazepam is popular) with or without paralysis. Propofol and midazolam have been used with success.
- Recently a continuous infusion of magnesium (to achieve a serum concentration of 2–4 mmol l^{-1}) has been used successfully to prevent spasms without sedation or paralysis, with the additional benefit of autonomic stability.
- Dantrolene (1 mg kg^{-1} over 3 h), chlorpromazine and intrathecal baclofen to prevent spasm have been reported.
- Tracheal intubation will be necessary if there is laryngospasm, uncontrolled generalised spasms, uncontrolled convulsions or severe dysphagia.
- Morphine, β- and α-adrenergic blockers, epidural local anaesthetics and clonidine have been used to treat 'autonomic storms'.
- Early enteral feeding should be introduced. Generally, critical care is not sufficiently prolonged to merit percutaneous enteral feeding.
- Active immunisation with tetanus toxoid, which should be administered at a site most distant from the tetanus immune globulin and repeated at 6–12 weeks. Tetanus infection does not confer immunity due to the low antigenicity of the organism.

PROLONGED INTENSIVE CARE:
- Recovery from severe phase in 2–4 weeks. Some patients take months for full recovery.
- Deep venous thrombosis prophylaxis
- Gastric protection if gastric feeding not feasible
- Early tracheostomy
- Prevention of infection
- Prevention of bed sores.

1

BIBLIOGRAPHY

Attygalle D, Rodrigo N. Magnesium as first line therapy of tetanus: a prospective study of 40 patients. Anaesthesia 2002; 57:811–817

Cook TM, Protheroe RT, Handel JM. Tetanus: a review of the literature. British Journal of Anaesthesia 2001; 87:477–487

CROSS-REFERENCES

Autonomic dysfunction
  Patient Conditions 1: 4

2

ENDOCRINE SYSTEM
G. Hall

Acromegaly

W. J. Fawcett

Acromegaly results from increased growth hormone (GH) secretion, leading to an overgrowth of bone, connective tissue and viscera. The effects are mediated directly by GH and by the release of insulin-like growth factor 1 (IGF-1). Regulatory factors for GH secretion include GH-releasing hormone (GRH), growth hormone-releasing peptide (Ghrerin), somatostatin and IGF-1. Treatment for the condition may be surgical (hypophysectomy) or medical (dopamine agonists or somatostatin analogues; e.g. octreotide).

PATHOPHYSIOLOGY

Acromegaly usually results from a pituitary adenoma, and rarely from ectopic GH-producing tumours. In addition to the effects of hypersecretion of GH, there may also be clinical features arising from local pressure effects (visual field defects) and/or from damage to normal pituitary tissue causing hypopituitarism. There is a higher mortality rate from malignancy, and also from respiratory, cardiovascular and cerebrovascular disease, in patients with acromegaly. The diagnosis may be confirmed by a random GH level > 5 ng ml^{-1} and by the failure of GH to fall in response to a 75-g oral glucose tolerance test. IGF-1 is also used as an indicator of GH activity because it has a longer half-life than GH.

CARDIOVASCULAR SYSTEM:
- Hypertension and cardiomegaly
- Cardiomyopathy
- Complications of diabetes mellitus.

NEUROMUSCULAR SYSTEM:
Proximal myopathy and nerve entrapment syndromes, kyphoscoliosis.

RESPIRATORY SYSTEM:
- Somnolence and sleep apnoea
- Partial upper respiratory tract obstruction resulting from soft tissue hypertrophy of the pharyngeal and nasal mucosa

- Voice changes, from vocal cord involvement (glottic stenosis, chondrocalcinosis or vocal cord paresis from recurrent laryngeal nerve involvement)
- Macroglossia and prognathism.

ENDOCRINE SYSTEM:
- Overgrowth of soft tissues and skeleton, particularly head, tongue, jaw, hands and feet
- Impaired glucose tolerance
- Hypercalcaemia and hypercalcuria
- Other related endocrine problems include:
  —nodular goitre, which may compress the trachea
  —hyperthyroidism and hypothyroidism
  —hypopituitarism
  —diabetes insipidus.

PREOPERATIVE ASSESSMENT

Careful assessment of the upper airway (stridor, snoring, sleep apnoea). Associated cardiovascular, neuromuscular and endocrine involvement is sought. Preparation should be made for a difficult intubation, including awake fibreoptic intubation. Arrangements should be made for postoperative respiratory monitoring in the ITU, especially with the coexistence of sleep apnoea.

Premedication should avoid respiratory depressant drugs in patients with upper airway involvement. A drying agent (glycopyrrolate) is useful if a fibreoptic intubation is contemplated. If glucose intolerance is present, a glucose and insulin infusion may be required. Somatostatin analogues are sometimes used before operation.

INVESTIGATIONS:
- Blood tests: urea and electrolytes, glucose, calcium, thyroid function tests.
- Neck radiography (for glottic involvement, pharyngeal tissue overgrowth).
- Indirect laryngoscopy may characterise vocal cord involvement.

- Cardiovascular investigations should include:
  - —chest radiography
  - —ECG
  - —echocardiography.
- Consider a baseline arterial blood gas estimation.

PERIOPERATIVE MANAGEMENT

AIRWAY

If intubation is required (and particularly if there is upper airway involvement) then skilled assistance is mandatory. A selection of long armoured tracheal tubes should be available. Awake fibreoptic intubation is probably safest in experienced hands. The oral route is preferred as the nasal mucosa may be thickened considerably. There may be difficulties obtaining an airtight fit with a face-mask. Without serious upper airway involvement, intravenous induction and intubation avoiding the pressor response to laryngoscopy (e.g. alfentanil 10 μg kg^{-1}) should be undertaken, ensuring that the patient can be ventilated before administering a non-depolarising neuromuscular blocking drug. In patients in whom direct or fibreoptic laryngoscopy is not possible, or in those with vocal cord involvement or a history of sleep apnoea, elective tracheostomy is indicated. Experience with the intubating laryngeal mask airway in this condition is limited.

MONITORING:

- Full monitoring in the anaesthetic room is necessary (including ECG, blood pressure and SpO_2). The patient's fingers may be too large for the SpO_2 probe.
- An arterial cannula for those undergoing prolonged operation, or who need respiratory care in the ITU afterwards.
- Central venous or pulmonary arterial catheterisation may be useful in those with significant cardiac disease.
- A peripheral nerve stimulator (there may be altered sensitivity to non-depolarising neuromuscular blocking drugs; e.g. neuromuscular abnormalities, hypercalcaemia).
- Serum glucose.

POSTOPERATIVE MANAGEMENT

Patients with airway involvement should be admitted to the ITU. Although extubation at the end of the procedure is normal, patients with serious upper airway problems may require a period of postoperative intubation or tracheostomy. Patients should receive humidified oxygen, with monitoring of arterial blood gases, and SaO_2. Caution is required in the use of opioid analgesics in the extubated patient. Acute pulmonary oedema secondary to airway obstruction is a recognised postoperative complication. The presence of sleep apnoea is associated with a high risk of perioperative airway problems, including airway obstruction.

In addition, patients undergoing hypophysectomy will also have a marked reduction in insulin requirements in the postoperative period. They may develop diabetes insipidus (permanent or temporary) needing treatment with DDAVP, and in the longer term need replacement with adrenocorticotrophic hormone (ACTH) and thyroid-stimulating hormone (TSH) (see hypopituitarism, p. 66). Some of the changes in clinical features may resolve following hypophysectomy (e.g. vocal cord changes, left ventricular hypertrophy), but this may take some weeks.

BIBLIOGRAPHY

Schmitt H, Buchfelder M, Radespiel-Troger M, Fahlbusch R. Difficult intubation in acromegalic patients: incidence and predictability. Anaesthesiology 2000; 93:110–114

Seidman PA, Kofke WA, Policare R, Young M. Anaesthetic complications of acromegaly. British Journal of Anaesthesia 2000; 84:179–182

Smith M, Hirsch NP. Pituitary disease and anaesthesia. British Journal of Anaesthesia 2000; 85:3–14

2

Adrenocortical insufficiency

A. Quinn

Primary adrenocortical insufficiency (Addison's disease) is a rare condition in which there is destruction of the adrenal cortex. Secondary insufficiency is due to inadequate ACTH production by any disease affecting the hypothalamus or pituitary. However, the commonest cause of this disorder results from exogenous steroid administration. The usual cause of primary insufficiency is an autoimmune disorder, and the patient may exhibit signs of other autoimmune diseases, such as pernicious anaemia, hypothyroidism or diabetes. Other causes are listed in Box 2.1. Assessment of the hypothalamic–pituitary–adrenal (HPA) axis is complicated: no single test of adrenal function satisfies all the criteria of efficacy, safety, simplicity and cost. However, common tests are random plasma cortisol levels, the short Synacthen test, the insulin tolerance test, circulating corticotrophin-releasing hormone (CRH) levels.

BOX 2.1

Causes of primary hypoadrenalism

- Autoimmune disease
- Tuberculosis
- Surgical removal
- Haemorrhage or infarction:
- Meningococcal septicaemia
- Venography
- Infiltration
- Malignant destruction
- Amyloid
- Schilder's disease (adrenal leukodystrophy)

PATHOPHYSIOLOGY

CARDIOVASCULAR SYSTEM

Mineralocorticoids act on the distal tubule to increase sodium reabsorption. Loss of this function leads to sodium and secondary fluid loss, resulting in hypovolaemia and hypotension. Glucocorticoids facilitate the action of nora-

drenaline on the arterioles; in their absence, vasodilatation exacerbates hypotension.

SKIN

ACTH is a pigmentary hormone. High levels present in Addison's disease may cause abnormal pigmentation in the mouth, on the hands, flexural regions or on recent scars.

BIOCHEMICAL OR METABOLIC:

- Hyponatraemia and high urinary sodium
- Hyperkalaemia (moderate)
- Hyperuricaemia
- Symptomatic hypoglycaemia as cortisol antagonises the effects of insulin; reduced gluconeogenesis and glycogenolysis
- Hypercalcaemia.

HAEMATOLOGICAL:

- Raised haematocrit
- Normochromic normocytic anaemia (after rehydration)
- Eosinophilia, leukocytosis.

PREOPERATIVE ASSESSMENT

HISTORY

The history is often insidious and includes anorexia, weight loss, nausea and vomiting, abdominal pain, diarrhoea or constipation, weakness and dizziness. The Addisonian crisis is usually associated with the stresses of illness, infection, surgery or trauma, and the patient may present in a moribund state.

INITIAL INVESTIGATIONS:

- Urea and electrolytes, blood glucose
- Full blood count
- ECG (peaked T waves, widened QRS)
- Chest radiography for evidence of tuberculosis
- Abdominal radiography (tuberculosis may cause calcified adrenals).

A patient presenting with an Addisonian crisis who requires emergency surgery should be managed in an ITU. Central venous, pulmonary artery and arterial cannulation enable rapid fluid replacement and frequent blood electrolyte sampling, and a urinary catheter is usually required to monitor urine output.

FLUID REPLACEMENT:
- Sodium chloride 0.9%, 1 litre rapidly, then more slowly
- Dextrose (50% i.v.) to correct hypoglycaemia
- Plasma volume expanders (e.g. gelofusine)
- Treat hyperkalaemia with insulin (added to the dextrose) and calcium gluconate (10 mmol).

HYPONATRAEMIA
Chronic hyponatraemia should be corrected with a 0.9% sodium chloride infusion. Correction of hyponatraemia in Addison's disease using hypertonic saline has been documented before emergency operation. However, this treatment is controversial as 'osmotic demyelination' may occur, associated with sudden deterioration, brain damage and death.

ADRENAL HORMONE REPLACEMENT
Acute presentation, cardiovascular collapse
Hydrocortisone hemisuccinate or phosphate (200 mg i.v.) followed by an infusion of 100 mg hydrocortisone in 0.9% saline over 24 h.

After the initial acute presentation
See adrenocortical insufficiency (p. 46) for steroid replacement regimen.

Oral maintenance for Addison's disease is cortisone 20–30 mg daily in divided doses plus fludrocortisone (0.1 mg once a day).

PERIOPERATIVE MANAGEMENT

MONITORING:
- ECG (arrhythmias)
- Capnography (hypocapnia will lower extracellular potassium concentration)
- Urine output
- Central venous pressure or pulmonary artery flotation catheter
- Arterial cannula (sodium, potassium, blood glucose levels).

GENERAL ANAESTHESIA
Induction of anaesthesia should be in theatre with full monitoring. There are no particular indications for any one anaesthetic technique: a careful conventional anaesthetic is appropriate.

These patients are susceptible to the depressant effects of many induction agents, narcotic analgesics and general anaesthetics. Ketamine was used successfully in a previously documented case. The induction agent etomidate inhibits the release of cortisol and is contraindicated. The importance of the adrenocortical responses to anaesthetic and surgical stress is unclear, particularly in view of the finding that patients may withstand surgery after the adrenocortical responses have been inhibited pharmacologically. Inadequate replacement of fluid and electrolytes is the more usual cause of perioperative hypotension.

LOCAL ANAESTHESIA
Cardiovascular instability may require additional intravenous fluid replacement and inotropic support.

POSTOPERATIVE MANAGEMENT

The patient should be monitored in the ITU:
- Fluid balance
- Electrolyte abnormalities (may have postoperative hypokalaemia)
- Renal function
- Steroid replacement.

BIBLIOGRAPHY

Herzberg L, Shulman MS. Acute adrenal insufficiency in a patient with acute appendicitis during anaesthesia. Anesthesiology 1985; 62:517–518

Kehlet H. A rational approach to dosage and preparation of parenteral glucocorticoid substitution therapy during surgical procedures. Acta Anaesthesiologica Scandinavica 1975; 19:260–264

Nicholson G, Burrin JM, Hall GM. Peri-operative steroid supplementation. Anaesthesia 1998; 53:1091–1104

Smith MG, Byrne AJ. An Addisonian crisis complicating anaesthesia. Anaesthesia 1981; 361:681

Weatherill D, Spence AA. Anaesthesia and disorders of the adrenal cortex. British Journal of Anaesthesia 1984; 56:741–749

2

CROSS-REFERENCES

Water and electrolyte disturbances
    Anaesthetic Factors 27: 624

Apudomas

J. Desborough

APUD describes groups of cells characterised by amine precursor uptake and decarboxylation, which results in the synthesis of biologically active amines and peptides. APUDomas are tumours of cells with APUD properties. The clinical manifestations of the tumour are characterised by overproduction of particular hormones and peptides. APUD cells are found in the pituitary, adrenal medulla, peripheral autonomic ganglia, gastrointestinal tract, pancreas, lung, gonads and thymus. Tumours may occur as part of multiple endocrine neoplasia (MEN) syndrome. The management of patients with phaeochromocytoma, insulinoma and carcinoid tumours is dealt with elsewhere.

GASTRINOMA

A very rare gastrin-producing tumour. Incidence is one case per million population per year. Second commonest functional islet cell tumour. Gastrin stimulates acid production from gastric parietal cells. Gastrinomas present with peptic ulcer disease; the Zollinger–Ellison syndrome is characterised by gastric acid hypersecretion with recurrent peptic ulceration and diarrhoea. Some 20–60% of patients with gastrinoma have coexisting MEN-1.

Sixty per cent of gastrinomas are malignant; 50% of patients have metastases at diagnosis.

PERIOPERATIVE MANAGEMENT
Elective surgery is considered if medical therapy does not suppress gastric acid hypersecretion. Therapy includes:
- Proton pump inhibitors (e.g. omeprazole)
- H_2 antagonists (e.g. ranitidine, cimetidine)
- Octreotide (octapeptide analogue of somatostatin).

Operation usually involves pancreatic resection of tumours. Preoperative and intraoperative tumour localisation is important. Patients with MEN-1 have multiple tumours with a tendency towards duodenal wall location.

Acute presentation may occur with gastrointestinal bleeding and perforation. Diarrhoea may lead to fluid volume depletion, electrolyte disturbance and dysrhythmias.

Invasive cardiovascular monitoring is required. The operation is prolonged.

POSTOPERATIVE MANAGEMENT:
- High-dependency unit or intensive care unit management
- Continue cardiovascular and biochemical monitoring
- Mortality rate is high for emergency procedures.

VIPomas

Extremely rare tumour that releases vasoactive intestinal peptide (VIP). Patients present with severe, large-volume secretory diarrhoea. Potassium and bicarbonate are lost from the gut resulting in hypokalaemia and metabolic acidosis. WDHA syndrome refers to the association of watery diarrhoea, hypokalaemia and achlorhydria.

PREOPERATIVE MANAGEMENT:
- Symptom control with octreotide and correction of electrolyte abnormalities
- Aggressive management of fluid volume status and metabolic acidosis.

PERIOPERATIVE MANAGEMENT:
- Invasive cardiovascular monitoring
- VIPomas are vascular tumours
- Frequent blood sampling for pH and electrolytes.

BIBLIOGRAPHY

Azimuddin K, Chamberlain RS. The surgical management of pancreatic neuroendocrine tumours. Surgical Clinics of North America W B Saunders 2001; 81:511–525

Owen R. Anaesthetic considerations in endocrine surgery. In: Lynn J, Bloom SR, eds. Surgical endocrinology. Oxford: Butterworth–Heinemann; 1993:71–84.

CROSS-REFERENCES

Water and electrolyte disturbances
    Anaesthetic Factors 27: 624

2

Conn's syndrome

A. Quinn

Aldosterone, the mineralocorticoid secreted by the zona glomerulosa of the adrenal cortex, promotes sodium reabsorption and potassium exchange in the renal tubules. Excess aldosterone production may be due to an adrenal adenoma (60%), bilateral adrenal hyperplasia (30%) or carcinoma. Conn's syndrome is rare, accounting for less than 1% of patients with hypertension.

PATHOPHYSIOLOGY
Biochemical or renal
Plasma renin levels are low; plasma aldosterone levels are high. Urinary potassium concentration is high despite a low total body potassium level, and serum sodium level may be raised. Renal function may be abnormal, and this is related to chronic potassium depletion and hypertension.

CARDIOVASCULAR SYSTEM:
- Hypertension may be severe, associated with renal and retinal damage.
- The ECG may show arrhythmias or T-wave flattening and U waves.
- Heart failure – aldosterone potentiates the effects of catecholamines and blocks noradrenaline uptake. It also causes myocardial fibrosis.
- Cardiomyopathy may be caused by chronic K^+ depletion.

METABOLIC:
- Hypokalaemic alkalosis from excessive tubular secretion of potassium and magnesium
- Abnormal glucose tolerance test in up to 50% of patients.

PREOPERATIVE ASSESSMENT

Differentiation of an adenoma from hyperplasia involves adrenal computed tomography (CT) or magnetic resonance imaging (MRI), complex biochemical testing and venous sampling. In Conn's syndrome, aldosterone levels are high only in the adrenal vein draining the tumour and are suppressed on the contralateral side. Surgical removal is recommended for unilateral adenoma only; bilateral hyperplasia responds better to medical treatment.

HISTORY
The common symptoms are weakness, nocturia, polyuria and polydipsia. Hypokalaemia may result in tetany. Quadriparesis has been described, and was reversed by potassium.

INVESTIGATIONS:
- Urea, electrolytes and blood glucose
- Arterial blood gases
- Increased plasma aldosterone and reduced renin levels
- ECG for arrhythmias, signs of hypokalaemia, left ventricular hypertrophy
- Chest radiograph may show cardiomegaly
- Blood cross-matching.

PREOPERATIVE MANAGEMENT
- Potassium infusion (e.g. 6–20 mmol h^{-1}) – at least 24 h may be required to restore potassium equilibrium
- ECG – hypokalaemia causes ST depression, flattened T waves, U waves
- Aldosterone antagonist (e.g. spironolactone 100 mg three times a day)
- Insulin infusion.

PERIOPERATIVE MANAGEMENT

PREMEDICATION
Moderate sedation with opioids or hypnotics.

INDUCTION AND MAINTENANCE
The anaesthetic technique should be tailored to avoid hypotensive or hypertensive events. A regional technique is often used, commonly a thoracic epidural continued in the postoperative period.

SPECIAL POINTS FOR ADRENALECTOMY

Adrenalectomy can be performed laparoscopically, or via an open incision, in the supine or lateral positions depending on tumour size, accessibility and surgical preference.

There may be marked intraoperative blood loss from nearby major blood vessels. Good muscle relaxation is important as surgical access may be difficult. Postoperative pneumothorax may occur.

MONITORING:

- Arterial cannula to monitor acid–base balance, blood glucose, haematocrit and direct arterial pressure
- Central venous line for monitoring fluid requirements
- ECG monitoring during induction and intubation; high risk of arrhythmia, ischaemia
- Capnography – hyperventilation exacerbates alkalosis
- Urinary catheter, as risk of renal failure
- Peripheral nerve stimulation – increased sensitivity to myoneural blocking agents (hypokalaemia and alkalosis)
- May have hypertensive surges during surgical manipulation; treat with, for example, labetalol (10–50 mg i.v.) or phentolamine (2.5–5 mg) every 5 min.

POSTOPERATIVE CARE

- Initial management should be on a high-dependency unit or intensive care unit
- Postoperative respiratory support – there may be a compensatory respiratory acidosis for the metabolic alkalosis and increased sensitivity to respiratory depressant drugs and muscle relaxants that the patient may require
- Postoperative arrhythmias
- Abnormal glucose tolerance
- Renal function
- Beware pneumothorax
- Thoracic epidural will provide good postoperative analgesia, particularly in open operations.
- After operation it may take a week for sodium and potassium levels to return to normal values, and hypertension may persist even longer
- Glucocorticoid or mineralocorticoid therapy should be required only if both adrenal glands are mobilised or removed.

BIBLIOGRAPHY

Weatherill D, Spence AA. Anaesthesia and disorders of the adrenal cortex. British Journal of Anaesthesia 1984; 56:741–749

Winship SM, Winstanley JH, Hunter JM. Anaesthesia for Conn's syndrome. Anaesthesia 1999; 54(6):569–574

CROSS-REFERENCES

Hypertension
    Patient Conditions 4: 151
Assessment of renal function
    Patient Conditions 6: 186

2

Cushing's syndrome

A. Quinn

This is the term used to describe the clinical state of increased free circulating glucocorticoid. It occurs most frequently as a result of exogenous corticosteroid administration; all the spontaneous forms are rare.

CAUSES OF CUSHING'S SYNDROME

ACTH-dependent disease (60–70%):
- Pituitary-dependent (Cushing's disease) producing bilateral adrenal hyperplasia
- Ectopic ACTH-producing tumours (bronchial, pancreatic carcinoma)
- ACTH administration.

Non-ACTH-dependent causes:
- Adrenal adenomas
- Adrenal carcinomas
- Glucocorticoid administration.

Other:
- Alcohol-induced pseudo-Cushing's syndrome

PATHOPHYSIOLOGY

The main actions of glucocorticoids are:
- Suppression of pituitary ACTH secretion
- Glycogen deposition, increased gluconeogenesis, fat deposition
- Increased protein catabolism and decreased synthesis
- Potassium loss, sodium retention, increased free water clearance and uric acid production
- Immunosuppression and increased circulating neutrophils.

PREOPERATIVE ASSESSMENT

Some patients require perioperative intensive care management for optimal treatment of diabetes, hypertension or cardiac failure, restrictive lung disease, fluid and electrolyte abnormalities (low potassium concentration, especially if diuretic therapy) and steroid requirements.

GENERAL:
- Assessment of airway in obese patient
- Careful positioning (osteoporosis and pathological fractures, obesity, easy bruising)
- Assessment of fragile veins and arteries
- Assessment of ease of local anaesthetic technique.

HISTORY
The following history may be elicited:
- *Metabolic* – diabetes
- *Cardiovascular* – hypertension, oedema
- *Skin and subcutaneous tissue* – centripetal obesity, acne, hirsutism, bruising, striae, pigmentation, thin skin, poor wound healing, skin infection, frontal balding pattern, moon face, plethora, buffalo hump
- *Bone* – osteoporosis, rib fractures, pathological fractures, vertebral collapse, kyphosis
- *Muscle* – proximal muscle wasting, proximal myopathy, weakness
- *CNS* – depression or psychosis
- *Children* – growth arrest.

INVESTIGATIONS:
- Full blood count
- Urea and electrolytes, blood glucose levels
- ECG (ischaemia, hypokalaemia)
- Chest radiography (kyphoscoliosis, osteoporosis, cardiac enlargement, left ventricular failure, lower lobe collapse, carcinoma of the bronchus)
- Lung function tests.

PERIOPERATIVE MANAGEMENT

The patient may present for adrenalectomy (see Conn's syndrome, p. 50) or pituitary surgery (usually transsphenoidal hypophysectomy), but more commonly for routine surgery.

The mortality rate following bilateral adrenalectomy in patients with Cushing's syndrome is 5–10%.

PREMEDICATION

Preoperative apprehension has little effect on plasma cortisol levels. Conventional premedication is used. May require steroid cover (see Iatrogenic adrenocortical insufficiency, p. 71). Concomitant medication commonly includes: antihypertensives, diuretics, insulin, antibiotics, antacids, inhibitors of cortisol synthesis (e.g. metyrapone, glutethimide, bromocriptine), H_2 antagonists and deep vein thrombosis (DVT) prophylaxis.

MONITORING

This should commence in the anaesthetic room and includes:

- Central venous pressure (CVP) and pulmonary artery pressure measurement (patients with Cushing's syndrome tend to have a bleeding tendency and a raised CVP)
- Arterial pressure monitoring
- Blood sampling for arterial blood gases, blood glucose, haematocrit
- ECG (CM_5 to detect myocardial ischaemia)
- Capnography, SpO_2
- Peripheral nerve stimulator
- Urine output.

INTRAOPERATIVE MANAGEMENT

No particular anaesthetic technique is indicated. However, anaesthetic agents should be administered slowly and carefully as these patients are sensitive to any cardiodepressant effects.

GENERAL ANAESTHESIA:

- Rapid sequence induction for obese patients
- Prepare equipment for difficult intubation
- Intermittent positive-pressure ventilation (IPPV)
- May require high F_{IO_2}
- Careful patient positioning is essential.

LOCAL ANAESTHESIA

This may lessen the stress response to surgery (e.g. epidural anaesthesia). Local anaesthesia may be technically difficult, but the advantages are that it produces good analgesia and enables minimal administration of opioids and rapid mobilisation. It may also reduce the incidence of thromboembolism.

POSTOPERATIVE MANAGEMENT

Patients should be admitted to the ITU after operation. Muscle weakness, obesity, kyphosis and frequent rib fractures make respiratory complications common. There is delayed wound healing and increased incidence of postoperative stroke, myocardial infarction, stress ulceration and pulmonary thromboembolism.

- Electrolyte abnormalities – avoid excessive administration of sodium-containing intravenous fluids because of the mineralocorticoid effect of excess cortisol
- Continuous humidified oxygen therapy
- Analgesia – opioid infusion, patient-controlled analgesia, epidural opioid or local anaesthetic
- Steroids – maintenance therapy after operation may be necessary for rest of life
- Insulin infusion
- Physiotherapy and early mobilisation
- DVT prophylaxis
- Vitamin D (treatment before operation may lead to hypercalcaemia and renal stones)
- Pancreatitis (after adrenalectomy).

BIBLIOGRAPHY

Mellor A, Harvey RD, Pobereskin LH, Sneyd JR. Cushing's disease treated by trans-sphenoidal selective adenomectomy in mid-pregnancy. British Journal of Anaesthesia 1998; 80(6):850–852

Weatherill D, Spence AA. Anaesthesia and disorders of the adrenal cortex. British Journal of Anaesthesia 1984; 56:741–749

CROSS-REFERENCES

Hypertension
    Patient Conditions 4: 151
Metabolic and degenerative bone disease
    Patient Conditions 8: 240
Water and electrolyte disturbances
    Anaesthetic Factors 27: 624
Iatrogenic adrenocortical insufficiency
    Patient Conditions 2: 71

2

Diabetes insipidus

W. J. Fawcett

Diabetes insipidus (DI) is a syndrome in which there is failure either of arginine vasopressin (AVP) production (neurogenic or cranial DI) or of the kidneys to respond to AVP (nephrogenic DI). AVP is usually released in response to increased serum osmolality or a reduction in plasma volume. Thus, there is failure to conserve water, leading to polydipsia and polyuria.

PATHOPHYSIOLOGY

Cranial DI
- Primary
- Secondary
  - trauma
  - postoperative (neurosurgery)
  - tumour (primary or secondary)
  - infection
  - vascular causes.

Nephrogenic DI
- Primary
- Secondary
  - hypercalcaemia
  - hypokalaemia
  - drugs (lithium, demeclocycline, glibenclamide, amphotericin B, methoxyflurane)

The hallmarks of the syndrome are large urine volumes (up to 1 l h^{-1}) with low urine osmolality (50–100 mOsm kg^{-1}). However, plasma osmolalities and sodium concentrations may be in the normal range if there is access to free water. If not, then hypovolaemia and hypernatraemia may rapidly follow. There is a wide range of severity, depending on whether or not there is a complete loss of osmoregulation, and whether or not the response to volume stimuli is intact. The syndrome is diagnosed by increased plasma osmolality (> 295 mOsm l^{-1}), hypotonic urine (< 300 mOsm l^{-1}) and polyuria (> 2 ml kg^{-1} h^{-1}) The ability to correct this is tested by giving DDAVP: in cranial DI there is a response; in nephrogenic DI there is no response.

PREOPERATIVE ASSESSMENT

The preoperative assessment will be directed principally towards the assessment of fluid balance and serum osmolality. Attention should be turned to the amount the patient is drinking and the fluid balance status. Look for signs of dehydration suggested by:
- Dry mouth, loss of skin turgor
- Tachycardia, low venous pressure and, eventually, hypotension
- In addition, in secondary DI there may be other problems, such as lung carcinoma.

INVESTIGATIONS:
- Serum urea, electrolytes and osmolality
- Serum calcium
- Urinary volumes and osmolality – the aim should be to have a serum osmolality of less than 290 mOsm l^{-1}.

No patient with uncontrolled DI should undergo surgery until the diabetes is corrected. This should be done in conjunction with an endocrinologist, and would usually include intranasal DDAVP (5–20 μg twice daily) or oral DDAVP (0.1–0.4 mg three times a day) for cranial DI. Other treatments used for partial cranial DI include chlorpropamide and carbamazepine, which probably sensitise the renal tubules to the endogenous AVP. Nephrogenic DI is treated with thiazides. Acute treatment of hypovolaemia should gradually reduce serum sodium concentration and osmolalities (over 48 h). Rapid correction with large amounts of hypotonic fluids, or overenthusiastic use of DDAVP, is to be condemned as there is a substantial risk of cerebral oedema and haemorrhage.

The patient should not undergo prolonged fasting without intravenous fluids. Patients need to be monitored in an ICU or HDU environment after operation.

2

PERIOPERATIVE MANAGEMENT

The principal aim is to maintain the patient's fluid balance. Thus, meticulous care is required to ensure that urine loss and other losses from surgery (insensible/blood) are accurately replaced.

Monitoring should include:

*   Urine output
*   Arterial cannula for major surgery
*   Central venous pressure
*   Serum and urine osmolalities need to be checked regularly (i.e. 2–4 hourly) in the acute situation.

In cranial DI, DDAVP would normally be given immediately before operation, with further amounts given if the serum osmolality exceeds 290 mOsm l^{-1}. In patients with some AVP production, the 'stress' response of surgery may produce adequate amounts of AVP, but this cannot be relied on.

POSTOPERATIVE MANAGEMENT

The patient will require continued management of fluid balance in the postoperative period, particularly after major surgery, or whilst blood loss is a problem.

BIBLIOGRAPHY

Smith M, Hirsch NP. Pituitary disease and anaesthesia. British Journal of Anaesthesia 2000; 85:3–14

CROSS-REFERENCES

Water and electrolyte disturbances
Anaesthetic Factors 27: 624

2

Diabetes mellitus type 1

R. Milaszkiewicz

An autoimmune disorder of the pancreas characterised by β-cell destruction.

CHARACTERISTICS:
- Onset usually in younger age group
- Absolute insulin deficiency
- Abrupt onset of symptoms
- Tendency to ketosis.

Diagnosed by consistently raised random plasma glucose concentration > 11.1 mmol l^{-1} (venous whole blood glucose > 10 mmol l^{-1}) or fasting plasma glucose > 7.0 mmol l^{-1} (blood glucose > 6.1 mmol l^{-1}).

COMPLICATIONS
Long term:
- Retinopathy
- Ischaemic heart disease – two to four times higher than in the general population
- Hypertension – blood pressure increased in 30–60% of diabetics
- Nephropathy – 30–40% of type 1 diabetics
- Neuropathy – peripheral and autonomic (autonomic found in up to 40% of type 1 diabetics)
- Respiratory disease - poor glycaemic control in type 1 diabetics has been associated with impaired lung function
- Stiff joint syndrome – may cause difficulty with intubation.

Short term:
- Hypoglycaemia
- Hyperglycaemia with metabolic disturbance – may be exacerbated by the 'stress response' during operation
- Gastric stasis is common, especially with hyperglycaemia and ketoacidosis.

PREOPERATIVE ASSESSMENT

HISTORY:
- Diabetes:
  —duration
  —control

—type, quantity and timing of insulin dosage.
- Assess presence of coexisting disease:
- Renal – nephropathy (mild–severe).
- Cardiovascular system:
  —ischaemic heart disease with decreased exercise tolerance
  —hypertension.
- Respiratory system.
- CNS – peripheral and autonomic neuropathy.
- Other drugs.

EXAMINATION
Full physical examination, with attention to cardiac, respiratory and renal disease according to any positive indicators in the history. Airway assessment should include the 'prayer sign', indicative of the stiff joint syndrome.

INVESTIGATIONS:
- Glycaemic control:
  —short-term – fasting blood glucose
  —long-term – glycosylated haemoglobin (HbA_1C). This should be within normal limits. An $HbA_1C > 9\%$ is indicative of poor control; hyperglycaemia, hypovolaemia and electrolyte abnormalities should be anticipated and corrected before operation.
- Full blood count.
- Renal function – urinalysis, plasma urea, creatinine and electrolyte concentration
- Chest radiography, if clinically indicated.
- ECG or exercise ECG – silent ischaemia.

$HbA1C > 7\%$ can be used as a predictor of coronary heart disease. If associated with other risk factors such as a poor exercise tolerance, age over 55 years, obesity or physical inactivity, a 'stress ECG' to evaluate for silent ischaemia may be indicated before major surgery. An inability to climb two flights of stairs has a positive predictive value of 89% for postoperative cardiopulmonary complications in these patients.

AIMS OF PERIOPERATIVE MANAGEMENT

MAINTENANCE OF NORMOGLYCAEMIA

Blood glucose should stay within the range $6-11$ mmol l^{-1}. Hyperglycaemia causes dehydration, electrolyte disturbance, acidosis, poor tissue perfusion and organ ischaemia, impaired wound healing and increased susceptibility to infection. Cerebral or myocardial ischaemia is aggravated by hyperglycaemia. Hypoglycaemia may cause cerebral damage.

APPROPRIATE MANAGEMENT OF COEXISTING DISEASE

Coexisting disease is a greater cause of morbidity than the diabetes itself. Cardiovascular drugs including beta-blockers should be continued in the preoperative period, as they may be protective. Fluid and electrolytes should be optimised before operation.

Autonomic neuropathy may cause cardiovascular instability during anaesthesia.

GENERAL PRINCIPLES OF MANAGEMENT

MAJOR SURGERY

Ideally, the patient is admitted 24 h before the operation. With the increasing use of preassessment clinics, advice can be given about the management of insulin before operation, and well controlled diabetic patients can be safely admitted on the evening before surgery, or even on the day of operation if this is in the afternoon. Long-acting insulins should be omitted the night before surgery. Ideally patients with diabetes should be operated on at the beginning of morning lists. If this is not possible, a sliding scale should be started in the morning.

Glucose

Glucose should be started when calories or fluids are required and cannot be obtained by the enteral route. Sufficient glucose is supplied to prevent hypoglycaemia and to provide basal energy requirements. It is recommended that glucose be given at a rate of $5-10$ g h^{-1}. For an average person, this usually works out at 5% dextrose given at about $100-200$ ml h^{-1}. For longer term infusions, 0.9% sodium chloride is also needed to prevent hyponatraemia.

Insulin

The morning dose of insulin should be omitted. However, if the patient is due to have surgery in the afternoon, either (a) set up an infusion of glucose + insulin + potassium in the morning, or (b) if allowed to eat, give half the usual dose of insulin with a light breakfast, then set up an infusion mid-morning when the effects of the insulin are wearing off.

Insulin should be given by an intravenous infusion, following a sliding scale regimen (see Table 2.1). Intravenous boluses have too short a half-life and they may cause deterioration of metabolic control. Absorption of subcutaneous insulin is variable, especially in the perioperative period, and this route is not recommended for patients undergoing major surgery. Strict monitoring of blood glucose must be performed.

Insulin may be also added to a bag of glucose (the Alberti regimen; see Box 2.2). The usual requirements are $0.25-0.35$ units per gram of glucose.

TABLE 2.1	
Sliding scale for insulin	
Blood glucose (mmol l^{-1})	Insulin infusion* (units h^{-1})
0–5	0–0.5
6–10	1–2
11–15	2–3
16–20	3–4
> 20	Medical intervention needed

*Infusion: make up 50 units insulin to 50 ml with saline (1 unit ml^{-1}). No need to add colloid, provided the first few millilitres are flushed through the giving set.

BOX 2.2	
The Alberti regimen	
Glucose 10%	500 ml
Insulin (soluble)	15 units
Potassium	10 mmol

- Add together
- Infuse this at 100 ml h^{-1}
- Blood glucose is monitored 2-hourly and insulin content of bag adjusted by 5 units if blood glucose level falls outside the range $6-11$ mmol l^{-1}.

2

Insulin requirements are increased with: steroid therapy, sepsis, liver disease, obesity and during cardiopulmonary bypass.

Potassium
Potassium should be added as required – usually fluid 20 mmol l^{-1}.

MINOR SURGERY AND DAY CASES
Type 1 diabetic patients are presenting for day-case surgery more frequently. There is no consensus regarding management and no agreement that these patients are suitable for such treatment. The procedure should be performed in the morning, should be minor, unlikely to cause much pain, and be associated with a low incidence of postoperative nausea and vomiting. Patients should be able to demonstrate a good understanding of how to alter their insulin dosage, and they must have good support at home to be accepted as day cases. The HbA$_1$C should be < 7%. Facilities must exist to admit these patients after operation, if necessary.

Either:
Omit the morning dose of insulin (except for long-acting insulins such as ultralente, which will not affect or be affected by the fasting in the perioperative period), and give a partial or full dose before the next meal, according to the patient's blood glucose level and the amount of carbohydrate consumed.

Or:
Omit the morning dose of insulin and start glucose–insulin–potassium infusions on admission.

Glucose and a sliding-scale insulin infusion should be started if the fasting glucose is outside the range 6–11 mmol l^{-1} or if there is any delay to the start of the operation, and should be started after operation if the patient suffers from nausea and vomiting. The infusion should then continue until a normal diet has been resumed. Nausea and vomiting may indicate the development of ketoacidaemia.

MONITORING
Both hypoglycaemia and hyperglycaemia are harmful. Under anaesthesia, symptoms of hypoglycaemia are masked.

Blood glucose
This should be checked every 0.5–1 h before operation and in theatre, depending on how brittle the diabetic control has been, both using stick tests, and periodically confirming with laboratory blood glucose determinations. After operation, check hourly until a normal diet has been established.

Potassium
Plasma potassium levels should be monitored 3–4 hourly, or more frequently if clinically indicated.

ANAESTHESIA
No technique has been shown to be superior. Regional techniques, where appropriate, are preferable to general anaesthesia, as they usually allow a swifter return to normal eating patterns. They may partially decrease the 'stress response' associated with surgery.

CROSS-REFERENCES
Water and electrolyte balance
Anaesthetic Factors 27: 624

Diabetes mellitus type 2

R. Milaszkiewicz

More common than type 1. Characterised by both hepatic and extrahepatic insulin resistance, probably due to decreased stimulation of glycogen synthesis in muscle by insulin, related to impaired glucose transport. Insulin secretion and/or insulin action are thought to be deficient, with excessive hepatic glucose production.

CHARACTERISTICS:
- Variable age of onset – usually a disease of adults
- Slow onset
- Unlikely to develop ketoacidosis.

COMPLICATIONS
There is an increased incidence of macrovascular disease, especially peripheral vascular and cardiovascular disease, irrespective of age at diagnosis. Silent ischaemia is common, particularly if there is poor glycaemic control and in the presence of other risk factors such as obesity, physical inactivity and age > 55 years.

Nephropathy is common and is associated with cardiovascular disease.

MANAGEMENT:
- Diet
- Exercise
- Drugs:
  —*Sulphonylureas* – increase pancreatic ß-cell sensitivity to glucose, thereby enhancing insulin release. Long-acting drugs may exacerbate hypoglycaemia during fasting. Highly protein bound. Metabolised by the liver; metabolites have some activity. Excreted by the kidneys.
  —*Biguanides* – several possible modes of action. Probably reduce hepatic glucose production. May enhance glucose uptake in muscles. Metformin is only available drug. Not protein bound. Not metabolised by liver. Excreted unchanged by kidneys.
  —*Thiazolidinediones* – improve peripheral glucose uptake in the muscle and fat. Inhibit hepatic glucose production. Not

associated with lactic acidosis. May cause hepatotoxicity.
  —*Prandial glucose regulators* – nateglinide and repaglinide. Stimulate release of insulin from the pancreas. Fast onset and short duration of action; therefore taken just before meals. Less likely to cause hypoglycaemia than sulfonylureas.
  —*Acarbose* – inhibits α-glucosidases in the brush border of small intestinal mucosa. Delays absorption of glucose.

PREOPERATIVE ASSESSMENT

Should follow the same lines as for type 1 diabetes mellitus.

PERIOPERATIVE MANAGEMENT

These patients are still able to secrete some insulin; however, they are insulin resistant.

MINOR SURGERY OR DAY SURGERY
Well controlled, diet-treated patients do not usually need special treatment – apart from monitoring of blood glucose levels. For those taking oral hypoglycaemic agents, there is still controversy. If on long-acting agents, such as chlorpropamide, ideally this should be changed to a shorter-acting drug 48 h before the operation. If this is not possible, continue as normal up to the day before surgery and then omit any oral hypoglycaemics on the day of operation. Ideally, operation should be undertaken in the morning: this may avoid the need to intervene. If the patient is scheduled for afternoon surgery, regular monitoring of blood glucose levels should take place. As most patients are allowed fluids for up to 2 h before operation, give glucose-containing drinks if the blood glucose concentration decreases. If blood glucose concentration is < 11 mmol l^{-1}, it is usually sufficient just to monitor the blood glucose level. Start a sliding-scale infusion of

insulin if the patient is an inpatient and the fasting blood glucose level is > 11 mmol l^{-1}.

The most important feature is careful, frequent monitoring of blood glucose concentration and early corrective measures if the blood glucose level goes outside the range of $6–11$ mmol l^{-1}.

MAJOR SURGERY
Treat as for patients with type 1 diabetes mellitus. Hyperosmolar, hyperglycaemic, non-ketotic coma may occur after operation.

FLUIDS
There is some evidence against the use of Hartmann's solution, but it is unlikely to be deleterious if given more slowly than $1 \, l \, h^{-1}$.

ANAESTHESIA
Many of these patients will be presenting for surgery for complications of their diabetes. Careful management of pre-existing medical problems is important. Anaesthesia should cause minimal metabolic disturbance. Regional techniques are usually preferable to general anaesthesia, unless there is severe cardiovascular disturbance.

BIBLIOGRAPHY

McAnulty GR, Robertshaw HJ, Hall GM. Anaesthetic management of patients with diabetes mellitus. British Journal of Anaesthesia 2000; 85(1):89–90

Scherpereel P. Perioperative care of diabetic patient. Minerva Anesthesiologica 2001; 67:258–262

Scherpereel PA, Tavernier B. Perioperative care of diabetic patients. European Journal of Anaesthesiology 2001; 18:277–294

CROSS-REFERENCES

Diabetes Mellitus type 1
    Patient Conditions 2: 56

2

Hyperparathyroidism

R. Edwards

Hyperparathyroidism is a syndrome resulting from increased secretion of parathyroid hormone (PTH) from the parathyroid glands. PTH acts both directly and indirectly to increase serum calcium levels (normal total serum calcium concentration $2.3–2.8$ mmol l^{-1}).

Hyperparathyroidism may be classified as primary, secondary or tertiary.

CAUSES OF HYPERPARATHYROIDISM
Primary hyperparathyroidism:
- Single adenoma (80%) or multiple gland hyperplasia (10–15%) of parathyroid
- Adenoma may be part of multiple endocrine adenoma (MEA) syndrome
- Carcinoma (1–3%)
- Ectopic PTH may be produced by carcinoma of the lung or kidney.

Secondary hyperparathyroidism:
- Increased PTH secretion as a physiological response to hypocalcaemia (e.g. chronic renal failure).

Tertiary hyperparathyroidism
- Occurs when chronic secondary hyperparathyroidism has led to an autonomous adenoma.

ACTIONS OF PTH:
- Directly increases renal tubular reabsorption of calcium and decreases tubular reabsorption of phosphate
- Increases calcium reabsorption from bone
- Controls hydroxylation of 25-hydroxycholecalciferol in the kidney, and therefore promotes the synthesis of 1,25-dihydroxycholecalciferol and increases calcium absorption from the gut.

METABOLIC ABNORMALITIES
Primary and tertiary hyperparathyroidism:
- Serum calcium level high
- Low serum phosphate level

- PTH concentration high
- Raised alkaline phosphatase level
- Mild hyperchloraemic acidosis.

Secondary hyperparathyroidism
- Serum calcium level low
- High serum phosphate level.

PATHOPHYSIOLOGY

Most of the signs and symptoms of hyperparathyroidism are due to hypercalcaemia, and their severity is related to the level of serum calcium. Patients with mild hypercalcaemia (serum calcium level < 3.0 mmol l^{-1}) are often asymptomatic.

SIGNS AND SYMPTOMS OF HYPERCALCAEMIA
General:
- Muscle fatigue and hypotonicity
- Psychosis and depression with severe, prolonged hypercalcaemia
- Calcium deposition in conjunctiva, usually medial limbus of eye
- Radiographs of hands, feet and teeth may show subperiosteal resorption, bone cysts and loss of lamina dura of teeth.

Renal system:
- Polyuria
- Polydipsia
- Dehydration
- Renal calculi, nephrocalcinosis and later renal failure.

Gastrointestinal tract:
- Anorexia
- Nausea and vomiting
- Abdominal pain
- Constipation
- Dyspepsia
- Peptic ulceration.

2

Cardiovascular system:
- Tachycardia
- Arrhythmias
- Hypertension.

PREOPERATIVE ASSSESSMENT

HISTORY

Review of symptoms associated with hypercalcaemia.

INVESTIGATIONS:

- Serum calcium, electrolytes and urea
- ECG (shortened PR or QT interval)
- Patients with severe hypercalcaemia may present with hypovolaemia and coma. Emergency treatment comprises: hydration, diuresis and phosphate repletion; emergency parathyroidectomy.

PERIOPERATIVE MANAGEMENT

- No special monitoring required.
- Care should be taken to protect the eyes from pressure or abrasion during operation.
- An armoured orotracheal tube avoids airway obstruction due to kinking of the tube.
- All airway connections should be secured before draping the patient, as access to the head and neck is limited when the operation has commenced.
- No advantage of any one anaesthetic agent over another has been demonstrated in these patients.

POSTOPERATIVE COMPLICATIONS

NERVE DAMAGE

Bilateral recurrent laryngeal nerve injury (due to trauma or oedema) leads to stridor and laryngeal obstruction due to unopposed adduction of vocal cords. With a partial lesion of the recurrent laryngeal nerve, the cord is adducted; in a complete lesion, the cord is half abducted. A partial lesion is therefore more serious than a complete lesion. Bilateral partial lesions require immediate intubation and tracheostomy until recovery occurs. Unilateral damage is often unnoticed because of compensatory overadduction of the opposite cord.

Oedema of the glottis and pharynx may occasionally follow parathyroid surgery.

METABOLIC ABNORMALITIES

Hypocalcaemia may occur due to insufficient residual parathyroid tissue, delay in recovery of normal tissue, operative trauma or ischaemia. There may be laryngeal spasm, convulsions, a positive Chovstek sign and/or a positive Trousseau sign.

Hypomagnesaemia or hypophosphataemia may also occur after operation. Correction of serum magnesium concentration is important, as a low level inhibits the secretion of PTH.

Serial determinations of serum calcium, phosphate, magnesium and PTH levels are required for several days after operation.

BIBLIOGRAPHY

Roizen MF. Diseases of the endocrine system. In: Katz J, Benumof JL, Kadis LB, eds. Anaesthesia and uncommon diseases. Philadelphia: WB Saunders; 1990:245–292

Sebel PS. Thyroid and parathyroid disease. In: Nimmo WS, Smith G, eds. Anaesthesia. Oxford: Blackwell Scientific; 1989:771–778

CROSS-REFERENCES

Multiple endocrine neoplasia
  Patient Conditions 2: 77
Water and electrolyte disturbances
  Anaesthetic Factors 27: 624

Hyperthyroidism

R. Edwards

This is a clinical syndrome resulting from excessive production of the thyroid hormones tri-iodothyronine (T3) and thyroxine (T4). The production of these hormones from the thyroid gland is regulated by thyroid-stimulating hormone (TSH) from the anterior pituitary, which is in turn influenced by thyrotrophin-releasing factor (TRF) from the hypothalamus. Diagnosis is confirmed by raised serum concentrations of free and total T4 and T3, and undetectable levels of serum TSH.

PATHOPHYSIOLOGY

In 90% of cases there is multinodular diffuse enlargement of the thyroid gland. In Graves' disease there is a toxic nodular goitre. Rarer causes include thyroid adenoma, choriocarcinoma, thyroiditis and pituitary adenoma.

CLINICAL FEATURES

GENERAL:
- Weight loss
- Heat intolerance
- Fatigue
- Anxiety.

CARDIOVASCULAR:
- Tachycardia
- Atrial fibrillation
- Increased cardiac output
- Cardiac failure
- Increased myocardial sensitivity to catecholamines (thyroid hormones increase the number of myocardial β-receptors)
- Elderly patients may present with heart failure.

GASTROINTESTINAL:
- Diarrhoea.

NEUROMUSCULAR:
- Muscle weakness
- Proximal myopathy.

HAEMATOLOGICAL:
- Anaemia
- Thrombocytopenia.

PREOPERATIVE ASSESSMENT

It is essential that patients be rendered euthyroid before operation, as the operative risk is greater in untreated patients. This is achieved with antithyroid drugs, usually carbimazole or propylthiouracil for 2–3 months. This may be followed by iodine for 10 days to reduce the vascularity of the gland. Propranolol alone, or in combination with the above regimen, may be used and is associated with rapid relief of symptoms and preoperative cardiovascular stability.

HISTORY AND EXAMINATION
Preoperative assessment should include systematic review of symptoms or signs to determine adequate control of thyroid function. The neck should be examined and position of the trachea noted. A history of dyspnoea, stridor or dysphagia suggests tracheal and/or oesophageal compression by goitre. A retrosternal goitre may obstruct the superior vena cava (SVC).

INVESTIGATIONS
Investigations should include determination of haemoglobin level, white cell and platelet count, urea and electrolytes, and ECG. Chest radiography and thoracic inlet views allow evaluation of the extent of compression or deviation of the trachea by a goitre. Indirect laryngoscopy is performed before operation by many surgeons to document vocal cord function.

CT and MRI are of value in some cases.

PREOPERATIVE MANAGEMENT

- Premedication may be necessary to reduce anxiety. Antithyroid drugs, including beta-blockers, should be continued on the day of operation.

2

- Although thyroidectomy may be performed under deep or superficial cervical plexus block, general anaesthesia is the usual practice.
- In the absence of cardiovascular instability, indirect arterial pressure monitoring is adequate. An oesophageal stethoscope is useful, as patient access is limited during operation.

AIRWAY MANAGEMENT

- Equipment for a difficult intubation should always be available.
- If no tracheal involvement is expected from preoperative assessment, a reinforced oral or nasal tracheal tube is used. An armoured tube is advisable to prevent kinking during surgical dissection. A laryngeal mask airway is an alternative, although dislodgement during operation is a risk.
- If tracheal involvement is suspected or known, awake fibreoptic intubation or inhalation induction may be used.
- The tip of the tube should be advanced beyond any area of tracheal compression.
- The tube should be firmly taped in position and all connections secured, as access to the airway is limited when the operation has commenced.
- There is no evidence that the choice of anaesthetic agent is important, although studies in rodents treated with T3 have demonstrated a higher incidence of hepatic necrosis with halothane anaesthesia.
- The patient is positioned with the neck fully extended and a head-up tilt to reduce venous bleeding. Venous air embolism is a potential complication in this position. Many surgeons infiltrate the site of incision with adrenaline (epinephrine)-containing local anaesthetic solutions. Care should be taken that the accepted dose is not exceeded.
- The eyes should be adequately protected and taped shut, especially in patients with proptosis and lid retraction associated with Graves' disease.

- Bradycardia and hypotension are a complication of carotid sinus manipulation. This ceases with cessation of surgery and administration of atropine. Infiltration of the area with lidocaine (lignocaine) helps to prevent recurrence.

POSTOPERATIVE COMPLICATIONS

THYROID STORM
- Low incidence but associated with a high mortality rate
- Occurs in untreated or partially treated patients, or those with intercurrent infection
- May occur up to 18 h after operation
- Symptoms are fever, tachycardia, cardiac failure and coma
- May be confused with malignant hyperthermia
- Treatment comprises intravenous propranolol, steroids, sodium iodide, fluids and surface cooling.

NERVE INJURY
Recurrent laryngeal nerve:
- Unilateral nerve injury is well tolerated as a result of compensation by the unaffected cord.
- Bilateral nerve injury causes airway obstruction and requires reintubation.
- Superior laryngeal nerve (sensory innervation to larynx and piriform fossa) – may remain undetected until patient takes first drink, when aspiration may occur

OTHER COMPLICATIONS
Haematoma formation: some advocate extubation while the patient is deeply anaesthetised to reduce the incidence of coughing and, therefore, the risk of haematoma. Stitch cutters or clip removers must be immediately available.
- Tracheal collapse
- Tracheal laceration
- Tracheo-oesophageal fistula
- Pneumothorax
- Phrenic nerve injury
- Pneumomediastinum
- Parathyroid damage leading to postoperative hypocalcaemia.

BIBLIOGRAPHY

Farling PA. Thyroid disease. British Journal of
Anaesthesia 2000; 85:15–28

Mercer DM, Eltringham RJ. Anaesthesia for thyroid
surgery. Ear, Nose and Throat Journal 1985;
64:375–378

Roizen MF. Diseases of the endocrine system. In: Katz
J, Benumof JL, Kadis LB, eds. Anaesthesia and
uncommon diseases. Philadelphia: WB Saunders;
1990:245–292

Sebel PS. Thyroid and parathyroid disease. In: Nimmo
WS, Smith G, eds. Anaesthesia. Oxford: Blackwell
Scientific; 1989:771–778

CROSS-REFERENCES

Difficult airway
    Anaesthetic Factors 28: 660
Complications of positions
    Anaesthetic Factors 31: 736

2

Hypopituitarism

W. J. Fawcett

There are six major hormones produced in the anterior pituitary:

- Growth hormone (GH)
- Prolactin
- Thyroid-stimulating hormone (TSH) or thyrotrophin
- Follicle-stimulating hormone (FSH)
- Leuteinising hormone (LH)
- Adrenocorticotrophic hormone (ACTH) – and related peptides such as lipoproteins, endorphins and melanocyte-stimulating hormone (MSH).

The anterior pituitary also secretes other peptides, such as vasoactive intestinal peptide, chorionic gonadotrophin, substance P and renin. Production and release of anterior pituitary hormones is under the control of the hypothalamus, usually by releasing or inhibiting hormones.

The posterior pituitary lobe stores and releases arginine vasopressin (AVP) and oxytocin. Deficiency of these two hormones is rare in lesions confined to the pituitary fossa, but occurs more commonly with hypothalamic disease and/or suprasellar extension of a pituitary tumour.

PATHOPHYSIOLOGY

Hypopituitarism commonly arises from a primary pituitary tumour (e.g. prolactinoma in adults, craniopharyngioma in children). Other causes include trauma, secondary tumours, infection, vascular causes (malformations, massive blood loss), postoperative or post-irradiation. The clinical features depend on the degree of disruption of the various hormones. Of major relevance to anaesthesia are ACTH and TSH deficiency from the anterior pituitary, and AVP deficiency from the posterior pituitary (to be considered elsewhere). It is noteworthy that when cortisol and AVP deficiency coexist there may not be any features of diabetes insipidus as cortisol deficiency reduces free water excretion. Diagnosis may be confirmed by no response of

GH to hypoglycaemia, and no response of TSH to thyrotrophin-releasing factor (TRH).

TSH DEFICIENCY

Thyrotrophin is the principal regulator of thyroid function. The patient will therefore be hypothyroid and there will be low circulating serum levels of thyroxine (T4) and TSH, and impaired response to TRH. The clinical features may include:

- Reduced cardiac output (secondary to reduced stroke volume and bradycardia); ischaemic heart disease
- Reduced respiratory reserve (due to a reduction in maximum breathing capacity and carbon monoxide transfer factor, and pleural effusions)
- Hoarseness, sleep apnoea and respiratory obstruction (related to mucopolysaccharide deposition on the vocal cords)
- Reduced response to both hypoxia and hypercarbia
- Abnormal baroreceptor function
- Reduction in plasma volume, anaemia and coagulopathy
- Hypoglycaemia and hyponatraemia.

ACTH DEFICIENCY

This will cause adrenal cortisol hyposecretion, but mineralocorticoid secretion should be normal (although not always). The classical picture is that of:

- Postural hypotension, hypovolaemia, hyponatraemia, hyperkalaemia and hypoglycaemia, and high serum urea concentration
- Normochromic, normocytic anaemia
- Nausea and vomiting, and diarrhoea
- Low serum cortisol and ACTH levels, but a response to Synacthen.

PREOPERATIVE ASSESSMENT

A thorough cardiovascular and respiratory system evaluation is required, looking for airway obstruction (snoring, sleep apnoea), cardiac failure and hypotension. In addition, the underlying cause of hypopituitarism should be known, and other systems evaluated as necessary, such as neurological assessment in patients with head injuries.

INVESTIGATIONS
Investigations include:
- Full blood count
- Clotting screen
- Serum urea and electrolytes, glucose, T4 and cortisol levels
- Chest radiography, ECG and echocardiography

Patients must have normal circulating T4 and cortisol values before undergoing elective surgery and, if necessary, the operation should be postponed until this is so. Treatment should be carried out in conjunction with an endocrinologist. Great care is required in the use of intravenous T3 and T4 (for myxoedematous coma) which may precipitate myocardial ischaemia. Replacement hormones should be continued throughout the perioperative period, especially T3 (which has a half-life of 1.5 days); this is less critical for T4 (half-life 5 days). Patients requiring steroid hormones would conventionally receive extra steroid 'cover'. Sedative premedication should be used sparingly, if at all, in patients with hypothyroidism.

PERIOPERATIVE MANAGEMENT

Patients with normal hormone levels but with no other problems (such as raised intracranial pressure) require no special treatment. However, it is sometimes necessary to operate on patients who do not have a normal hormone profile. There may be a number of problems:
- Patients who are hypothyroid will be very sensitive to all sedative agents (opioids, benzodiazepines and anaesthetic agents) and, in addition, will have reduced metabolism and excretion of these agents.
- Induction must be undertaken with extreme care: cardiac arrest has been reported at induction for both hypothyroidism and hypoadrenalism. Moreover, these patients may be very resistant to resuscitation with catecholamine therapy.
- Avoid etomidate in those with impaired cortisol secretion.
- Hypothermia may be a problem, and active measures should be taken to reduce heat loss (warming of intravenous fluids, warming mattress).
- Patients who are cortisol deficient will need cortisol to cover surgery (hydrocortisone 25 mg i.v. at induction, followed by 100 mg per 24 h). In addition, these patients are likely to be dehydrated, and will require careful titration of both saline and glucose to maintain serum sodium and glucose levels within normal limits. Hypothyroid patients may have adrenocortical insufficiency and therefore require hydrocortisone.

MONITORING
In addition to standard monitoring:
- Arterial and central venous cannulae in patients with cardiac impairment and/or fluid balance problems. The use of oesophageal Doppler or pulmonary artery catheters may also be useful.
- Temperature
- Urine output
- Serum glucose level should be monitored and, if low (< 4 mmol l^{-1}), 10 ml 50% glucose given.

If unexplained hypotension occurs, cardiac filling pressures should be checked first. Fluids and/or hydrocortisone (which has a permissive effect on endogenous catecholamines) and occasionally fludrocortisone (which is usually for primary adrenocortical insufficiency) may be required.

POSTOPERATIVE MANAGEMENT

Patients with hypopituitarism following major surgery warrant ITU/HDU management. Particular emphasis should be placed on:
- The airway (in those with vocal cord involvement)
- Cardiovascular status
- Temperature control
- Urine output
- Biochemistry, particularly electrolytes and glucose.

Maintenance hormones should be continued into the postoperative period, as should steroid cover, if used. Many cases of postoperative collapse in patients with a disrupted hypophyseal–pituitary–adrenal axis are probably not related to insufficient steroids, but to other factors, particularly hypovolaemia or, more rarely, sepsis. This should be borne in mind as these patients have little physiological reserve and tolerate these conditions poorly.

BIBLIOGRAPHY

Farling PA. Thyroid disease. British Journal of Anaesthesia 2000; 85:15–28

Smith M, Hirsch NP. Pituitary disease and anaesthesia. British Journal of Anaesthesia 2000; 85:3–14

CROSS-REFERENCES

Diabetes insipidus
    Patient Conditions 2: 54
Hypothyroidism
    Patient Conditions 2: 69
Anaesthesia for trans-sphenoidal hypophysectomy
    Surgical Procedures 10: 301

2

Hypothyroidism

R. Edwards

This is a clinical syndrome resulting from a deficiency of the thyroid hormones tri-iodothyronine (T3) and thyroxine (T4). The diagnosis is confirmed by demonstrating a low serum concentration of T4 and raised level of thyroid-stimulating hormone (TSH), unless the hypothyroidism is secondary to TSH deficiency.

PATHOPHYSIOLOGY

Causes of hypothyroidism:
* Autoimmune thyroiditis (Hashimoto's disease)
* Iatrogenic – surgical or medical radio-iodine therapy for thyrotoxicosis
* Iodine deficiency
* Drugs (e.g. lithium, amiodarone)
* Congenital
* Secondary hypothyroidism – pituitary disease, idiopathic thyrotrophin-releasing hormone (TRH) deficiency.

CLINICAL FEATURES

GENERAL:
* There is a reduction in basal metabolic rate leading to lethargy, reduced mental function, weight gain and cold intolerance.
* Hypothermia is a risk, especially in the elderly.
* There is increased sensitivity to narcotics and anaesthetic agents.

CARDIOVASCULAR SYSTEM:
* There is both bradycardia and reduced stroke volume, producing a reduction in cardiac output.
* Pericardial effusion may be present.

RESPIRATORY SYSTEM:
* There is a reduction in the ventilatory response to hypoxia and hypercapnia.
* Maximum breathing capacity and carbon monoxide transfer factor may be reduced.

* Pleural effusions may occur, further reducing ventilatory capacity.

SKIN:
* There is dryness, alopecia and vitiligo.
* Mucopolysaccharide deposition beneath the skin causes non-pitting oedema ('myxoedema') and in the vocal cords causes hoarseness and even acute respiratory obstruction.

HAEMATOLOGICAL:
* Anaemia (normochromic, normocytic or macrocytic)
* There is an association with pernicious anaemia.

GASTROINTESTINAL TRACT:
* Constipation
* Ileus
* Ascites.

Untreated hypothyroidism culminates in myxoedema coma, which is characterised by hypothermia, shock, acidosis, hyponatraemia, hypoglycaemia and, finally, coma and death.

PREOPERATIVE ASSESSMENT

HISTORY AND EXAMINATION
Symptoms and signs of hypothyroidism should be sought. Patients should be rendered euthyroid before operation with thyroxine (50–200 μg daily). In the previously undiagnosed patient, tri-iodothyronine is effective in a few hours ($t_{1/2}$ 1.5 days) and may be given intravenously in an emergency. This must be done in the intensive care unit with full monitoring.

A history of hoarseness is important as it indicates vocal cord involvement. Assessment of goitre should be thorough, as for patients with hyperthyroidism.

INVESTIGATIONS:
* Haemoglobin
* Serum urea and electrolyte concentrations

2

- ECG – slow voltage with flattened or inverted T waves in untreated hypothyroidism
- Chest radiography – cardiomegaly, pleural effusion
- Radiograph of thoracic inlet for tracheal involvement by goitre.

PERIOPERATIVE MANAGEMENT

Hypothyroidism is usually coincidental to surgery, unlike hyperthyroidism. The treated hypothyroid patient does not present a particular problem. Untreated hypothyroidism is associated with adrenocortical insufficiency, and steroid supplements should be administered before operation.

If premedication is necessary, narcotics and sedatives should be used with care because of increased sensitivity and the risk of respiratory depression. Cardiac output is decreased owing to a reduction in both heart rate and stroke volume. Blood volume is also reduced, so myocardial depression and blood loss are poorly tolerated. Induction agents should be administered cautiously, with ECG and arterial pressure monitoring.

Airway management in the presence of goitre is the same as that described for the hyperthyroid patient. Arterial pressure, ECG, respiratory variables and temperature should be closely monitored from induction through to the postoperative period. Controlled ventilation should be used because the respiratory response to hypoxia and hypercarbia is reduced. A reduction in thyroid hormone secretion results in a reduced basal metabolic rate and a reduced ability to maintain core temperature. Facilities for warming the patient should be available to avoid hypothermia. Intravenous fluids and gases should be warmed.

POSTOPERATIVE MANAGEMENT

Opioids are associated with prolonged respiratory depression and there is the possibility of delayed recovery, whatever anaesthetic technique is employed. Intensive care facilities should be available for these patients after operation.

Reduced free water excretion may result in postoperative hyponatraemia.

BIBLIOGRAPHY

Farling PA. Thyroid disease. British Journal of Anaesthesia 2000; 85:15–28

Hobbiger HE, Allen JG, Greatorex RG, Denny NM. The laryngeal mask airway for thyroid and parathyroid surgery. Anaesthesia 1996; 51:972–974

Ladenson PW, Levin AA, Ridgeway EC, Daniels GH. Complications of surgery in hypothyroid patients. American Journal of Medicine 1984; 77:261–266

Murkin JM. Anaesthesia and hypothyroidism: a review of thyroxine physiology, pharmacology and anesthetic implications. Anaesthesia and Analgesia 1982; 61:371–383

Singh V, Catlett JP. Hematologic manifestations of thyroid disease. Endocrinologist 1998; 8:87–91

CROSS-REFERENCES

Adrenocortical insufficiency
    Patient Conditions 2: 46
Hypopituitarism
    Patient Conditions 2: 66
Failure to breathe or wake up
    Anaesthetic Factors 31: 740

2

Iatrogenic adrenocortical insufficiency

A. Quinn

Synthetic glucocorticoids are used for many non-endocrine conditions:

- Respiratory disease:
  - —asthma, chronic bronchitis and emphysema
  - —sarcoidosis
  - —hay fever (usually topical).
- Gastrointestinal disease:
  - —ulcerative colitis
  - —Crohn's disease.
- Neurological disease:
  - —cerebral oedema.
- Tumours:
  - —Hodgkin's lymphoma
  - —other lymphomas.
- Renal disease:
  - —some nephrotic syndromes
  - —glomerulonephritis.
- Rheumatological disease:
  - —rheumatoid arthritis
  - —systemic lupus erythematosus
  - —polymyalgia rheumatica.
- Skin disease.
- Transplantation:
  - —immunosuppression.

Short-term use carries little risk of adrenal suppression. However, daily oral doses of prednisolone (7.5 mg), or the equivalent of an alternative steroid, for a period longer than 1 month will suppress the hypothalamic–pituitary–adrenal (HPA) axis, as may lower doses in patients with a chronic disease (e.g. rheumatoid arthritis). Suppression may also occur after topical, oral, parenteral, nebulised or inhaled preparations.

Table 2.2 gives the potency ratios of some commonly used steroids relative to cortisol.

PATHOPHYSIOLOGY

The patient receiving exogenous glucocorticoid may exhibit many of the signs and symptoms of Cushing's syndrome and have suppression of the HPA axis. The adverse effects of particular

TABLE 2.2

Potency ratios of commonly used steroids

Steroid	Glucocorticoid	Mineralocorticoid
Cortisol (hydrocortisone)	1	1
Prednisolone	4	0.7
Dexamethasone	40	2
Aldosterone	0.1	400
Fludrocortisone	10	400

importance to the anaesthetist are diabetes, obesity and hypertension.

Adverse effects of corticosteroid therapy include:

- *Cardiovascular system* – hypertension
- *Renal* – polyuria, nocturia
- *CNS* – depression, euphoria, psychosis, insomnia
- *Gastrointestinal tract* – peptic ulcer, pancreatitis
- *Eyes* – cataracts
- *Increased susceptibility to infection* – septicaemia, tuberculosis, skin (e.g. fungi)
- *Skin* – thinning, easy bruising
- *Endocrine* – weight gain, diabetes, impaired growth, amenorrhoea
- *Bone and muscle* – osteoporosis, proximal myopathy, wasting, aseptic necrosis of the hip, pathological fractures.

PREOPERATIVE ASSESSMENT

HISTORY

See appropriate sections on the assessment of problems associated with obesity (p. 174), hypertension (p. 151), diabetes (p. 54) and Cushing's syndrome (p. 52).

DEGREE OF ADRENAL SUPPRESSION

Perioperative steroid requirements are difficult to assess. The adverse sequelae of excessive

2

corticosteroid therapy include delayed healing, increased susceptibility to infection and gastrointestinal haemorrhage, and attempts should be made to rationalise steroid supplementation for surgical patients at risk of having adrenocortical insufficiency. In some cases, however, it may be imperative to continue high-dose steroid treatment, for instance in patients with severe immunological conditions such as systemic lupus erythematosus (SLE) or glomerulonephritis.

The following tests may be useful in assessing adrenal suppression:
- Plasma cortisol level > 500 nmol l^{-1} indicates the adrenal to be free from significant suppression.
- The short Synacthen test.
- The insulin tolerance test measures the cortisol response to hypoglycaemia. This is the 'gold standard' diagnostic test, but is difficult and potentially dangerous to perform.

PERIOPERATIVE MANAGEMENT

PREMEDICATION:
- Concomitant medication commonly includes: antihypertensives, diuretics, insulin, antibiotics, antacids, H$_2$ antagonists and deep vein thrombosis (DVT) prophylaxis
- Steroid replacement regimens (see Table 2.3).

MONITORING:
- Arterial cannula
- Blood glucose concentration
- Capnography, Sp_{O_2}
- Urine output.

INTRAOPERATIVE ANAESTHESIA
There are no particular indications for any one anaesthetic technique for this disorder. However, anaesthetic agents should be administered slowly and carefully as these patients are sensitive to any cardiodepressant effects.

General anaesthesia:
- Rapid sequence induction for obese patients
- Prepare equipment for difficult intubation
- Intermittent positive-pressure ventilation (IPPV); may require high F_{IO_2} and positive end-expiratory pressure (PEEP)
- Careful positioning, because of susceptibility to bruising and fractures
- Hypotension – usually reflects inadequate fluid replacement.

TABLE 2.3

Steroid treatment regimens

	Treatment regimen
Patients taking steroids	
< 10 mg daily	Assume normal HPA response; additional cover not required
> 10 mg daily	
Minor surgery	25 mg hydrocortisone at induction
Moderate surgery	Usual preoperative steroids + 25 mg hydrocortisone at induction + 100 mg hydrocortisone over next 24 h
Major surgery	Usual preoperative steroids + 25 mg hydrocortisone at induction + 100 mg hydrocortisone daily for 48–72 h
High-dose immunosuppression	Usual immunosuppressive dose in perioperative period
Patients who have stopped taking steroids	
< 3 months	Treat as if on steroids
> 3 months	No perioperative steroids necessary

Local anaesthesia
Subarachnoid, epidural block, regional blocks, etc. These may be technically difficult but have the advantages of good analgesia, enabling minimal administration of opioids and rapid mobilisation, and may also reduce the incidence of thromboembolism.

POSTOPERATIVE MANAGEMENT

These patients may require postoperative ventilatory support and there are often problems with delayed wound healing.
- High-dependency unit
- Continuous humidified oxygen therapy
- Analgesia – opioid infusion, patient-controlled analgesia, epidural opioid/local anaesthetic
- Steroids – start on oral steroids once gastrointestinal function resumed
- Insulin infusion, DVT prophylaxis
- Renal function
- Physiotherapy and early mobilisation.

BIBLIOGRAPHY

Kehlet H. A rational approach to dosage and preparation of parenteral glucocorticoid substitution therapy during surgical procedures. Acta Anaesthesiologica Scandinavica 1975; 19:260–264

Nicholson G, Burrin JM, Hall GM. Peri-operative steroid supplementation. Anaesthesia 1998; 53:1091–1104

CROSS-REFERENCES

Asthma
   Patient Conditions 3: 86
Rheumatoid disease
   Patient Conditions 8: 242
Sarcoidosis
   Patient Conditions 3: 103

2

Insulinoma

J. Desborough

Insulinoma is the commonest type of pancreatic islet cell tumour. Most of these lesions are benign (90%), intrapancreatic, small and solitary. Up to 10% are multiple, associated with multiple endocrine neoplasia (MEN). The incidence is four cases per million population per year.

Tumours secrete insulin or pro-insulin, producing hypoglycaemia. If undiagnosed, or symptoms uncontrolled, patients may present with:

- Cerebral dysfunction, focal neurological deficits
- Abnormal behaviour, confusion
- Visual disturbance, weakness, sweating.

PREOPERATIVE ASSESSMENT

Most cases are diagnosed and the patient is prepared for operation. Assessment for other endocrine tumours (MEN) should be made. Patients may be obese and hypertensive.

Medical therapy includes:

Drug	Effect
Diazoxide	Inhibits release of insulin from tumour
Diuretic	Treats oedema associated with use of diazoxide
Glucagon infusion	Maintenance of blood sugar levels
Beta-blockers	Antihypertensive
Calcium antagonists	Antihypertensive
Cytotoxic drugs	Antitumour

Tumour localisation may be undertaken before and during operation to allow selective adenomectomy and avoid blind subtotal pancreatectomy. Techniques include spiral CT, endoscopic and intraoperative ultrasonography, angiography and selective venous hormone sampling. Bimanual palpation of the pancreas at operation is useful.

PERIOPERATIVE MANAGEMENT

Patients having wide fluctuations in blood glucose concentration may require dextrose infusion up to 2–3 h before surgery.

- Generous premedication
- Prepare for major laparotomy
- Direct cardiovascular monitoring
- Continuous or intermittent glucose, insulin and potassium sampling
- 50% glucose available to treat hypoglycaemic response to tumour manipulation
- Likely intraoperative tumour localisation
- Continue glucose and insulin monitoring after operation.

BIBLIOGRAPHY

Azimuddin K, Chamberlain RS. The surgical management of pancreatic neuroendocrine tumours. Surgical Clinics of North America; W B Saunders; 2001; 81:511–525

Owen R. Anaesthetic considerations in endocrine surgery. In: Lynn J, Bloom SR, eds. Surgical endocrinology. Oxford: Butterworth–Heinemann; 1993:71–84

CROSS-REFERENCES

Multiple endocrine neoplasia
    Patient Conditions 2: 77
Diabetes Mellitus type 1
    Patient Conditions 2: 56

Malignant hyperthermia

J. Dinsmore

Malignant hyperthermia is a potentially fatal, pharmacogenetic disorder of skeletal muscle. It is triggered in susceptible individuals by all volatile anaesthetic agents and suxamethonium. The reported incidence varies considerably, but is about 1 in 40 000 with a higher incidence in children.

PATHOPHYSIOLOGY

The exact aetiology is unknown, but the primary defect is believed to lie in the skeletal muscle calcium release channel, known as the ryanodine receptor (RYR1). Human malignant hyperthermia is a greatly heterogeneous disorder, but gene mutations on the short arm of chromosome 19 are thought to be responsible for the condition in about 50% of families.

Malignant hyperthermia is a hypermetabolic condition, characterised by increased skeletal muscle metabolism. Triggering agents cause a sustained increase in myoplasmic calcium levels, producing myofibrillar contraction, an increased metabolic rate, increased oxygen consumption, and increased carbon dioxide and heat production. The clinical features are shown in the Table 2.4.

PERIOPERATIVE MANAGEMENT

PREOPERATIVE ASSESSMENT

Identification of individuals susceptible to malignant hyperthermia is difficult, as they appear entirely normal until exposed to triggering agents and may even have undergone uneventful anaesthesia previously. Patients with a history of a malignant hyperthermia-like reaction, or a family history, should be investigated before anaesthesia. Susceptibility is diagnosed by a standardised *in vitro* muscle contracture test (IVCT). This measures the contracture response of fresh muscle to caffeine and halothane. It is invasive, but testing based on

TABLE 2.4

Clinical features of malignant hyperthermia

Signs	Investigations
Masseter spasm[a] and muscle rigidity	$\downarrow$ pH, $\uparrow$ $P\text{co}_2$, $\uparrow$ base deficit, $\downarrow$ $P\text{o}_2$
Rising $Fe^1\text{co}_2$ and tachypnoea	Hyperkalaemia
Tachycardia and cardiac arrhythmias	Creatine kinase
Hypertension	Myoglobinuria
Mottled cyanosis	
Increasing body temperature	

[a]Only 50% of patients who develop masseter spasm will be susceptible to malignant hyperthermia by contracture testing. The safest course of action is to abandon surgery and monitor for other signs of malignant hyperthermia. The patient should be referred for further investigation, especially if there is corroborative evidence.

DNA markers can be offered only to families where linkage with chromosome 19 mutations has been shown to exist.

Various neuromuscular disorders and stress syndromes have been linked to malignant hyperthermia. The association is strong in the case of central core disease. Duchenne muscular dystrophy and King–Denborough syndrome are possibly associated. There is little evidence for an association with other disorders.

PREMEDICATION

Opinion is divided regarding prophylaxis with dantrolene, but there is little evidence to support its routine use. Malignant hyperthermia reactions are reputed to have occurred despite pretreatment and dantrolene may be associated with significant side-effects.

2

THEATRE PREPARATION

If a general anaesthetic is to be given, a volatile-free anaesthetic machine is needed. This is achieved by removal of the vaporisers, flushing with oxygen at 8 l min⁻¹ for 20 min and the use of new tubing. Dantrolene should be available with facilities for resuscitation.

MONITORING

This should be commenced in the anaesthetic room and include:

- Arterial cannula for direct blood pressure monitoring and blood gas sampling
- ECG
- Sao_2
- $Fe^{1}co_2$
- Temperature
- CVP
- Urine output

ANAESTHESIA

Many drugs have been implicated, but the only agents proven to trigger malignant hyperthermia are suxamethonium and volatile agents. All other drugs may be presumed safe. Provided a volatile-free anaesthetic machine is used and trigger agents are avoided, general anaesthesia should pose no problem. All local anaesthetics are considered safe. However, it has been proposed on theoretical grounds that amide local anaesthetics and sympathetic vasoconstrictors should be avoided during an acute episode of malignant hyperthermia.

POSTOPERATIVE CARE

Malignant hyperthermia may present in the recovery room or even later after operation, and facilities should be available for extended postoperative monitoring. It has been suggested that straightforward cases might be done as day cases. All suspected cases of malignant hyperthermia should be followed, and family members screened.

MANAGEMENT OF AN ACUTE MALIGNANT HYPERTHERMIA REACTION

- Stop trigger agents and terminate the operation as soon as possible. Maintain anaesthesia with non-triggering drugs such as propofol, midazolam or opioids.
- Establish monitoring as recommended above and ventilate with 100% oxygen (up to three times the minute volume may be necessary).

- Dantrolene 1–10 mg kg⁻¹. Most malignant hyperthermia reactions are reversed by dosages of 2–3 mg kg⁻¹.
- Correct acidosis with sodium bicarbonate as necessary.
- Correct hyperkalaemia with insulin and glucose. Consider early haemodiafiltration.
- Vigorous rehydration with intravenous fluids (Hartmann's solution is best avoided because it contains lactate).
- Treat dysrhythmias as appropriate.
- Encourage diuresis after fluid loading.
- Cooling if required (surface cooling is largely ineffective).
- Admit to ITU for further management.

OUTCOME

With better early recognition of the clinical signs and prompt treatment, the mortality rate associated with malignant hyperthermia has fallen from more than 80% to less than 7% in recent years. However, this is still regarded as unacceptably high. The reasons for this clinical discrepancy include preoccupation with the name hyperthermia, leading to delays in diagnosis, and preoccupation with non-specific therapy such as cooling. Neurological and renal damage contribute to the morbidity resulting from the acute episode in survivors, particularly if body temperature exceeds 43°C.

BIBLIOGRAPHY

Jurkat-Rott K, McCarthy T, Lehmann-Horn F. Genetics and pathogenesis of malignant hyperthermia. Muscle Nerve 2000; 23:4–17

Maclennan DH, Phillips MS. Malignant hyperthermia. Science 1992; 256:789–793

Nelson TE. Malignant hyperthermia: a pharmacogenetic disease of Ca²⁺ regulating proteins. Current Molecular Medicine 2002; 2:347–369

Rosenberg H, Shutack JG. Variants of malignant hyperthermia. Special problems for the paediatric anaesthesiologist. Paediatric Anaesthesia 1996; 6:87–93

CROSS-REFERENCES

Malignant hypothermia
   Anaesthetic Factors 31: 764

Multiple endocrine neoplasia

J. Desborough

This condition occurs when tumours involve two or more endocrine organs. The usual tumour sites in the various subtypes of multiple endocrine neoplasia (MEN) are as follows:
- MEN-1 – rare, complex, dominant inheritance
  —Parathyroid
  —Pancreatic islets
  —Anterior pituitary.
- MEN-2 – autosomal dominant inheritance, incomplete penetrance, variable expression
  —Medullary thyroid carcinoma (MTC)
  —Adrenal (phaeochromocytoma)
  —Parathyroid.
- MEN-2A
  —Tumour sites as above
  —Affected patients have normal physical appearance.
- MEN-2B
  —Thyroid
  —Adrenal (phaeochromocytoma)
  —Patients have marfanoid habitus, mucosal neuromas, gut ganglioneuromatosis.
- MTC only

PERIOPERATIVE MANAGEMENT

Presentation depends on the clinical syndrome resulting from particular tumours involved. Usually patients are diagnosed and prepared for major surgery. In emergency operations, the possibility of endocrine tumours should be remembered.
- Generous premedication
- Invasive cardiovascular monitoring
- Frequent blood sampling for hormones, glucose, electrolytes, etc.
- Continue cardiovascular and biochemical monitoring after operation.

BIBLIOGRAPHY

Gagel R. Multiple endocrine neoplasia. Endocrinology and Metabolism Clinics of North America; W B Saunders; 1994; 23:1–228

Owen R. Anaesthetic considerations in endocrine Surgery. In: Lynn J, Bloom SR, eds. Surgical endocrinology. Oxford: Butterworth–Heinemann; 1993:71–84

2

Muscular dystrophies

P. Newman

The muscular dystrophies are a group of genetically determined primary degenerative myopathies. They are best classified by their mode of inheritance.

- X-linked:
  —Duchenne's (most common and most severe)
  —Becker's.
- Autosomal recessive:
  —Limb girdle
  —Childhood
  —Congenital (?associated with arthrogryposis).
- Autosomal dominant:
  —Facioscapulohumeral
  —Oculopharyngeal.

All the above show atrophy and weakness of muscle to differing degrees. The onset and groups of muscles involved vary according to the specific dystrophy; fortunately, their names often define the muscles involved. Involvement of organs other than muscles is uncommon except in Duchenne's muscular dystrophy, which is by far the most common and severe. In view of this, the information given below refers mainly to Duchenne's dystrophy.

PATHOPHYSIOLOGY

Duchenne's dystrophy affects striated, smooth and cardiac muscle fibres.

RESPIRATORY SYSTEM
Respiratory failure is common as a result of:
- Muscle weakness
- Oropharyngeal muscle weakness allowing repeated aspiration
- Spinal deformities, causing restrictive lung disease.

CARDIOVASCULAR SYSTEM
Obstructive cardiomyopathy occurs, but failure is often masked because of the patient's immobility. Arrhythmias are common; tachycardia and ventricular fibrillation have been reported on induction. Severe bradycardia may occur in the facioscapulohumeral variant. There is a particular ECG pattern with Duchenne's dystrophy:
- Sinus tachycardia
- Tall R in V_1
- Deep Q in lateral leads
- Short PR interval.

GASTROINTESTINAL TRACT
Hypomotility of the gastrointestinal tract and weak pharyngeal muscles predispose to aspiration. Acute gastric dilatation has been reported.

MUSCULOSKELETAL
Pseudohypertrophy of affected muscles occurs and contractures can be problematic. Kyphoscoliosis occurs early in the disease and further diminishes respiratory reserve. There may be an association with malignant hyperthermia; a malignant hyperthermia-like syndrome has been reported following suxamethonium and halothane administration.

PREOPERATIVE ASSESSMENT

HISTORY:
- Review of respiratory function
- Previous anaesthetic history (possibility of malignant hyperthermia)
- Swallowing difficulties.

INVESTIGATIONS:
- Respiratory function tests
- Arterial blood gases
- ECG
- Echocardiography if significant cardiovascular disease
- Chest radiography (aspiration, cardiac failure).

PREMEDICATION:
- Avoid respiratory depressants
- Acid aspiration prophylaxis and at least 6 h starvation

- If positive history of malignant hyperthermia -type reaction, use non-triggering anaesthetic agents.

PERIOPERATIVE MANAGEMENT

MONITORING:
- ECG
- $EtCO_2$
- Temperature
- Peripheral nerve stimulator (PNS).

INDUCTION AND MAINTENANCE
Positioning may be difficult due to contractures and kyphoscoliosis.

The association with malignant hyperthermia is unproven, and suxamethonium and volatile agents have been given uneventfully. However, suxamethonium has been associated with hyperkalaemia, cardiac arrest, muscle rigidity and rhabdomyolysis, and should be avoided. If there is significant cardiovascular disease, minimal volatile agent should be used with opioids. Total intravenous anaesthesia provides a safe alternative to a volatile anaesthetic technique. Sensitivity to non-depolarising muscle relaxants has been reported; small doses of vecuronium seem to be safe with continued monitoring with a PNS. Watch $EtCO_2$, ECG and temperature for early signs of malignant hyperthermia, and have dantrolene available in theatre.

Local or regional techniques will avoid the risks of general anaesthesia, but may be difficult because of contractures and kyphoscoliosis.

A nasogastric tube should be passed as a precaution against gastric dilatation.

POSTOPERATIVE MANAGEMENT

- Observation on ITU/HDU for at least 24 h.
- Ventilate prophylactically if any doubt about respiratory function.
- Physiotherapy will reduce postoperative respiratory complications.
- Acute gastric dilatation occurs up to 48 h after operation, so leave nasogastric tube *in situ*.

BIBLIOGRAPHY

Sethna NF, Rockoff MA, Worthen HM, Rosnow JM. Anesthesia related complications in children with Duchenne's muscular dystrophy. Anesthesiology 1988; 68:462–465

Smith CL, Bush GH. Anaesthesia and progressive muscular dystrophy. British Journal of Anaesthesia 1985; 57:1113–1118

CROSS-REFERENCES

2

Myasthenia gravis and Eaton–Lambert syndrome

P. Newman

Myasthenia gravis is an autoimmune disease of the neuromuscular junction, resulting from the production of antibodies against the postjunctional acetylcholine (ACh) receptors. Clinically there is muscle weakness and fatigability on repeated muscle use. The incidence is 1 in 20 000 adults with a 2 : 1 female : male ratio. In 10% of cases there is an associated thymic tumour (thymoma). The Eaton–Lambert syndrome is an acquired myasthenic disorder associated with cancer, particularly small cell cancer of the lung. Muscle weakness improves with exercise.

PATHOPHYSIOLOGY

There may be respiratory complications due to weakness of muscles of respiration and bulbar muscles, leading to aspiration. It may be associated with other autoimmune diseases:
- Thyroid hypofunction
- Rheumatoid arthritis
- Systemic lupus erythematosus (SLE).

Patients presenting for surgery for lung cancer may have Eaton–Lambert syndrome.

PREOPERATIVE ASSESSMENT

TREATMENT:
- *Anticholinesterase drugs* – neostigmine and pyridostigmine. These provide symptomatic relief only; may need atropine concurrently to block muscarinic effects. Useful for diagnosis.
- *Plasmapheresis* – short term, but effective and useful in myasthenic crisis or for preoperative preparation.
- *Immune suppression* – azathioprine, cyclosporin and steroids eliminate the antibodies. Now first-line treatment.
- *Thymectomy* – complete removal of thymus leads to remission in many patients. This is best performed by the sternal route for more complete removal, but the

transcervical route is less invasive. Thymectomy is increasingly the early method of treatment, even for the less severe cases (see sternotomy/thymectomy).

HISTORY:
- Involvement of bulbar and respiratory muscle
- Drug treatment.

INVESTIGATIONS AND PREPARATION:
- Preoperative optimisation regimen before thymectomy. This may mean an increase in, or addition of, any of the above treatments.
- Respiratory function tests, including arterial blood gases.
- Preoperative chest physiotherapy.

PREMEDICATION:
- Continue steroids (see Iatrogenic adrenocortical insufficiency, p. 71)
- Minimal sedative premedication due to lack of respiratory reserve
- Acid aspiration prophylaxis if bulbar involvement
- Intramuscular atropine guards against potentiated vagal responses
- Discussion of possibility of postoperative ventilation is wise.

There remains controversy as to the timing of discontinuation of anticholinesterase therapy. A recent review suggests continuing until the evening of surgery. Respiratory monitoring will reveal impending respiratory failure due to myasthenic crisis.

PERIOPERATIVE MANAGEMENT

MONITORING
Peripheral nerve stimulator.

INDUCTION AND MAINTENANCE
The major problem with myasthenic patients is the unpredictable response to suxamethonium and sensitivity to non-depolarising relaxants. In

view of problems with muscle relaxants, intubation and muscle relaxation with inhalational anaesthesia is the preferred technique for some anaesthetists. If this is used, cardiovascular and respiratory depression may be a problem.

Resistance to suxamethonium occurs due to blockade of ACh receptors, so increased doses are often needed for rapid sequence induction (NB: bulbar weakness). Extreme sensitivity to non-depolarising relaxants occurs due to reduced numbers of ACh receptors; one-tenth the normal dose will provide adequate relaxation. Atracurium and vecuronium have both been used safely in myasthenics and can be completely reversed. Neuromuscular monitoring is mandatory for titration of relaxants. Reversal of residual block with neostigmine and atropine is safe, but excessive doses above those that the patient is taking orally may precipitate a cholinergic crisis.

30 mg oral = 1 mg i.v. neostigmine
120 mg oral = 4 mg i.v. pyridostigmine

High thoracic epidural anaesthesia, with opioid and local anaesthetic agent, and light inhalational anaesthesia have been used for thymectomy, and provide particularly good postoperative pain relief.

POSTOPERATIVE MANAGEMENT

- Ensure adequate respiratory function before extubation:
  —FVC > 15 ml kg^{-1}
  —Peak occlusion pressure > 30 cmH$_2$O.
- If any doubt about respiratory function, ventilate after operation.
- Chest physiotherapy to clear secretions.

- Monitoring on ITU/HDU for 24 h.
- Restart anticholinesterases in reduced doses; intravenous or intramuscular doses may need to be given if oral medication is difficult.
- In myasthenic crisis, careful postoperative cardiovascular monitoring and access to pacing is important as asystole has been reported in a recent series of patients. Plasmapheresis or immunoglobulins can be useful in the management of crises.
- Myasthenic or cholinergic crises may occur.
- Pain relief is important after thymectomy; opioids must be administered with care and with constant respiratory monitoring.

BIBLIOGRAPHY

Baraka A. Anaesthesia and myasthenia gravis. Canadian Journal of Anaesthesiology 1992; 39:476–486

Berrouschot.J, Baumann I, Kalischewski P et al. Therapy of myasthenic crisis. Critical Care Medicine 1997; 25:1228–1235.

Saito Y, Sakura S, Takatori T, Kosaka Y. Epidural anesthesia in a patient with myasthenia gravis. Acta Anaesthesiologica Scandinavica 1993; 37:513–515

CROSS-REFERENCES

2

Myotonia

P. Newman

Myotonia is the sustained contraction of a muscle that persists after the cessation of voluntary effort or stimulation. It is an abnormality of muscle rather than the neuromuscular junction. It appears in three hereditary syndromes, all of which are of autosomal dominant inheritance:

- Dystrophia myotonica
- Myotonia congenita
- Paramyotonia.

The latter two are essentially benign myotonic disorders of skeletal muscle only, which do not shorten life. Dystrophia myotonica (myotonic muscular dystrophy or myotonia atrophica) is a form of muscular dystrophy with myotonic symptoms which precede atrophy and weakness. However, atrophy and weakness, particularly of facial, sternomastoid and distal muscles, are the major complaints. Incidence is 1 in 20 000, with onset between the second and fourth decades. The diagnosis is often made late in the clinical course.

PATHOPHYSIOLOGY

RESPIRATORY

Respiratory failure is common due to:

- Muscle weakness and myotonia
- Central nervous system-mediated respiratory failure
- Oropharyngeal muscle weakness allowing repeated aspiration.

There is a reduced response to carbon dioxide.

GASTROINTESTINAL TRACT

Smooth muscle involvement leads to difficulty in swallowing and decreased gastric motility, both predisposing to aspiration. There is a high incidence of gallstones.

EYES

Presenile cataracts can be the earliest presenting feature.

CARDIOVASCULAR SYSTEM:

- Rhythm and conduction abnormalities both occur; first-degree heart block is the commonest, leading to Stokes–Adams attacks.
- Cardiomyopathy has been noted and arterial pressure is usually low but rises with worsening congestive heart failure.
- Cor pulmonale may occur due to respiratory failure.

ENDOCRINE SYSTEM

Abnormal glucose tolerance tests are common.

PREOPERATIVE ASSESSMENT

HISTORY:

- Review of respiratory disease
- Swallowing difficulties
- Cardiovascular history (pacemaker for heart block?)
- Drugs for myotonia: quinine, procainamide, phenytoin, steroids.

INVESTIGATIONS:

- Respiratory function tests and arterial blood gases
- Chest radiography (bronchiectasis/infection from aspiration)
- Fluoroscopy will detect diaphragmatic myotonia
- ECG and 24-h tape if rhythm disorder suspected
- Echocardiography if significant cardiovascular system (CVS) involvement.

PREMEDICATION:

- Avoid respiratory depressants.
- Acid aspiration prophylaxis is advisable.
- Intravenous potassium supplementation may make myotonia worse.

PERIOPERATIVE MANAGEMENT

MONITORING
This must commence in the anaesthetic room:
- ECG
- Arterial cannula for pressure and blood gas monitoring is desirable
- Invasive CVS monitoring is advisable if there is significant CVS impairment
- Peripheral nerve stimulator (NB: may give false sense of security regarding muscle power)
- Temperature.

INDUCTION AND MAINTENANCE
Cardiovascular and respiratory depression may be profound with the induction of anaesthesia. A minimal dose of induction agent should be used. Inhalational induction may be preferable.

Pulmonary ventilation is usually required and tracheal intubation will protect the airway. Due to muscle atrophy, intubation can usually be performed without muscle relaxation. Suxamethonium should be avoided as widespread myotonia may occur, making intubation very difficult. Short-acting non-depolarising muscle relaxants may provide relaxation, but often do not; minimal doses with close monitoring should be used. Reversal of non-depolarising block with neostigmine may increase myotonia, so it is safest to allow the block to wear off spontaneously. Opioids should be restricted because of respiratory depression.

Normothermia should be maintained to decrease postoperative shivering, which will increase myotonia.

Myotonia may occur with diathermy and surgical handling. This will be refractory to neuromuscular blockade and to both regional and peripheral nerve blockade. Myotonia may be treated with intravenous procainamide (NB: heart block) or phenytoin. Intravenous regional anaesthesia or direct infiltration of the muscle with local anaesthetic may reduce the myotonia.

REGIONAL TECHNIQUES
These avoid general anaesthesia and its complications; unfortunately myotonia is not abolished and paralysis of the abdominal muscles may precipitate respiratory failure. Epidural block may be helpful for pain relief, particularly after upper abdominal surgery, and avoids the need for opioids after operation.

Local anaesthetic injected directly into the muscle will relieve myotonia and may be used at the surgical site.

POSTOPERATIVE MANAGEMENT

- Patients should be closely monitored in the ITU/HDU.
- Postoperative ventilation is advisable.
- Controlled oxygen therapy should be used in those with chronic hypoxic drive.
- Early physiotherapy.
- Tracheostomy or minitracheostomy may be required if bronchial secretions are troublesome.
- ECG monitoring should be continued, as arrhythmias and sudden death have been reported.

BIBLIOGRAPHY

Imison AR. Anaesthesia and myotonia – an Australian experience. Anaesthesia and Intensive Care 2001; 29:34–37

Russell SH, Hirsch NP. Anaesthesia and myotonia. British Journal of Anaesthesia 1994; 72:210–216

2

CROSS-REFERENCES

3

RESPIRATORY SYSTEM
N. Soni

Asthma

N. Soni

Asthma is a respiratory disorder which may be defined as recurrent attacks of paroxysmal dyspnoea, characterised by variable airflow obstruction and increased bronchial hyper-responsiveness to a range of stimuli. Aetiology, pathology and clinical presentation are all heterogeneous, but an underlying inflammatory response is usually present. There is an immense range of clinical pathology, from children with reversible bronchospasm through to elderly patients in whom the broncho-spasm is superimposed on chronic respiratory disease.

EPIDEMIOLOGY

The geographical distribution is variable; about 5% of the population as a whole is affected, but up to 10% of children.

MORBIDITY

There is an increased risk of postoperative respiratory complications, especially in the older patient with chronic airways disease, in whom cardiac problems may also be present.

PATHOPHYSIOLOGY

Non-specific hyperresponsiveness is a common feature. This may be demonstrated by increased response to methacholine, exercise, histamine, cold air challenge or hyperventilation. Airway obstruction is due to constriction of airway smooth muscle, mucus secretion and oedema of the airway wall. Mechanisms include neural and cellular pathway activation. The neural pathway involves afferent irritant receptors in airways, causing reflex stimulation of postganglionic parasympathetic fibres, resulting in smooth muscle constriction and mucus secretion. C-fibre stimulation releases local neuropeptides; substance P changes membrane permeability and mucus secretion, while neurokinin A causes bronchoconstriction. Cellular pathway activation is known to involve immunoglobin E-mediated histamine release from mast cells, but eosinophils, neutrophils, macrophages and lymphocytes may also release mediators.

Mediators include the leukotrienes (LTB_4) and the cysteinyl leukotrienes (CysLTs). LTB_4 is a proinflammatory mediator that acts as a potent neutrophil chemotaxin, whereas CysLTs are potent bronchoconstrictors that increase vascular permeability, cause mucus secretion, mucociliary dysfunction, stimulate eosinophil recruitment and increase bronchial responsiveness. At a cellular level, smooth muscle tone is controlled by intracellular levels of cyclic adenosine monophosphate (cAMP) and possibly cyclic guanosine monophosphate (cGMP), low levels leading to bronchoconstriction. The effect on ventilatory function is V/Q mismatch leading to hypoxia, and air trapping leading to hypercapnia.

An early acute phase leads into a late-phase reaction, which is associated with cellular infiltration and may be sustained for several days.

PREOPERATIVE ASSESSMENT

If asthma is known to be present, the severity in terms of frequency of attacks, hospital

Mediator	Bronchospasm	Oedema	Mucus secretion
Histamine	+	+	+
Prostaglandin	+	+	
Leukotrienes C_4, D_4, E_4	+	+	+
Thromboxane	+	+	
Platelet-activating factor	+	+	

admissions, exercise tolerance and current medication required, as well as any trigger factors, must be established. A history of atopy or a family history of asthma should also alert the anaesthetist to the possibility of intra-operative bronchospasm. Patients with chronic obstructive airway disease (COAD) may have a significant reversible or asthmatic component to their chest problems. On physical examination the presence of wheezes might indicate inadequate control and that current medication requires review. The presence of a respiratory tract infection is a relative contraindication to anaesthesia.

INVESTIGATIONS:

- Chest radiography may show elements of hyperinflation. In the older patient, chronic lung changes or concomitant cardiac problems may be identified. Look for evidence of right ventricular predominance, suggesting long-standing and major problems.
- An ECG may also provide evidence of long-standing right ventricular hypertrophy or cor pulmonale in patients with chronic disease. These patients constitute a very high-risk group.
- Lung function tests: forced expiratory volume in 1 s (FEV_1) reduced more then forced vital capacity (FVC) (FEV_1 normally 50 ml kg^{-1}, and 70–80% FVC).
- Blood gases: baseline blood gases in asthmatics with COAD may be of value in postoperative management.

MAINTENANCE DRUGS

The most significant change in the management of asthmatics over the past few years is the range of agents that can maintain control of the asthma (Table 3.1). Many of these are now long acting. Patients should continue on maintenance therapy throughout their hospital stay, if possible.

PREMEDICATION

Sedation is often useful as anxiety may provoke an attack in some patients. Atropine will inhibit vagally mediated spasm. If an intramuscular opioid is required, pethidine is probably the least undesirable. An additional dose of bronchodilator may be given by inhaler or nebuliser with the premedicant drugs. Patients taking high-dose steroids (> 1500 μg daily in adults,

TABLE 3.1

Agents used to maintain control of asthma

Drug	Comment
Stabilising agents	
Sodium cromoglycate	
Bronchodilators	
Salbutamol	β_2-agonist
Terbutaline	β_2-agonist
Salmeterol	Long-acting β_2-agonist
Aminophylline	Phosphodiesterase inhibitor
Ipratropium	Anticholinergic agent
Steroids	
Beclomethasone dipropionate	
Fluticasone propionate	High potency, low toxicity
Budesonide	
Prednisolone	

less in children) may have adrenal suppression and will require perioperative replacement.

CHOICE OF ANAESTHESIA

Regional anaesthesia may be both feasible and acceptable to the patient, but anxiety can trigger bronchospasm and so patient acceptance is important. If general anaesthesia is necessary, avoid stimulation of the respiratory tract and, where possible, drugs known to cause bronchospasm. The advent of sevoflurane has made inhalational induction a possibility.

INDUCTION

Theoretically, induction agents that may release histamine should be avoided. Thiopental can release histamine and fail to block airway reflexes, but is usually a safe agent to use. Propofol has been used in asthma and its apparent effect on airway reflexes may be beneficial. Etomidate is safe to use. Ketamine has been used to treat status asthmaticus and is unlikely to trigger bronchospasm. It is not an ideal induction agent, but has a place in the asthmatic patient with bronchospasm requiring emergency anaesthesia.

INTUBATION

Although spraying the larynx with lidocaine (lignocaine) prior to intubation has its advocates, some reports and studies confirm the ability of sprayed lidocaine to stimulate bronchospasm

3

(not histamine mediated). The place of the laryngeal mask has yet to be established. Nebulised salbutamol preintubation has been reported to be helpful.

MAINTENANCE

The volatile agents halothane, enflurane and isoflurane are all potent bronchodilators and have been used in the treatment of refractory asthma. Sevoflurane has been used in asthmatics and has good bronchodilator properties at 3–5%.

MUSCLE RELAXANTS

Suxamethonium is a potent histamine releaser and should be avoided if possible. Older relaxants such as curare with potent histamine-releasing properties are contraindicated. Pancuronium is devoid of such problems, but is long acting and generally requires an anticholinesterase for reversal, and these may induce spasm. Atracurium can cause histamine release, but does have the advantage of Hofmann degradation which reduces the need for anticholinesterase. With its short duration of action and low histamine-releasing potency, vecuronium is probably the relaxant of choice.

ANALGESIA

Local and regional techniques are recommended, but are not always feasible. Morphine and diamorphine release histamine and so should be avoided. There is controversy as to the histamine-releasing potential of pethidine, but it has been widely used. Fentanyl and alfentanil are probably the safest of the opioids commonly used. Aspirin is known to cause bronchospasm in one group of asthmatic patients and is best avoided. The place of other non-steroidal anti-inflammatory drugs (NSAIDs) is less clear.

Anticholinesterases can induce bronchospasm, although the atropine given concurrently should inhibit this.

POSTOPERATIVE MANAGEMENT

Analgesia must be effective, whether using systemic drugs or regional techniques. The problems of chronic asthmatics refer to the problems of chronic lung disease. Effective analgesia and the ability to tolerate physio-

therapy and cough adequately prevent the development of atelectasis. Warm, humidified air and the use of bronchodilators should minimise the impact of mucus retention and plugging.

THE EMERGENCY CASE WITH SYMPTOMATIC BRONCHOSPASM

This is a potentially disastrous situation, but fortunately rare. Surgery must be absolutely essential. The normal methods for treating bronchospasm should be employed aggressively, with the use of steroids if indicated. There is potentially a role for magnesium sulfate (2 g i.v.), which may assist bronchodilatation. The induction agent of choice is probably ketamine. Suxamethonium does release histamine in some patients, but its use may be difficult to avoid. An opiate such as fentanyl can be used. Inhalational agents such as isoflurane or halothane are effective in treating bronchospasm and should assist induction. Once induced and deep on these agents, the patient may be better controlled than prior to induction. Continued bronchospasm with high airway pressure may require the use of β-agonists and, if required, adrenaline (epinephrine), either by nebuliser or intravenously.

Ventilation may pose problems, as airway pressures are likely to be high. Manipulation of tidal volume, rate and I/E ratios can be used to minimise peak airway pressure with due attention to the maintenance of an adequate minute ventilation. Permissive hypercapnia has sometimes been employed from necessity, and is reasonably tolerated. The possibility of a pneumothorax must be considered throughout the case. Postoperative management should be in an ITU.

DEVELOPMENT OF INTRAOPERATIVE ASTHMA

It must be remembered that not all wheezing is necessarily asthma. Tube placement at the carina or in a main bronchus can produce wheezing. Airway obstruction may result from tube blockage, secretions or blood, and aspiration, tension pneumothorax or an anaphylactic or anaphylactoid reaction may all produce spasm. Treatment consists of eliminating these possibilities and the use of deep inhalational anaesthesia and bronchodilators to gain relief of the problem.

3

Salbutamol (2–5 μg kg^{-1} slowly i.v.) or aminophylline (5 mg kg^{-1}). Steroids or hydrocortisone (100 mg) will not have immediate effect but may assist in gaining control. Airway pressures may have been very high (see above), so beware of pneumothorax developing.

DRUGS TO AVOID

- Curare
- Morphine, diamorphine and other histamine-releasing opiates
- Beta-blockers
- Aspirin, and probably other NSAIDs that are prostaglandin mediated.

BIBLIOGRAPHY

Busse W. Asthma in the 1990s. Postgraduate Medicine 1992; 92:177–190

Hirshman CA. Perioperative management of the asthmatic patient. Canadian Journal of Anaesthesia 1991; 38:R26–R32

CROSS-REFERENCES

Iatrogenic adrenocortical insufficiency
    Patient Conditions 2: 71
Pulmonary hypertension
    Patient Conditions 4: 138
Intraoperative bronchospasm
    Anaesthetic Factors 31: 750

3

Bronchiectasis

N. Soni

Bronchiectasis is a chronic lung disease characterised by permanent abnormal dilatation of the bronchi, accompanied by chronic inflammation and expectoration of purulent sputum. The prevalence of bronchiectasis has been declining since the advent of antibiotics, and the life expectancy of bronchiectatic patients has improved considerably. Bronchiectasis is now diagnosed by high-resolution computed tomography (CT) of the lung rather than bronchography under general anaesthesia, and treatment by surgical resection of the affected lobes has been replaced by medical management; consequently, anaesthesia for investigation or treatment of the primary condition is uncommon.

PATHOPHYSIOLOGY

Many cases of bronchiectasis are the long-term sequelae of childhood pulmonary infections, but there are several congenital conditions that predispose to bronchiectasis.

CAUSES OF BRONCHIECTASIS:
- Following childhood pneumonia
- Congenital:
  —cystic fibrosis
  —bronchial cartilage deficiency
  —abnormal ciliary motility
  —hypogammaglobulinaemia.
- Distal to bronchial obstruction:
  —inhaled foreign body
  —tumour.

Bronchiectasis usually affects only part of the lung. The clinical features and severity of symptoms vary with the cause and extent of the disease. Severe bronchiectatics produce up to 500 ml purulent sputum per day, with worse exacerbations. Self-limiting haemoptyses occur because of extensive collateral circulation from bronchial and intercostal arteries. In severe cases, pulmonary hypertension and cor pulmonale may occur as a result of destruction of

lung tissue and systemic–pulmonary collateral circulation. Amyloidosis and lung or distant abscess formation are rare complications.

The conservative treatment of bronchiectasis is based on percussive chest physiotherapy and postural drainage, with either prophylaxis or early treatment of exacerbations with antibiotics. *Haemophilus influenzae* or *Pseudomonas aeruginosa* are common infecting organisms.

PREOPERATIVE ASSESSMENT

LUNG FUNCTION
Helpful:
- History, especially the patient's assessment of how they are compared with their 'best'
- Arterial blood gases as a baseline for postoperative management
- High-resolution CT to define the extent of the disease.

Not helpful:
- Spirometry
- Plain chest radiography.

CARDIOVASCULAR SYSTEM
- Clinical examination and an ECG will elicit signs of cor pulmonale.
- Right ventricular function can be examined with echocardiography.

PERIOPERATIVE MANAGEMENT

PREPARATION OF THE PATIENT
Admit the patient to hospital several days before operation for extensive chest physiotherapy with postural drainage. Give amoxicillin (3 g daily) if needed to control bronchial sepsis.

PREMEDICATION
Avoid anticholinergics as they may make bronchial secretions more viscid. Respiratory depressant drugs should be used with caution.

MONITORING

Monitoring should be started in the anaesthetic room and should include pulse oximetry and ECG. In severe cases an arterial line will assist intraoperative and postoperative management.

ANAESTHETIC MANAGEMENT

The choice of anaesthetic will be determined by the type and site of operation. In general, a regional or local anaesthetic technique is preferred. If general anaesthesia is used, artificial ventilation should be employed.

RESPIRATORY MANAGEMENT DURING ANAESTHESIA:

- Maintain adequate gas exchange:
  —Adjust oxygen to maintain 90% or greater SaO_2.
  —The $EtCO_2 : PaCO_2$ difference may be widened, as in all patients with chronic lung disease.
- Avoid retention of sputum and infected material:
  —Use humidified anaesthetic gases, either a heater/humidifier or a passive heat and moisture exchanger
  —Employ frequent tracheal suction (catheters that can be directed into the left or right bronchi are useful)
  —On-table positioning to assist postural drainage, if possible
  —Perioperative flexible bronchoscopy to help clear sputum.
- Avoid contamination of non-bronchiectatic areas with infected sputum – in severe cases the bronchiectatic area must be isolated from the unaffected lung using a left endobronchial tube or a bronchial blocker placed under rigid bronchoscopy.

POSTOPERATIVE MANAGEMENT

- Give immediate postural drainage and physiotherapy; this will require good analgesia with patient-controlled devices, epidural analgesia or non-steroidal anti-inflammatory drugs (NSAIDs).
- Entonox may be useful during physiotherapy.
- Humidified oxygen should be used.
- Intravenous antibiotics may be required for exacerbations.
- There is no place for elective postoperative ventilation, except for rewarming.

BIBLIOGRAPHY

Hopkin JM. The suppurative lung diseases. In: Weatherall DJ, Ledingham JGG, Warrell DA, eds. Oxford textbook of medicine. 2nd edn. Oxford: Oxford University Press; 1987:15.100–15.103

Katz J. Anaesthesia and uncommon paediatric diseases. Philadelphia: WB Saunders; 1987:83–84

CROSS-REFERENCES

Pulmonary hypertension
    Patient Conditions 4: 138
Lobectomy
    Surgical Procedures 15: 402

3

Bronchogenic carcinoma

Neil Soni

Cancer of the lung now kills more people than any other tumour. The most common tumour is bronchogenic carcinoma (Table 3.2).

Bronchogenic carcinoma is almost unknown among non-smokers. The peak incidence is in men aged 50–60 years. It is a tumour of the bronchial epithelium, 75% occurring at the carina or the first-, second- or third-order bronchus. The tumour may break through the epithelium into the bronchial lumen, ultimately causing obstruction and lung collapse, or it may spread along peribronchial tissues invading other mediastinal organs.

Lymphatic involvement and haematological spread to distant organs is common. Adrenal glands, brain and bone are frequently involved.

PREOPERATIVE ASSESSMENT

Presenting symptoms include:
- Cough
- Haemoptysis
- Chest pain
- Dyspnoea (pleural effusion)
- Metastases
- Hoarseness
- Ectopic hormonal activity.

TABLE 3.2

Lung cancer and its incidence

Tumour	Incidence (%)
Bronchogenic carcinoma	90
Squamous cell carcinoma	63
Adenocarcinoma	9
Undifferentiated carcinoma	18
Large cell	11
Oat or small cell	7
Alveolar cell carcinoma	2
Bronchial adenoma	5
Mesenchymal and other tumours	3

Physical examination of the chest may well be unremarkable. Grossly abnormal physical signs such as lobar collapse, consolidation, pleural effusion or superior vena caval obstruction indicate late presentation. Signs of coincident obstructive airway disease are common. It is worthwhile assessing general muscle mass and strength as peripheral neuropathy and neuromuscular transmission problems (Eaton–Lambert syndrome) are sequelae of bronchial carcinoma.

Physical examination may reveal ectopic hormone activity by bronchogenic cancer. Virtually any polypeptide hormone may be produced, usually by the histologically small cell variety of tumour. These hormones, of anaesthetic importance, include antidiuretic hormone (ADH), adrenocorticotrophic hormone (ACTH), parathyroid hormone (PTH), insulin and glucagon. Bronchial adenomas are usually carcinoid tumours capable of 5-hydroxytryptamine (5-HT, serotonin) secretion, clinically manifest as the carcinoid syndrome.

INVESTIGATIONS:
- Chest radiography – posteroanterior and lateral – may or may not reveal the tumour. However, it will be helpful in assessing coincident disease such as the increased anterior–posterior diameter and flattened diaphragms of chronic obstructive airway disease. Pleural effusion will be obvious. Enlarged heart shadow may mean pericardial effusion and mediastinal invasion.
- ECG may be useful as atrial fibrillation commonly complicates thoracic surgery.
- Estimation of serum levels of electrolytes is indicated as ectopic ADH may cause a remarkably low serum level of sodium, clinically expressed as confusion and weakness.
- Ectopic ACTH can lead to features of hypercortisolaemia, particularly hypokalaemia. Clinical features of Cushing's

syndrome rarely develop because the overall 5-year survival rate is 9%, and for small (oat) cell tumours the 2-year survival rate is only 6%.

- Adrenocortical failure (Addison's disease) may occur with metastatic carcinoma invasion of the gland, and hyperkalaemia – with or without hyponatraemia – can be a clue.
- Ectopic PTH can cause raised serum calcium levels, resulting in renal problems and shortening of the PR interval on the ECG. Widespread bony metastases will have similar consequences.
- Ectopic ACTH, glucagon and insulin may cause glucose metabolism problems.
- Lung function tests are mandatory if lung resection is considered. Forced expiratory volume in 1 s (FEV_1) and forced vital capacity (FVC) are most commonly available and useful. Arterial blood gases on air are valuable as a preoperative baseline.
- CT of the thoracic cavity is routinely performed to help assess operability of lung tumours, particularly mediastinal lymph gland enlargement.

Signs of inoperability in advanced disease:
- Obstruction of the superior vena cava (SVC)
- Left recurrent laryngeal nerve palsy
- Carinal or tracheal involvement
- Phrenic nerve palsy
- Oesophageal mucosal invasion
- Cardiac and great vessel involvement
- Pancoast's syndrome – apical carcinoma invading the eighth cervical and first thoracic nerves, causing pain and wasting in the upper limb plus stellate ganglion involvement giving features of Horner's syndrome (ptosis, enophthalmos, miosis, impaired sweating on face).
- Vertebral involvement.

PREOPERATIVE PREPARATION

- Optimise respiratory function
- Physiotherapy
- Bronchodilators
- Pleural effusion drainage
- Correct anaemia or electrolyte disturbance
- Antibiotic cover and treatment of respiratory infections.

Although all patients should be cross-matched before operation, the use of blood transfusion in patients with cancer has recently been reviewed. Several investigators have described an adverse outcome in those who have received perioperative transfusion; this has led to consideration of anaesthetic techniques designed to reduce the requirement of transfusion.

PREMEDICATION
Any premedication that includes a drying agent will be suitable.

ANAESTHETIC TECHNIQUE
Controlled ventilation is preferable in all but the briefest of procedures.

Neuromuscular monitoring is essential, and short- to medium-acting agents, which do not accumulate, should be used.

Bronchodilating anaesthetic techniques including volatile anaesthetic agents avoid possible intraoperative bronchoconstriction.

POSTOPERATIVE CARE
Although many patients are treated in a high-dependency area in the initial postoperative phase, more intensive treatment, especially postoperative ventilation, often implies a much greater severity of respiratory disease. Although postoperative respiratory failure is not common, these patients frequently do not survive the initial postoperative period.

ANALGESIA
Respiratory function will be enhanced when diaphragmatic splinting due to pain is reduced to a minimum, and the use of epidural analgesia is common in patients with respiratory disease.

BIBLIOGRAPHY

Hirschler CJ, Hylkeman BS, Meyer RW. Mechanical ventilation for acute postoperative respiratory failure after surgery for bronchial carcinoma. Thorax 1985; 40:387–390

O'Neill JH, Murray NM, Newson-Davis J. Lambert–Eaton syndrome. A review of 50 cases. Brain 1988; III:577–596

Schreimer PA, Longnecker DE, Mintz PD. The possible immunosuppressive effects of perioperative blood transfusion in cancer patients. Anesthesiology 1988; 68:422–428

Small S, Ali HH, Lennon VA, Brown RH, Carr DB, De Armendi A. Anesthesia for an unsuspected Lambert–Eaton myasthenic syndrome with autoantibodies and occult small cell lung carcinoma. Anesthesiology 1992; 76:142–145

3

CROSS-REFERENCES

Lobectomy
    Surgical Procedures 15: 402
Pneumonectomy
    Surgical Procedures 15: 408
One lung anaesthesia
    Anaesthetic Factors 30: 710
Intraoperative bronchospasm
    Anaesthetic Factors 31: 750
Preoperative assessment of pulmonary risk
    Anaesthetic Factors 27: 638

3

COPD and anaesthesia

N. Soni and J. C. Goldstone

PATHOPHYSIOLOGY

Obstruction to airflow is the hallmark of this common respiratory disease, which affects thousands of patients and is responsible for 10% of absence from work and 10% of bed occupancy in general hospitals. Airflow obstruction results in:

- Raised residual volume
- Hyperinflation of the thorax
- Decrease in inspiratory capacity (respiratory muscle shortening).

Clinically, two patterns of disease often present (Table 3.3).

It is common that these clinical extremes overlap. In general, oxygen therapy, general anaesthesia and the effect of sleeping are more problematic in the 'blue bloater' type. The presence of cor pulmonale is an insidious sign, especially in emphysema.

PREOPERATIVE ASSESSMENT

The necessity for preoperative pulmonary function tests may be assessed in part from the preoperative history of:

- Breathlessness
- Cough
- Sputum production
- Exercise limitation.

In the presence of symptomatology, peak flow, FEV_1 and mid-expiratory flow rate (MEFR) can be assessed (Table 3.4). This can be performed at the bedside with hand-held spirometers or calculated from a Vitalograph tracing.

In chronicity, poor pulmonary function leads to hypercapnia and this should be excluded by performing arterial blood gas analysis while breathing room air (Table 3.5). Additionally, the degree of hypoxaemia can be assessed as well as any acute decompensation.

The development of heart failure is ominous, with a 30% 5-year survival rate. The likelihood of postoperative ventilation is related to the severity of disease; patients with hypercapnia are a particular at-risk group. Some attention should be given to the feasibility of postoperative oxygen therapy.

PERIOPERATIVE MANAGEMENT

- Cessation of cigarette smoking
- Preoperative physiotherapy
- Optimisation of bronchodilator therapy
- Additional bronchodilator therapy if persistent wheezing
- Caution with sedative drugs in patients with hypercapnia or severe obstruction.

3

TABLE 3.3

Patterns of disease

Chronic bronchitis ('blue bloaters')	Emphysema ('pink puffers')
Thickening of bronchial wall and excessive mucus production leading to: —increased airway resistance —reduced expiratory airflow	Destruction of lung tissue leading to: —decrease in elastic recoil —narrowing and collapse of airway during expiration
Severe hypoxaemia	Severe breathlessness
Hypercapnia	Normoxaemic or slightly hypoxaemic
Cor pulmonale	Normocapnic

TABLE 3.4

FEV_1 and MEFR

	FEV_1 (% predicted)	$MEFR_{25-75}$ (% predicted)
Asymptomatic	65–80	60–75
Moderate	50–64	45–59
Marked	35–49	30–44

TABLE 3.5

Investigations on sequelae of airflow obstruction

Important further sequelae of airflow obstruction	Investigations
Cor pulmonale	ECG
	Echocardiography
Sleep apnoea	Overnight oximetry in obstructive lesions
	Formal sleep study if central apnoea present
Polycythaemia	Full blood count

Cessation of smoking may be helpful acutely by reducing carboxyhaemoglobin levels. A reduction in postoperative morbidity occurs if abstinence is greater than 8 weeks. In all but those patients who have a fixed, non-reversible obstruction, preoperative broncho-dilatation with a nebulised β_2-agonist is a usual preparation.

ANAESTHETIC TECHNIQUE

The maintenance of spontaneous breathing and an awake patient unaffected by centrally acting drugs is an attractive feature of regional anaesthesia, and this is the preferred technique in many peripheral procedures. Of practical significance is the effect of dyspnoea on patient position and the duration of the operation. Obstructive lung disease is characterised by expiratory muscle hypertrophy and prolongation of expiratory flow. Extensive regional techniques that reduce expiratory muscle strength are likely to decompensate patients, and motor loss above T8 may not be tolerated.

GENERAL ANAESTHESIA
General anaesthesia may be indicated when neuromuscular paralysis is required or when a procedure is not likely to be tolerated, for example in the severely dyspnoeic patient. A spontaneously breathing technique has many advantages:
- Avoids excessive positive intrathoracic pressure
- Avoids auto-peep induced by mechanical ventilation
- May avoid tracheal intubation.

Bronchodilatation is enhanced by volatile anaesthetic agents, and, experimentally, halothane and isoflurane are of equal efficacy. Recently, little difference was found between volatile and propofol-based general anaesthesia in COPD in terms of intraoperative lung mechanics or outcome, suggesting an alternative to this traditional approach. It is suggested that propofol may have bronchodilating properties in addition to its sedating effects.

CONTROLLED VENTILATION
Airway control, avoidance of respiratory depression and further hypercapnia, and difficulties with volatile uptake are all advantages of controlled ventilation. Of particular note is:
- Auto-peep
- Barotrauma.

POSTOPERATIVE CARE

ANALGESIA
Effective analgesia without respiratory depression is the indication for postoperative epidural analgesia for abdominal or thoracic surgery. This should be monitored in the setting of a high-dependency area that permits further monitoring of ventilatory status. Peripheral nerve blocks, especially as a continuous technique via a catheter, may also be advantageous.

RESPIRATORY MONITORING
Although oxygenation may be monitored by pulse oximetry, an indwelling arterial cannula allows frequent arterial blood gas analysis. Rapid shallow breathing may indicate decompensation. Knowledge of preoperative arterial blood gas status is essential when interpreting postoperative changes.

POSTOPERATIVE VENTILATION
Hypercapnic patients with severe airflow obstruction may not easily resume spontaneous ventilation, and difficulties with weaning may be anticipated. Continuance of controlled ventilation into the postoperative period merely postpones trials of weaning and is seldom beneficial, contrasting to maintenance of controlled ventilation in patients with decompensated cardiovascular disease. In order to breathe, such patients require an adequate central drive, no reduction in respiratory muscle strength and an optimised load : strength ratio. It may not be possible to achieve this immediately after operation, although this should be the goal.

OUTCOME

Hypercapnia denotes decompensation and distinguishes a more severely affected group of patients who are likely to require postoperative support and ITU admission. Postoperative complications are common when FEV_1 is low. Unfortunately, preoperative pulmonary function testing alone does not select those patients at risk; rather, general indicators such as American Society of Anesthesiologists (ASA) status and duration of operation are significant factors.

BIBLIOGRAPHY

Conti G, DellUtri D, Vilardi V et al. Propofol induces bronchodilation in mechanically ventilated chronic obstructive pulmonary disease (COPD) patients. Acta Anaesthesiologica Scandinavica 1993; 37:105–109

DeSouza G, DeLisser EA, Turry P, Gold MI. Comparison of propofol with isoflurane for maintenance of anaesthesia in patients with chronic obstructive pulmonary disease; use of pulmonary mechanics, peak flow rates and blood gases. Journal of Cardiothoracic and Vascular Anaesthesia 1995; 9:24–28

Wong DH, Weber EG, Schell MJ, Wong AB, Anderson CT, Barker SJ. Factors associated with postoperative pulmonary complications in patients with severe chronic obstructive pulmonary disease. Anaesthesia and Analgesia 1995; 80:276–284

CROSS-REFERENCES

Polycythaemia
    Patient Conditions 7: 223
Intraoperative bronchospasm
    Anaesthetic Factors 31: 750
Weaning from controlled ventilation
    Anaesthetic Factors 31: 803
Preoperative assessment of pulmonary risk
    Anaesthetic Factors 27: 638

3

Cystic fibrosis

N. Soni

Cystic fibrosis (CF) is a congenital disease of Caucasians affecting 1 in 1500 births, currently with an estimated 5200 patients in England and Wales. It presents between birth and early infancy and, despite advances in treatment, still progresses to multisystem failure and death during early adult life. Patients with CF require surgery more frequently than normal (Table 3.6) and involvement of the cardiorespiratory system renders anaesthesia hazardous. However, the mortality rate associated with surgery in patients with CF has decreased from 27% in the 1950s to 0.5% in 1987 (Fig. 3.1).

TABLE 3.6

Operative procedures associated with cystic fibrosis

Age group	Procedure
Neonates and infants	Meconium ileus or obstruction
Teenagers	Nasal polyps, bronchoscopy
Age over 20 years	Pleurodesis, lobectomy, gastrostomy, feeding lines, lung or heart–lung transplant

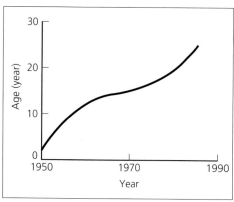

Fig. 3.1 Average survival of patients with cystic fibrosis.

PATHOPHYSIOLOGY

The CF gene and the protein for which it codes have both been identified, which may possibly lead to a gene therapy cure for CF. The transport of chloride and sodium in mucosal cells is defective, causing the production of abnormal mucus resulting in impaired ciliary function, infection and, ultimately, organ damage (Table 3.7).

In the lung the pathological process leads to:

- Type 1 respiratory failure (normal or low Pa_{CO_2})
- Low V/Q ratios
- Increased alveolar to arterial oxygen difference
- Hypoxic respiratory drive
- Hyperreactive bronchioles.

TABLE 3.7

Organ pathology resulting from CF

Organ system	Disease process
Lung	Obstruction, emphysema, bronchiectasis, fibrosis
Heart	Pulmonary hypertension, right heart failure
Liver	Obstructive jaundice, biliary cirrhosis, coagulopathy
Pancreas	Diabetes mellitus, malabsorption (vitamins A, E, K)
Bowel	Obstruction, malabsorption and cachexia

PREOPERATIVE MANAGEMENT

ASSESSMENT

Clinical evaluation to assess the various disease processes involved in CF is essential. The usual preoperative investigations are performed.

Reduced forced vital capacity (FVC), hypoxaemia and dyspnoea at rest are associated with postoperative ventilation.

PREPARATION

Before operation vigorous efforts are required to optimise the patient's condition, including:
- Physiotherapy
- Bronchodilators
- Hydration (consider intravenous fluids)
- Antibiotics for respiratory infections
- Parenteral vitamin K (if not on oral treatment).

PREMEDICATION

Opioids are not advisable and drying agents should not be given before surgery. Benzodiazepines may be used for particularly anxious patients.

PERIOPERATIVE MANAGEMENT

REGIONAL ANAESTHESIA

Regional anaesthesia is preferable to general anaesthesia in terms of both respiratory function and postoperative analgesia. Unfortunately, the age of patients with CF and the likely operation performed are not ideal for regional techniques.

INDUCTION

Preoxygenation followed by intravenous induction is preferable in all age groups, with an anticholinergic agent given at this time if required.

MAINTENANCE

A high FiO_2 may be needed and nitrous oxide is contraindicated in patients with pneumothorax, bullous pulmonary disease or neonatal obstruction. A volatile agent technique is therefore preferable to opioid–nitrous oxide for maintenance. The following measures should be considered throughout the procedure, but particularly before extubation:
- Effective humidification
- Frequent tracheal suctioning
- Tracheal instillation of normal saline
- Chest physiotherapy.

AIRWAY

Tracheal intubation with paralysis and intermittent positive-pressure ventilation (IPPV)

is advisable in almost all cases. This allows control of the airway and respiration as well as facilitating effective tracheobronchial toilet and preventing coughing during surgery.

MONITORING

In addition to the usual monitoring the following are useful in patients with CF:
- Airway pressure (to detect pneumothorax, bronchospasm or mucous plugs)
- $EtCO_2$
- Arterial blood gases (keep $PaCO_2$ at the preoperative value)
- Blood glucose level
- Transcutaneous oxygen in neonates.

POSTOPERATIVE CARE

RESPIRATORY CARE

Before return to the recovery area, patients should have normal neuromuscular function and be able to cough well. Humidified oxygen of controlled FiO_2 should be given and intensive chest physiotherapy must begin in the recovery area and continue until the patient is discharged. After a major operation, monitoring of the respiratory system (e.g. pulse oximetry) should continue for a few days, particularly at night, and oxygen given as necessary.

Facial or nasal continuous positive airway pressure (CPAP) may be useful after operation. If possible IPPV should be avoided in patients with CF because of the risk of barotrauma. Weaning from ventilation may be prolonged due to uncompliant lungs and chronic malnutrition.

ANALGESIA

When feasible, regional analgesia is the method of choice even in small children (caudal injections) and thoracic procedures (thoracic epidurals or intercostal nerve blocks). Provided that renal and pulmonary function allow, NSAIDs may be used and should be commenced before or during the operation. Finally, in many cases opioids are still required and should be used in carefully titrated doses with close monitoring of the patient, for instance in a high-dependency unit.

3

BIBLIOGRAPHY

Cole RR, Cotton RT. Preventing postoperative complications in the cystic fibrosis patient. International Journal of Pediatric Otorhinolaryngology 1990; 18:263–269

Lamberty JM, Rubin BK. The management of anaesthesia for patients with cystic fibrosis. Anaesthesia 1985; 40:448–459

Nunn JF, Milledge JS, Chen D, Dore C. Respiratory criteria for fitness for surgery and anaesthesia. Anaesthesia 1988; 43:543–551

3

Restrictive lung disease

N. Soni

Restrictive lung disease is characterised by a reduced vital capacity, usually with a small resting volume and normal airway resistance. Relevant conditions include:

- Chest wall or respiratory muscle disease – kyphoscoliosis, myasthenia gravis, Guillain–Barré syndrome, poliomyelitis
- Pleural thickening – tumour, inflammation
- Space-occupying lesions – tumour, pleural effusion, pneumothorax
- Lung resection
- Pulmonary infiltration:
  —known causes – asbestos, radiation, drugs (chemotherapy, etc.)
  —Unknown causes – idiopathic infiltration, collagen vascular disease, amyloidosis, sarcoidosis.

This section discusses mainly pulmonary infiltration. Although symptoms and signs of the other conditions are different, the relevant investigations are similar. Restrictive and obstructive lung disease commonly coexist.

PATHOPHYSIOLOGY

- Thickened alveolar interstitium and irregular fibrosis
- 'Honeycomb' destruction of alveoli
- Desquamation of macrophages in alveolar spaces.

Anaesthetic risk is presented by:
- Limited alveolar gas transfer
- Variable ventilation–perfusion mismatch
- Inability to respond to stress or exercise
- Superadded lung infection.

Coexistent medical conditions present their own risks.

PREOPERATIVE ASSESSMENT

HISTORY
- Dyspnoea, with rapid shallow breathing
- Early dyspnoea on exertion
- Dry irritating cough

- Ankle oedema and other evidence of cor pulmonale
- Recurrent chest infections may also occur.

EXAMINATION
- Cyanosis, especially on exertion
- Fine crackles on auscultation (without oedema)
- Finger clubbing may be seen in long-standing cases
- Signs of cor pulmonale
- Signs of superadded chest infection.

INVESTIGATIONS
- Evidence of specific conditions as above.
- Chest radiography may show a ground glass haziness, small lung fields, basal collapse and raised diaphragm(s).
- Chest infection may be visible.
- Spirometry reveals decreased vital capacity, decreased FEV_1, but perhaps increased FEV_1/FVC ratio; the spirogram may show a square initial waveform.
- Total lung volume, functional residual capacity and residual volume may fall.
- Pressure–volume curves are flattened and displaced downwards.
- Lung diffusion capacity reduced.
- Arterial blood gas analysis:
  —reduced PaO_2 and $PaCO_2$
  —normal pH
  —PaO_2 falls early in stress conditions
  —$PaCO_2$ rises with progressing disease.
- Cardiac output is limited by raised pulmonary vascular resistance; raised cardiac output may not increase oxygen uptake because of V/Q mismatch.

PREOPERATIVE PREPARATION

- Drainage of interpleural fluid and/or air
- Treatment of coincident reversible airflow limitation – bronchodilators, steroids if indicated

3

- Attention to superadded chest infection – antibiotics, physiotherapy for sputum clearance
- Optimisation of cardiac failure – diuretics, antihypertensives, vasodilators
- Preparation for recovery – respiratory exercises.

PERIOPERATIVE MANAGEMENT

PREMEDICATION
Respiratory depressant drugs should be used with caution. Anticholinergic agents should be given if intubation is anticipated as difficult.

AIRWAY
Bony chest wall deformity may pose problems with tracheal intubation. Preoxygenation and rapid sequence induction may be necessary.

CONTROLLED VENTILATION
Assisted ventilation is advisable because the work of breathing is increased, and airway recruitment may be useful. Nevertheless, positive-pressure ventilation may not improve oxygen uptake beyond preoperative levels owing to impaired alveolar diffusion and irregular ventilation–perfusion mismatch. There is a risk of pneumothorax with positive airway pressure in interstitial lung disease; attention to high inflation pressures and oxygen desaturation is necessary.

REGIONAL ANAESTHESIA
Respiratory failure may occur if extradural anaesthesia reaches levels higher than the T10 segment. Head-down positioning contraindicates spontaneous breathing.

INTRAOPERATIVE MONITORING:
- ECG
- Blood pressure
- SaO_2
- $EtCO_2$
- Fluid balance.

POSTOPERATIVE CARE
These patients are at risk of basal lung collapse and retention of sputum. Late extubation is advisable, and at least a brief period of ventilation in a recovery or high-dependency area should be considered to optimise weaning from support. Analgesia with drugs that are not depressant to ventilation is preferable. Monitoring of SaO_2 during recovery is essential, and supplementary oxygen is required.

LATER POSTOPERATIVE CARE
Respiratory physiotherapy and close attention to postoperative chest infection are most important.

BIBLIOGRAPHY

Hughes JM, Lockwood DN, Jones HA, Clark RJ. DLCO/QAM diffusion limitation at rest and on exercise in patients with interstitial fibrosis. Respiratory Physiology 1983; 2:155–166

West JB. Restrictive diseases in pulmonary pathophysiology – the essentials. 3rd edn. Baltimore: Williams & Wilkins; 1987:92–111

3

Sarcoidosis

N. Soni

Sarcoidosis is a systemic granulomatous disease characterised by spontaneous and complete remissions in the early stages and by a slowly progressive course if the disease persists. The aetiology of sarcoidosis is unknown and the condition occurs in almost all races and all regions of the world. There is a slightly higher prevalence among women between the ages of 20 and 40 years.

The diagnosis is usually made by a combination of clinical, radiographic and histological findings. The Kveim–Siltzbach skin test is an intradermal injection of a heat-treated suspension of a sarcoidosis spleen extract which is then biopsied 4–6 weeks later. This yields sarcoidosis-like lesions in 70–80% of individuals with sarcoidosis, with less than 5% false-positives. The level of angiotensin-converting enzyme is raised in the serum in approximately two-thirds of patients with sarcoidosis, but false-positives and false-negatives are common. An increased 24-h urine calcium level is consistent with the diagnosis, but is not specific.

PATHOPHYSIOLOGY

Although sarcoidosis can affect almost every system in the body, the areas of most concern to anaesthetists are the respiratory, cardiovascular, renal, neurological and metabolic systems.

RESPIRATORY SYSTEM
Some 90% of patients with sarcoidosis will have an abnormal chest radiograph at some time during their illness (bilateral hilar lymphadenopathy being the most common abnormality). Overall, approximately 50% develop permanent pulmonary abnormalities and 5–15% have progressive fibrosis of the lung parenchyma. Sarcoidosis of the lung is primarily an interstitial lung disease leading to a restrictive defect with an associated fall in diffusing capacity. Occasionally, the large airways may be involved to a degree sufficient to cause an obstructive defect. Rarely, the larynx may be involved, usually presenting as hoarseness and dyspnoea, but may possibly cause complete obstruction.

CARDIOVASCULAR SYSTEM
The incidence of clinical cardiac sarcoid is low (1.5%). The common patterns of presentation in order of frequency are complete heart block, ventricular extrasystoles or ventricular tachycardia, myocardial disease with failure, supraventricular arrhythmias, mitral valve dysfunction and pericarditis.

Once the clinical symptoms of cardiac sarcoid become evident, the risk of sudden death increases. Additionally, more than 25% of patients with sarcoidosis have clinically silent myocardial involvement.

RENAL SYSTEM
Renal impairment in sarcoidosis is often nephrocalcinosis, resulting from prolonged hypercalcaemia. This occurs in about 1% of patients and is a late and serious problem because it can lead to pyelonephritis, fibrosis and intractable chronic renal failure. Rarely, massive granulomatous infiltration may occur, also resulting in renal failure.

NEUROLOGICAL SYSTEM
Any part of the nervous system may be affected, and overall 7% of patients show evidence of neurological involvement. Peripheral neuropathies tend to occur with acute-onset sarcoidosis. Dysphagia may complicate sarcoidosis due to involvement of the glossopharyngeal and vagus nerves. Chronic sarcoidosis can be involved with granulomatous changes or space-occupying nodular lesions in the brain, spinal cord and meninges. This may present with signs of raised intracranial pressure, obstructive hydrocephalus or focal epilepsy.

3

PREOPERATIVE MANAGEMENT

RESPIRATORY SYSTEM

Chest radiography and estimation of arterial blood gases are advisable in patients with or without clinical respiratory involvement (Table 3.8). If abnormal, additional formal pulmonary function tests should be requested.

The larynx should be assessed formally if involvement is suspected. Late-onset respiratory tract involvement may occur up to 36 h after extubation. This may require treatment with steroids and nebulised adrenaline (epinephrine).

CARDIOVASCULAR SYSTEM

A preoperative ECG should be obtained in all cases (Table 3.8). However, as more than 25% of patients with sarcoidosis have silent myocardial involvement, continuous observation is required. If any signs of conduction defects are present, preoperative pacing should be considered. Heart block may occur during anaesthesia as the first sign of cardiac involvement, requiring permanent pacing. Echocardiography for mitral valve dysfunction may be required if sudden signs of failure occur.

RENAL AND METABOLIC SYSTEM

Electrolytes should be checked before operation (Table 3.8). The level of calcium is often raised but usually responds to simple measures such as rehydration. Patients with renal impairment should be treated according to the degree of impairment.

NEUROLOGICAL SYSTEM

The extent of involvement needs to be evaluated. The presence of neuropathy or a space-occupying lesion would dictate the use or avoidance of depolarising blockers and spinal anaesthesia respectively.

PERIOPERATIVE MANAGEMENT

Respiratory premedication may worsen subclinical hypoxaemia and should be used judiciously. Supplementary oxygen should be prescribed after premedication. Steroids may already be prescribed. However, if not, they should be discussed, because respiratory and cardiovascular symptoms and signs are often ameliorated.

ANAESTHETIC TECHNIQUE

The technique is dependent on the degree of involvement of the various systems, for example awake intubation in the presence of laryngeal involvement.

In general, intubation and ventilation are preferable to spontaneous respiration. Higher inspiratory oxygen concentration should be administered. It should be remembered that respiratory function, especially diffusing capacity, is usually worse than clinically apparent and that conduction defects may become apparent for the first time during anaesthesia.

POSTOPERATIVE MANAGEMENT

Administer supplementary oxygen after operation. Close monitoring is required for 24–36 h after surgery if upper respiratory tract involvement is suspected.

TABLE 3.8	
Preoperative investigations in patients with sarcoidosis	
Investigations	Results (if system involved)
Chest X-ray	Bilateral hilar lymphadenopathy, reticulonodular shadowing, pleural effusions, cardiomegaly, atelectasis
ECG	Conduction defects, ventricular hypertrophy
Arterial blood gases	Reduced Pa_{O_2} on room air
Lung function tests	Restrictive or obstructive defects
Electrolytes	Raised calcium and potassium levels
Echocardiography	Ventricular hypokinesis, mitral valve involvement, septal thickening and bright echoes (consistent with fibrogranulomatous infiltration)

3

BIBLIOGRAPHY

Miller A, Brown LK, Sloane MF et al. Cardiorespiratory responses to incremental exercise in sarcoidosis patients with normal spirometry. Chest 1995; 107:2

Silverman KJ, Grover GM, Buckley BH. Cardiac sarcoid: a clinicopathological study of 84 unselected patients with systemic sarcoidosis. Circulation 1978; 58:1204–1211

Thomas DW, Mason RA. Complete heart block during anaesthesia in a patient with sarcoidosis. Anaesthesia 1988; 43:578–580

Valentine H, McKenna WJ, Nihoyannapoulos P. Sarcoidosis: a pattern of clinical and morphological presentation. British Heart Journal 1987; 57:256–263

Wills MH, Harris MM. An unusual airway complication with sarcoidosis. Anaesthesiology 1987; 66:554–555

3

Smoking and anaesthesia

N. Soni

Smoking has been described as a dangerous addiction. It is one of the many factors that predispose to postoperative complications. This risk is lessened the longer that smoking is stopped before operation. A history of smoking is a standard part of any preoperative assessment.

PATHOPHYSIOLOGY

RESPIRATORY SYSTEM:
- Mucus hypersecretion
- Impairment of mucociliary clearance
- Small airway narrowing
- Increased bronchial reactivity and epithelial permeability
- Reduced pulmonary surfactant and compliance
- Ventilation–perfusion mismatch.

CARDIOVASCULAR SYSTEM:
- Nicotine causes a pressor response, resulting in increased levels of catecholamines, tachycardia and vasoconstriction with raised systolic and diastolic blood pressure at blood levels of 15–50 ng l^{-1} found in smokers.
- Carbon monoxide has a great affinity for haemoglobin, reducing the oxygen supply to tissues by up to 15% in smokers.
- The oxygen dissociation curve is shifted to the left by carboxyhaemoglobin.
- Carbon monoxide exerts a negative inotropic effect.

HAEMATOLOGICAL SYSTEM:
- Increased red blood cell mass to compensate for chronic tissue hypoxia (overall oxygen content may be equal to that in non-smokers)
- Increased incidence of arterial thromboembolism
- Decreased platelet survival time and increased aggregation potential.

IMMUNE SYSTEM:
- Tobacco smoke attracts alveolar macrophages causing excessive proteolysis with resulting damage to alveolar interstitium (NB: emphysema); exhaustion of supply means the patient is unable to combat infection.
- IgE levels increased.
- Altered T-cell activity.

PREOPERATIVE ASSESSMENT

- Discourage smoking, even on the day of the operation (the perioperative period is in many ways an ideal time to abandon the smoking habit permanently)
- Exclusion of commonly associated medical conditions
- Systematic review of likely chronic diseases; excessive alcohol consumption is often associated with heavy smoking
- Chest physiotherapy is recommended together with deep-breathing exercises (postoperative respiratory complications are commoner in the smoker).

INVESTIGATIONS
See Table 3.9.

TABLE 3.9	
Preoperative investigations in smokers	
Investigation	Result
Full blood count	Increased red cell mass
	Increased haematocrit
	Raised white cell count
ECG	Ischaemic heart disease
Chest radiography	Chronic airway limitation
	Malignancy
Arterial blood gases	Hypoxaemia
Lung function tests	Decreased FEV_1
	Diminished FVC
	Decreased PEFR

PREMEDICATION

Withdrawal syndrome from smoking is a potential hazard. This may manifest itself as irritability, headache, nausea, sleep disturbance and anxiety. However, there can be no case for continuation of smoking up to the time of surgery.

Consider an anxiolytic, bronchodilator, anticholinergic agent, anticoagulant and antibiotics. Avoid histamine-releasing drugs.

PERIOPERATIVE MANAGEMENT

- Preoxygenation and increased inspired oxygen concentration throughout the operation.
- The combined effects of carbon monoxide and nicotine on the cardiovascular system result in less oxygen being available when more is demanded (NB: ischaemic heart disease and/or acute blood loss perioperatively).
- Altered drug handling due to liver enzyme induction (e.g. opiates, lidocaine (lignocaine), propranolol, theophylline, warfarin); dosage and frequency of drugs administered may need to be increased because of accelerated metabolism
- Antacids and H_2 blockers are less effective in smokers.

REGIONAL ANAESTHESIA
Ideal for the prevention of coughing and to encourage deep breathing after operation.

AIRWAY
Intubation may show an exaggerated pressor response in the presence of nicotine, but a tracheal tube allows bronchial toilet to be performed. Lidocaine (lignocaine) spray to the glottis and carina reduces coughing.

Mechanical ventilation may be preferred to avoid deep anaesthesia in the spontaneously breathing patient and to prevent coughing.

MONITORING:
- ECG
- Non-invasive blood pressure
- $EtCO_2$
- SaO_2 (an overestimation of saturation by pulse oximetry of the order of several per cent is possible because of the effect of carbon monoxide).

POSTOPERATIVE MANAGEMENT

- Stop smoking – the benefits from giving up smoking are both immediate and long term (Table 3.10)
- Physiotherapy
- Humidified oxygen by mask for up to 24 h
- Analgesic requirements may be increased because of liver enzyme induction and anxiety through not smoking.

OUTCOME

In 1944, Morton reported a sixfold increase in the incidence of postoperative respiratory morbidity in smokers over non-smokers. These findings have been confirmed in several other studies more recently. Every opportunity should be taken to discourage smoking in the perioperative period.

TABLE 3.10		
Benefits of stopping smoking in the perioperative period		
Time before operation	Benefit	
2 h	Nicotine blood levels fall	
12 h	Carbon monoxide blood levels fall	
Days	Sputum volume reduced; haematocrit falls	
Weeks	Ciliary activity restored towards normal; epithelial permeability returns towards normal	
Months	Immune system recovery; drug metabolism restored towards normal	

3

BIBLIOGRAPHY

Chodoff P, Margand PMS, Knowles CL. Short term
abstinence from smoking: its place in preoperative
preparation. Critical Care Medicine 1975; 3:131–133

Egan TD, Wong KC. Perioperative smoking cessation
and anesthesia: a review. Journal of Clinical
Anesthesia 1992; 4:63–72

Forrest JB, Rehder K, Cahalan MK, Goldsmith CH.
Multicentre study of general anaesthesia. III.
Predictors of severe perioperative adverse outcomes.
Anesthesiology 1992; 76:3–15

Pearce AC, Jones RM. Smoking and anaesthesia:
preoperative abstinence and peroperative morbidity.
Anesthesiology 1984; 61:576–584

CROSS-REFERENCES

COPD and anaesthesia
    Patient Conditions 3: 95

3

4

CARDIOVASCULAR SYSTEM
B. J. Pollard and C. Morgan

General considerations

B. J. Pollard and C. Morgan

Goldman et al, in a classical work of 1977, identified nine risk factors associated with life-threatening or fatal postoperative cardiac complications (Box 4.1). Important valvular aortic stenosis was the only valve lesion found to be a significant risk factor. Mitral valve disease in itself was not an independent risk factor. However, advanced mitral valve disease is invariably associated with some of the identified risk factors. Not infrequently, a third heart sound or a raised jugular venous pressure is present in patients with mitral valve disease. Surprisingly variables such as smoking, diabetes mellitus, hypertension, stable angina and cardiomegaly were not found to be significant risk factors. Of the nine risk factors, four are potentially treatable or controllable. Heart failure can be treated, the patient who has had a recent infarct can have his or her operation delayed, abnormal rhythms can be treated and the general medical condition of a patient can be improved.

BOX 4.1

Cardiac complications – risk factors

- Signs of heart failure
- Recent myocardial infarction
- Atrial arrhythmia
- Premature ventricular contractions
- Major surgery planned
- Age > 70 years
- Aortic stenosis
- Emergency
- Poor general condition

More recently, Jackson et al (1990) reviewed risk factors in valvular heart disease (VHD) and came to broadly the same conclusions as Goldman et al. They noted that there is a correlation between the severity of the patient's preoperative symptoms and the perioperative risk of cardiac morbidity and mortality. Thus, in VHD an accurate assessment of risk can be made without resorting to expensive invasive and non-invasive investigations.

While, in general, the severity of symptoms in patients with VHD helps to quantify the underlying inotropic state of the myocardium, heart failure may imply an imbalance between the inotropic state of the myocardium and the pressure and volume loads on the heart. An example of this is seen in pregnancy in a patient who, with previously well compensated mitral stenosis, presents in heart failure. A second example may be seen in a patient with an acute septic condition, such as cholecystitis, who develops heart failure.

One in five patients with VHD will show new or increased heart failure following surgery.

PATHOPHYSIOLOGY

Valvular heart disease causes either abnormal volume or abnormal pressure loads on the heart.

Pressure loads (e.g. aortic stenosis) cause concentric hypertrophy of the myocardium with a greatly increased ventricular wall thickness. While there is a considerable increase in the myocardial muscle mass, the overall size of the heart is not increased. This type of hypertrophy imposes an increased demand on the systolic function of the heart.

In contrast, volume loads cause an eccentric hypertrophy when the heart becomes grossly dilated (e.g. aortic regurgitation, mitral regurgitation). During diastole an increased volume of blood flows through the regurgitant valves. This imposes an increased demand on diastolic function.

Both the systolic and diastolic functions of the myocardium consume energy. In all varieties of VHD there are increased energy demands. Therefore, patients with ischaemic heart disease and VHD are more prone to cardiac decompensation.

4

ANAESTHETIC MANAGEMENT

PREMEDICATION

In all patients with VHD one should avoid heavy premedication. This will ensure that the balance between preload and afterload is maintained and that myocardial function is not depressed. Premedication that causes undue respiratory depression may precipitate respiratory failure or, in susceptible patients, aggravate pulmonary hypertension.

Temazepam (10 mg orally) or morphine (5–10 mg) combined with hyoscine (0.2–0.3 mg intramuscularly) will be effective and safe in most adults.

ANAESTHESIA

A full range of resuscitation drugs including both vasopressors and vasodilators should be readily available.

Appropriate monitoring is essential in every case. In general, this should be at a higher level than in patients without VHD, and in major cases may include invasive systemic arterial pressure monitoring, central venous pressure (CVP) monitoring, and pulmonary artery and wedge pressure monitoring.

Agents that depress the myocardium should be avoided. Of all the commonly used intra-venous induction agents, etomidate is least likely to depress the myocardium.

CONCLUSION

Safe anaesthesia depends on an understanding of:
- The abnormal volume and pressure loads caused by abnormal valves
- The secondary effects, both on the heart and other organs, particularly the lungs
- The compensatory mechanisms adopted by the heart.

If risk factors are present that can be treated, anaesthesia and surgery should be delayed unless the indications for surgery are life threatening.

BIBLIOGRAPHY

Braunwald E. Valvular heart disease. In: Braunwald E, ed. Heart disease. Philadelphia: WB Saunders; 1988

Goldman L, Caldera DL, Nussbaum SR et al. Multifactorial index of cardiac risk in non-cardiac surgical procedures. N Engl J Med 1977; 297:845

Jackson JM, Klein PS, Thomas SJ. Preoperative assessment of the patient with valvular heart disease. In: Mangano DT, ed. Preoperative cardiac assessment. Philadelphia: JB Lippincott; 1990:57–83

4

Adult congenital heart disease

B. Keogh

This section considers some of the troublesome adult congenital heart disease (CHD) conditions that may present for non-cardiac anaesthesia. General principles, as discussed in the previous section, are clearly relevant to the management of these individual conditions.

EBSTEIN'S ANOMALY

This is the most common form of congenital tricuspid regurgitation, representing 0.5% of congenital heart disease. Clinical relevance includes potential for profound hypoxia but also late presentation in adult life. Such patients may present undiagnosed for surgical procedures.

ANATOMY
The tricuspid valve is displaced downwards into the right ventricle and the effective right ventricular chamber is small. The degree of tricuspid regurgitation is variable, as is the often associated tricuspid stenosis. Most patients have an atrial septal defect with potential for a right-to-left shunt.

CLINICAL SPECTRUM
Patients may be essentially asymptomatic or severely cyanosed. Many present late in life with dyspnoea, fatigue, palpitations and cyanosis. Some are unrecognised and diagnosed at autopsy.

PATHOPHYSIOLOGY
Tricuspid regurgitation and variable degree of tricuspid stenosis result in reduced cardiac output. Dilatation of the right atrium predisposes to a wide variety of arrhythmias. Recurrent cyanotic attacks suggest paroxysmal tachycardia.

ANAESTHETIC IMPLICATIONS
The limited cardiac output may be difficult to manipulate due to diminished right ventricle capacity. Tachyarrhythmias are common and badly tolerated due to decrease in diastolic filling time. Right ventricular function may be poor; if inotropic support is required, consider phosphodiesterase inhibitors, but excess chronotropy with any inotropes may be counterproductive. Consider pulmonary vasodilators (nitric oxide, prostacyclin), but effects are limited and unpredictable.

Assessment of preload is difficult. Such patients require an adequate preload, but CVP is misleading. Pulmonary artery catheters are useful only for assessing flow (pulmonary arterial and left atrial pressures should be low) and their use is not advised because of arrhythmia potential and exacerbation of tricuspid valve dysfunction. Volume titration with fluid challenges is used to establish adequate preload, and can be facilitated by non-invasive cardiac output assessment techniques.

Aim for cardiovascular stability; for example, etomidate, fentanyl or alfentanil and vecuronium are suitable. Patients with Ebstein's anomaly also tolerate bradycardia badly, so with deep anaesthesia there may be a need for rate support, either with intermittent low doses of atropine or very low-dose isoprenaline (less than $0.01\ \mu g\ kg^{-1}\ min^{-1}$).

EISENMENGER'S SYNDROME

This rare condition, characterised by pulmonary hypertension and a significant intracardiac right-to-left shunt, has substantial and grave implications for the anaesthetist. Its incidence is decreasing with improved neonatal and paediatric intervention, but such patients continue to present for general procedures.

ANATOMY
Eisenmenger's syndrome is a functional rather than purely anatomical diagnosis, occurring after the unprotected pulmonary circulation is exposed to high blood flow. Pulmonary hypertension develops and results in either a reversal of shunt to right-to-left, or a decrease in pulmonary blood flow and increasing cyanosis.

Common associations include untreated ventricular septal defect (VSD) and complex anomalies, but it can even occur with large atrial septal defect (ASD) and even patent ductus arteriosus, and particularly a combination of both.

PATHOPHYSIOLOGY

Patients with Eisenmenger's syndrome who previously had left-to-right shunts become cyanotic as the pulmonary vascular resistance (PVR) increases and a bidirectional shunt occurs through intracardiac connections. Changes in PVR and systemic vascular resistance (SVR) can then influence the relative degree of each directional shunt, but in reality PVR in these patients is essentially fixed. The most common event witnessed clinically is an increase in cyanosis associated with a decrease in SVR.

ANAESTHETIC IMPLICATIONS

These patients represent a very high-risk group. They may present at any stage, including in cardiac decompensation. The fundamental principle of management is maintaining the balance of PVR and SVR. As PVR is essentially fixed, agents that avoid systemic vasodilatation are preferable, and vasoconstrictor infusions are commonly necessary. Recent epidemiological data suggest that enhanced understanding of, and aggressive manipulation of, the pathophysiology of the syndrome has resulted in improved outcome; referral of these patients to specialist centres is recommended.

INDUCTION

Aim for cardiovascular stability; for example, etomidate, vecuronium and narcotics are suitable. Ketamine has been used in such patients, even though there is a potential risk of increased PVR. In practice, the benefits of SVR maintenance may outweigh any small increase in PVR. It is advisable to have vasoconstrictors available at induction, and many cardiac anaesthetists prefer to induce such patients on a background of low-dose noradrenaline (norepinephrine) (0.01–0.03 $\mu g\ kg^{-1}\ min^{-1}$).

MAINTENANCE

Both inhalational and intravenous techniques are applicable and vasoconstrictor infusions, such as noradrenaline (norepinephrine) 0.01–0.1 $\mu g\ kg^{-1}\ min^{-1}$, should be used to counteract SVR fall. Controlled ventilation is virtually mandatory with high FiO_2 and hyperventilation to $PaCO_2$ 3.5–4.0 kPa. Pulmonary vasodilators tend not to be effective but nebulised prostacyclin or nitric oxide is often applied speculatively. Intravenous prostacyclin may increase cyanosis due to predominant effects on SVR.

MONITORING

SpO_2 monitoring is mandatory, as is an arterial line, inserted under local anaesthesia before induction, for any but the shortest procedures. Central venous access for vasoactive drugs and volume titration is recommended. A pulmonary artery catheter may be impossible to insert and, depending on the anatomy, may provide little useful information. Even if correctly sited, such catheters are notoriously difficult to wedge in severe pulmonary hypertension. Non-invasive cardiac output monitoring should ideally be employed. $EtCO_2$ monitoring, although an inaccurate indicator of $PaCO_2$ due to increased physiological deadspace, reflects trends in effective pulmonary blood flow and, with unchanged ventilatory settings, will decrease when right-to-left shunting occurs.

EISENMENGER'S SYNDROME IN OBSTETRICS

This is an extremely difficult area when fetal requirements are added to the equation. Discussions relating to the advisability of allowing labour as opposed to caesarean section are ongoing in the literature. Success has been reported with both general and epidural anaesthesia for caesarean section, and there are proponents of both approaches. The maternal mortality rate unfortunately remains high and, despite best practice with either technique, remains in the region of 40%. Such patients are at risk of severe exacerbation of pulmonary hypertension in the postnatal period; this may occur late (up to 7–10 days after the birth) and is of uncertain aetiology.

SPECIFIC TREATED CONDITIONS

It is impossible to consider all the possibilities that may be encountered. However, several conditions will be encountered regularly and deserve consideration.

SURGICAL PROCEDURES FOR TRANSPOSITION OF THE GREAT ARTERIES

The therapy of choice is complete correction in the neonatal period with transection and appropriate reconnection of the great arteries (arterial switch). Such patients should, with a good surgical result, have normal life expectancy. Outflow tract obstruction may occur and should be assessed by preoperative echocardiography.

The Mustard procedure – an intra-atrial baffle to redirect systemic and pulmonary venous return at atrial level – is undertaken if patients present late or the anatomy is unsuitable for switch. These patients have a morphologically right systemic ventricle, are prone to obstruction of either venous return and to arrhythmias, have a shortened lifespan and may present in cardiac failure. The morphological right ventricle is likely to require inotropic support.

PROCEDURES FOR TRICUSPID ATRESIA OR UNIVENTRICULAR HEART

The ideal is to separate the systemic and pulmonary blood flow. This is achieved by the Fontan operation or total cavopulmonary connection (TCPC) operation, where the systemic venous return is connected directly to the pulmonary arteries without a pumping ventricle. An increasing number of such patients will be encountered in the community. The Glenn procedure, anastomosis of the superior vena cava to the pulmonary artery, may be an early stage of this approach. Pulmonary blood flow in both situations is passive and requires adequate preload. CVP measurement is mandatory in all but the simplest procedures, remembering that this represents pulmonary artery pressure. An ideal level of CVP (mean pulmonary artery pressure in this context) is 18 mmHg, although a lower level is acceptable if systemic output is maintained. Higher levels lead to systemic venous congestion with ascites and pleural effusions, but may be necessary in the short term. Patients with the Glenn procedure, and those with TCPC in whom a small fenestration into the systemic atrium is left in order to allow decompression of excess pulmonary artery pressures if PVR rises, are cyanosed, although patients with a complete TCPC are not. Both groups have limited cardiac output and tolerate tachyarrhythmias poorly. Manipulation of the circulation involves adequate preload and pulmonary vasodilatation. Inotropes tend to be ineffective and their effect on the under-filled, hypertrophied systemic ventricle may be adverse. If inotropes are required, the phosphodiesterase inhibitors with their positive lusitropic effects are probably those of choice. Such patients are physiologically at an advantage with spontaneous respiration, but if intermittent positive-pressure ventilation (IPPV) is

necessary it should be performed with low intrathoracic pressures.

Because of the particular anatomy, such patients are greatly advantaged by the maintenance of sinus rhythm. This may be because the right atrium is incorporated as a pumping chamber in the pulmonary circuit. If the right atrium is not in circuit, sinus rhythm is still favourable for systemic cardiac function and decreasing systemic atrial pressure (hence enhancing the hydrostatic gradient for pulmonary blood flow). Loss of sinus rhythm under anaesthesia should be treated with cardioversion. If the rhythm proves refractory, consider amiodarone (loading dose is 5 mg kg^{-1} over at least 20 min followed by an infusion of approximately 10 mg kg^{-1} day^{-1}). If more rapid injection is required, beware the substantial negative inotropic effects.

BIBLIOGRAPHY

Ammash NM, Connolly HM, Abel MD, Warnes CA. Noncardiac surgery in Eisenmenger's syndrome. Journal of the American College of Cardiology 1999; 33:222–227

Cohen AM, Mulvein J. Obstetric anaesthetic management in a patient with the Fontan circulation. British Journal of Anaesthesia 1994; 73:252–255

Lowe DA, Stayer SA. Abnormalities of the atrioventricular valves. In: Lake CL, ed. Paediatric cardiac anaesthesia. 2nd edn. Norwalk: Appleton & Lange; 1993:325–346

Martin JT, Tautz TJ, Antognini JF. Safety of regional anesthesia in Eisenmenger's syndrome. Regional Anesthesia and Pain Medicine 2002; 27:509–513

Yentis SM, Steer PJ, Plaat F. Eisenmenger's syndrome in pregnancy: maternal and fetal mortality in the 1990s. British Journal of Obstetrics and Gynaecology 1998; 105:921–922

CROSS-REFERENCES

Cardiac conduction defects
    Patient Conditions 4: 120
Pulmonary hypertension
    Patient Conditions 4: 138

Aortic valve disease

M. Scallan

AORTIC STENOSIS

PATHOPHYSIOLOGY
Systolic function is affected by the increase in pressure load and leads to hypertrophy of the left ventricle. With progression of the disease, the ventricle becomes stiff and diastolic function is impaired. There is a decrease in diastolic compliance.

CLINICAL FEATURES
Patients with aortic stenosis may remain asymptomatic for 30 or 40 years. However, when symptoms develop there is a rapid deterioration over the next 1–2 years.

The symptoms of aortic stenosis are angina (Box 4.2), syncope and heart failure. Heart failure is a late symptom in this disease. Any of these symptoms are contraindications for non-cardiac surgery unless the indications for surgery are life-threatening.

ANAESTHESIA
It is essential that the balance between preload and afterload is maintained. A decrease in the preload may impair filling of the poorly compliant left ventricle. Monitoring by pulmonary artery catheter and/or transoesophageal echocardiography will assist in the maintenance of this balance.

If the systemic diastolic pressure is allowed to fall, coronary perfusion will be impaired. For this reason an α-agonist should be available in the event of a fall in the diastolic pressure. Both metaraminol and phenylephrine, which must be given cautiously, are effective in this situation.

Because of the risk of myocardial ischaemia, glyceryl trinitrate should be available. However, it should be used with caution because it may decrease the diastolic pressure and adversely affect myocardial oxygen supply.

As a result of the poor compliance of the left ventricle, atrial contraction contributes 40% of left ventricular filling. The normal contribution is 20%. For this reason the anaesthetist should avoid agents that may cause arrhythmias. If arrhythmias arise they should be treated. Cardioversion by DC shock may be necessary.

Tachycardias should be avoided because they will aggravate myocardial ischaemia. In addition, the shorter diastole seen in tachycardias will decrease the filling of the stiff left ventricle.

> **BOX 4.2**
>
> Causes of angina in aortic stenosis
>
> - A greatly increased muscle mass of the left ventricular wall has an increased basic oxygen requirement.
> - To overcome the obstruction caused by the aortic valve, the wall tension of the left ventricle is increased.
> - Systolic emptying is prolonged. This shortens the diastolic time and, therefore, the time available for coronary artery blood flow. It is during diastole that most coronary blood flow takes place.
> - Owing to the poor ventricular compliance, the left ventricular end-diastolic pressure is increased. This impairs coronary blood flow through the subendocardial region of the myocardium.
> - There is an increased incidence of coronary artery disease in patients with aortic stenosis.
> - A jet of blood passing through the stenotic aortic valve may cause a Venturi effect in the proximal aorta. As this is where the coronary arteries are sited, this may impair coronary blood flow during systole.

AORTIC REGURGITATION

PATHOPHYSIOLOGY:
- There is both systolic and diastolic volume overload of the left ventricle.

- There is eccentric enlargement of the left ventricle with an increase in size of the left ventricular cavity and some thickening of the wall.
- Left ventricular stroke volume is increased and cardiac output is well maintained in the early years of the disease. Peripheral vasodilatation is common and this aids cardiac output.
- Although the left ventricular end-diastolic volume is increased, in the early phase of the disease the left ventricular end-diastolic pressure remains normal.
- In the latter phase of the disease when cardiac decompensation is near, the left ventricular end-diastolic pressure is increased, the cardiac output falls and an increase in the peripheral vascular resistance is seen.
- Due to stretching of the mitral valve orifice by the dilated left ventricle, mitral regurgitation may arise.

CLINICAL FEATURES

Patients with aortic regurgitation may remain asymptomatic for 20 years. Symptoms are not usually seen until the regurgitant fraction is greater than 40%. Dyspnoea and tiredness are the usual presenting features.

Unlike aortic stenosis, angina is not a feature of aortic regurgitation. This is in spite of the low systemic diastolic pressure. Relatively little energy is required for the fibre shortening of the volume-overloaded ventricle. This is in contrast to the considerable energy required for pressure generation in aortic stenosis.

Tachycardia may develop as a late sign. The short diastole associated with tachycardia will decrease the regurgitation.

ANAESTHESIA

Vasodilators should be used with caution because they may decrease the diastolic pressure. However, if the SVR is raised, regurgitation would be aggravated. In this situation, afterload reduction would be of benefit. Thus a balance must be maintained. Monitoring by pulmonary artery catheter and/or transoesophageal echocardiography will assist in the maintenance of this balance. Bradycardia increases regurgitation. A heart rate between 80 and 100 beats per min is beneficial.

BIBLIOGRAPHY

Grayboys TB, Cohn PF. The prevalence of angina pectoris and abnormal coronary arteriograms in severe aortic valvular disease. American Heart Journal 1977; 93:683

Rappaport E. Natural history of aortic and mitral valve disease. American Journal of Cardiology 1975; 35:221

CROSS-REFERENCES

4

Atrial septal defect

M. Barnard

EMBRYOLOGY

The atrial septum is derived from the septum primum and the septum secundum. The septum primum develops initially and joins the endocardial cushions inferiorly. The ostium primum is formed by its lower free edge. Perforations form superiorly in the septum and coalesce to form the ostium secundum. The septum secundum then arises from an infolding of the right atrial wall following its incorporation of the left sinus horn. The septum secundum forms the valve of the foramen ovale by covering the ostium secundum. Persistence of the ostium primum is due to faulty fusion of the anterior and posterior endocardial cushions, and is often associated with a cleft in the anterior leaflet of the mitral valve. An unusually large ostium secundum or failure of the septum secundum to approximate with the septum primum results in a secundum defect. A sinus venosus defect results from abnormal fusion of the sinus horn (the primitive venous collecting chamber) with the right atrium.

ANATOMICAL TYPES (BOX 4.3)

Ostium primum forms of ASD occur early and may be associated with defects of the heart valves.

Defects of the septum secundum can be classified into:

- Patent foramen ovale
- Ostium secundum
- Sinus venosus.

PATHOPHYSIOLOGY

The degree of shunting of blood across an ASD is related to the relative compliance of the two ventricles and the cross-sectional area of the defect. In the neonate right- and left-sided cardiac pressures are approximately equal, and

---

BOX 4.3

Atrial septal defects

Ostium primum

Usually large and leads to early manifestation of symptoms. The atrial septum may be entirely absent, which results in a single atrial chamber. This lesion is associated with endocardial cushion defects and is a type of partial atrioventricular canal defect.

Patent foramen ovale

Frequently other cardiac defects; 40% of patients with a ventricular septal defect have an associated patent foramen ovale.

Ostium secundum

Accounts for 80% of all atrial defects. Comprises an opening in the atrial wall (which may be fenestrated) due to resorption of the septum primum, defective septum secundum development, or a short septum primum that fails to close the foramen ovale.

Sinus venosus

The defect is rare; it occurs high in the septal wall above the fossa ovalis close to the junction of the right atrium with the superior vena cava. Commonly associated with anomalous pulmonary venous drainage.

---

little or no shunting occurs. As PVR falls, left-to-right shunting develops. Symptoms are related to the ratio of the pulmonary to systemic flow (Qp/Qs). A ratio of less than 1.5 is well tolerated with minimal symptoms, whereas a ratio greater than 3 results in fatigue, dyspnoea and heart failure. An increase in pulmonary blood flow leads to increased pulmonary artery pressures and PVR. This, in turn, results in right ventricular hypertrophy and further increased in pulmonary artery pressures. Eventually the ventricular pressures may equalise, which produces bidirectional shunting across the defect. Uncommonly in severe cases the raised PVR can cause right-to-left shunting. This manifests as cyanosis, and is a type of Eisenmenger syndrome. Surgery will halt the progression to cyanotic disease, but if it is delayed until PVR is fixed and irreversible, closure can precipitate acute right heart failure.

NATURAL HISTORY

ASDs do not often close spontaneously.

Small, haemodynamically insignificant defects have no effect on lifespan, although there is a small increase in infective endocarditis and paradoxical embolism.

Moderate defects are usually well tolerated into adulthood, when left-to-right shunt and right ventricular volume overload may manifest in the third or fourth decade.

- 14% of adults with large ASDs manifest signs of congestive heart failure
- 20% exhibit dyshrythmias.

Large defects cause pulmonary vascular disease and decrease life expectancy.

Operative closure of ASDs prevents late complications and increases life expectancy. Closure is preferably carried out at 4–5 years of age. Patients who have defects repaired after 40 years of age have decreased survival compared with controls.

DIAGNOSIS AND PREOPERATIVE EVALUATION

Uncomplicated defects are asymptomatic and are detected by auscultation of pulmonary flow murmurs and echocardiography (Box 4.4). Significant defects are associated with frequent respiratory infections in children and fatigue

---

BOX 4.4

Investigations used for evaluation

- ECG – right ventricular hypertrophy and incomplete right bundle branch block
- Chest radiography – increased peripheral vascularity and heart size
- Transthoracic echocardiography – detects primum and secundum defects with 89% sensitivity
- Transoesophageal echocardiography – necessary for identification of sinus venosus defects

---

and dyspnoea in adults. Patients with large defects present in early infancy with symptoms of increased pulmonary flow and heart failure, whereas smaller defects may remain undetected until adulthood. Examination reveals a pulmonary systolic murmur and fixed splitting of the second heart sound. There may be a tricuspid flow murmur.

Cardiac catheterisation is not necessary for the preoperative evaluation of ASD repair and is rarely carried out before other surgery. If it has been performed, an increase in oxygen saturation will be apparent at the atrial level. There may be a small systolic gradient in the right ventricular outflow tract due to increased blood flow.

ASD AND EISENMENGER'S SYNDROME

Patients with right-to-left shunts will appear cyanosed and have finger clubbing. Auscultation reveals an increased pulmonic component to the second heart sound. Pulmonary regurgitation, if present, will cause a decrescendo diastolic murmur. Chest radiography shows right ventricular hypertrophy, prominent pulmonary arteries and increased lung markings. Cardiac catheterisation will confirm increased right ventricular and pulmonary artery pressures.

ANAESTHETIC TECHNIQUE

Choice of premedication assumes importance only in patients with significant heart failure, low cardiac output and right-to-left shunting. In these patients caution with sedatives is necessary as profound decompensation may occur with small doses.

The alveolar concentration of moderately soluble agents (e.g. halothane) increases more rapidly in patients with left-to-right shunts during induction. Insoluble agents, such as nitrous oxide, are little influenced by the shunt.

Intravenous induction is relatively slower due to the additional dilution by recirculating blood. An increased dose of induction agent may be necessary, with attention paid to the risks of overdosage. However, these theoretical concerns on the rate of induction are of relatively minor clinical importance compared with the nature of premedication and the adequacy of alveolar ventilation. Standard hypnotic agents (thiopental, propofol) are used for intravenous induction. Opioids, such as fentanyl, are preferred for patients with advanced disease. Inhalational agents are usually used for maintenance of anaesthesia. Children may be satisfactorily induced with halothane inhalation. Potent inhalational agents depress cardiac output and decrease systemic vascular resistance, and could potentially reverse a left-to-right shunt. However, this is unusual in the absence of marked pulmonary hypertension, when intravenous agents may be preferable.

The monitoring required does not differ from that appropriate for patients without ASDs. Invasive monitoring is indicated for repair of the defect itself.

COMPLICATIONS

There is a constant hazard of air or particulate matter in all patients with ASDs, including those with left-to-right shunting. Intravenous tubing and connectors must be checked rigorously for the presence of air. Bubbles tend to adhere to sites where there are changes in the diameter of the lumen of the tubing. Small bubbles can come out of solution over time and coalesce, making rechecking of apparatus important.

The prevention of infective endocarditis is guided by local microbiological protocols, which take into account differences in bacterial prevalence and sensitivities. Isolated secundum defects are considered low risk, and many authorities do not consider that antibiotic prophylaxis is necessary. The risk of endocarditis is related to the velocity of blood flow, impact on cardiac structures, shear rate and likelihood of bacteraemia. Nasotracheal intubation is significantly more likely than orotracheal intubation to cause bacteraemia. A typical antibiotic prophylaxis regimen is outlined in Box 4.5.

BOX 4.5

Typical antibiotic prophylaxis regimen

Low-risk procedure

- Amoxicillin 3 g orally 1 h before procedure plus amoxicillin 3 g orally 6 h after surgery, *or*
- Amoxicillin 1 g i.v. at induction plus 500 mg orally at 6 h
- *Penicillin allergic*: clindamycin 600 mg orally 1 h before procedure

High-risk procedure

- Amoxicillin 1 g i.v. at induction plus gentamicin 120 mg i.v. plus amoxicillin 500 mg orally 6 h after surgery
- *Penicillin allergic*: vancomycin 1 g i.v. 2 h before procedure plus gentamicin 120 mg i.v. at induction

BIBLIOGRAPHY

Baum VC, Perloff JK. Anaesthetic implications of adults with congenital heart disease. Anesthesia and Analgesia 1993; 76: 1342–58

Lake CL, ed. Pediatric cardiac anesthesia. 2nd edn. Norwalk: Appleton & Lange; 1993

Konstantinedes S, Geibel A, Olschewski M et al. A comparison of surgical and medical therapy for atrial septal defect in adults. New England Journal of Medicine 1995; 333:469–473

CROSS-REFERENCES

Adult congenital heart disease
    Patient Conditions 4: 112
Pulmonary hypertension
    Patient Conditions 4: 138

4

Cardiac conduction defects

B. J. Pollard

WOLFF–PARKINSON–WHITE SYNDROME

PATHOPHYSIOLOGY

Wolff–Parkinson–White (WPW) syndrome is one of the pre-excitation syndromes in which activation of accessory atrioventricular conduction pathways leads to early and rapid ventricular contractions. The ECG typically shows a short P-R interval (< 0.12 s), a wide QRS (> 0.12 s) and a delta wave. The dysrhythmia commonly associated with WPW syndrome is paroxysmal supraventricular tachycardia.

PERIOPERATIVE MANAGEMENT

The patient's antidysrhythmic drugs should be continued. Monitoring should consist of at least continuous ECG and pulse oximetry. A defibrillator should be in the room and the ECG leads connected to the patient. During operation the goals are to avoid increases in heart rate and in sympathetic nervous system activation. Therefore, vagolytic drugs should be avoided, and adequate depth of anaesthesia needs to be obtained prior to laryngoscopy and during surgical stimulation.

TREATMENT OF SUPRAVENTRICULAR TACHYCARDIA DUE TO PRE-EXCITATION SYNDROMES

Avoid digoxin and calcium channel blockers, as in the acute setting these drugs may decrease the refractory period of the accessory pathways and, paradoxically, increase the ventricular response rate.

- If haemodynamically unstable, synchronous cardioversion with 25, 50, 100 J
- If haemodynamically stable:
  —Adenosine (6 mg followed by 12 mg i.v. push), which may convert the rhythm to sinus, *or*
  —Esmolol (250–500 μg kg^{-1} followed by an infusion of 50–300 μg kg^{-1} min^{-1}), *or*
  —Propranolol (0.025 mg kg^{-1}) to control rate, *then*

—Procainamide (10 mg kg^{-1} load followed by 1–4 mg min^{-1}) to convert the rhythm to sinus.

PROLONGED QT INTERVAL

CONGENITAL LONG QT INTERVAL SYNDROME

Pathophysiology

There are four types of congenital long QT interval syndrome that are all characterised by a QT interval greater than 0.44 s. The congenital prolonged QT syndromes may or may not be associated with congenital neural deafness, epilepsy or a family history of sudden death. This syndrome is an important cause of sudden death in the young patient and has a mortality rate of up to 73% in untreated patients. The basic abnormality is still not fully understood, but the most accepted theory is that the syndrome results from an asymmetrical adrenergic stimulus to the heart. The result of this alteration in sympathetic tone is to delay repolarisation of the ventricles (producing the prolonged QT interval) which then increases the susceptibility of the heart to dysrhythmias, most commonly ventricular tachycardia and fibrillation.

Treatment

Because of the high mortality rate, treatment is essential. Beta-blockers shorten the QT interval in patients with congenital long QT syndrome (beta-blockers prolong the QT interval in normal patients) and decrease the mortality rate from 73% to 6%. Other drugs that may have a role include phenytoin, phenobarbital, primidone, digoxin, verapamil and bretylium. Other treatment options include left stellate ganglion block, surgical ganglionectomy or sympathectomy if medical therapy has failed.

Preoperative management

The main anaesthetic goal in the management of congenital long QT syndrome is to avoid excessive sympathetic nervous system discharge during the entire preoperative, intraoperative and postoperative period. Patients who respond to beta-blockade alone appear to have a low risk of developing malignant dysrhythmias. Patients who require more than beta-blockers or who are unresponsive to beta-blockade are at high risk of life-threatening dysrhythmias during operation. These patients may benefit from preoperative left stellate ganglion blockade.

Premedication with a hypnotic agent on the night before surgery, and a narcotic and benzodiazepine on the morning of surgery, are recommended. Antiarrhythmic drugs, a defibrillator, transcutaneous pacing device and temporary transvenous pacemaker should be immediately available in the operating room. There appears to be no difference between general and regional anaesthesia with respect to the development of arrhythmias. If local anaesthesia is used, adrenaline (epinephrine) should be avoided.

Perioperative management
- *Induction*:
  —Avoid ketamine.
- *Intubation*:
  —The patient must be deeply anaesthetised.
- *Muscle relaxants*:
  —Avoid pancuronium
  —Succinylcholine can be used with caution
  —Vecuronium probably safest.
- *Reversal of relaxants*: neostigmine plus atropine or glycopyrolate do not affect the QT interval.
- *Maintenance*:
  —Avoid halothane
  —Narcotics, nitrous oxide and isoflurane are safe.
- *Emergence*: Extubate deep, or prevent hypertension and tachycardia if planning to extubate awake.
- *Postoperative care*:
  —Adequate analgesia is paramount
  —Resume preoperative medications
  —24–48 h of monitoring on the ICU.

Treatment of intraoperative arrhythmias
Ventricular dysrhythmias in patients who respond to beta-blockers are usually responsive to further beta-blockade. Primidone, bretylium or verapamil may be used in those who do not respond to beta-blockade. In both groups, premature ventricular contractions usually respond to lidocaine (lignocaine). Left stellate ganglion block may also be used. Standard advanced cardiac life support protocols, with the possible exception of using adrenaline (epinephrine) last, should be followed for ventricular tachycardia or fibrillation.

ACQUIRED LONG QT INTERVAL SYNDROME
Pathophysiology
Acquired long QT interval syndrome is a separate syndrome, but is still associated with malignant dysrhythmias, especially torsade de pointes. It can be caused by:
- Cardiac disease
- Thermal and electrolyte abnormalities
- Drugs, especially antidysrhythmics
- Neurological disease
- Endocrine and metabolic disturbances.

Preoperative management
Correct the underlying cause. Remove or adjust drugs if syndrome is drug induced.

Perioperative management
Avoid hypothermia, hypocalcaemia, hypokalaemia and hypomagnesaemia. Thiopental and succinylcholine prolong the QT interval in normal patients and may increase it in patients with acquired long QT syndrome. Vagotomy and head and neck procedures can prolong the QT interval.

Treatment of intraoperative arrhythmias
Follow established advanced cardiac life support guidelines initially. If the dysrhythmia does not respond, isoprenaline (which shortens the QT interval) may be useful. Temporary use of a pacemaker has also been described.

SICK SINUS SYNDROME

This is often caused by degenerative changes in the sinoatrial node that lead to inappropriate episodes of sinus bradycardia and supraventricular tachycardia. Patients with this disorder should have had a recent evaluation by a cardiologist to address the need for a transvenous pacemaker.

FIRST-DEGREE ATRIOVENTRICULAR HEART BLOCK

This is caused by a delay in conduction through the atrioventricular node which results in a P-R interval greater than 0.2 s. This may be caused by ageing, ischaemia, myocarditis, cardiomyopathy, aortic regurgitation or any cause of increased vagal tone. This heart block is usually asymptomatic, and can easily be treated with atropine or glycopyrrolate.

SECOND-DEGREE ATRIOVENTRICULAR HEART BLOCK

Mobitz type I (Wenckebach) is caused by a delay in conduction through the atrioventricular node and is characterised by progressive prolongation of the P-R interval until there is a dropped beat. This rhythm is usually asymptomatic and requires no specific therapy.

Mobitz type II, however, is caused by a block below the atrioventricular node (usually in the His–Purkinje fibres). The ECG shows sudden block of conduction without progressive elongation of the P-R interval. Because this may suddenly progress to complete heart block, a pacemaker is usually placed, even in patients without symptoms.

RIGHT BUNDLE BRANCH BLOCK

Right bundle branch block (RBBB), characterised by a QRS of more than 0.1 s and RSR complexes in V_1–V_3, is found in 1% of all hospitalised adults and does not always imply serious cardiac disease. The right bundle branch is usually supplied by a small septal branch of the left anterior descending branch (LAD) of the left coronary artery. There are no special anaesthetic concerns for patients with RBBB.

LEFT BUNDLE BRANCH BLOCK

The left bundle branch is made up by the smaller anterior fascicle with blood supply from the septal branches of the LAD and the larger posterior fascicle, which usually has a dual blood supply from the LAD and the right coronary artery.

Left anterior hemiblock is block of the anterior fascicle which shows left-axis deviation of more than – 60° with minimal prolongation of the QRS complex. Left posterior hemiblock is a block of the posterior fascicle which on the ECG shows right-axis deviation greater than 120° with minimal prolongation of the QRS complex. The hemiblocks are associated with coronary artery disease, so patients should have a thorough preoperative evaluation.

Complete left bundle branch block (LBBB) shows a QRS of more than 0.12 s, with notched R waves in all leads. Incomplete LBBB shows a similar pattern of wide R waves in all leads, but the QRS complex is 0.10–0.12 s. These two blocks are also associated with coronary artery disease.

Because placement of pulmonary artery catheters can cause RBBB, especially in patients with known coronary artery disease, this can lead to complete heart block in patients with prior hemiblocks or LBBB. Thus it is reasonable to have a transcutaneous pacemaker attached to the patient before placement of the pulmonary artery catheter, or to use a pacing pulmonary artery catheter.

BIFASCICULAR HEART BLOCK

Bifascicular heart block is defined as a hemiblock and RBBB. This is also associated with coronary artery disease, and this block may over time progress to complete heart block. However, in the absence of symptoms there no evidence to support the placement of a prophylactic pacemaker prior to elective surgery with general or regional anaesthesia.

THIRD-DEGREE (COMPLETE OR TRIFASCICULAR) ATRIOVENTRICULAR HEART BLOCK

This is present when there is no conduction from the atria to the ventricles. If the block is above the atrioventricular node, the rate is 45–55 beats min^{-1} and the QRS complex is normal. If the block is below the atrioventricular node, the rate will be 30–40 beats min^{-1} and the QRS complex will be wide in all leads. This block should always be treated with a temporary or permanent pacemaker. Isoprenaline (1–4 μg kg^{-1} min^{-1}) may be used while the pacemaker is being placed.

ATRIOVENTRICULAR DISSOCIATION

Atrioventricular dissociation is not a diagnosis, but a symptom that is due to one of four causes:
- Slowing of the dominant pacemaker of the heart, which allows the escape of a latent pacemaker
- Acceleration of a latent pacemaker that takes over control of the ventricles
- Block that prevents normal impulse conduction and allows the ventricles to beat under the control of a secondary pacemaker

- Any combination of the above three.

The treatment and anaesthetic management of atrioventricular dissociation will depend on the underlying cause of the rhythm and can range from:

- Atropine administration to patients with sinus bradycardia with ventricular escape beats
- Lidocaine (lignocaine) administration for ventricular tachycardia
- Pacemaker insertion for patients with complete heart block.

BIBLIOGRAPHY

Galloway PA, Glass PSA. Anesthetic implications of prolonged QT interval syndromes. Anesthesia and Analgesia 1985; 64:612–620

Hurst WJ, Schlaut RC, Reekle CE et al, eds. Cardiac arrhythmias and conduction disturbances. In: The heart. 7th edn. New York: McGraw-Hill; 1990

Stoelting RK, Dierdorf SF. Abnormalities of cardiac conduction and cardiac rhythm. In: Anesthesia and co-existing disease. 4th edn. New York: Churchill Livingstone; 2002:117–126

CROSS-REFERENCES

Iatrogenic adrenocortical insufficiency
    Patient Conditions 2: 71
Assessment of renal function
    Patient Conditions 6: 186

4

Cardiomyopathy

W. Aveling

The cardiomyopathies are a group of conditions characterised by progressive failure of ventricular function not caused by ischaemic, valvular or hypertensive heart disease. A variety of conditions (e.g. viral infection, alcohol toxicity, sarcoidosis) may be the cause, but many are idiopathic.

CLASSIFICATION

Classification by morphology and haemodynamic factors helps one understand the pathophysiology (Table 4.1).

PATHOPHYSIOLOGY

DILATED CARDIOMYOPATHY

This is characterised by progressive dilatation of both ventricles leading to intractable heart failure. The ejection fraction is low (< 40%) and arrhythmias are a frequent problem. Death is either sudden, due to dysrhythmia, or a result of cardiac failure.

RESTRICTIVE AND OBLITERATIVE CARDIOMYOPATHIES

These conditions are similar with markedly decreased ventricular compliance resulting in a picture like that of constrictive pericarditis or tamponade. Decreased diastolic filling and low cardiac output lead to congestive failure, with dysrhythmias again a problem.

HYPERTROPHIC CARDIOMYOPATHY

This is frequently hereditary. Hypertrophic cardiomyopathy is very different from the other types. It is characterised by uneven myocardial hypertrophy which is usually greatest in the interventricular septum. This may cause left ventricular outflow obstruction – hypertrophic obstructive cardiomyopathy (HOCM). The obstruction can mimic aortic stenosis but can be variable, which makes it such an intriguing anaesthetic problem.

Outflow obstruction is increased by:
- Increased myocardial contractility – β stimulation, catecholamines, digoxin, tachycardia
- Decreased preload – hypovolaemia, vasodilators, tachycardia
- Decreased afterload – hypovolaemia, vasodilators, hypotension.

Outflow obstruction is decreased by:
- Decreased myocardial contractility – β blockade, calcium antagonists, volatile anaesthetic agents
- Increased preload – volume loading, bradycardia

TABLE 4.1

Classification of cardiomyopathies

	Dilated	Restrictive	Obliterative	Hypertrophic
Morphology	Biventricular dilatation	↓Ventricular compliance	Thickened endocardium	Hypertrophy: Left ventricular ± septum
Ventricular volume	↑↑	→↑	↓	→↓
Ejection fraction	↓↓	→↓	→↓	↑↑
Ventricular compliance	→↑	↓↓	↓↓	↓↓
Ventricular filling pressure	↑↑	↑↑	↑	→↑
Stroke volume	↓↓	→↓	→↓	→↑

4

- Increased afterload – volume loading, α stimulation.

PREOPERATIVE ASSESSMENT

It is important to know which kind of cardiomyopathy one is dealing with because management of HOCM is so different from the others. Specialist cardiological opinion is needed here.

PERIOPERATIVE MANAGEMENT

DILATED, RESTRICTIVE AND OBLITERATIVE CARDIOMYOPATHIES

The aim should be to avoid drug-induced myocardial depression, to maintain adequate filling pressures and to reduce afterload. Full invasive monitoring including a pulmonary artery catheter may be required. High-dose opiates (e.g. fentanyl) are the mainstay of anaesthesia; the addition of nitrous oxide will be depressant, but isoflurane can be used to decrease afterload without depression. Inotropes may be needed to improve cardiac output.

HYPERTROPHIC CARDIOMYOPATHY

In complete contrast to the above, efforts are directed at reducing outflow obstruction and avoiding factors that increase it (see Box 4.1). Premedication to reduce anxiety and sympathetic drive is valuable, and atropine should be avoided. Intravenous induction (not ketamine), followed by volatile agents producing mild cardiac depression (e.g. halothane) and filling to increase preload, will all help to reduce obstruction. If systemic pressure falls this should be treated with α agonists (e.g. phenylephrine) not inotropes or β agonists.

BIBLIOGRAPHY

Stoelting RK, Dierdorf SF. Anesthesia and co-existing disease. 4th edn. New York: Churchill Livingstone; 2002

CROSS-REFERENCES

Preoperative assessment of pulmonary risk
   Anaesthetic Factors 27: 638

4

Children with congenital heart disease – for non-cardiac surgery

B. J. Pollard

Appropriate anaesthetic management of children with congenital heart disease undergoing non-cardiac surgery requires an understanding of the pathophysiology of the child's anomalies and the changes imposed by the surgical procedure.

PATHOPHYSIOLOGY

SHUNT LESIONS

With large defects, the direction and magnitude of shunting is determined by the ratio of pulmonary and systemic vascular resistances. As defects become smaller, shunting becomes largely independent of changes in vascular resistance and is determined primarily by defect size.

Right-to-left shunts:
• Cyanosis – decreased pulmonary blood flow, mixing
• Increased cardiac work
• Decreased cardiac reserve
• Polycythaemia with increased risk of cerebral or renal thrombosis
• Increased blood volume and viscosity
• Coagulopathy with impaired platelet aggregation
• Alveolar hyperventilation
• Neovascularisation.

Left-to-right shunts:
• Pulmonary overperfusion
• Volume overload
• May progress to pulmonary hypertension and congestive heart failure
• Increased risk of pulmonary hypertensive crisis
• Decreased cardiopulmonary reserve.

OBSTRUCTIVE LESIONS:
• Fixed cardiac output
• Cardiac hypertrophy
• Potential myocardial ischaemia, especially subendocardium

• Inability to compensate for changes in vascular resistance
• Congestive heart failure
• Sudden serious arrhythmias
• Complete obstructive lesions are dependent upon patency of ductus arteriosus.

COMPLEX SHUNT LESIONS:
• Outflow obstruction(s) plus central communication(s)
• Obstruction may be fixed or dynamic
• Resistance of obstruction is additive to that of corresponding side of circulation.

PREOPERATIVE ASSESSMENT

In addition to determining the nature of the cardiac anomaly, the patient's present status must be assessed to determine the need for optimisation or referral to a specialised facility. Patients may present with unrepaired, palliated or repaired lesions. Repairs may be physiological, but not anatomical, and may be followed by residual problems (see below).

In the history and physical examination, special attention should be directed toward cyanosis, dyspnoea, symptoms and signs of congestive heart failure (see list below), as well as exercise intolerance, repeated pulmonary infections, medications, and acute or chronic concurrent problems. Investigations should be directed by the history and physical findings, and may include haematocrit, electrolytes, oximetry, electrocardiography, cardiology consultation, echocardiography, and possible cardiac catheterisation. Patient assessment also requires consideration of the physiological trespass imposed by anaesthesia and surgery.

Children undergoing major procedures, as well as those with congestive heart failure, pulmonary hypertension or complex congenital heart disease, are best managed in a specialised facility.

RESIDUAL PROBLEMS FOLLOWING CARDIAC SURGERY:

- Arrhythmias, especially atrial repairs
- Conduction disturbance
- Ventricular dysfunction
- Residual shunts
- Valvular stenosis or regurgitation
- Pulmonary hypertension, especially in Down's syndrome.

SIGNS AND SYMPTOMS OF CONGESTIVE HEART FAILURE:

- Poor feeding
- Perspiring while feeding
- Failure to thrive
- Hepatomegaly
- Tachypnoea
- Peripheral oedema.

PERIOPERATIVE MANAGEMENT

PREMEDICATION

Suitable antibiotic prophylaxis should be used, except in children with an isolated atrial septal defect secundum, or an atrial septal defect secundum, ventricular septal defect or patent ductus arteriosus that has been repaired more than 6 months previously. The utility of sedative premedication should be assessed on an individual basis. While it may be beneficial in certain instances (e.g. tetralogy of Fallot), it may be hazardous in children with decreased cardiopulmonary reserve. Dehydration due to prolonged fasting should be avoided in children with polycythaemia (haematocrit > 45%) to decrease the risk of thrombotic complications.

INDUCTION

Induction should be smooth (minimal crying or struggling), with the choice of agents dictated by the patient's pathophysiology and the availability of vascular access. Thiopental, ketamine, halothane, opioids and combinations of these have all been used safely. A reduced dosage and careful titration of intravenous agents is required, especially in patients with decreased cardiac reserve or right-to-left shunts. Experience with propofol in this patient population is limited, and its use is not recommended in critically ill patients. Inhalation induction may be delayed in patients with right-to-left shunts. Non-depolarising muscle relaxants have a slower onset of action with both left-to-right and right-to-left shunts. An increased dose of muscle relaxants may be required if the circulatory time is prolonged. Secure intravenous access should be established as soon as possible and care taken to avoid bubbles in the intravenous fluid (the risk of systemic emboli is extremely high in patients with right-to-left shunts).

MAINTENANCE

The method of maintaining anaesthesia should be based on both the patient's pathophysiology and the destabilising effects of the procedure. Volatile anaesthetics are suitable in children with less severe disease. Ketamine or opioids may be used in children at risk of excessive myocardial depression with volatile anaesthesia. Careful fluid management is essential. Hypotension will lead to hypoxaemia in patients with pulmonary artery bands or those dependent on shunts for pulmonary perfusion.

INTRAOPERATIVE MONITORING

Standard paediatric anaesthetic monitoring is used. In children with cyanotic congenital heart disease, the $EtCO_2$ underestimates arterial carbon dioxide, and the difference between the two is not stable. Invasive monitoring is indicated for children with advanced disease or for major surgery.

AIRWAY AND VENTILATION

Ventilation should be adjusted to maintain an optimum pulmonary vascular resistance by control of lung volume, end-expiratory pressure, carbon dioxide and oxygen tensions. A 'pulmonary steal' phenomenon can occur in some left-to-right shunt lesions.

EMERGENCE

Similar to induction, emergence should be smooth and well managed.

TREATMENT OF HYPERCYANOTIC SPELLS

In patients with tetralogy of Fallot, increased catecholamine levels secondary to stress or stimulation may cause right ventricular outflow tract spasm and right-to-left shunting. Treatment consists of:

- Deepening anaesthesia or sedation
- Hyperventilation with 100% oxygen
- Phenylephrine
- Aortic constriction
- Beta-blockers.

POSTOPERATIVE MANAGEMENT

Monitoring and supplemental oxygen administration should be used until the child has fully recovered. The provision of adequate analgesia and careful fluid management are essential.

4

Elective admission to a paediatric ICU should be considered for major procedures and for children with advanced cardiac disease or complex medical problems.

BIBLIOGRAPHY

Dajani AS, Bisno AL, Chung KJ et al. Prevention of bacterial endocarditis. Recommendation of the American Heart Association. Journal of the American Medical Association 1990; 264:2919

Ekert H, Sheers M. Preoperative and postoperative platelet function in cyanotic congenital heart disease. Journal of Thoracic and Cardiovascular Surgery 1974; 67:184–190

Hickey PR. Anesthesia for children with heart disease. In: International Anesthesia Research Society Review Course Lectures, 1988:86–90

Laishley RS, Burrows FA, Lerman J, Roy WL. Effect of anesthetic induction regimens on oxygen saturation in cyanotic congenital heart disease. Anesthesiology 1986; 65:673–677

Lazzell VA, Burrows FA. Stability of the intraoperative arterial to end-tidal carbon dioxide partial pressure difference in children with congenital heart disease. Canadian Journal of Anaesthesia 1991; 38:859–865

Lebovic S, Reich DL, Steinberg LG, Vela FP, Silvay G. Comparison of propofol versus ketamine for anesthesia in pediatric patients undergoing cardiac catheterization. Anesthesia and Analgesia 1992; 4:490–494

CROSS-REFERENCES

Pulmonary hypertension
    Patient Conditions 4: 138
The failing heart
    Patient Conditions 4: 146
Polycythaemia
    Patient Conditions 7: 223

4

Coronary artery disease

W. Davies

The incidence of coronary artery disease (CAD) is 3–4% of the population.

Approximately 10–15% of myocardial infarctions are silent. CAD and its consequences are the main cause of death in anaesthesia and surgery. The mortality rate following perioperative myocardial infarction is high (Table 4.2), although with aggressive monitoring and intervention it may be reduced. Previous successful percutaneous balloon angioplasty (PTCA) and/or coronary artery bypass grafting (CABG) may lower the perioperative mortality rate associated with non-cardiac surgery to 0–1.2%. Thoracic, upper abdominal, major aortic or other vascular surgery increases the risk by 2–3-fold. The mortality rate following reinfarction is 50–70% (90% of deaths occurring within 48 h of reinfarction).

PATHOPHYSIOLOGY

STABLE ANGINA

Defined as angina with no change in precipitating factors, frequency or duration of pain for at least the previous 2 months, and generally relieved by glyceryl trinitrate.

UNSTABLE ANGINA

Defined as angina with a changing pattern indicative of impending infarction, e.g. more frequent, longer duration of pain, pain not relieved by glyceryl trinitrate, or pain at rest. Silent infarction does not evoke angina.

CORONARY ARTERY DISEASE

CAD usually means more than 50% obstruction of the lumen of one or more coronary arteries by atheromatous plaque. Moderate reductions in diameter can produce considerable reductions in flow; eccentricity of lesions is also an important consideration. Ischaemia develops if myocardial oxygen demand exceeds supply. In stable disease, atheromatous plaque comprises a constant proportion of the arterial lumen. In unstable disease, intra-arterial thrombosis or acute plaque disruption is superimposed on plaque fissuring, causing total or subtotal obstruction. Sudden death is usually due to an ischaemia-induced arrhythmia.

Risk factors for developing CAD:
- Increasing age (e.g. > 40 years)
- Male sex
- Cigarette smoking
- Genetic predisposition
- Hypertension
- Diabetes
- Obesity
- Hypercholesterolaemia (increased low-density lipoproteins)
- Sedentary lifestyle.

Increased perioperative morbidity:
- Recent myocardial infarction (within the last 6 months)
- Congestive heart failure
- High-risk surgery (e.g. thoracic or upper abdominal surgery, or major vascular surgery on the aorta).

TABLE 4.2

Incidence of perioperative myocardial infarction following non-cardiac surgery

	%
Overall	0–0.7
With known CAD	0–1.1
With known triple vessel disease (left anterior descending, circumflex and right coronary artery) (> 70% stenosis)	6
History of previous myocardial infarction	
> 6 months ago	6
> 3 but < 6 months ago	10–15
< 3 months ago	20–37

4

CLINICAL HISTORY

- Previous myocardial infarction.
- Angina (stable or unstable).
- Associated diseases:
  —diabetes
  —congestive heart failure
  —syncope
  —transient ischaemic episodes or stroke
  —peripheral vascular disease
  —renal disease
  —obstructive airway disease.
- Exercise tolerance: Can the patient climb two to three flights of stairs? Is it limited by chest pain, breathlessness or other factors?
- Orthopnoea and paroxysmal nocturnal dyspnoea
- Drug history:
  —nitrates
  —beta-blockers
  —calcium channel blockers
  —antiplatelet agents
  —digoxin.

CLINICAL EXAMINATION

In particular, look for:
- Raised jugular venous pressure
- S_3 gallop rhythm
- Dyspnoea or basal crackles on chest auscultation
- Pulsatile hepatomegaly
- Presence of peripheral pulses
- Resting blood pressure and heart rate.

SPECIFIC INVESTIGATIONS

CHEST RADIOGRAPHY:
- Cardiomegaly is associated with a decreased ejection fraction
- Venous engorgement.

ECG:
- Rate
- Rhythm
- Ischaemia: > 1 mm S-T depression measured 60–80 ms after J point when slope of S-T segment is down-going, or 1.5 mm when S-T segment is up-going, suggests significant ischaemia
- Infarction
- Dysrhythmias.

EXERCISE ECG
Standard or automated 24-h Holter ECG (with S-T segment analysis). Look for evidence of ischaemia, dysrhythmia or hypotension.

ECHOCARDIOGRAPHY:
- Predicts ejection fraction
- Wall motion abnormalities – hypokinesia, dyskinesia, akinesia.

MULTIPLE GATED ACQUISITION (MUGA) SCAN
Measures ejection fraction and detects wall motion abnormalities.

DIPYRIDAMOLE THALLIUM SCANNING
Accurately highlights areas with poor or no perfusion.

ANGIOGRAPHY
Used to assess left ventricular function and document extent of CAD. Mortality rate 0.01–0.1%.

Use the above data to assess ventricular function as shown in Table 4.3.

EJECTION FRACTION
With an ejection fraction of less than 0.35, the incidence of perioperative myocardial infarction in high-risk surgery is 75–85%, whereas if the ejection fraction is greater than 0.35 the perioperative risk is reduced to approximately 20%.

RISK OF POSTOPERATIVE ISCHAEMIC EVENT
In patients with known ischaemic heart disease, some useful predictors of developing a postoperative ischaemic event are:
- Left ventricular hypertrophy on preoperative ECG
- History of hypertension
- Preoperative diabetes
- Confirmed CAD
- Preoperative digoxin therapy.

TABLE 4.3		
Ventricular function		
	Good function	Poor function
Ejection fraction	> 0.55	< 0.4
LVEDP (mmHg)	< 12	> 18
Cardiac Index (l min^{-1} m^{-2})	> 2.5	< 2
Dyskinesia	None	Ventricular

4

Risk of postoperative myocardial ischaemia in high-risk surgery increases progressively with the number of predictors present, for example 22% with none, 31% with one, 46% with two, 70% with three, 77% with four predictors.

ANAESTHESIA AND CAD

UNSTABLE DISEASE:
- Postpone surgery if at all possible, and consider further assessment such as coronary angiography with a view to improving current medical therapy and/or consider PTCA or CABG first.
- Exclude recent infarct by serial ECG or serial determination of cardiac enzyme levels if possible.

URGENT SURGERY
Optimise medical therapy:
- Aspirin or other antiplatelet agent – to reduce intravascular thrombosis.
- Consider transdermal nitrate patch (with premedication) to:
  —reduce left ventricular end-diastolic pressure (LVEDP)
  —reduce preload
  —improve collateral flow
  —dilate stenotic areas
  —decrease systemic blood pressure.
- Beta-blockers (e.g. atenolol 50–100 mg daily) – to reduce contractility and heart rate.
- Calcium channel blockers (e.g. diltiazem 60 mg t.d.s.) to:
  —reduce SVR
  —relieve coronary spasm.

CONDUCT OF ANAESTHESIA

Continue preoperative drug therapy, but consider stopping angiotensin-converting enzyme (ACE) inhibitors 24 h before operation, as they may potentiate 'induction' hypotension.

PREMEDICATION
Aim to provide adequate sedation and reduce apprehension, whilst continuing optimal medical therapy and oxygen therapy (benzodiazepine, hyoscine, opiate is satisfactory).

Before surgery instigate invasive monitoring and insert large-bore venous access under local anaesthesia and/or sedation. (direct arterial blood pressure, central venous pressure line, pulmonary artery catheter), depending on assessment of patient.

Attach appropriate non-invasive monitoring, e.g. ECG CM_5/V_5/lead II, oximetry, non-invasive blood pressure.

INDUCTION:
- Preoxygenation
- Moderate doses of potent opioids:
  —fentanyl (25–50 µg kg^{-1})
  —sufentanil (10–15 µg kg^{-1})
  —alfentanil (50–100 µg kg^{-1}; infusion 0.5–1.0 g kg^{-1} min^{-1})
- Induction agent: etomidate > thiopental > propofol or midazolam
- Choice of relaxant is dependent on desired haemodynamic effect and length of operation (e.g. vecuronium, atracurium, pancuronium).

MAINTENANCE
IPPV with volatile agent, relaxant or further opioid. Combined general and regional anaesthesia may be a useful technique.

REVERSAL:
- Edrophonium is preferable to neostigmine.
- Glycopyrrolate is preferable to atropine.

MONITORING
The severity of disease and the magnitude of surgery will determine degree of monitoring:
- Invasive blood pressure monitoring is mandatory for high-risk surgery
- ECG – lead II and V_5 (or CM_5), with continuous S-T analysis if available
- Oximetry
- Capnography
- CVP
- Pulmonary artery flotation catheter
- Core temperature
- Urethral catheter
- Transoesophageal echocardiography (TOE)
- Transoesophageal Doppler echocardiography.

Optimal myocardial oxygen supply–demand balance is achieved when the heart rate is slow (maximal diastolic time), the heart size is small (reduced wall tension) and the heart is well perfused (adequate coronary perfusion pressure) (Box 4.6). A reduction in contractility may be beneficial to reduce demand, depending on left ventricular function.

The choice of agent or technique may have little or no influence on cardiac outcome. Avoid tachycardia, sympathetic stimulation, pain and hypoxaemia. Aim to keep cardiovascular parameters at or near to preoperative values (± 20%). Use nitrates or calcium channel blockers as coronary vasodilators, inotropes to maintain

BOX 4.6

Factors affecting myocardial oxygen delivery and demand

Factors increasing oxygen requirement

- Sympathetic stimulation
- Pain
- Tachycardia
- Systolic hypertension
- Increased myocardial contractility
- Increased afterload

Factors decreasing oxygen delivery

- Decreased coronary perfusion pressure
- Decreased carbon dioxide
- Tachycardia
- Diastolic hypotension
- Coronary artery spasm
- Decreased oxygen content:
  —anaemia
  —arterial hypoxaemia
  —shift of oxygen dissociation curve to the left
  —increased preload

ventricular performance, and beta-blockers to control heart rate.

OUTCOME

SPECIFIC GOALS:

- Treat hypertension associated with tachycardia with labetalol, opioids or increased depth of anaesthesia.
- Treat hypertension without tachycardia with increased depth of anaesthesia, opioids, hydralazine, nicardipine or glyceryl trinitrate.
- Treat hypotension with fluid, if hypovolaemic; with vasoconstrictors (e.g. phenylephrine or ephedrine), if vasodilated; with an inotrope (e.g. dobutamine), if reduced contractility.
- Actively treat metabolic acidosis with inotropes, vasodilators and appropriate fluid replacement.
- If persistent ischaemia develops despite the above measures, consider the use of a perioperative intra-aortic balloon pump.

POSTOPERATIVE CARE:

- ITU/HDU stay for minimum of 48–72 h.
- Continue aggressive monitoring, intervention and oxygen therapy for 48–72 h after surgery.
- Adequate analgesia (ventilate if necessary).
- Treat hypothermia; avoid shivering.

- Actively and aggressively treat:
  —hypotension
  —hypertension
  —acidosis
  —hypercarbia
  —hypocarbia
  —hypoxaemia
  —arrhythmias.
- Aim for a packed cell volume (PCV) of 33%.
- Increase oxygen delivery, until oxygen consumption plateaus and is therefore no longer supply-dependent.
- Aim to keep parameters within 20% of the preoperative baseline.

Overall morbidity and mortality rates may be reduced with appropriate invasive monitoring and aggressive treatment of adverse cardiovascular parameters, which should be continued into the postoperative period. Definitive treatment of unstable CAD should precede non-urgent non-cardiac surgery.

BIBLIOGRAPHY

Anderson WG. Anaesthesia for patients with cardiac disease. Postoperative care. British Journal of Hospital Medicine 1987; 37:411, 414–418

Ballard P. Anaesthesia for patients with cardiac disease. Intraoperative management. British Journal of Hospital Medicine 1987; 37:398–404, 407, 410

Fleisher LA, Barash P. Preoperative cardiac evaluation: a functional approach. Anesthesia and Analgesia 1992; 74:586–598

Masey SA, Burton GW. Anaesthesia for patients with cardiac disease. Preoperative management. British Journal of Hospital Medicine 1987; 37:386–396

Thomas SJ, Kramer JL. Manual of cardiac anaesthesia. 2nd edn. Edinburgh: Churchill Livingstone

Walter SN, Rowbotham DJ, Smith G. In: Reiz S, Mangano DT, Bennett S, eds. Anaesthesia, vol 2. 2nd edn. Oxford: Blackwell Scientific; 0000:1212–1263

West JNW, Gammage MD. Angina: strategies for management. Current Anaesthesia and Critical Care 1993; 4:124–134

CROSS-REFERENCES

Carotid endarterectomy
    Surgical Procedures 20: 509
Coronary artery bypass grafting
    Surgical Procedures 25: 574

Mitral valve disease

M. Scallan

MITRAL STENOSIS

PATHOPHYSIOLOGY

In mitral stenosis, owing to the chronic under-filling of the left ventricle there is a decrease in both left ventricular end-diastolic pressure and left ventricular end-diastolic volume. In the early stages left ventricular function is preserved, but with time chronic underfilling leads to a decrease in contractility and the development of cardiomyopathy.

When right heart failure occurs there may be a shift of the interventricular septum, which produces an additional impairment of left ventricular function.

The increase in the left atrial pressure causes atrial distension, which in turn leads to a decrease in the left atrial contractility.

Later, sinus rhythm is lost and replaced by atrial fibrillation. Loss of atrial systole leads to an increase in the patient's symptoms, as atrial systole contributes approximately 30% to left ventricular filling in patients with mitral stenosis. A normal atrial contribution is 20%.

Atrial fibrillation causes a tachycardia. Because of the shorter diastolic time, a greater gradient across the valve is necessary to maintain filling of the left ventricle. This further increases the left atrial pressure. The chronic increase in left atrial pressure may cause pulmonary vascular disease. Thrombi may form within the cavity of the atrium or its appendage, with a risk of systemic embolisation.

CLINICAL FEATURES

Patients with mitral stenosis remain asymptomatic for 20 years. Thereafter their symptoms become rapidly progressive and they will have a severe disability at 7 years.

The main symptoms of mitral stenosis are dyspnoea, paroxysmal nocturnal dyspnoea, fatigue, pulmonary oedema and atrial fibrillation.

ANAESTHESIA:

- Avoid agents that impair ventricular contractility.
- Maintain preload but avoid excess fluid as this may precipitate pulmonary oedema.
- Tachycardias have a detrimental effect on left ventricular filling.
- If pulmonary vascular disease is present, hypercarbia, acidosis and hypoxia should be avoided at all times. Nitrous oxide should probably not be used because it increases pulmonary vascular resistance.
- Pulmonary artery catheters are of value during the perioperative management of patients with mitral stenosis (Box 4.7). TOE should be considered as an alternative or in addition to pulmonary artery catheters if haemodynamic instability is anticipated.
- Many patients will benefit from a period of postoperative IPPV.

MITRAL REGURGITATION

PATHOPHYSIOLOGY

In the early stages there is an increase in left ventricular end-diastolic volume and concentric

BOX 4.7

Pulmonary artery catheters in mitral stenosis

- There is an increased risk of pulmonary artery rupture.
- The catheter has a greater distance to travel, which may make its insertion more difficult.
- The catheter may 'loop' within the enlarged right ventricle.
- Arrhythmias may occur during the insertion of catheters.
- In the presence of pulmonary hypertension, the pulmonary artery diastolic pressure may not be a true reflection of left atrial pressure.
- The monitored waveforms may be distorted by left atrial pressure events – interpretation may be difficult.

4

hypertrophy of the myocardium. The considerable increase in left ventricular stroke volume ensures that the forward flow to the aorta is maintained.

In the later stages forward flow is diminished and is associated with fatigue. There is a large increase in the volume of the left atrium.

The pressure in the left atrium is not increased in the early stages of the disease.

As in mitral stenosis, atrial fibrillation and pulmonary hypertension may occur.

CLINICAL FEATURES

Patients with chronic mitral regurgitation may remain asymptomatic for 20–40 years.

The symptoms associated with this disease are dyspnoea, orthopnoea, fatigue, pulmonary oedema and atrial fibrillation.

ANAESTHESIA:

- While the preload should be maintained, excess fluid should be avoided as this may cause further dilatation of the mitral valve ring.
- Agents that impair ventricular contractility should be avoided.
- Bradycardia should be avoided as this will increase regurgitation.

- An increase in the SVR should be avoided as this will increase the regurgitant fraction.
- If pulmonary vascular disease is present, steps should be taken to avoid increases in the PVR. Postoperative mechanical ventilation may be required.
- Monitoring by pulmonary artery catheter and/or TOE should be considered.

BIBLIOGRAPHY

Rappaport E. Natural history of aortic and mitral valve disease. American Journal of Cardiology 1975; 35:221

CROSS-REFERENCES

Marfan's syndrome
    Patient Conditions 8: 238
Aortic valve surgery
    Surgical Procedures 25: 580
Mitral valve surgery
    Surgical Procedures 25: 583
Preoperative assessment of pulmonary risk
    Anaesthetic Factors 27: 638

4

Patients with permanent pacemakers *in situ*

N. Curzen

Permanent pacemakers (PPMs) are fitted with increasing frequency to treat a variety of brad-yarrhythmias as well as a few types of tach-yarrhythmia. Modern systems are becoming more complex, but also safer.

PREOPERATIVE ASSESSMENT

ELECTIVE CASES

Preoperative assessment should provide enough information to establish:

- The type of pacemaker present and its basic mode of operation
- Where it is sited – to minimise the chance of iatrogenic damage
- Whether there is evidence that the unit is currently working
- Whether other factors are present that may influence the PPM function.

PACEMAKER CODE

Produced by a combined working party of the North American Society of Pacing and Electrophysiology (NASBE) and the British Pacing and Electrophysiology Group (BPEG), the pacemaker code (Box 4.8) takes the form of a four-letter code to describe the PPM function in a systematic way.

FACTORS THAT CAN AFFECT PACING FUNCTION PERIOPERATIVELY

These factors can alter pacing threshold or make the myocardium more irritable (Table 4.4). For all but emergency cases it is important to know this information and, ideally, to have the unit fully checked by a PPM clinic, especially because a significant proportion of PPM units will be sensing most of the time, and there will be little evidence on the resting ECG as to whether they are functioning. In addition, it is not always possible to identify the specific programme in which a unit is set (e.g. rate response) unless it is formally interrogated. There are some settings that would be better altered before general anaesthesia, but this deci-

sion is necessarily patient specific and should be made by an expert.

HISTORY:

- When and where was the unit fitted? Were there later box or lead changes?

BOX 4.8

Pacemaker code

First letter	Paced chamber	A	atrium
		V	ventricle
		D	both
Second letter	Sensed chamber	A	atrium
		V	ventricle
		D	both
		O	none
Third letter	Mode of response to sensed events	I	inhibited
		T	triggered
		D	inhibited and triggered
		O	no response
Fourth letter	Rate	R	responsiveness

TABLE 4.4

Factors that can affect pacing function perioperatively

	Clinical finding
Electrolytes	Hypokalaemia, hyperkalaemia
Acid–base balance	Acidosis, alkalosis
Myocardial	Ischaemia, acute infarction
Drugs	Digoxin toxicity, catecholamines, antiarrhythmic agents (e.g. lidocaine (lignocaine))
Metabolic	Hypothermia and thyroid disturbances

4

- When was the PPM last checked? Were the technicians happy or did they ask for follow-up earlier than normal?
- Is the patient carrying a PPM card, which details unit and programme?
- Any recent symptoms to suggest malfunction (e.g. syncope, dizzy spells)?

EXAMINATIONS:

- Bradycardia; hypotension
- Where is the pacemaker generator (left, right, abdominal)?

INVESTIGATIONS:

- Electrolytes
- Chest radiography:
  —Dual or single chamber?
  —Where is the generator?
- ECG:
  —What is the current rate and rhythm?
  —Is there evidence of satisfactory pacing?
  —If mode is known, is the PPM performing in that mode?
- Whenever possible, has there been a satisfactory pacing check before elective surgery?

EMERGENCY SURGERY

Even in these cases it will be possible to establish where the generator is and whether the patient is pacing or not. If there is doubt as to the functional integrity of the unit then:

- Place a magnet over the pacemaker generator (see Magnet mode).
- If this fails to induce pacemaker activity, it may be advisable to request the placement of a temporary pacing wire.

MAGNET MODE

This should reprogramme all commonly used units to the VOO, DOO or AOO mode (i.e. they pace the chamber(s) indicated at a fixed rate with no sensing of intrinsic activity) at rates that depend on the manufacturer and the unit, but are most often 70–90 beats min^{-1}. The magnet works in most modern PPM units by closing a reed switch and the PPM will remain in this setting until the magnet is removed, when it will revert to its previous mode. This property can therefore be useful:

- To confirm that the PPM is working, *or*
- To overcome sensing problems that may be causing pacing failure.

INTRAOPERATIVE MANAGEMENT

MONITORING

The ECG monitor will not identify malfunctions such as failure to capture. It is essential to have a system that monitors the blood pressure or arterial waveform every beat (i.e. oximeter or arterial line) rather than just electrical activity, and this should ideally be accompanied by auditory output.

DIATHERMY

This is the equipment that interferes with PPM function most commonly. Most PPMs will revert to asynchronous (non-sensing mode; e.g. VOO) when exposed to continuous electromagnetic interference (EMI). This may not occur with intermittent EMI, such as that generated by diathermy, and this can cause failure to pace. The major manufacturers recommend that diathermy is relatively contraindicated and that it is not used near to the generator.

- When unipolar electrocautery is used, keep the apparatus (especially the grounding plate) away from the generator and leads.
- Use bipolar electrocautery if possible.
- Use as little diathermy as possible.
- The procedure should be followed by a formal PPM check.

ELECTRICAL CARDIOVERSION/ DEFIBRILLATION:

- Use the lowest possible energy level
- Paddles should be as far away from the generator as possible (not less than 10 cm)
- Paddles should be placed at right angles to the line between the generator and the lead tip
- The procedure should be followed by a formal PPM check.

MYOPOTENTIAL INHIBITION

This occurs when the PPM senses skeletal myopotentials, which may be generated by:

- Mechanical ventilation
- Drug-induced myoclonic movements (e.g. propofol, ketamine, etomidate)
- Drug-induced fasciculation (e.g. depolarising muscle relaxants).

Myopotention inhibition can present with pacing failure, in which case application of a magnet should restore fixed rate pacing (see Magnet mode). It is more commonly a problem with unipolar systems.

MAGNETIC RESONANCE IMAGING

This can affect PPM function in a number of ways, such as conversion to asynchronous mode, or even pacing failure. Because of this, MRI is contraindicated in pacing-dependent patients, and can damage the PPM of those who are not. It should be performed only if absolutely essential – and then only after planning by a pacing expert.

POSTOPERATIVE MANAGEMENT

It is advisable to have the function of any PPM checked after surgery; checking is essential following high-risk procedures including:
• Electrical cardioversion
• Diathermy.
Malfunction of the PPM in this period should be fully investigated. Possible contributory factors are included in Table 4.4.

BIBLIOGRAPHY

Atlee J. Cardiac pacing and electroversion. In: Kaplan JA, ed. Cardiac anaesthesia. 3rd edn. Philadelphia: WB Saunders; 0000

Bloomfield P, Bowler GM. Anaesthetic management of the patient with a permanent pacemaker. Anaesthesia 1989; 44:42–46

Furman S, Hayes DL, Holmes DR. A practice of cardiac pacing. 2nd edn. New York: Futura; 1989

Hayes DL, Vlietstra RE. Pacemaker malfunction. Annals of Internal Medicine 1993; 119:828–835

4

Pulmonary hypertension

B. Keogh

The definition of pulmonary hypertension is not clear. Generally accepted values include a pulmonary artery pressure greater than 35/15 mmHg or mean pulmonary artery pressure above 20 mmHg. The condition may be primary or secondary; in the latter case the primary condition may greatly influence both health and relevance to anaesthesia. Mild pulmonary hypertension is of little anaesthetic consequence, whereas pulmonary artery pressures approaching systemic levels represent a significant anaesthetic risk.

CLINICAL FINDINGS

MODERATE PULMONARY HYPERTENSION:
- Right ventricular heave
- Loud P2 heart sound
- Exertional dyspnoea
- Finger clubbing may be present.

ADVANCED PULMONARY HYPERTENSION:
- Raised jugular venous pressure (JVP)
- 'v' waves secondary to tricuspid regurgitation on the JVP
- Central cyanosis (may occur early)
- Oedema
- Hepatomegaly and later ascites.

ECG:
- Right ventricular hypertrophy, usually right-axis deviation
- P pulmonale (P > 2 mm tall in lead 2).

CHEST RADIOGRAPHY:
- Bilaterally enlarged pulmonary arteries
- Changes related to the original cause if secondary pulmonary hypertension.

BLOOD
Secondary polycythaemia.

AETIOLOGY

PRIMARY
Pulmonary hypertension is rare and of unknown cause. It typically occurs in young females. The condition is advanced at presentation, and patients die from right ventricular failure within 2–5 years.

SECONDARY:
- Cardiac factors – mitral or aortic valve disease, left ventricular failure
- Congenital heart disease
- Chronic thromboembolic disease
- Pulmonary veno-occlusive disease
- Parenchymal pulmonary diseases
  —chronic obstructive pulmonary disease (COPD), pulmonary fibrosis, granulomatous disease
  —collagen and generalised vasculitic diseases
  —secondary to kyphoscoliosis, or 'pickwickian'.

COR PULMONALE

This is a confusing term. It is defined (World Health Organisation classification) as: right ventricular enlargement secondary to diseases of lung parenchyma or vasculature, excluding congenital and left-sided cardiac disease. Thromboembolic and veno-occlusive diseases are variously included or omitted from this group. Such patients have high right-sided pressures with low left atrial pressure and left ventricular end-diastolic pressure. By far the most common presenting group is those with COPD.

RECENT DEVELOPMENTS IN THERAPY FOR PULMONARY HYPERTENSION

Despite the overall poor prognosis of pulmonary hypertension, recent therapeutic advances have shown some promise. Prostacyclin and its analogues have been used by inhalation and latterly subcutaneous infusion with some effect. Most promising is bosentan, an endothelin receptor antagonist which may act both by a reduction in vascular tone and by initiating vascular remodelling. Sildenafil has also been reported to have a beneficial effect in some patients. These agents are currently being investigated in patients with pulmonary hypertension of varying aetiologies, and their efficacy – and indeed their relevance to anaesthesia – is yet to be established.

ANAESTHETIC IMPLICATIONS

The response of pulmonary hypertension patients to anaesthesia depends on the aetiology of the disease, disease progression and the degree of decompensation. In many patients the underlying cause will bear greater relevance to anaesthesia than the pulmonary hypertension itself.

GENERAL PRINCIPLES:
- High F_{IO_2}; normocarbia, if possible.
- Maintain right ventricular preload.
- Orientation to cardiac output and oxygen delivery rather than Pa_{O_2}.
- Vasodilators give disappointing results in established pulmonary hypertension. Options are:
  —prostacyclin (2.5–20 ng kg^{-1} min^{-1} i.v.)
  —prostacyclin (5–10 ng kg^{-1} min^{-1} nebulised)
  —nitroglycerin (0.5–3 µg kg^{-1} min^{-1} i.v.)
  —sodium nitroprusside (0.2–3 µg kg^{-1} min^{-1} i.v.)
  —inhaled nitric oxide (2–50 p.p.m.).
- All systemic vasodilators may decrease right ventricular preload.
- Right ventricular inotropy:
  —phosphodiesterase inhibitors (e.g. milrinone 0.25–0.75 mg kg^{-1} min^{-1}) lower PVR
  —dobutamine has a variable effect on PVR.
- Right ventricular relaxation:
  —phosphodiesterase inhibitors
  —may decrease tricuspid regurgitation.
- Switch oral anticoagulants to intravenous heparin.

NB: Systemic vasoconstrictors may be required. An imbalance of oxygen supply–demand to the right ventricle can occur, resulting in right ventricular failure, when systemic pressure falls and right ventricular systolic and diastolic pressures remain increased in the presence of fixed, raised PVR. Suggest noradrenaline (norepinephrine) (0.01–0.1 µg kg^{-1} min^{-1}), which has little effect on PVR in this context (higher dose may be required if in combination with phosphodiesterase inhibitors).

PULMONARY HYPERTENSION SECONDARY TO CARDIAC DISEASE
Pulmonary hypertension secondary to left heart dysfunction mandates a high left atrial pressure. Anaesthesia for left ventricular failure requires both preload and afterload reduction, e.g. by nitrate therapy or phosphodiesterase inhibitors. Specific therapy of valve lesions is discussed elsewhere. IPPV may have favourable effects on left ventricular function. In pulmonary hypertension, right ventricular preload must be maintained and may be difficult to optimise due to effects of tricuspid regurgitation. Direct arterial pressure monitoring, pulmonary artery catheters and TOE are usually indicated. A prudent anaesthetic approach to such patients includes induction with etomidate, fentanyl and vecuronium (a narcotic-based anaesthetic), followed by elective postoperative ventilation and full monitoring in the postsurgical and weaning phase. Epidural and spinal anaesthesia has little to offer in such patients. In very severe cases, perioperative intra-aortic balloon counterpulsation should be considered to provide mechanical support to the failing left ventricle during the perioperative period.

COR PULMONALE
Preoperative assessment
See COPD section (p. •)
- Pulmonary function tests mandatory
- Pulmonary circulation
  —direct, by pulmonary artery catheter
  —indirect, by Doppler echocardiography – assessment of right ventricular function, degree of tricuspid regurgitation and reasonable assessment of peak pulmonary artery pressure and pulmonary blood flow.

Choice of anaesthesia
Choice of anaesthesia will probably be dictated by the underlying aetiology:
- Primary pulmonary hypertension and chronic thromboembolic disease is probably best managed by 'cardiac'-type general anaesthesia.
- In pulmonary parenchymal disease, regional techniques with judicious attention to right ventricular preload and maintenance of

systemic vascular resistance are likely to offer an advantage over general anaesthesia, especially if the right ventricle is coping.

- If there is clear evidence of right ventricular decompensation with gross peripheral oedema and ascites, the patient is at extremely high risk, whatever technique is applied. The author still believes that general anaesthesia is the preferable option in this case.

Pharmacological manipulation

Vasodilators (as listed above) with attention to SVR maintenance, if necessary. The phosphodiesterase inhibitors have a particularly favourable pharmacological profile for use in patients with pulmonary hypertension. The increase in cyclic adenosine monophosphate (cAMP) levels and resultant inotropy is independent of β-receptor activity (often downregulated in chronic cardiac disease). In addition, lusitropic effects should enhance biventricular function.

Facilities for prolonged ventilation

Patients are clearly at risk due to protracted recovery. The availability of postoperative ventilation facilities is mandatory and a low threshold for their use should be adopted.

Postoperative analgesia

A key factor in recovery. Epidural analgesic techniques may be particularly beneficial. The risks associated with epidural anaesthesia in some anticoagulated patients may need to be balanced against the perceived advantages, particularly in the presence of poor pulmonary function.

BIBLIOGRAPHY

Maloney JP. Advances in the treatment of secondary pulmonary hypertension. Current Opinion in Pulmonary Medicine 2003; 9:139–143

Widlitz A, Barst RJ. Pulmonary arterial hypertension in children. European Respiratory Journal 2003; 21:155–176

Severe congenital heart disease in adult life

B. Keogh

Approximately 70% of patients with congenital heart disease (CHD) reach adulthood, most of them after corrective or palliative surgery. Such patients are likely to present for non-cardiac surgical procedures. Many have associated abnormalities as part of the syndrome complex. There may be associated intellectual impairment (40% of patients with trisomy 21 have CHD).

PATHOPHYSIOLOGY

Enormous variability in anatomy and resultant dysfunction is observed, and this is compounded by varying success in surgical intervention. An understanding of the direction and quantity of blood flow is key to understanding individual physiology.

ADULT CHD PATIENT GROUPS:
- Corrected patients:
  —non-cyanotic
  —risk of valve and conduit dysfunction with degeneration over time
  —may have limited cardiac output.
- Palliated patients:
  —commonly limited pulmonary blood flow
  —often aortopulmonary shunts
  —usually cyanotic; limited exercise tolerance with age
  —may progress to congestive cardiac failure.
- Untreated patients:
  —balanced physiology
  —usually moderately cyanotic.
- All-groups risk:
  —arrhythmias, increasing with age
  —infective endocarditis.

MANIPULATION OF CARDIAC SHUNTS AND PULMONARY BLOOD FLOW

General principles are shown in Table 4.5.

DECREASE PVR:
- $F_{IO_2} = 1$
- Hyperventilate to $Pa_{CO_2} = 3.5$ kPa

TABLE 4.5

General principles of changes in SVR and PVR and the effects on flow and shunt

SVR	PVR	Pulmonary blood flow	Shunt direction
↓		↓	R → L
↑		↓	L → R
	↓	↑	L → R
	↑	↓	R → L

- Short inspiratory time; no positive end-expiratory pressure (PEEP)
- Prostacyclin (2–20 ng kg^{-1} min^{-1} i.v.; 3–15 ng kg^{-1} min^{-1} nebulised)
- Inhaled nitric oxide (suggest 2–40 p.p.m.).

INCREASE PVR:
- $F_{IO_2} = 0.21$–0.3
- Hypoventilate to $Pa_{CO_2} > 7$ kPa
- Long inspiratory time; moderate PEEP levels.

INCREASE SVR:
- Phenylephrine (0.25–0.5 µg kg^{-1})
- Metaraminol (0.5–1 µg kg^{-1})
- Noradrenaline (norepinephrine) (0.01–0.20 µg kg^{-1} min^{-1} infusion).

DECREASE SVR:
- Sodium nitroprusside (infusion)
- Phentolamine (10 µg kg^{-1} bolus).

APPROACH TO ADULT PATIENTS WITH CHD

- Identify basic congenital anatomy
- Consider functional effect of repair
- Consider associated medical conditions
- Always consider endocarditis
- Maintain antiarrhythmic therapy
- Remember potential for paradoxical emboli.

4

ANAESTHETIC MANAGEMENT

The majority of patients with CHD who have stable cardiopulmonary physiology will tolerate anaesthesia without significant instability. Owing to extreme patient variability, it is difficult to construct a strict framework for anaesthetic management. In general it is advisable to maintain the pre-existing balance between SVR and PVR.

GENERAL PRINCIPLES:

- Avoid injection of air, clot, precipitates
- Ensure adequate hydration; avoid prolonged fasting
- Rarely isovolaemic venesection may be considered if haematocrit is > 60%
- Switch anticoagulants to intravenous heparin
- Antithrombotic measures – thromboembolism-deterrent (TED) stockings.

ANTIBIOTIC PROPHYLAXIS

Recommendations vary regionally and with the contemplated surgery. The regimen should include anti-staphylococcal agents (e.g. flucloxacillin, teicoplanin or vancomycin) with broad-spectrum cover (e.g. gentamicin or second-generation cephalosporin).

INDUCTION:

- Many options; cardiovascular stability is the key
- Suggest etomidate, fentanyl or alfentanil, vecuronium
- Ketamine useful to maintain SVR but infrequently used in adults
- Ketamine (i.m.) in patients with intellectual impairment
- Inhalational anaesthesia is possible, but is unpredictable due to variable pulmonary blood flow.

MAINTENANCE

Volatile or intravenous agents are equally acceptable. Marked decreases in SVR should be avoided. Tachycardia associated with isoflurane may be troublesome in some patients. In general, the balance between PVR and SVR is altered little by potent narcotics such as fentanyl, alfentanil and sufentanil. There is a theoretical risk when using nitrous oxide in patients with right-to-left shunts, in that the bubble size of inadvertently injected air will increase with nitrous oxide, which should probably be avoided in such patients.

MONITORING

Arm blood pressure monitoring may underestimate the true systemic blood pressure in patients who have had previous aortopulmonary shunts involving the subclavian artery. Peripheral SpO_2 is mandatory, in addition to basic monitoring. Interpretation of $EtCO_2$ tracing is complex. $EtCO_2$ does not necessarily reflect $PaCO_2$, but trends in $EtCO_2$ can indicate variations in pulmonary blood flow. A low threshold for arterial line and central venous pressure line placement is appropriate. Pulmonary artery catheterisation is likely to yield valuable information in relatively few patients, and is anatomically impossible in a considerable number. Newer options for non-invasive cardiac output estimation should be employed in complex cases or in low-output states. Intraoperative TOE by a skilled operator is also desirable in complex cases, particularly if the proposed operation is complex or prolonged.

HAEMODYNAMIC SUPPORT

This is a complex area and depends greatly on the anatomy. In addition to the manipulation of intracardiac shunt (see above), inotropic support of either ventricle may be required. The phosphodiesterase inhibitors milrinone ($0.25–0.75$ µg kg^{-1} min^{-1}) and enoximone ($5–10$ µg kg^{-1} min^{-1}) have proved useful in the cardiac sphere in view of associated pulmonary vasodilatation and positive ventricular relaxation, which can improve filling of often restrictive ventricles. Isoprenaline ($0.02–0.05$ µg kg^{-1} min^{-1}) is useful for rate support, but does decrease SVR. Noradrenaline (norepinephrine) ($0.02–0.20$ µg kg^{-1} min^{-1} – higher after cardiac surgery) may be employed to modulate the reduction of SVR seen with vasodilating inotropes. Adenosine ($4–12$-mg bolus) may successfully treat a troublesome tachycardia. In a desperate situation, adrenaline (epinephrine) ($0.01–0.2$ µg kg^{-1} min^{-1} or even higher doses) tends to be the drug of choice.

REGIONAL ANAESTHESIA

Cardiac anaesthetists, regularly confronted with such patients, rarely consider epidural or spinal regional techniques. The decrease in SVR may be troublesome in some patients, but can be counteracted by vasoconstrictor infusions. Many patients are anticoagulated, representing a relative contraindication.

DAY-CASE ANAESTHESIA

The presence of CHD alone does not preclude day-case surgery. Patients with stable cardiopulmonary physiology undergoing limited surgical procedures may be considered suitable.

CARDIOPULMONARY RESUSCITATION

This may be difficult because of the anatomy. External cardiac compression is ineffective in some patients, for example those with a right ventricle to pulmonary artery conduit that lies behind the sternum and is blocked by compression. Systemic vasoconstrictors are useful in many circulations, and in a deteriorating situation may improve pulmonary blood flow and avoid the need for cardiopulmonary resuscitation.

GENERAL COMMENTS

Polycythaemic patients with decreased plasma volume have an increased bleeding tendency and require extra haematological support. Patients with relatively simple lesions (e.g. ASD), who have not had access to medical therapy and may present quite late in the disease process, are at risk of acute decompensation. Discussion with the congenital cardiothoracic centre staff is advisable before undertaking anaesthesia, especially if the cardiopulmonary connections are difficult to understand.

4

Tetralogy of Fallot

B. Keogh

Tetralogy of Fallot accounts for 10% of congenital heart disease. Early surgical correction (< 6 months) is now generally favoured, although a palliative aortopulmonary shunt followed by later definitive correction is acceptable in children who have difficult anatomy or are subject to severe hypercyanotic spells. Only 5% of untreated patients survive beyond the age of 25 years.

ANATOMY

- Ventricular septal defect (VSD)
- Pulmonary stenosis
- Right ventricular hypertrophy
- Aorta overriding VSD.

CLINICOPATHOPHYSIOLOGICAL FEATURES

- Right-to-left shunt
- Cyanosis and clubbing
- Polycythaemia
- Dyspnoea on exertion.

HYPERCYANOTIC SPELLS

These intermittent cyanotic episodes are characteristic of children with tetralogy of Fallot. Right ventricular infundibular (subpulmonary but supra-VSD) muscle spasm increases right-to-left shunt, resulting in profound hypoxaemia. Children squat in response to this phenomenon, resulting in increased SVR and decreased venous return, both of which decrease the right-to-left shunt. Propranolol therapy is indicated to control spells.

COMPLICATIONS AND SEQUELAE

- Increasing dyspnoea with age
- Arrhythmia

- Infective endocarditis
- Paradoxical emboli
  —cerebral thrombosis
  —cerebral abscess
- Ischaemic cardiomyopathy.

INVESTIGATIONS

CHEST RADIOGRAPHY
'Boot shaped' heart and oligaemic lung fields.

ECG
Right ventricular hypertrophy and right-axis deviation.

BLOOD
Polycythaemia (haematocrit > 50%) and thrombocytopenia (uncommon).

Sa_{O_2}
Range 70–90%.

ANAESTHETIC MANAGEMENT

Anaesthesia for the correction of tetralogy of Fallot lies within the province of the cardiothoracic anaesthetist. Palliated or uncorrected patients may present at any age for non-cardiac or, particularly, emergency surgery. Relevant issues are discussed below.

PREOPERATIVE ISSUES

- Sedative premedicants are indicated in younger patients.
- Avoid prolonged starvation period; consider intravenous hydration.
- Continue beta-blockers and antiarrhythmics perioperatively.
- Antibiotic prophylaxis is mandatory.
- Switch anticoagulation to intravenous heparin.
- General antithrombotic measures (TED stockings).

- Reduced plasma volume (may need coagulation support).
- Venesect if haematocrit is greater than 60%; replace with albumin in children.

INDUCTION

Inhalational induction is commonly used in children, but may precipitate a hypercyanotic spell. Inhalational induction may be slower in patients with tetralogy because of limited pulmonary blood flow, especially during a hypercyanotic spell. Sevoflurane is most commonly used.

Intravenous induction (after local anaesthetic cream) allows induction to be achieved with little patient awareness, potentially decreasing the risk of a hypercyanotic spell. Ketamine (intramuscular or intravenous) maintains SVR with little increase in PVR in these patients, thus decreasing the right-to-left shunt, but is popular in a few centres. Increased right-to-left shunt with routine induction agents due to decreased SVR may be antagonised by vasoconstrictors (e.g. phenylephrine $0.5 \mu g\ kg^{-1}$ i.v. or metaraminol $1 \mu g\ kg^{-1}$ i.v.). In practice, vasoconstrictors are rarely required, but noradrenaline (norepinephrine) infusion ($0.02–0.10 \mu g\ kg^{-1}\ min^{-1}$) may be commenced before surgery in a child with severe hypercyanotic spells, bearing in mind that a severe hypercyanotic spell generates myocardial ischaemia and should be avoided if possible.

MONITORING

Besides ECG, monitoring of peripheral SpO_2 is mandatory in a right-to-left shunt, and $EtCO_2$ trends can reflect variations in pulmonary blood flow. A low threshold for direct intravascular monitoring of arterial pressure and CVP is appropriate. Pulmonary artery catheterisation is unhelpful, technically difficult and, in fact, contraindicated owing to the risk of generating right ventricular infundibular spasm.

MAINTENANCE

Volatile or intravenous techniques are equally appropriate as long as marked falls in SVR are avoided. Low-dose noradrenaline (norepinephrine) infusion (typically $0.01–0.05 \mu g\ kg^{-1}\ min^{-1}$) can control SVR changes. Potent narcotics (e.g. alfentanil) may ablate undesired cardiovascular responses. Spontaneous respiration may be employed for minor cases. Adequate fluid replacement is vital.

MANAGEMENT OF A HYPERCYANOTIC SPELL UNDER ANAESTHESIA

The drug of choice is intravenous propranolol; a dose of $0.05–0.1\ mg\ kg^{-1}$ decreases infundibular spasm. Resistant spells require vasoconstrictors by bolus and by infusion (see doses above). In addition, extra sedatives (e.g. opiates), aggressive hyperventilation and correction of the cause of metabolic acidosis are indicated. The use of sodium bicarbonate is, as always, controversial. Paradoxically, children who have required propranolol in association with cardiac surgery may require ongoing inotropic support after correction.

OTHER SPECIAL CONSIDERATIONS

There is a substantial risk of paradoxical embolus through the VSD. Injection of air, drug precipitates or clots in lines must be avoided.

REGIONAL ANAESTHESIA

Reduced SVR due to spinal and epidural anaesthesia is likely to increase right-to-left shunt. Fluid resuscitation will exacerbate this effect. If regional techniques are considered truly preferable to general anaesthesia, manipulation of SVR with a vasoconstrictor infusion is integral to the safety of an unpredictable technique.

POSTOPERATIVE FACTORS

The same general principles apply, but in addition avoid the oxygen consumption demands of excessive shivering. Treatment of spells is as described above. Arrhythmias are common; amiodarone is useful in these patients and is often prescribed prophylactically in adult patients undergoing definitive repair.

UNCORRECTED, PALLIATED AND CORRECTED PATIENTS

Uncorrected patients are severely at risk of complications and adverse haemodynamic sequelae. Palliated patients, while at risk of paradoxical emboli and consequences of polycythaemia, do not exhibit hypercyanotic spells as pulmonary blood flow is maintained by the aortopulmonary shunt. The presence of residual intracardiac shunts should be determined by echocardiography in patients who have had correction of tetralogy of Fallot. Antibiotic prophylaxis is indicated. The vast majority of patients who have undergone successful repair can be expected to exhibit normal cardiopulmonary interactions.

4

The failing heart

W. Aveling

The presence of a failing heart in a patient presenting for non-cardiac surgery is known to increase mortality and morbidity rates. Patients fall into two categories:
- Treated, not likely to improve further
- Untreated or undertreated.

As always, the problem in untreated or undertreated patients is to balance the risk of delaying surgery against the benefit of medical improvement.

PATHOPHYSIOLOGY

The factors affecting ventricular performance are described below.

PRELOAD
The Frank–Starling relationship (Fig. 4.1) describes how stroke volume increases as end-diastolic volume (i.e. cardiac muscle fibre length) increases within limits. End-diastolic pressure is easier to measure and can be substituted for volume. Preload can easily be manipulated to produce maximum cardiac output by judicious filling of the circulation.

AFTERLOAD
The tension that the left ventricle must develop to move blood forward depends on the state of the aortic valve (fixed) and the SVR. Reducing resistance by vasodilatation can increase output in the failing heart.

INOTROPIC STATE
The force of contraction for a given fibre length can be increased by sympathetic stimulation (intrinsic) or β-sympathomimetic drugs. In heart failure there is a depletion of catecholamines and a decreased density of β receptors, resulting in decreased response to β stimulation.

RATE

$$\text{Cardiac output} = \text{Stroke volume} \times \text{Rate}$$

So, one might expect an increase in rate to increase cardiac output. However, at high rates, diastole is reduced, and with it coronary perfusion. Manipulation of rate by chronotropic agents is helpful only in bradycardia.

PREOPERATIVE ASSESSMENT

- History – exercise tolerance and dypsnoea.
- Right ventricular function – raised JVP and oedema are early signs.
- Left ventricular function – tachycardia, basal crepitations and a third heart sound.
- Chest radiography – upper lobe diversion (early), bat's wing shadowing (late).
- Many cardiological investigations:
  —Ejection fraction is a simple and useful guide (< 50% impaired; < 30% poor; < 10% very poor)
  —A pulmonary artery catheter can be used to measure cardiac output
  —Wedge pressure reflects left atrial pressure
  —Full cardiac catheterisation gives most information – left ventricular end-diastolic pressure increases to more than 12 mm in left ventricular failure.
- Renal and liver function are not often impaired.

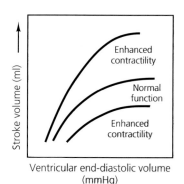

Fig. 4.1 The Frank–Starling relationship.

4

PREOPERATIVE TREATMENT

Where time permits, cardiac function should be optimised.

- *Vasodilatation* to offload the ventricle. ACE inhibitors are now the first-line treatment, but they have to be given orally (e.g. captopril 25–75 mg). If time presses, intravenous infusion of nitroprusside (0.5–5 $\mu g\ kg^{-1}\ min^{-1}$, venous and arteriolar) or nitroprusside (0.5–5 $\mu g\ kg^{-1}\ min^{-1}$, mainly arteriolar) or isosorbide (2–40 $mg\ kg^{-1}\ min^{-1}$, venous and arteriolar). Dosage is limited by hypotension.
- *Adjustment of filling pressures* requires at least central venous pressure monitoring. It is better to use a pulmonary artery catheter so that cardiac output and pressures can be measured in response to aliquots of 200 ml colloid.
- *Inotropes.* Digoxin is still useful, but even when given intravenously it takes 30 min for an effect. Dobutamine (5–20 $\mu g\ kg^{-1}\ min^{-1}$) can be used for an immediate effect.
- *Phosphodiesterase inhibitors* increase cAMP levels. Known as 'inodilators', they can be of benefit in intractable failure (e.g. milrinone 50 $\mu g\ kg^{-1}$ bolus, then 0.4–0.75 $\mu g\ kg^{-1}\ min^{-1}$ infusion).
- *Intra-aortic balloon counterpulsation* – this can be inserted percutaneously before operation in severe cases.

ANAESTHESIA

The haemodynamic consequences of extensive blockade make regional analgesia a hazardous choice. General anaesthesia with minimum cardiovascular disturbance is preferred.

MONITORING:
- Arterial and central venous lines
- Urine output
- Consider placing a pulmonary artery catheter.

PREMEDICATION
Premedication is either minimal or not required.

INDUCTION
Ketamine, etomidate or midazolam plus an opiate (i.v.).

MAINTENANCE
Opiates are the mainstay of maintenance. Use fentanyl (10–20 $\mu g\ kg^{-1}$) or alfentanil (50 $\mu g\ kg^{-1}$ bolus, then 50 $\mu g\ kg^{-1}\ min^{-1}$ infusion). Note that nitrous oxide depresses myocardial function in the presence of opiates.

POSTOPERATIVE MANAGEMENT

Continue monitoring in the ITU.

BIBLIOGRAPHY

Stoelting RK, Dierdorf SF. Congestive heart failure. In: Anaesthesia and co-existing disease. 4th edn. New York: Churchill Livingstone; 2002:105–116

CROSS-REFERENCES

Preoperative assessment of pulmonary risk
  Anaesthetic Factors 27: 638

4

Surgery in heart transplant recipients

B. J. Pollard

BACKGROUND

The most common reason why an anaesthetist will manage a heart transplant recipient is that the patient is requiring surgery for some other procedure. In the 10 years to 1992 there was a tremendous growth in the number of proce-dures performed yearly (Fig. 4.2). Continually improving survival (Fig. 4.3) has meant that many heart transplant patients are receiving surgical treatment at hospitals that are not transplant centres. Surgical procedures per-formed on these patients are usually due to the complications of the transplant surgery or

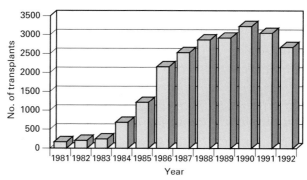

Fig. 4.2 Number of heart transplants performed worldwide between 1981 and 1992. More than 2500 transplants have been performed yearly since 1987, and 87% of all transplants performed have occurred since 1984. (From the registry of the International Heart and Lung Transplantation Society 1993.)

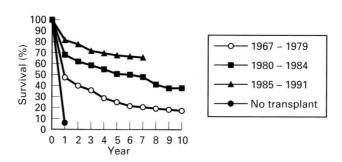

Fig. 4.3 Survival following heart transplantation in patients transplanted during three periods. Patients in the no-transplant group were selected for transplantation but no sutiable donor could be found. Most recent data reflect improved survival associated with the introduction of ciclosporin and the growth of the numbers of centres performing transplantation.

chronic immunosuppression. Surgery may be needed for mediastinal bleeding, late infection such as an abscess, or joint replacement for aseptic necrosis. Two reviews of surgery in heart transplant patients found that cholecystectomy was the commonest general surgical procedure and may be related to altered bile metabolism caused by ciclosporin (Yee et al 1990, Melendez et al 1991).

PATHOPHYSIOLOGY

The two main concerns for the anesthesiologist are:
- The denervated heart
- The consequences of chronic immunosuppressive therapy (Kanter & Samuels 1977, Shaw et al 1991).

The denervated heart responds to stress by increasing cardiac output from increased preload and later by direct effects of circulating catecholamines. Changes in heart rate are late and occur from the direct effects of catecholamines. The denervated heart is preload dependent, making regional anaesthesia potentially problematic, and making the heart rate an unreliable guide to the patient's volume status and the adequacy of anaesthesia. Vasodilators can be hazardous, because they may cause a fall in cardiac output without an increase in heart rate. Myocardial depressants should also be used with care as the denervated heart typically increases cardiac output by increasing stroke volume rather than rate. When treating bradycardia and hypotension in these patients, direct-acting drugs such as isoprenaline are more efficacious than indirect agents such as atropine or drugs with mixed effects such as ephedrine. The transplanted heart typically has a high resting heart rate because it is denervated from its vagal tone. It also has a higher density of α and β receptors due to denerva-

tion upregulation. Despite this experimental finding, there is no clinical evidence of hypersensitivity to catecholamines. Dysrhythmias are not common in transplanted hearts; however, they are more common in the first 6 months and are associated with episodes of rejection. Hypertension is not uncommon in heart transplant recipients. Ciclosporin is nephrotoxic and many patients have mild renal insufficiency and hypertension, and are often on vasodilating agents. Myocardial ischaemia will probably be painless, and transplanted hearts are prone to atherosclerosis. Ventricular function is generally good, unless there is rejection.

THE EFFECT OF DRUGS

Drugs that have direct actions on the heart are not affected by the presence of a transplanted heart. Drugs that have indirect actions (mediated by the autonomic nervous system) will not have their ordinary effects on the transplanted heart. Drugs with mixed actions (both direct and indirect) will have their full effects attenuated by the absence of innervation. Phenylephrine has no direct cardiac effects; however, it has a direct effect on the peripheral vessels. In the normal circulation, vagal innervation slows the heart when the pressure increases due to vasoconstriction. In the transplant patient, phenylephrine results in increased blood pressure, but no reflex decrease in heart rate (Table 4.6).

PREOPERATIVE ASSESSMENT

The heart transplant patient should be evaluated carefully for evidence of rejection, especially before elective surgical procedures. Most transplant patients undergo frequent evaluations of the function of their heart, and often

TABLE 4.6

Effect of various drugs on the normal and transplanted heart

	Action	Heart rate		Pressure	
		Normal	Transplant	Normal	Transplant
Atropine	Indirect	Increase	None	None	None
Neostigmine	Indirect	Decrease	None	None	None
Ephephrine	Both	Increase	Small increase	Increase	Small increase
Adrenaline (epinephrine)	Direct	Increase	Increase	Increase	Increase
Phenylephrine	Direct	Decrease	None	Increase	Increase

present with extensive information. Endo-myocardial biopsies are performed regularly, and most centres perform yearly coronary angiography to look for new coronary disease. Both liver and renal function should be evaluated before surgery, in addition to routine blood tests, chest radiography and ECG.

PERIOPERATIVE MANAGEMENT

Strict sterile technique needs to be observed at all times. Virtually all anaesthetic techniques have been used with success in heart transplant recipients. Despite concerns about the preload dependence of the denervated heart, conduction anaesthesia has been used successfully in conjunction with administering a moderate amount of intravenous fluids prior to the block (Melendez et al 1991, Shaw et al 1991). Thiopental and propofol are not contraindicated, but the dose should be reduced. Isoflurane has been advocated for maintenance of anaesthesia owing to its absence of significant myocardial depression. However, other inhalational agents have also been used successfully.

Fluids are used to maintain preload. Most patients are haemodynamically stable during surgery, as long as they are not undergoing acute rejection. The major haemodynamic differences that can be observed are the absence of immediate haemodynamic response to tracheal intubation and surgical incision, as well as a slowly progressive increase in heart rate during surgery, which is probably secondary to increasing levels of circulating catecholamines (Melendez et al 1991). Invasive monitoring is therefore not needed due to the presence of a transplanted heart *per se*, but is dictated by the procedure being performed.

Several studies have suggested that ciclosporin may have effects both on sedative drugs as well as neuromuscular blocking agents. However, clinical observations of delayed awakening from anaesthesia have not been described, despite this experimental concern. Care must be taken, however, in the use of muscle relaxants, because the preservative in ciclosporin potentates the block and may make reversal difficult if normal doses are given. Reduced doses and careful monitoring are used. If careful monitoring is used, this complication can also be avoided (Melendez et al

1991). The chronic use of steroids means that prophylactic stress doses of steroids are necessary. OKT-3 has no known interactions with anaesthetic agents. Azathioprine may cause resistance to muscle relaxants; however, the effects of ciclosporin are more relevant and overdose is more commonly seen than resistance to neuromuscular blocking agents. Common anaesthetic problems must be watched for in these patients. Ventilation and oxygenation must be maintained, and cannot be lost sight of while worrying about the transplanted heart.

POSTOPERATIVE PERIOD

- Prompt extubation of trachea.
- Resume immunosuppression (Shaw et al 1991):
  —oral, if possible, at preoperative doses
  —intravenous if nil-by-mouth
  —azathioprine – same as oral dose
  —ciclosporin – 25% of oral dose twice daily over 6 h
  —methylprednisolone – 0.8 of oral dose of prednisolone.

Ciclosporin blood levels should be monitored carefully, aiming for blood levels of 150–250 mg ml^{-1}.

BIBLIOGRAPHY

IHLTS. The registry of the International Heart and Lung Transplantation Society: tenth official report – 1993. Journal of Heart and Lung Transplantation 1993; 12:541–548

Kanter SF, Samuels SI. Anesthesia for major operations on patients who have transplanted hearts. A review of 29 cases. Anesthesiology 1977; 46:65–68

Melendez JA, Delphin E, Lamb J, Rose E. Noncardiac surgery in heart transplant recipients in the cyclosporin era. Journal of Cardiothoracic and Vascular Anesthesia 1991; 5:218–220

Shaw IH, Kirk AJB, Conacher ID. Anaesthesia for patients with transplanted hearts and lungs undergoing non-cardiac surgery. British Journal of Anaesthesia 1991; 67:772–778

Yee J, Petsikas D, Ricci MA, Guerraty A. General surgical procedures after heart transplantation. Canadian Journal of Surgery 1990; 33:185–188

4

Hypertension

M. Y. Aglan

DEFINITION

Systemic hypertension is diagnosed by the physical finding of an increase in blood pressure.

INCIDENCE

Hypertension is a silent killer. It afflicts nearly one-third of the adult population and half of the elderly. Nearly 30% of patients undergoing non-cardiac surgery have a history of hypertension.

AETIOLOGY

- 95% primary or essential hypertension
- 5% secondary hypertension, e.g.:
  —chronic renal failure
  —endocrine – adrenocortical hyperfunction, phaeochromocytoma.

SIGNIFICANCE

Major concerns for the anaesthetist:
- Hypertension affects end organs – heart, kidney and brain

- Association with other atheromatous artery disease – cerebral, coronary and peripheral
- Antihypertensive drug interactions, with each other and with anaesthetic agents
- Role of the anaesthetist as a screen for the patient.

PATHOPHYSIOLOGY

Sustained rise in blood pressure leads to adaptive muscular hypertrophy in both the arterioles and left ventricle. Following LaPlace's law, this results in two major pathophysiological changes: high systemic vascular resistance (SVR) and left ventricular hypertrophy (LVH) (Fig. 4.4).

SHOULD ELECTIVE SURGERY BE POSTPONED?

For rational guidelines, five important debatable questions need to be addressed.

1. IS THE PATIENT HYPERTENSIVE?
There is no physiological dividing line between normotension and hypertension.
- The WHO criterion is blood pressure grater than 160/90 mmHg.

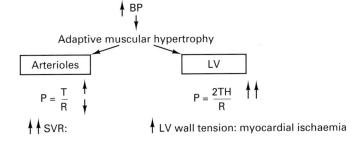

Fig. 4.4 Physiological effects of hypertension.

- A good definition is the level at which the benefits of action exceed the risks of inaction.

Considering this, the Fourth Joint National Committee on Detection, Evaluation and Treatment of High Blood Pressure classified hypertension as:

- Mild: diastolic BP 90–104 mmHg
- Moderate: diastolic BP 104–114 mmHg
- Severe: diastolic BP > 115 mmHg.

The Committee also stressed the significance of systolic BP. However, systolic BP increases progressively with age (Fig. 4.5). Good rules of thumb are:

Age + 110 = Upper limit of normal
Age + 130 = Significantly high systolic BP

2. ARE HYPERTENSIVES AT HIGHER RISK?

- Dagnino & Prys-Roberts (1989) have shown that the incidence of postoperative myocardial infarction or reinfarction in hypertensive patients was almost consistently double that observed in normotensives.
- Systolic BP increases are a better determinant of risk (strokes, myocardial infarction) than diastolic BP.

3. DOES TREATMENT MATTER?

- *Severe* untreated hypertensive patients have greater variations in BP and a greater incidence of myocardial ischaemia and dysrhythmias.
- *Mild or moderate* untreated hypertension is more controversial. However, it seems that the presence of end-organ involvement increases the risk, and controlling treatment does matter.

- *Mild* untreated hypertension is associated with a high incidence of myocardial ischaemia during intubation and emergence from anaesthesia.

4. IS SHORT-TERM 'COSMETIC' THERAPY SUFFICIENT?

Acute treatment with vasodilatation reduces the BP reading but does not alter the reactivity of blood vessels. Treatment should be given for several weeks to bring the regression of the curve back to normal (Fig. 4.6).

5. IS LOCAL ANAESTHESIA A SAFE ALTERNATIVE?

- Spinal or epidural – untreated hypertensives respond with a greater and unpredictable decrease in BP than do treated patients.
- Local infiltration or nerve block – this seems to be a simpler and safer technique; however, the possibility of inadequate block should be borne in mind.

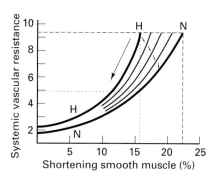

Fig. 4.6 Is short-term therapy sufficient?

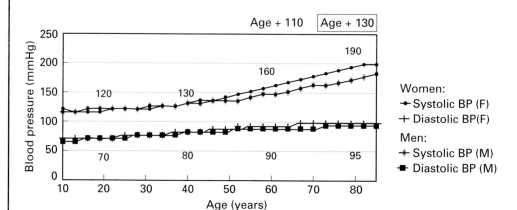

Fig. 4.5 Age- and sex-adjusted blood pressure.

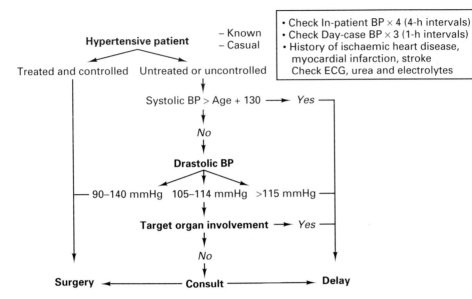

Fig. 4.7 Plan of action.

PLAN OF ACTION

See Figure 4.7.
- Confirm that it is *sustained high BP* (you need at least three abnormal readings) and not 'white coat syndrome':
  —Inpatient: four BP measurements at 4-h intervals
  —Day case: three BP measurements at 1-h intervals.
- Look for *evidence of end-organ involvement*:
  —History of ischaemic heart disease, myocardial infarction, transient ischaemic attack or stroke.
  —Check ECG for left ventricular hypertrophy, and urea and electrolyte levels for renal involvement.
- Assess the *severity of systolic BP* – a better determinant of risk.
- Assess the *severity of diastolic BP* – for moderate uncontrolled group with no end-organ involvement, the decision will depend on:
  —Experience of the anaesthetist
  —Duration and type of operation
  —Other medical conditions – obesity, diabetes mellitus, chronic obstructive airway disease.
- *Delay* the operation:
  —Educate – the disease can be treated to improve quality of life
  —Consult a cardiologist to investigate and control BP
  —Inform the general practitioner.

MANAGEMENT

AIM
Optimise perfusion so that end-organ ischaemia does not occur.

PREOPERATIVE:
- Continue antihypertensive medication, even during fasting period
- Adequate rehydration, as patients are relatively volume deficient.

PREMEDICATION:
- Anxiolytic
- Beta-blocker or clonidine may protect against myocardial ischaemia.

PERIOPERATIVE:
- Avoid stress response to laryngoscopy, intubation and extubation – intravenous opioid, lidocaine (lignocaine) or esmolol
- Control BP and heart rate within the range of adequate preoperative values
- Avoid hypoxaemia, hypercapnia, hypothermia and haemodynamic fluctuations.

POSTOPERATIVE:
- Adequate analgesia
- Continue monitoring (on HDU) for severe uncontrolled hypertension
- Resume medication as soon as possible.

BIBLIOGRAPHY

Dagnino J, Prys-Roberts C. Strategy for patients with hypertensive heart disease. Bailliere's Clinical Anaesthesiology 1989; 3:261–289

Goldman L, Caldera DL. Risks of general anaesthesia and elective operation in hypertensive patients. Anesthesiology 1979; 50:285–292

Hulyakar AR, Miller ED. Evaluation of the hypertensive patient. In: Rogers MC, Tinker JH, Covino BG, Longnecker DE, eds. Principles and practice of anesthesiology. St Louis: Mosby-Year Book; 1993:155–167

CROSS-REFERENCES

Preoperative assessment of pulmonary risk
    Anaesthetic Factors 27: 638
Preoperative assessment of cardiovascular risk
    27: 634

4

5

GI TRACT
B. J. Pollard

Carcinoid syndrome

B. J. Pollard

Carcinoid syndrome is caused by peptides, particularly serotonin (5-hydroxytryptamine or 5-HT) and bradykinin, which reach the systemic circulation in abnormally high concentrations after release by carcinoid tumours. It occurs in approximately 8 per 100 000 population.

PATHOPHYSIOLOGY

Carcinoid tumours are derived from argentaffin cells and may occur in several locations, such as bronchus and pancreas, although 75% are found in the gastrointestinal tract, most commonly in the appendix. Appendiceal tumours are usually benign and non-secreting. The amines and peptides responsible for the symptoms of carcinoid syndrome are produced by malignant tumours. Up to 20 peptides and amines have been isolated examples are serotonin, bradykinin (which is derived from kallikrein), histamine, somatostatin, prostaglandins, vasoactive peptide and substance P. However, only about 7–18% of people with carcinoid tumours exhibit carcinoid syndrome, because peptides are produced by only 25% of malignant tumours and these are normally cleared from the portal circulation by the liver if the tumour is in the gastrointestinal tract. Carcinoid syndrome is usually associated with ileal tumours with liver secondaries which secrete peptides directly into the hepatic veins. Bronchial tumours release peptides that bypass the portal circulation, resulting in symptoms at an earlier stage.

PREOPERATIVE EVALUATION

Patients should have had computed tomography (CT) or magnetic resonance imaging (MRI) to determine the site of the tumour and the possible existence of metastases. Symptoms are caused by:
- The primary tumour:
  —intestinal obstruction
  —haemoptysis.
- Right heart valve lesions.
- The systemic effects of peptides released by the tumour.

Serotonin:
- Watery diarrhoea (75% of patients) associated with cramps may be severe, resulting in dehydration, hyponatraemia, hypokalaemia and hypochloraemia. Malabsorption with steatorrhoea and hypoproteinaemia is less common.
- Pallor.
- Hypertension – 5-HT stimulates the release and inhibits the uptake of noradrenaline (norepinephrine) and potentiates the response of α_1-adrenoreceptors to catecholamines.
- Tachycardia – 5-HT is a positive chromotrope.
- Hyperglycaemia.
- Right heart failure (33% of patients) due to pulmonary stenosis and tricuspid regurgitation resulting from subendocardial fibrosis.
- Raised urinary 5-hydroxyindoleacetic acid (5-HIAA) levels, which are diagnostic of carcinoid syndrome. A 24-h urinary collection is usually undertaken.

Bradykinin:
- Flushing (90% of patients) of the face and upper body increases in duration as the disease progresses.
- Hypotension.
- Bronchospasm (20% of patients), especially in previous asthmatics and in the presence of cardiac disease.

Histamine
Particularly in some patients with gastric carcinoid:
- Flushing
- Hypotension
- Bronchospasm.

PREOPERATIVE DRUG THERAPY

Preoperative drug therapy is aimed at antagonising the mediators of carcinoid syndrome or preventing their release from carcinoid tumours.

Serotonin antagonists:
- Cyproheptadine and methysergide are effective against gastrointestinal manifestations.
- Ketanserin blocks the effects of serotonin mediated by the 5-HT$_2$ receptor: vasoconstriction, bronchoconstriction and platelet aggregation. It also has adrenergic antagonist activity and reduces central sympathetic outflow, and is therefore used to treat hypertension in patients with carcinoid.

Bradykinin antagonists:
- Aprotinin inhibits the kallikrein cascade. By infusion it is used to control flushing and treat hypotension.
- Steroids (e.g. methylprednisolone) reduce the synthesis of prostaglandins, which mediate the action of bradykinin.

Histamine antagonists
H$_2$ antagonists or combination antihistamines are more effective than H$_1$ blockers on their own.

Inhibitors of mediator release by tumours:
- Somatostatin inhibits the release of mediators from carcinoid tumours. It has a short half-life and must be given by infusion.
- Octreotide, a long-acting synthetic octapeptide somatostatin analogue, has been used as a sole agent to treat diarrhoea, hypertension, hypotension and bronchospasm in patients with carcinoid syndrome. It reduces the plasma levels of mediators by inhibiting their release from carcinoid tumours.

ANAESTHETIC CONSIDERATIONS

- Hypovolaemia and electrolyte abnormalities may be significant in patients with severe diarrhoea.
- Prevent the release of mediators, i.e. somatostatin and somatostatin analogues.
- Avoid factors that can trigger carcinoid crisis by causing the release of mediators:
  —catecholamines, which may release peptides from carcinoid tumours
  —anxiety, hypercapnia, hypothermia and hypotension, which release catecholamines
  —drugs that release histamine (e.g. morphine, atracurium, suxamethonium)
  —hypertension, which causes the release of bradykinin.
- Prepare for carcinoid crisis – i.e. resistant bronchospasm and sudden variations in arterial pressure, particularly at induction of anaesthesia and when the tumour is handled.

PREOPERATIVE MANAGEMENT

- Correct fluid and electrolyte abnormalities secondary to severe diarrhoea, and consider nutritional support if malabsorption is severe.
- Echocardiography may be valuable to investigate right heart and tricuspid valve function.
- Octreotide, 100 μg subcutaneously two or three times a day for 2 weeks prior to surgery followed by 100 μg intravenously at induction of anaesthesia and a slow postoperative wean over a few days, reduces mediator release.
- Continue antagonists of serotonin, bradykinin and histamine to minimise symptoms and maintain haemodynamic stability.
- All antimediator drugs (e.g. ketanserin, cyproheptadine, somatostatin, antihistamines and aprotinin) should be available for immediate administration if required perioperatively.
- Premedication should include an anxiolytic drug and a sedative antihistamine, for example a benzodiazepine and promethazine.

PERIOPERATIVE MANAGEMENT

Monitoring starts prior to induction and should include:
- Intra-arterial blood pressure
- ECG
- Central venous pressure (CVP)
- Blood gases
- Blood sugar
- Airway pressure
- In patients with right-sided heart lesions, pulmonary hypertension must be avoided and pulmonary artery catheterisation should be considered.

5

Regional anaesthesia is relatively contraindicated, because hypotension may occur. General anaesthesia should be induced with drugs that maintain haemodynamic stability, obtund the hypertensive response to laryngoscopy and tracheal intubation, and do not release histamine. Suxamethonium and ketamine should be avoided. Volatile agents may delay recovery and cause myocardial depression, but are often used. Therefore, a technique including high-dose narcotics may be indicated for maintenance. A flow-generating ventilator may be required to overcome bronchospasm.

Hypotension should be treated with fluid guided by the CVP or with an infusion of aprotinin. Angiotensin and vasopressin have also been used. Catecholamines should not be given as they cause the release of peptides. Hypertension is controlled with intravenous ketanserin and cyproheptadine. Adrenergic receptor antagonists and clonidine have also been used, but may precipitate hypotension. Somatostatin and its analogues prevent preoperative and perioperative episodes of hypertension, hypotension and bronchospasm that may be resistant to other forms of drug therapy. An intravenous dose of octreotide may be useful in the treatment of an intraoperative carcinoid crisis.

POSTOPERATIVE MANAGEMENT

As recovery from anaesthesia in this group of patients may be delayed and close monitoring should continue, the patient should be sent to the HDU or ITU in the immediate postoperative period. If octreotide was used before operation, it should be reduced slowly over the first postoperative week.

CONCLUSION

In patients with carcinoid syndrome the severity of symptoms does not predict the severity of perioperative complications, so that patients with minor preoperative symptoms may have significant intraoperative complications. Perioperative preparation and vigilance is of great importance in the anaesthetic management of these patients. The introduction of somatostatin and its analogues has shifted the emphasis of treating perioperative carcinoid crises from antagonising mediators that have been released to inhibiting their release from carcinoid tumours altogether.

BIBLIOGRAPHY

Holdcroft A. Hormones and the gut. British Journal of Anaesthesia 2000; 85:58–68

Hughes EW, Hodkinson BP. Carcinoid syndrome: the combined use of ketanserin and octreotide in the management of an acute crisis during anaesthesia. Anaesthesia and Intensive Care 1989; 17:367–370

Quinlivan JK, Roberts WA. Intraoperative octreotide for refractory carcinoid-induced bronchospasm. Anesthesia and Analgesia 1994; 78:400–402

Veall GR, Peacock JE, Bax ND, Reilly CS. Review of the anaesthetic management of 21 patients undergoing laparotomy for carcinoid syndrome. British Journal of Anaesthesia 1994; 72:335–341

5

Chronic liver disease

R. Alcock

There are numerous causes of chronic hepatic dysfunction, but cirrhosis is the most common and its incidence is increasing. These patients present an extreme risk for surgery. Cirrhosis is the end-stage of a number of conditions including excess alcohol intake, chronic viral hepatitis, haemochromatosis and primary biliary cirrhosis.

PATHOPHYSIOLOGY

GASTROINTESTINAL TRACT:
- Portal hypertension and associated oesophageal varices
- Ascites, causing increased intra-abdominal pressure
- Delayed gastric emptying and hyperacidity
- Poor hepatocellular function with decreased drug clearance and increased free drug concentration.

CARDIOVASCULAR SYSTEM:
- Vascular shunts – arteriovenous, intrapulmonary, pleural, portosystemic
- Hyperdynamic circulation with decreased peripheral vascular resistance and increased cardiac output
- Increased circulating volume
- Low incidence of coronary artery disease.

RESPIRATORY
Patients with cirrhosis, particularly end-stage disease, have arterial hypoxaemia, due to:
- Intrapulmonary shunts (not corrected with supplementary oxygen)
- Ventilation–perfusion mismatch (correctable with supplementary oxygen)
- Restrictive defects due to pleural effusions and ascites
- Smokers (chronic obstructive airway disease).

NERVOUS SYSTEM
Encephalopathy, aggravated by sedatives and diuretics.

RENAL AND METABOLIC:
- Increased sodium and water retention
- Metabolic alkalosis with obligatory kaliuresis
- Susceptible to renal failure; acute tubular necrosis and hepatorenal failure.

BLEEDING AND CLOTTING
There are numerous causes of coagulopathy in patients with end-stage liver disease:
- Decreased production of vitamin K-dependent factors
- Decreased production of non-vitamin K-dependent factors
- Thrombocytopaenia
- Abnormal platelet function
- Hyperfibrinolysis.

PREOPERATIVE ASSESSMENT

HISTORY AND EXAMINATION:
- Associated disease – cardiomyopathy, chronic obstructive airway disease
- Degree of ascites
- Degree of encephalopathy – caution with sedatives
- Bleeding varices and Sengstaken tube
- Neomycin – may prolong neuromuscular blockade
- Cimetidine – may prolong action of drugs (e.g. fentanyl)
- Peripheral oedema
- Nutritional status.

INVESTIGATIONS:
- ECG.
- Arterial blood gases:
  —PaO_2 (if low, see whether corrected with oxygen)
  —acid–base status.
- Renal function – urea, creatinine, creatinine clearance.
- Full blood count:
  —haemoglobin
  —white cell count – look for infection
  —platelet count.

5

- Chest radiography – pleural effusions, heart size.
- Lung function – restrictive or obstructive defects.
- Biochemistry – dilutional hyponatraemia, low potassium, low albumin, raised liver enzyme levels.
- Coagulopathy:
  —prothrombin time (PT)
  —partial thromboplastin time (PTT)
  —bleeding time.
- Assess infection risk – hepatitis B and C antigens.

PREOPERATIVE PREPARATION

- Ascites should be controlled in consultation with a hepatologist.
- Improve poor nutritional status and optimise coexisting disease.
- Have adequate blood cross-matched, especially for abdominal surgery. The need for fresh frozen plasma (FFP) and cryoprecipitate should be anticipated.
- Give vitamin K for several days before operation.
- Start an intravenous infusion from the point of starvation.

PREMEDICATION

Opioids are not well tolerated. Avoid intramuscular premedication if there is a coagulopathy, and avoid drugs that rely on phase I liver metabolism. Oral lorazepam is an effective anxiolytic. Anticholinergic drugs can be prescribed if necessary. Acid aspiration prophylaxis should be given.

PERIOPERATIVE MANAGEMENT

MONITORING
Routine:
- ECG
- Pulse oximetry
- Temperature
- Urinary catheter (hourly urine output)
- Blood pressure – non-invasive or direct
- Capnography
- Neuromuscular monitoring.

All but minor surgery:
- Arterial line:
  —hourly arterial blood gases
  —haemoglobin

  —sodium and potassium
  —glucose
  —calcium
  —clotting studies.
- CVP/pulmonary artery catheter may be useful.

INDUCTION
Appropriate prophylactic antibiotics should be given before surgery. Thiopental, etomidate or propofol are all satisfactory for induction.

The action of suxamethonium may be prolonged in severe disease, but avoidance must be weighed against the increased risk of aspiration in these patients. Use suxamethonium if necessary.

MAINTENANCE
Intubation and ventilation for all but minor procedures, avoiding hypocapnia. If using a technique based around volatile agents, desflurane or isoflurane is satisfactory. Propofol infusion is a suitable alternative. Pharmacokinetics remain normal except in patients with severe cirrhosis, where dosage must be titrated against effect. Supplement cautiously with fentanyl or alfentanil. Remifentanil is a useful alternative. Nitrous oxide is best avoided during abdominal procedures as bowel distension can make surgery more difficult. Atracurium and cisatracurium are ideal muscle relaxants.

URINE OUTPUT
Maintenance of urine output is of paramount importance:
- Aim to maintain output at above 50 ml h^{-1} in adults.
- Crystalloid infusion during surgery (5% dextrose or dextrose–saline). Avoid excessive volumes of saline solutions.
- 100-ml boluses of 20% mannitol.
- Loop diuretics should be used with caution.

COAGULOPATHY
During major surgery with marked blood loss, regular assessment of clotting should guide replacement therapy. Laboratory tests such as PT, PTT and platelet count may be used, but thromboelastography has also been found to be a reliable and effective guide to blood product requirements.

Blood product usage can be reduced by giving intraoperative aprotinin, which decreases the hyperfibrinolysis seen in these patients. Aprotinin is given as a loading dose of 2 million units intravenously, followed by an infusion of 500 000 units per h.

TABLE 5.1

Pugh's modification of Child's classification of risk for cirrhotic patients undergoing surgery: low risk < 6 points, moderate risk 7–9 points, high risk > 10 points

Clinical and biochemical measurements	Points scored for increasing abnormality		
	1	2	3
Encephalopathy (grade)	None	1 or 2	3 or 4
Ascites	Absent	Controlled	Not controlled
Albumin (g l^{-1})	> 35	28–35	< 28
Prothrombin time, prolonged (s)	1–4	4–6	> 6
Bilirubin (μmol l^{-1})	< 40	40–50	> 50

TEMPERATURE

Avoid hypothermia. The use of a warming mattress and warm air blanket, and the warming of all fluids, is vital.

POSTOPERATIVE MANAGEMENT

- Analgesia – opiates are best administered intravenously either by infusion or via a patient-controlled system. Regional analgesia is worth considering, provided there is no coagulopathy. Non-steroidal analgesics are not currently recommended, although cyclo-oxygenase (COX) 2 inhibitors may prove to be safe.
- Elective ventilation should be considered for:
  —prolonged surgery
  —severe blood loss
  —continuing haemorrhage
  —hypothermia.

Careful monitoring of urine output, coagulation, and the administration of analgesia and supplementary oxygen is best carried out in a HDU.

OUTCOME

The leading causes of death in the surgical patient are:

- Infection
- Liver failure
- Renal failure
- Haemorrhage.

There have been few studies on survival not involving surgery for portosystemic shunts or bleeding oesophageal varices. The Pugh score divides patients into three groups, classifying them as good, moderate and poor surgical risks (Table 5.1).

Other factors associated with a high mortality rate include:

- Respiratory failure
- Cardiac failure
- Infection, particularly intra-abdominal
- Emergency surgery.

BIBLIOGRAPHY

Mallett S, Cox D. Thromboelastography. British Journal of Anaesthesia 1992; 69:307–313

Pugh RNH, Murray-Lyon IM, Dawson JL, Pietroni MC, Williams R. Transection of the oesophagus for bleeding oesophageal varices. British Journal of Surgery 1973; 60:646–649

CROSS-REFERENCES

The full stomach
    Patient Conditions 5: 164

5

Disorders of the oesophagus and of swallowing

B. J. Pollard

Disorders of the oesophagus and the swallowing mechanism present hazards to the patient undergoing anaesthesia because mechanisms to clear the pharynx of foreign material and keep it clear may be compromised.

PATHOPHYSIOLOGY

ANATOMICAL:
- *Hiatus hernia* results in compromise to the functional integrity of the lower oesophageal sphincter.
- *Pharyngeal pouch and other diverticulae* in the oesophagus may contain solid food particles or fluid for many hours after ingestion. They may also contain partially putrefied food. Discharge of the contents of the pouch may occur with changes in posture, or unexpectedly, and present an aspiration risk.
- *Tracheo-oesophageal fistula* – a direct communication between the trachea and oesophagus.
- *Tumours of the oesophagus* usually present with dysphagia, which may be partial or complete at the time of surgery. Residual food particles may remain in the oesophagus, as may liquid in the case of complete aphagia. Where obstruction is complete, the patient will not be able to clear saliva.
- *Achalasia of the cardia* is characterised by a hypertrophy of the muscular layer at the lower end of the oesophagus, resulting in increasing obstruction to the passage of material into the stomach. Although the risk of regurgitation is very low in these patients, the oesophagus may be greatly dilated above the obstruction and may contain significant volumes of swallowed material. This may be demonstrated on a preoperative barium swallow. The dilated oesophagus does not contain stomach acid.

PHYSIOLOGICAL:
- *Oesophageal motility* is reduced in scleroderma. The lower oesophageal sphincter is functionally incompetent in these patients, and this may result in reflux of gastric contents into the oesophagus. A history of heartburn can often be elicited, but is absent in patients taking omeprazole.
- *Neurogenic cerebrovascular accident*.

PREOPERATIVE ASSESSMENT

The history should determine whether or not obstruction of the oesophagus is present and whether the patient can swallow liquid without regurgitation. A history of regurgitation of solid material hours after food suggests the presence of either a diverticulum or a dilatation above an obstruction. In the case of a pharyngeal pouch, the patient may be able to prevent filling of the pouch or empty it by pressure on the neck. Prolonged avoidance of solid food allowing free fluids may help to clear solid material. A nasogastric tube placed in the oesophagus may be useful in achalasia of the cardia.

PREMEDICATION

Antacids are of no value in oesophageal obstruction. However, where surgery relieves an obstruction, reflux of stomach acid may occur after operation.

Drying agents are beneficial if the patient is unable to swallow saliva.

ANAESTHETIC MANAGEMENT

- Rapid sequence induction of anaesthesia is required where the oesophagus may not be empty at the time of induction.

- In the case of pharyngeal pouches, the source of the risk is above the cricoid cartilage and cricoid pressure is of no value. Induction of anaesthesia in the lateral position should be considered with the pouch dependent.
- Intubation of the trachea with a cuffed tube is required for protection of the airway. For oesophageal tumour resections, a double-lumen tube may be required.
- If the patient is unable to swallow saliva, induction in the lateral position should be considered.

POSTOPERATIVE MANAGEMENT

- Extubate the trachea with the patient awake and in the lateral position, as the risk to the airway may persist into the postoperative period.
- After intubation of an oesophageal tumour, reflux of stomach acid may occur through the tube.
- Surgery for achalasia of the cardia may render the lower oesophageal sphincter incompetent and be followed by acid reflux in the postoperative period.
- Full competence of the protective laryngeal reflexes may take several hours to return.

5

The full stomach

B. J. Pollard

The avoidance of aspiration of gastric contents into the airway is of paramount importance during the administration of anaesthesia. Aspiration of solid material may cause obstruction of the airway, leading to asphyxia, lobar pneumonia or lung abscess formation. Irritation of the vocal cords during light anaesthesia by regurgitated material may cause laryngeal spasm, and aspiration of as little as 25 ml liquid of pH < 2.5 may cause bronchospasm, pneumonitis, bronchopneumonia and adult respiratory distress syndrome.

PATHOPHYSIOLOGY

Both the active process of vomiting and the passive process of regurgitation of gastric contents present a hazard in a patient with a full stomach. Vomiting is a hazard at induction, during recovery, and when anaesthesia is light. Regurgitation is a hazard immediately after induction and throughout maintenance, and may occur silently. Regurgitation is predisposed to by a full stomach and any reduction in the functional integrity of the lower oesophageal sphincter (LOS).

FAILURE OF PREPARATION
The rate of emptying of the stomach after oral intake is variable. No patient can ever be assumed to have a completely empty stomach. In general, for a normal healthy patient, stomach emptying is complete within 6 h after food, 4 h after most liquids and 2 h after water.

DELAYED GASTRIC EMPTYING:
- Obstruction of the gastrointestinal tract:
  —pyloric stenosis
  —tumours.
- Ileus:
  —postoperative
  —metabolic.
- Peritonitis of any cause.
- Pain.
- Fear or anxiety.

- Pregnancy (third trimester).
- Drugs:
  —opiates
  —alcohol.

REFLUX OF MATERIAL FROM THE BOWEL
In prolonged intestinal obstruction, feculent material may enter the stomach retrogradely.

LOWER OESOPHAGEAL SPHINCTER:
- Increased pressure zone (not anatomically distinct)
- Pinch-cock action of the diaphragm
- Mucosal one-way valve.

PREOPERATIVE ASSESSMENT

HISTORY:
- Last oral intake of food/drink, especially alcohol
- Possibility of swallowed blood
- Factors known to delay gastric emptying
- History of reflux, heartburn or hiatus hernia
- Drugs known to reduce LOS tone:
  —alcohol, opiates
  —anticholinergics
  —tricyclics
  —dopamine
  —β agonists.

PREPARATION
Delay surgery where possible to allow time for the stomach to empty. Induction of vomiting is not normally practical, and residual emetic tendency at the time of induction is dangerous. Passing a nasogastric tube and aspirating gastric contents may not be fully effective, but in the case of liquid contents will reduce intragastric pressure and thus the tendency to regurgitate. At the time of induction the presence of the tube may compromise the function of the LOS, and gastric contents may leak past it and enter the oesophagus. Administration of a non-particulate acid-neutralising drug (sodium citrate) offers protection from the effects of

acid aspiration, but does not protect against regurgitation. Administration of an H_2-blocking drugs or a proton pump inhibitor may offer protection only if the acid in the stomach has already been neutralised. Administration of prokinetic drugs such as metoclopramide may increase the rate of gastric emptying. Metoclopramide also increases the LOS tone. Anticholinergic drugs do not reliably increase gastric pH.

PERIOPERATIVE MANAGEMENT

PREMEDICATION
Avoid opiates and anticholinergics – both reduce LOS tone and delay gastric emptying.

ANAESTHETIC MANAGEMENT
Management of the induction of anaesthesia depends on the cause of the full stomach and clinical circumstances. Intubation of the trachea with a cuffed tube in order both to secure and to protect the airway is required.

In most cases a rapid sequence induction with full preoxygenation and cricoid pressure is preferred. In the case of blood in the stomach where bleeding into the airway is responsible (e.g. post-tonsillectomy bleeding) an inhalation induction with the patient in the lateral position and tilted head-down is safest. (NB: Although suxamethonium increases intragastric pressure, it also increases LOS tone.) Head-up tilt may reduce the incidence of regurgitation, but predisposes to aspiration of any material in the pharynx into the lungs. Emptying of the stomach during anaesthesia with a gastric tube should be considered. Emergence from anaesthesia carries the same potential hazards as induction, and the patient should be placed in the lateral position before anaesthesia is terminated. The trachea should be extubated only on return of protective airway reflexes.

POSTOPERATIVE MANAGEMENT

- Risk continues until larynx is competent
- Gastric emptying is delayed by pain and opiates
- Maintain lateral position
- Avoid sedative agents.

BIBLIOGRAPHY

Maltby JR. Preoperative Fasting. Current Anaesthesia and Critical Care 1996; 7:276–280

5

Hiatus hernia

B. J. Pollard

Hiatus hernia is a condition caused by migration of a portion of the stomach through the oesophageal hiatus in the diaphragm. It is common, particularly in later life.

Two forms are usually described: the sliding type (85% of cases), in which the gastro-oesophageal junction passes into the thorax, and the rolling type, where the stomach itself migrates into the thorax, the gastro-oesophageal junction remaining in the abdomen.

A higher incidence of hiatus hernia is associated with the following:

- Increasing age
- Obesity
- Pregnancy.

Although often associated with symptoms of reflux oesophagitis, a hiatus hernia may be symptomless. Equally, reflux oesophagitis may occur in the absence of hiatus hernia. Reflux is associated with decreased pressure in the lower oesophageal sphincter (LOS).

TABLE 5.2

Drugs affecting lower oesophageal sphincter pressure

Increase LOS pressure	Decrease LOS pressure
Antiemetics:	Anticholinergics:
Metoclopramide	Atropine
Prochlorperazine	Glycopyrrolate
Domperidone	Thiopental
Anticholinesterases:	Opioids
Neostigmine	Alcohol
Edrophonium	Nicotine
α-Receptor agonists	Dopamine
Histamine	α-Receptor antagonists
Suxamethonium	β-Receptor agonists
	Tricyclic antidepressants
	Ganglion blockers

LOWER OESOPHAGEAL SPHINCTER

The LOS is an anatomically indistinct area of the oesophagus found around the diaphragmatic hiatus, 3–5 cm long, detectable as a high-pressure zone by manometry. It is usually closed at rest. The important variable is not LOS tone, but barrier pressure (LOS pressure – gastric pressure). Reflux is unlikely to occur if barrier pressure is greater than 13 cmH$_2$O, although there is wide variation between individuals.

The normal response to an increase in gastric pressure is an increase in LOS pressure, but this adaptation is lost in those who develop reflux. The response is decreased by atropine, vagotomy, and in symptomatic pregnant women at term. Drugs affecting LOS pressure are shown in Table 5.2.

Of greater anaesthetic relevance is symptomatic evidence of gastric reflux rather than the presence of a hiatus hernia.

PREOPERATIVE ASSESSMENT

HISTORY:

- Epigastric or retrosternal pain and heartburn, promoted by bending or lying down, pregnancy or obesity, relieved by antacids (sliding type)
- Discomfort or 'crushing' chest pain due to distension of the stomach with food (rolling type – symptoms of reflux are unusual)
- Waterbrash and reflux of bitter fluid into the pharynx and mouth
- Dysphagia – rare, and usually denotes oesophageal stenosis; may prevent further regurgitation and therefore produces a reduction in symptoms
- Nocturnal cough – suggesting regurgitation and aspiration; may lead to aspiration pneumonitis.

INVESTIGATIONS:

- Full blood count – chronic blood loss is common, resulting in iron deficiency anaemia

- Chest radiography – to exclude aspiration pneumonia
- Barium studies.

PERIOPERATIVE MANAGEMENT

PREMEDICATION
Consideration should be given to the preoperative use of antacids, proton pump inhibitors or H_2- receptor antagonists, if not already prescribed. If the patient is symptomatic, opioids should be used with caution. As anticholinergic drugs cause a reduction in LOS pressure, which may make regurgitation more likely, careful consideration must be given to their use as part of premedication. Metoclopramide or domperidone will increase LOS pressure and negate the effects of anticholinergic drugs.

AIRWAY
If the patient is asymptomatic, if there are no factors present likely to increase the risk of regurgitation, and if the operation itself is short and does not require tracheal intubation, then spontaneous ventilation using a laryngeal mask following antacid premedication may be considered.

However, if there is any doubt about the patient's safety, full precautions to prevent regurgitation and aspiration of stomach contents must be employed, i.e. preoxygenation, rapid sequence induction with cricoid pressure, and tracheal intubation. This is mandatory when the hiatus hernia is symptomatic.

EMERGENCE
Ensure emergence and extubation with the patient in the lateral position.

POSTOPERATIVE MANAGEMENT

Semirecumbent or sitting position, when practical.

BIBLIOGRAPHY

Pollard BJ, Lipscomb GR. Gastrointestinal disorders. In: Vickers MD, Power I, eds. Medicine for anaesthetists. 4th edn. 1999, Oxford: Blackwell; 1999:175–191

Stoelting RK, Dierdof SF. Anaesthesia and co-existing disease. 4th edn. New York: Churchill Livingstone; 2002

CROSS-REFERENCES

Obesity
  Patient Conditions 5: 173

5

The jaundiced patient

B. J. Pollard

In the jaundiced patient presenting for surgery, liver disease may be divided into:
- Hepatocellular
- Cholestatic (obstructive).

Causes of hepatocellular jaundice include toxins, viruses and drugs. Surgery in this group carries a poor prognosis and must be avoided – emergency procedures only.

Cholestasis may be extrahepatic – obstruction commonly caused by calculus, stricture and cancer – or intrahepatic. Viral hepatitis may mimic intrahepatic obstruction (hence the importance of serology). Drugs may cause a hypersensitivity hepatitis (e.g. chlorpromazine, carbamazepine, erythromycin, imipramine, azathioprine) or present a pure intrahepatic cholestatic picture (e.g. synthetic oestrogens). Presentation for surgery is not uncommon. Aetiology is difficult to ascertain clinically.

Complications of surgery increase with:
- Haematocrit < 30% on presentation
- Plasma bilirubin level > 200 mmol l^{-1}
- Presence of malignancy
- Duration of jaundice – secondary biliary cirrhosis develops.

ASSOCIATED PROBLEMS

ACUTE OLIGURIC RENAL FAILURE
Occurs in 9% of all jaundiced patients undergoing surgery, with a mortality rate of 50%; 75% will have a fall in glomerular filtration rate after operation. Factors implicated include:
- Hypovolaemia and hypotension
- Presence of bile salts
- Bilirubin
- Endotoxins.

Glomerular and peritubular fibrin deposition has been demonstrated in affected kidneys. Hepatorenal syndrome may occur, associated with deterioration of hepatic function.

COAGULOPATHY
Vitamin K deficiency reduces clotting factors 2, 7, 9 and 10 (exacerbated by cholestyramine) and prolongs prothrombin time (> 4 s above control is abnormal), but hepatocellular coagulopathy is refractory to vitamin K administration. Disseminated intravascular coagulation (DIC) is associated with secondary biliary tract infection (and possibly endotoxaemia) and increases mortality.

ALTERED DRUG HANDLING
Drugs excreted via the biliary system have a prolonged elimination half-life in cholestasis. Increased volume of distribution and reduced clearance produces initial pancuronium resistance. Repeated dosing is associated with prolongation of action. Atracurium is the drug of choice for paralysis. Narcotics may produce spasm in the sphincter of Oddi (biliary colic and difficulty with cholangiography).

Pseudocholinesterase has a very long half-life, and suxamethonium apnoea is not a feature, even in fulminant liver failure, although the duration of action of a dose of suxamethonium may be longer than expected.

GASTROINTESTINAL TRACT
Stress ulceration occurs, with gastrointestinal haemorrhage demonstrated in 16% of cases.

WOUND HEALING
This is significantly reduced, and correlates closely with degree of malnutrition and the presence of sepsis and malignancy.

PREOPERATIVE ASSESSMENT

HISTORY AND CLINICAL EXAMINATION
Look for malnutrition, malignancy, anaemia, dehydration, deep jaundice, pyrexia, signs of drug abuse, concomitant diseases.

INVESTIGATIONS:
- Haemoglobin – at presentation and current
- White cell count – cholangitis, isolates and sensitivities

- Platelet count – reduced with severe infection and DIC
- Clotting screen – note effect of vitamin K administration
- Urea, electrolytes, creatinine, glucose – creatinine clearance if poor or deteriorating renal function
- Serum bilirubin – beware if less than 200 mmol l⁻¹
- Serum albumin, calcium and magnesium
- Serum transaminases – raised in hepatocellular dysfunction
- Blood gases – respiratory alkalosis and hypoxaemia
- Serology – consider risks to staff
- Biopsy – pattern and degree of damage.

PREOPERATIVE PREPARATION

Depends on severity of disease. Commonly required preparation involves:
- Rehydration
- Appropriate cross-match and preoperative transfusion
- Perioperative antibiotic administration
- Administration of vitamin K
- If PT remains abnormal, arrange clotting factors
- H_2 antagonist drugs
- Urinary catheter early
- Optimisation of concurrent disease
- Percutaneous drainage – symptoms improve, prognosis unaltered.

Administration of taurocholate and selective gut decontamination are controversial.

PREMEDICATION:
- Anxiolysis is useful; if there is coagulopathy avoid intramuscular route
- With hepatocellular disease, consider duration of action of drugs
- Avoid sedatives in encephalopathy
- Continue H_2 antagonist and vitamin K.

PERIOPERATIVE MANAGEMENT

Poor prognosis may relate to reduction in hepatic blood flow associated with general anaesthetics, and total hepatic necrosis may occur. Renal insult must be avoided. Therefore, stable anaesthesia avoiding hypotension is essential. Preserve cardiac output with fluid loading. Adequate circulating volume and haematocrit are essential. Isoflurane does not have a major deleterious effect in animal models of hepatic circulation. Hyper-

carbia produces sympathetic activation; intermittent positive-pressure ventilation (IPPV) to $PaCO_2$ of 35–40 mmHg would be advisable. Altered drug metabolism depends on high and low extraction ratio and is therefore difficult to predict. Acid–base disturbance may occur; alterations in electrolytes may contribute to encephalopathy and should be monitored.

Preservation of urine output with mannitol (0.5 g kg⁻¹) and diuretics has been advocated. This should not be at the expense of circulating volume. Replace massive diuresis. Aggressive replacement of blood loss is essential. Hypoglycaemia may occur (with severe injury); monitor and treat.

In all cases a low threshold for invasive monitoring is to be recommended. In the presence of hepatocellular disease, it is essential. If resuscitation is required, a Swan–Ganz catheter sited before operation is advisable. Dopamine may be beneficial in preservation of renal function perioperatively.

Hypothermia worsens coagulopathy. Therefore, warm fluids, humidify respiratory gases, use warming blanket or warm air overblanket, and reduce body surface heat losses.

POSTOPERATIVE MANAGEMENT

Consider intensive care. Hypoxaemia is common. Drain losses should be aggressively replaced; hepatocellular disease may require additional clotting factors. Monitoring with thromboelastography is helpful. Replace urine losses appropriately. Continue dopamine until cardiovascularly stable. Catecholamines may reduce hepatic and renal blood flow. Epidural analgesia can be considered in the absence of coagulopathy. Intramuscular opiate administration is inappropriate in all but minor cases.

OUTCOME

Relates to severity of disease. Minor worsening of liver function is not uncommon; morphological change is. The following may worsen jaundice after surgery:
- Blood transfusion.
- Haemolysis.
- Hepatocellular damage:
  —postoperative cholestasis
  —circulatory failure
  —drug induced
  —exacerbated chronic disease.

5

- Extrahepatic obstruction:
  —duct stone
  —bile duct injury
  —postoperative pancreatitis.

Laparotomy in the presence of hepatocellular disease has been associated with a perioperative mortality rate of 9.5% and a morbidity rate of 12%. Approximately 25% of jaundiced patients undergoing surgery for relief of biliary obstruction have subsequently been demonstrated to have hepatocellular disease. A combination of anaemia at presentation, serum bilirubin level > 200 mmol l^{-1} and presence of malignancy carries a mortality rate of 60%.

BIBLIOGRAPHY

Dixon JM, Armstrong CP, Duffy SW, Davies GC. Factors affecting morbidity and mortality after surgery for obstructive jaundice a review of 373 patients. Gut 1983; 24:845–852

Wilkinson SP, Moodie H, Stamatakis JD et al. Endotoxaemia and renal failure in cirrhosis and obstructive jaundice. British Medical Journal 1976; 2:1415–1418

CROSS-REFERENCES

Acute renal failure
    Patient Conditions 6: 184
Open cholecystectomy
    Surgical Procedures 16: 419

5

Malnutrition

B. J. Pollard

Malnutrition occurs when protein or calorie supplies are inadequate to meet requirements; it is found in approximately 50% of surgical patients, resulting in an increased incidence of postoperative complications.

Malnutrition is defined as:

- Moderate: 15% loss of ideal bodyweight
- Severe: 30% loss of ideal bodyweight

Calculation of ideal bodyweight (IBW) (Broca's index):

- For men: IBW (kg) = Height (cm) – 100
- For women: IBW (kg) = Height (cm) – 105

PATHOPHYSIOLOGY

GENERAL EFFECTS

These include rapid weight loss; muscle wasting and fatigue; delayed ambulation following surgery, with an increased incidence of postoperative respiratory complications; bed sores and wound infections.

PULMONARY FUNCTION:

- Diaphragmatic muscle mass falls in a linear fashion with bodyweight. There is a fall in vital capacity and maximal ventilatory volume, an increased incidence of postoperative respiratory failure, and difficulty in weaning from mechanical ventilation.
- Decreased surfactant production and emphysematous changes in the lung causes alveolar atelectasis.
- Increased incidence of chest infection results from a depressed immune response, alveolar atelectasis and an ineffective cough.
- The ventilatory response to hypoxia is markedly depressed.
- The work of breathing is increased.

VISCERAL PROTEIN DEFICIENCY:

- Depletion of serum proteins, enzymes, immunoglobulins and vital organs
- Reduced cardiac output, stroke volume, contractility and reserve
- Hypoalbuminaemia results in interstitial and pulmonary oedema, and reduced binding of metabolites, drugs and toxins
- Anaemia – folate or iron deficiency, or mixed
- Low serum transferrin
- Low T lymphocyte count and function
- Impaired antibody response
- Low serum IgA
- Pseudocholinesterase deficiency in severe malnutrition (serum albumin level < 2 g dl^{-1}).

PREOPERATIVE ASSESSMENT

NUTRITIONAL ASSESSMENT

Many of the indices of malnutrition (Table 5.3) lack specificity and are poor predictors of perioperative morbidity and mortality. Immunological changes and loss of hand grip power, however, do predict those patients likely to have an increased risk of perioperative problems. Patients who demonstrate anergy at 48 h to the intradermal injection of several antigens (*Candida*, mumps, *Trichophyton*) have a marked increase in postoperative morbidity and mortality, and may benefit from preoperative nutritional support.

CLINICAL ASSESSMENT:

- Evidence of fat and muscle wasting (e.g. weight loss, fatigue, hypothermia)
- Symptoms of vitamin deficiency, such as anaemia (vitamin E) and bleeding tendency (vitamin K)
- Reduced pulmonary function (e.g. shortness of breath)
- Heart failure (e.g. peripheral oedema, orthopnoea)

5

TABLE 5.3

Nutritional evaluation

| | | Degree of malnutrition | | | |
	Normal value	Mild	Moderate	Severe	Cause of error
Weight (%)	100	80–90	70–79	< 70	
Weight loss (%)	< 0	10	10–20	> 20	Dehydration
Fat reserves					
Triceps skin fold (%)	100	80–90	60–79	< 60	Oedema
Somatic protein					
Arm muscle circumference (%)	100	80–90	60–79	< 40	Oedema
Weight (% of ideal)	100	80–90	70–79	< 70	Dehydration
Weight (% of usual)	100	90–95	80–89	< 80	Dehydration
Creatine/height index (%)	100	60–80	40–59	< 40	Renal disease
Visceral protein					
Serum albumin (g dl^{-1})	3.5–5.0	2.8–3.4	2.1–2.7	< 2.1	Liver disease
Serum transferrin (mg dl^{-1})	175–300	150–175	100–150	< 100	Trauma, surgery
Retinol-binding protein (mg dl^{-1})	3–6	2.7–3.0	2.4–2.7	< 2.4	State of hydration
Prealbumin (mg dl^{-1})	15.7–29.6	10–15	5–9.9	< 5	Increased protein loss or demand (e.g. trauma)
Total lymphocytes (mm^{-3})	1500–5000	1200–1500	800–1200	< 800	Abnormal white cell count
Cell-mediated immunity		Reactive	Relative energy	Non-reactive	Steroids, immune deficiency

- Arrhythmias
- Increased frequency of infection.

INVESTIGATIONS:
- ECG – AV block, prolonged QT interval
- Echocardiography – reduced myocardial contractility
- Pulmonary function tests – forced vital capacity 50 ml kg^{-1} in the absence of obvious lung disease; reduced maximal ventilatory volume.

PREOPERATIVE MANAGEMENT

Preoperative nutrition should be discussed with surgeons and dieticians. Enteral and total parenteral nutrition (TPN) are equally beneficial.

Examine patient for the complications associated with TPN (Box 5.1) and correct serum electrolytes and blood glucose abnormalities. TPN must not be stopped suddenly, as rebound hypoglycaemia may occur. It should be either:

BOX 5.1

Complications of TPN

- Catheter related
- Improper central line placement
- Infection
- Fluid overload
- Especially in the elderly and patients with heart failure
- Metabolic
- Hyperglycaemia
- Hypercarbia
- Hypokalaemia
- Hypomagnesaemia
- Hypophosphataemia

- Continued at the same rate, controlling hyperglycaemia perioperatively as in the diabetic patient
- Weaned to half the maintenance rate over 12 h before surgery

- Replaced by 10% glucose infused at the same rate (in unstable patients).

Blood transfusion for anaemia and correction of clotting abnormalities may be required. The impact of a low plasma albumin level and its correction with albumin solutions on postoperative outcome in the malnourished patient has yet to be shown. Endogenous albumin production should be encouraged with nutritional support. Exogenous albumin actually reduces the amount of albumin production by the liver. The effect of preoperative albumin infusions on increasing plasma oncotic pressure is ill defined, although they may play an important role as a result of increasing the binding of metabolites, drugs and toxins. Controversy exists over the routine use of albumin solutions.

PERIOPERATIVE MANAGEMENT

Monitoring includes measurement of:
- CVP
- Blood sugar
- $EtCO_2$.

Careful positioning of the patient and aseptic line placement reduces the incidence of sepsis and injury.

Controlled ventilation is indicated by preoperative pulmonary function tests. Ability to sustain head raise, forced vital capacity greater than 15 ml kg^{-1} and maximum inspiratory force greater than -25 cmH$_2$O indicate adequate muscle strength prior to extubation. The malnourished heart functions at the peak of the Starling curve, and so cardiac output may fall with increased diastolic filling, precipitating cardiac failure. Judicious fluid management with CVP monitoring may be required.

There is an increased sensitivity to:
- Intravenous induction agents
- Suxamethonium in severe malnutrition (albumin < 2.0 g dl^{-1}), as pseudocholinesterase deficiency may exist
- Non-depolarising neuromuscular blockers in the presence of hypocalcaemia, hypophosphataemia and hypomagnesaemia
- Drugs bound to albumin (e.g. diazepam)
- Drugs bound to skeletal muscle (e.g. digoxin).

POSTOPERATIVE MANAGEMENT

- ITU or HDU in patients with severely reduced cardiorespiratory reserve.

- Mechanical ventilation in the case of:
  - —fatigue
  - —increased carbon dioxide production due to glucose feed
  - —impaired response to hypoxaemia.
- Supplemental oxygen on the ward.
- Physiotherapy.
- Analgesia to allow an effective cough.
- Restart nutritional support slowly over 12–24 h after operation.
- Monitor blood glucose and serum potassium levels, and avoid hypophosphataemia.

OUTCOME

Several studies have shown an increased incidence of postoperative complications in the malnourished patient, for example respiratory complications, wound infections and bed sores. The role of preoperative and postoperative nutritional support in the malnourished patient is poorly defined. Both reduce postoperative complications and improve pulmonary function in patients with fistulae, short bowel syndrome, burns and acute renal failure, and may have a place in patients who have lost more than 20% of their usual bodyweight. For maximum nutritional benefit, feeding (whether enteral or parenteral) should be started 1 week to 10 days after surgery.

BIBLIOGRAPHY

Hill GL, Pickford I, Young GA et al. Malnutrition in surgical patients: an unrecognised problem. Lancet 1977; i:689–692

Meakins JL, Pietsch JB, Bubenick D et al. Delayed hypersensitivity: indicator of aquired failure to host defences in sepsis and trauma. Annals of Surgery 1977; 186:241–250

Meguid MM, Campos AC, Hammond WG. Nutritional support in surgical practice. American Journal of Surgery 1990; 159:345–358

Rochester DF, Arora NS. Respiratory muscle failure. Medical Clinics of North America 1983; 67:573–597

5

CROSS-REFERENCES

Pseudocholinesterase deficiency 31: 784

Obesity

J. C. Goldstone

Obesity is a chronic nutritional disorder characterised by hypertension, cardiovascular and respiratory disease, diabetes, cirrhosis and hiatus hernia. Although medical morbidity is correlated with weight, few prospective studies have been performed relating obesity and anaesthetic outcome (Fig. 5.1).

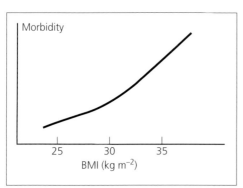

Fig. 5.1 Relationship between body mass index (BMI) and morbidity.

5

Obesity may be defined in a number of ways:

- Simple: Weight greater than 30% of ideal
- Morbid: Weight greater than 100% of ideal
             or
             Weight 45 kg in excess of ideal

Calculation of ideal bodyweight (IBW) (Broca's index):

- For men: IBW (kg) = Height (cm) − 100
- For women: IBW (kg) = Height (cm) − 105

Calculation of body mass index (BMI):

- BMI = Weight (kg)/Height^2 (m^2)

Patients with BMI > 25 are regarded as overweight
Patients with BMI > 30 are regarded as obese
Patients with BMI > 39 are morbidly obese

PATHOPHYSIOLOGY

CARDIOVASCULAR SYSTEM

In the absence of ischaemic heart disease, obesity raises end-diastolic ventricular volume, increases stroke volume, and thereby increases cardiac output. Left ventricular work rises, in part due to the increased systemic vascular resistance, and is compensated for by biventricular hypertrophy. Filling pressure and cardiac output rise promptly with exercise, which includes moving body position in the morbidly obese.

RESPIRATORY SYSTEM

Obesity acts to impose a load on the chest wall, such that the work of breathing is raised, although lung compliance, in the absence of coexisting disease, is normal. Lung volume is reduced, and falls further with recumbency. In the morbidly obese, tidal breathing falls within the closing volume range. Arterial hypoxaemia is common and increases pulmonary vascular resistance. In some morbidly obese patients (8%) the response to carbon dioxide is diminished – the obesity hypoventilation syndrome.

GUT

Both gastric acid and fasting gastric volume are raised in the obese. Abdominal pressure increases linearly with weight gain, and the incidence of hiatus hernia is high.

ENDOCRINE SYSTEM

Glucose tolerance in the obese is impaired and frank diabetes is common.

COAGULATION

Laboratory evidence of hypercoagulability is slight, although some clinical reports suggest that the incidence of deep venous thrombosis is raised.

PREOPERATIVE ASSESSMENT

MORPHOLOGICAL:
- Assessment of veins and arteries
- Airway – mouth, jaw, dentition, neck
- Posture for epidural, if appropriate
- Transportation to theatre.

HISTORY:
- Systematic review of associated cardiovascular and respiratory disease
- Obesity hypoventilation syndrome:
  —day-time somnolence, poor concentration
  —night-time respiratory obstruction
  —nightmares and restlessness.
- Right ventricular failure
- Smoking history.

INVESTIGATIONS
See Table 5.4.

TABLE 5.4

Investigations

Investigation	Result
ECG	Ventricular hypertrophy
	Ischaemia
	Evidence of pulmonary hypertension
Echocardiography	Right or left chamber enlargement
Spirometry (standing or supine)	Flow limitation
	Reduced vital capacity
	Reduced functional residual capacity (FRC)
Blood gas analysis (standing or supine)	Hypoxaemia when standing; falls when supine

PERIOPERATIVE MANAGEMENT

PREMEDICATION
Respiratory depressant drugs should be used with caution, and morbidly obese patients at risk of obesity hypoventilation syndrome should be monitored (Sao_2) and receive face-mask oxygen after premedication. Acid aspiration prophylaxis should be administered. Anticholinergic agents should be given when intubation is anticipated as being difficult.

MONITORING
This should commence in the anaesthetic room:

- ECG (lead CM5)
- Arterial cannula for invasive blood pressure
- Sao_2.

AIRWAY
Spontaneous respiration is contraindicated. Obese patients deoxygenate three to five times quicker than non-obese controls. Both face-mask ventilation and intubation may be impossible. There is an increased incidence of difficult intubation in obese patients. Controlled ventilation through a tracheal tube should be used for all procedures, including those of short duration.

When weight exceeds 75% of ideal, a suggested plan is to perform direct laryngoscopy under topical anaesthesia in the anaesthetic room prior to theatre. If the larynx cannot be seen, awake fibreoptic intubation is the safest approach.

When intubation is possible, a rapid sequence intubation should be performed. A range of intubating equipment should be available, including the polio blade. Obese patients have increased plasma levels of pseudocholinesterase, and may require increased doses of suxamethonium.

CONTROLLED VENTILATION:
- May require a volume preset constant flow generator
- Oxygenation may be impaired despite high inspired oxygen tensions and positive end-expiratory pressure (PEEP)
- Head-up tilt to reduce the abdominal pressure on the diaphragm.

Metabolism of inhaled agents is increased, and isoflurane or desflurane is therefore theoretically advantageous. The usefulness of nitrous oxide may be limited by the need for high inspired oxygen tensions.

Cardiovascular depression is likely during general anaesthesia, leading to rises in filling pressure and declining cardiac output. Aortocaval compression may occur in the supine posture, increasing systemic vascular resistance and decreasing venous return. Left ventricular function has been shown to continue to decline in the postoperative phase, in comparison with the non-obese.

Physical positioning and lifting may be impossible in the morbidly obese, requiring modifications to the theatre to accommodate heavy lifting equipment. Severe cases may require a 'dry run' to ensure that facilities are adequate.

5

REGIONAL ANAESTHESIA

Although this may be technically difficult if the bony landmarks are obscured, subarachnoid and epidural anaesthesia have been advocated in the morbidly obese. Dose requirements are generally reduced compared with those in the non-obese (75–80%). Cardiovascular decompensation has been reported in cases where the sympathetic block was variably higher than the somatic blockade. Motor blockade of the respiratory muscles limits the height of blockade to T7.

POSTOPERATIVE CARE

- Semirecumbent or sitting position
- Do not leave morbidly obese patients lying supine
- Continuous oxygen therapy
- Humidification
- Physiotherapy and early mobilisation
- Analgesia
- Deep venous thrombosis therapy
- ITU or HDU for the morbidly obese and those with cardiorespiratory disease.

OUTCOME

Although epidemiological studies have shown obesity to correlate with mortality, this is not the case with anaesthetic mortality. From the limited literature available, a similar mortality rate has been recorded for hysterectomy (1%) and gastric bypass (1.2%) when these results have been matched to non-obese controls. This is attributable to improvements in anaesthetic technique.

BIBLIOGRAPHY

Ashbaugh DG, Bigelow DB, Petty TL, Levine BE. Acute respiratory distress in adults. Lancet 1967; ii:319–323

Collighan NT, Bellamy MC. Anaesthesia for the obese patient. Current Anaesthesia and Critical Care 2001; 12:261–266

Vaughan RW, Bauer S, Wise L. Effect of position on postoperative oxygenation in markedly obese patients. Anesthesia and Analgesia 1976; 55:37–41

5

Previous liver transplant

B. J. Pollard

The first human orthotopic liver transplant (OLT) was performed in 1963. The procedure was recognised as a therapeutic procedure for end-stage liver disease in 1983. Improvements in organ preservation, surgical and anaesthetic techniques, and immunosuppression (ciclosporin initially) led to an exponential increase in centres and number of cases performed over the next decade. In 1993, more than 3500 OLTs were performed in the USA and 700 in the UK. Today, there are many thousands of patients alive who have had a successful OLT. The 1-year survival rate is 75–85% and the 5-year survival rate approaches 65%.

PATIENT CHARACTERISTICS

- Age ranges from infants to 70 years and over; the majority are 30–60 years old.
- Medical status is generally good:
  —reversal of cardiovascular and pulmonary effects of chronic liver disease (hyperdynamic circulation and shunting) reported within 3 months of OLT
  —increased incidence of renal insufficiency in OLT patients (preoperative and intraoperative factors and ciclosporin)
  —high incidence of hypertension reported after OLT.
- Normal liver function unless there is rejection, sepsis or recurrence of original disease.
- Immunosuppression increases susceptibility to infection.

SPECIFIC COMPLICATIONS OF OLT

- *Early* – vascular occlusion, bleeding and primary non-functional graft
- *Late* – biliary leak and duct stenosis requiring reconstruction.

These will usually be dealt with at a primary transplant centre and are not considered further here.

PREOPERATIVE ASSESSMENT AND INVESTIGATIONS

- Full systemic review for intercurrent or chronic problems and any evidence of infection
- Formal clinical and biochemical assessment of liver function – chronic rejection, recurrent disease, biliary obstruction
- Arrange conversion of immunosuppression from oral to intravenous administration
- Steroid cover intraoperatively
- Liaise with transplant centre if any queries.

INVESTIGATIONS:
- Full blood count – Haemoglobin, white blood cells (may be low with azathioprine)
- Liver function tests
- Chest radiography
- Urea and electrolytes, plasma creatinine and creatinine clearance
- Coagulation: PT, activated PTT, platelets ± bleeding time
- ECG.

PERIOPERATIVE MANAGEMENT: LAPAROTOMY

The aim is to avoid any deterioration or compromise in:
- *Liver function* – by optimising hepatic oxygenation and blood flow. Maintain PaO_2 above 15 kPa, normal $PaCO_2$ and pH, and normovolaemia at all times. CVP and direct arterial monitoring is therefore desirable.
- *Renal function* – by optimising volume status and using low-dose dopamine ($1-3$ μg kg^{-1} min^{-1}) and, if patient jaundiced, mannitol infusion.
- Be aware of *increased infection risk* – all invasive monitoring must be inserted with 'no touch' aseptic technique.

5

ANAESTHESIA:

- Isoflurane and desflurane are the agents of choice – minimal metabolism and best preservation of hepatic arterial and mesenteric flow.
- Avoid halothane
- Atracurium for neuromuscular relaxation
- Maintain normocapnia and normal acid–base status to minimise effects on liver blood flow
- Analgesia – epidural ideal for postoperative analgesia (NB: check coagulation). If liver function is deranged, fentanyl is the safest choice intraoperatively.

BLEEDING RISK

May be increased because:
- Previous surgery with possibility of vascular adhesions
- Abnormal liver function:
  —deranged coagulation
  —obstructive jaundice (vitamin K-dependent factors)
  —decreased synthesis of clotting proteins.

MANAGEMENT:

- Correct prolonged PT with fresh frozen plasma prior to surgery and invasive procedures.
- If platelet count is less than 80×10^9 l^{-1}, have platelets available for operation.
- Drugs such as DDAVP and aprotinin (Trasylol) are useful in reducing blood loss resulting from platelet dysfunction and fibrinolysis; aprotinin also decreases 'ooze' from vascular adhesions.
- Coagulation monitoring – thrombelastography and/or serial clotting screens.

POSTOPERATIVE MANAGEMENT

- For major procedures these patients will require HDU care for a minimum of 24 h.
- Postoperative analgesia:
  —epidural opiates or low-dose bupivacaine infusion
  —intravenous opiate infusion or patient-controlled analgesia pump
- Continue to ensure good oxygenation and optimise haemodynamics and volume status
- Renal dose of dopamine for 24 h after surgery
- Antibiotic prophylaxis
- Continue immunosuppression and steroid cover.

OUTCOME

Increasing numbers of patients have successful liver transplants and may present months to years later with unrelated surgical problems. Careful preoperative assessment is essential, especially in relation to liver and kidney function. Perioperative management is directed to avoiding any factors that might compromise hepatic and renal function, and minimising the infection risk with antibiotic prophylaxis and careful aseptic techniques.

BIBLIOGRAPHY

Cottam S, Jenkins S. Anaesthetic principles in liver transplantation. Current Anaesthesia and Critical Care 1999; 10:291–298

Hawker F. Liver transplantation. In: Park G, ed. The liver. Philadelphia: WB Saunders; 1993:196–249

Mallett SV, Cox DJA. The monitoring and treatment of coagulopathy during major surgery. British Journal of Anaesthesia 1992; 69:307–313

Stock PG, Payne WD. Liver transplantation. Critical care of the transplant patient. Critical Care Clinics 1990; 6:911–926

CROSS-REFERENCES

Liver transplantation
  Surgical Procedures 21: 522

Porphyria

I. T. Campbell

Porphyria is a group of diseases related to defects in the synthesis of haem, which functions in several systems concerned with the transport and utilisation of oxygen: haemoglobin, myoglobin, and mitochondrial and microsomal enzymes, including hepatic cytochrome P450 (Fig. 5.2).

Haem is essential to life. Its synthesis is regulated by the feedback mechanism of haem itself on the enzyme δ-aminolaevulinic acid (ALA) synthase – the first, and rate-limiting, step in the haem synthetic pathway. ALA activity can be induced directly by:

- Barbiturates
- Steroids
- Alcohol.

In addition, the cytochrome P450 enzyme system in the liver is the main hepatic consumer of haem; induction of the P450 system stimulates ALA synthesis via the resultant fall in haem concentration.

CLINICAL FEATURES

Clinical features are largely neurological. The reasons for this are uncertain. ALA or products of porphyrin may be neurotoxic. ALA also resembles the neurotransmitter α-aminobutyric acid, and so might compete for γ-aminobutyric acid (GABA) receptor sites.

Symptoms are non-specific, comprising scattered lesions in the central and autonomic nervous systems. There are few, or no, physical signs:

- Abdominal pain, possibly colicky
- Vomiting
- Constipation
- Dehydrated or hypovolaemic
- Base disturbances
- Acid–base sensory motor or autonomic abnormalities
- Pain syndromes
- Psychological disturbances
- Impairment of consciousness
- Bulbar palsy
- Convulsions.

Symptoms are provoked by pregnancy, alcohol, dietary restriction and a wide variety of drugs (see below).

ACUTE INTERMITTENT PORPHYRIA (SWEDEN)

All of the above features are seen, precipitated by lipid-soluble drugs. Diagnosis is by the ALA and porphobilinogen concentrations in urine.

VARIEGATE PORPHYRIA (SOUTH AFRICA)

As above, but 80% of cases have photosensitivity or skin fragility, possibly due to photosensitive porphyrins in the skin.

HEREDITARY COPROPORPHYRIA

This is very rare. It is similar to the acute intermittent form and is diagnosed by a pattern of porphyria and porphyrin precursors in urine. Symptoms may also be precipitated by stress, infections, fasting and endogenous hormonal fluctuations.

DIAGNOSIS OF PORPHYRIA

Diagnosis is made on the basis of blood and urinary levels of:

5

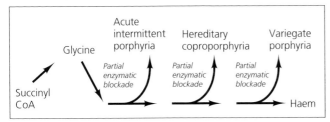

Fig. 5.2 Deficiencies in three enzymes give rise to three types of porphyria. A total block in one or other of these enzymes would be fatal, but the partial block leads to an accumulation of the various metabolites proximal to the block. CoA, coenzyme A.

- ALA
- Porphobilinogen
- Total porphyrin.

ANAESTHETIC TECHNIQUE

The porphyrogenicity of drugs is determined by using various types of cell culture and laboratory animals rendered porphyric by infusion of diethoxycarbonylophydrocollidine.

Anaesthetic drugs are high on the list of those that may precipitate an acute attack. No ideal anaesthetic technique has yet been determined; reports about the dangers of different agents are inconsistent and dependent on animal work and clinical experience. Various lists have been produced at various times of drugs that, with uncertain degrees of reliability, have been thought to precipitate or not to precipitate attacks. Recently published lists are reproduced in Box 5.2.

BOX 5.2

Safety of commonly used drugs in patients with porphyria

Safe	Possibly safe	No data	Unsafe or probably unsafe
Gases and vapours	*Induction agents*	*Gases and vapours*	*Induction agents*
Nitrous oxide	Propofol	Isoflurane	Barbiturates
Cyclopropane			Etomidate
Diethyl ether	*Neuromuscular*	*Neuromuscular*	
	blocking agents	*blocking agents*	*Gases and vapours*
Neuromuscular	Vecuronium	Atracurium	Enflurane
blocking agents			
Suxamethonium	*Benzodiazepines*	*Opiates*	*Neuromuscular*
Curare	Midazolam	Alfentanil	*blocking agents*
	Lorazepam	Sufentanil	Alcuronium
Local anaesthetics			
Procaine	*Other*	*Parasympathetic*	*Local anaesthetics*
Procainamide	Metoclopramide	*agents*	Mepivacaine
		Glycopyrronium	Tetracaine (amethocaine)
Opiates	Naloxone		
Pethidine	Corticosteroids	*Antidysrhythmia*	*Vasoactive agents*
Fentanyl		*agents*	Tilidine
Morphine	**Contentious**	Mexiletine	Verapamil
Buprenorphine	*Induction agents*	Bretylium	Nifedipine
	Ketamine		Diltiazem
Oral analgesics		*Vasoactive agents*	Hydralazine
Paracetamol	*Gases and vapours*	β Agonists	Phenoxybenzamine
Temazepam	Halothane	α Agonists	
			Opiates
Major tranquillisers	*Neuromuscular*	*Vasodilators*	Pentazocine
Droperidol	*blocking agents*	Sodium	
Phenothiazines	Pancuronium	nitroprusside	*Other*
			Aminophylline
Adrenergic agonists	*Local anaesthetics*		Cimetidine
and antagonists	Lidocaine (lignocaine)		
Beta-blockers	Prilocaine		
Adrenaline	Bupivacaine		
(epinephrine)			
Phentolamine	*Benzodiazepines*		
Salbutamol	Diazepam		
	Triazolam		
	Oxazepam		
Other			
Atropine	*Other*		
Neostigmine	Disopyramide		
Domperidone	Ranitidine		

The major problem has been the choice of induction agent. Numerous recent case reports have indicated that propofol may be safe. All the amide local anaesthetics have at various times been implicated, but a recent report has described the successful and uneventful use of bupivacaine in epidural anaesthesia for caesarean section.

BIBLIOGRAPHY

Harrison GG, Meissner PN, Hift RJ. Anaesthesia for the porphyric patient. Anaesthesia 1993; 48:417–421

McNeill MJ, Bennet A. Use of regional anaesthesia in a patient with acute porphyria. British Journal of Anaesthesia 1990; 64:371–373

Meissner PN, Harrison GG, Hift RJ. Propofol as an IV anaesthetic induction agent in variegate porphyria. British Journal of Anaesthesia 1991; 66:60–65

5

6

GU TRACT
P. R. Saunders

Acute renal failure

P. R. Saunders

This condition can be defined as an acute decline in renal function sufficient to result in the retention of nitrogenous end-products of metabolism, which is not reversible by manipulation of extrarenal factors. Patients are not necessarily oliguric.

CAUSES:
- Prerenal – inadequate perfusion
- Renal – intrinsic renal disease
- Postrenal – obstructive uropathy.

The most common situation is the development of 'acute tubular necrosis', due to ischaemia or, occasionally, renal toxins.

ACUTE TUBULAR NECROSIS (ATN)

CAUSES:
- *Hypoperfusion* – decreased intravascular volume, sepsis, cardiogenic shock, cardiac tamponade.
- *Embolic occlusion* of the renal arteries.
- *Severe hypoxia* will also contribute to ischaemic damage.
- *Drugs*:
  —aminoglycosides
  —amphotericin B
  —radiocontrast agents
  —non-steroidal anti-inflammatory drugs
  —furosemide (frusemide).
- *Endogenous toxins*:
  —haemoglobin after a transfusion reaction
  —myoglobin from rhabdomyolysis of massive trauma
  —abnormal reaction to succinylcholine
  —myeloma renal damage.

PREVENTION OF PRERENAL CAUSES OF ATN
Preoperative assessment
This must begin before operation, i.e. may require an intravenous infusion the night before surgery.

ASSESSMENT OF HIGH-RISK STATES
- Preoperative renal disease
- Preoperative 'shock' states
- Cirrhosis
- Biliary obstruction
- Sepsis
- Multiple system trauma
- Multiple organ failure
- Cardiac failure
- Extracellular fluid volume deficit
- Elderly patients
- Aortorenal vascular disease

Perioperative and postoperative management
Prevention of the development of renal failure in the perioperative period involves avoiding manoeuvres that lead to a reduction in renal blood flow and pharmacological means to support renal function:
- Maintain oxygenation
- Maintain normocarbia
- Maintain renal perfusion pressure (>80 mmHg)
- Optimise intravascular volume and cardiac output
- Drug therapy.

Furosemide (frusemide) is controversial; if patients respond, they are certainly easier to treat.

Dopamine increases renal blood flow.

Mannitol administered before an ischaemic insult will reduce renal damage, probably by its action as a free-radical scavenger.

If acute renal failure occurs in the perioperative period, the mortality rate is very high (60–75%), which probably reflects the severity of the insult. Although mortality is high, few patients die as a result of the renal disease.

An abnormal urine output does not preclude the presence of renal failure. Beware the blocked urinary catheter. Acute tubular necrosis may recover and be followed by a period of polyuria, usually after 1–2 weeks.

ACUTE RENAL FAILURE – ESTABLISHED

ANAESTHETIC ASSESSMENT

A full history is taken, with particular attention to previous renal disease, infection, stones or prostatism. Examination includes the state of fluid balance, i.e. evidence of postural hypotension, reduced skin turgor, poor circulation, weight and thirst. Patient must have a urinary catheter and central venous pressure monitor.

INVESTIGATIONS:

- Serum levels of urea, creatinine and electrolytes
- Ratio of urine : blood osmolality; a value greater than 1.5 : 1 suggests hypovolaemia
- Urine.

When oliguria is due solely to hypovolaemia, the specific gravity is grater than 1015 and the urea concentration is above 2 g 100 ml^{-1}.

Intrinsic renal failure leads to a fixed specific gravity of 1010 and a urea concentration of less than 600 mg ml^{-1}.

PERIOPERATIVE AND POSTOPERATIVE MANAGEMENT:

- Avoid drugs that require renal function for elimination.
- Maintain renal perfusion pressure.
- Monitor any urine output.

BIBLIOGRAPHY

Byrick RJ, Rose DK. Pathophysiology and prevention of acute renal failure: the role of the anaesthetist. Canadian Journal of Anaesthesia 1990; 37:457–467

Gokhale YA, Marathe P, Patil RD et al. Rhabdomyolysis and acute renal failure following a single dose of succinylcholine. Journal of the Association of Physicians India 1991; 39:968–970

CROSS-REFERENCES

Water and electrolyte balance
Anaesthetic Factors 27: 624
Assessment of renal function
Patient Conditions 6: 186

6

Assessment of renal function

P. R. Saunders

An assessment of renal function aids in an overall estimate of the degree of physiological derangement and reserve of the individual.

FACTORS AFFECTING RENAL FUNCTION TESTS

- Intrinsic renal disease
- Intravascular and extravascular fluid status
- Cardiovascular function
- Neuroendocrine factors

Perioperative acute renal failure accounts for 50% of all patients requiring dialysis and is associated with a high mortality rate (oliguric 50–80%, non-oliguric 20–40%). Before operation it is important to try to identify those patients at risk and to take measures to protect them from developing renal complications after surgery. There is no single comprehensive test of renal function; all results should be viewed together with any significant history and examination.

BASIC FUNCTIONS OF THE KIDNEY:

- Glomerular
- Tubular
- Endocrine.

The glomeruli are responsible for filtration and subsequent excretion of nitrogenous wastes. Tubular function involves the movement of water and sodium, and the maintenance of fluid balance, along with the excretion or re-absorption of hydrogen ions in acid–base homeostasis. The endocrine activity involves the metabolism of vitamin D, prostaglandins and erythropoietin.

NORMAL VARIABLES

Cardiac output	5000 ml min-1
Renal blood flow	1250 ml min-1
Renal plasma flow	750 ml min-1
Glomerular filtration rate	125 ml min-1
Urine flow	2 ml min-1

HISTORY AND EXAMINATION

SYMPTOMS:
- Polyuria
- Polydipsia
- Fatigue
- Dysuria
- Oedema.

SIGNS:
- Long-standing hypertension
- Hypovolaemic signs if overdialysed.

MEDICATION:
- Diuretics
- Potassium supplements
- Immunosuppressive agents
- Antihypertensive therapy
- Dialysis schedule.

INVESTIGATIONS

PLASMA:

Sodium	140 mmol l^{-1}
Potassium	3.5–5.0 mmol l^{-1}
Chloride	95–105 mmol l^{-1}
Osmolality	280–295 mOsm^{-1}
Urea (blood urea nitrogen; BUN)	2.5–7.0 mmol l^{-1}
Creatinine	40–120 mmol l^{-1}
Bicarbonate (HCO_3^-)	21–25 mmol l^{-1}
Calcium	2.1–2.8 mmol l^{-1}
Magnesium	0.7–1.0 mmol l^{-1}

URINE:

Sodium	50–200 mmol 24 h^{-1}
Potassium	30–100 mmol 24 h^{-1}
Chloride	100–300 mmol 24 h^{-1}
Osmolality	300–1000 mOsm^{-1}
Specific gravity (SG)	1003–1030
Creatinine	9.0–18 mmol l^{-1}
Creatinine clearance	110–130 ml min^{-1}
Urea clearance	60–95 ml min^{-1}
H$^+$	60 mEq 24 h^{-1}

6

URINALYSIS

As a sole investigation, urinalysis is sufficient screening in patients with no history of renal or systemic disease.

APPEARANCE
- Gross – bleeding, infection.
- Microscopic – casts, bacteria, cell forms.

PH
Normally urine is acidic. Acidification is therefore a measure of function.

SPECIFIC GRAVITY
Specific gravity refers to the concentration of solutes in urine; the ability to concentrate is a measure of tubular function. This is, however, non-specific.

SUBSTANCES AND CONDITIONS AFFECTING SPECIFIC GRAVITY

- Protein
- Glucose
- Mannitol
- Diuretics
- Extremes of age
- Antibiotics (carbenicillin)
- Temperature
- Hormonal imbalance (pituitary, adrenal and thyroid disease).

OSMOLALITY

Osmolality = No. of osmotically active particles/Unit solvent

Osmolality is more specific than specific gravity and is helpful at extreme values:
- Oliguria + Osmolality >500 suggests prerenal azotaemia
- Oliguria + Osmolality <350 likely to be ATN.

Oliguria itself also affects the osmolality value. Determination of osmolality is useful only in low urine output states, coupled with a low specific gravity. An osmolality <350 mOsm kg^{-1} suggests an inability to concentrate urine and excrete electrolytes.

PROTEIN:
- *<150 mg 24 h^{-1}* – excretion in health (exercise and standing can increase this)
- *>750 mg 24 h^{-1}* – specific indicator of renal parenchymal disease
- *Massive* – glomerular damage.

GLUCOSE
Freely filtered and reabsorbed. Glycosuria occurs when an abnormally heavy load is presented to the tubules (e.g. diabetes mellitus, intravenous glucose.).

BUN AND CREATININE
Indicators of general function, urea being filtered at the glomerulus and 33% reabsorbed when the urine flow <2 ml min^{-1}. There is a steady production of creatinine (proportional to body mass) which is never reabsorbed. BUN and creatinine values vary widely, and do not increase despite a fall in glomerular and tubular function by as much as 50%.

Creatinine >180 mmol l^{-1} indicates renal failure.

NON-RENAL VARIABLES AFFECTING BUN AND CREATININE LEVELS

- Increased nitrogen absorption
- Increased nitrogen waste production
- Diet
- Body mass
- Activity
- Hepatic disease
- Diabetic ketoacidosis
- Large haematoma
- Gastrointestinal bleeding
- Drugs (steroids)

CREATININE CLEARANCE
Measures the glomerular filtration of creatinine, which approximates to glomerular filtration rate.

Creatinine clearance = (Urine creatinine × Urine volume)/ Plasma creatinine

Creatinine clearance <25 ml min^{-1} indicates severe renal failure; 50–80 ml min^{-1} indicates mild renal dysfunction.

Creatinine clearance = [140 − Age × Weight (kg)]/ (72 × Plasma creatinine)

This approximation overestimates values in females by 15%, and is invalid in gross renal failure.

PLASMA ELECTROLYTES
Sodium, potassium, chloride and bicarbonate levels remain normal until disease is advanced, when a hyperkalaemic, hyperchloraemic acidosis is seen. These changes will exacerbate

6

dysrhythmias and compromise resuscitation. Frank renal failure results in hypocalcaemia, hyperphosphataemia and hypermagnesaemia.

HAEMATOLOGY:

- End-stage renal failure: Hb = 3–9 g dl^{-1}
- White cell count and platelets are deranged if the patient is immunosuppressed or has a coagulopathy.

CHEST RADIOGRAPHY

It is important to look for signs of hypertensive cardiovascular disease, pericardial–pleural effusions and, rarely, uraemic pneumonitis.

ECG

Toxic effects of:
- Hyperkalaemia:
  —tall, peaked T waves
  —ST depression
  —QRS widening
  —ventricular dysrhythmias.
- Hypocalcaemia.
- Signs of hypertension.
- Signs of ischaemic heart disease.

ECHOCARDIOGRAPHY

In the presence of symptoms and signs of heart failure, left ventricular dysfunction should be evaluated. If present, the patient is at increased risk of developing renal failure following major surgery.

CONCLUSION

At present, the measurement of creatinine clearance is the most sensitive test of renal function. However, it is time consuming, has an inherent delay factor, and does not offer the anaesthetist a simple, single-shot assessment of renal reserve. One relies on electrolytes, BUN and creatinine levels, which are not reliable indices of glomerular or tubular function.

BIBLIOGRAPHY

Burton AW, Mazze RI, Prough DS. Renal diseases. In: Benumof JL, ed. Anaeshesia and Uncommon Diseases, 4th edn. Philadelphia: WB Saunders 1998:Ch. 5; 123–146

Kellen M, Aronson S, Roizen MF, Barnard J, Thisted RA. Predictive and diagnostic tests of renal function: a review. Anesthesia and Analgesia 1994; 78:134–142

Prough DS, Foreman AS. Anesthesia and the renal system. In: Barash, Cullen, Stoelting, eds. Clinical anesthesia. 4th edn. Philadelphia: JB Lippincott; 1998

Thompson FD. Modern tests of renal function and drugs affecting the kidney. In: Kaufman L, ed. Anaesthesia review, vol 7. Edinburgh: Churchill Livingstone; 1990:ch 4, 67–74

6

Chronic renal failure

P. R. Saunders

Chronic renal failure results from a reduction in renal function by a chronic disease process, which causes retention of nitrogenous waste products and inability of the kidneys to maintain fluid, electrolyte and acid–base homeostasis in the face of normal variations of fluid and dietary intake and of physical activity. It is characterised by uraemia.

Anaesthesia in this condition is complicated by a number of factors. Each patient may have a widely varying cardiovascular status, blood volume and biochemical profile. Consideration needs to be given to other associated medical conditions, such as diabetes, to their often multiple medications and to their treatment requirements (i.e. peritoneal or haemodialysis).

AETIOLOGY:
- Chronic pyelonephritis
- Chronic glomerulonephritis
- Essential (primary) malignant hypertension
- Polycystic disease
- Systemic lupus erythematosus
- Diabetes mellitus
- Amyloidosis
- Gout
- Analgesic nephropathy
- Nephrocalcinosis.

PATHOPHYSIOLOGY

BIOCHEMICAL:
- Uraemia
- High serum creatinine level (>180 mmol l^{-1})
- Hyperkalaemia
- Hyponatraemia
- Metabolic acidosis.

CARDIOVASCULAR:
- Hypertension
- Fluid overload (unless dialysed)
- Cardiac failure (secondary to hypertension and increased cardiac output)
- Pericarditis pericardial effusion.

HAEMATOLOGICAL:
- Anaemia ($3–9$ g dl^{-1})
- Bleeding tendency (abnormal platelet function).

IMMUNOLOGICAL:
- Tendency to acquire infections.

NEUROLOGICAL:
- Drowsiness, convulsions and coma (uraemia)
- Peripheral and autonomic neuropathies, especially if diabetic.

GASTROINTESTINAL:
- Autonomic neuropathy may lead to delayed gastric emptying and risk of aspiration.

SKELETAL:
- Bone disease leading to pathological fractures.

PREOPERATIVE ASSESSMENT

HISTORY:
- Drug history:
  —immunosuppression
  —antihypertensives
  —hypoglycaemics.
- Systematic review of cardiovascular disease.
- Method and time of last dialysis.

EXAMINATION:
- Signs of fluid overload
- Weight (in relation to dialysis record)
- Location of any arteriovenous fistula sites.

INVESTIGATIONS:
- Full blood count (normochromic, normocytic anaemia)
- Clotting studies (including bleeding time)
- Full biochemical screen
- ECG
- Chest radiography.

6

PREMEDICATION

Premedication with sedative drugs and opioids is unpredictable and potentially dangerous. The decreased tolerance to these drugs is due to abnormal levels of plasma proteins and the effect of altered blood pH on their pharmacokinetics.

PERIOPERATIVE MANAGEMENT

Patients should be preoxygenated and monitored before induction. Avoid using venous and arterial access that may compromise the use of vessels for future arteriovenous fistulae formation.

Central venous access should be established for monitoring fluid balance.

INDUCTION

Propofol and etomidate are safe to use for induction. Thiopentone should be used with caution and in lower dosage because of the patient's requirement of a high cardiac output to maintain oxygen delivery, in the face of chronic anaemia and low levels of plasma proteins, leading to an increased percentage of free drug during the initial bolus effect.

Avoid suxamethonium when the serum potassium level exceeds 5 mmol l⁻¹ or when there is peripheral neuropathy.

For neuromuscular blockade, atracurium and cisatracurium are preferred because of their rapid elimination and independence of renal metabolism and excretion. Mivacurium is also suitable provided there is no deficiency in plasma cholinesterase levels. Neuromuscular blockade with vecuronium and rocuronium has a longer duration of action, and is best used as a single dose, not by infusion.

MAINTENANCE:

- Maintain blood volume and blood pressure whilst monitoring filling pressures to prevent overload.
- Monitor urine output, if indicated.
- Regional techniques such as brachial plexus blocks for fistula formation may be employed, but watch for bleeding tendencies. Bupivacaine and lidocaine (lignocaine) may be used safely and have been shown to have a shorter duration of action with no accumulation. Levobupivacaine has a similar pharmacokinetic profile to the racemic mixture.
- Total intravenous anaesthesia (TIVA) with propofol and remifentanil can be used. Remifentanil has an active metabolite (1/1000 potency), which in practice has not been shown to cause problems.
- Isoflurane and desflurane are ideal inhalational agents, with minimal metabolism and good muscle relaxation. The use of enflurane is controversial because of the potential accumulation of fluoride ions, usually <15 μmol l⁻¹. Nephrotoxicity is seen when levels are in excess of 50 μmol l⁻¹. Sevoflurane lacks renal toxicity and is safe to use, probably due to its relative insolubility and site of metabolism.

ANALGESIA

Use morphine and pethidine with caution, as their metabolites (morphine-6-glucuronide, norpethidine) tend to accumulate.

POSTOPERATIVE MANAGEMENT

- Watch fluid balance closely, whilst monitoring filling pressures and urine output, if any.
- Oxygen therapy to maximise carrying capacity.
- Monitor electrolytes.
- Avoid transfusion, unless excessive blood loss.

THE LATER POSTOPERATIVE PERIOD:

- Bleeding may occur.
- Patients may require many further anaesthetics, usually for vascular access surgery for dialysis, or for transplantation.

6

BIBLIOGRAPHY

Bedford RF, Ives HE. The renal safety of sevoflurane. Anesthesia and Analgesia 2000; 90:505–508

Chauvin M, Sandouk P, Scherrmann JM, Farinotti R, Strumza P, Duvaldestin P. Morphine pharmacokinetics in renal failure. Anesthesiology 1987; 66:327–331

Dyson D. Anesthesia for patients with stable end-stage renal disease. Veterinary Clinics of North America, Small Animal Practice 1992; 22:469–471

McLeod GA, Burke D. Levobupivacaine. Anaesthesia 2001; 56:331–341

Moore EW, Hunter JM. The new neuromuscular blocking agents: do they offer any advantages? British Journal of Anaesthesia 2001; 87(6):912–925

Rice AS, Pither CE, Tucker GT. Plasma concentrations of bupivacaine after supraclavicular brachial plexus blockade in patients with chronic renal failure. Anaesthesia 1991; 46:354–357

Smith I, Nathanson M, White PF. Sevoflurane – a long-awaited volatile anaesthetic. British Journal of Anaesthesia 1996; 76:435–445

CROSS-REFERENCES

Hypertension
    Patient Conditions 4: 151
Diabetes Mellitus type 1
    Patient Conditions 2: 56

6

Goodpasture's syndrome

P. R. Saunders

Although originally described in an 18-year-old man who developed haemoptysis and died following an influenza-type illness, it was not until later that the term Goodpasture's syndrome was used to describe the entity of pulmonary haemorrhage and glomerulonephritis.

The pathogenetic mechanism appears to involve the development of antibodies to pulmonary and glomerular basement membranes, with an ensuing autoimmune process accounting for the renal lesions (crescentic glomerulonephritis), and pulmonary alveolitis resulting in haemoptysis.

Antiglomerular basement membrane antibodies (anti-GBM) and antineutrophil cytoplasmic autoantibodies (ANCA) can be assayed by immunofluorescence, allowing for a more rapid and accurate diagnosis than was possible in the past. It must be stressed that the term Goodpasture's syndrome refers to the clinical situation of glomerulonephritis with pulmonary haemorrhage, and therefore includes diseases that are also antibody negative, such as:

- Polyarteritis nodosa
- Wegener's syndrome
- Primary crescentic glomerulonephritis
- Following treatment with penicillamine
- Systemic lupus erythematosus.

PATHOPHYSIOLOGY
History:
- Male preponderance 2 : 1
- Caucasians
- HLA/DRA association (possibly inherited?).

PRESENTING FEATURES:
- *Pulmonary features* appear early:
  —dyspnoea
  —haemoptysis (rusty sputum to massive bleed).
- *Renal*:
  —haematuria
  —nephrotic picture
  —oliguria or anuria
  —hypertension.

CLINICAL COURSE AND OUTCOME
Once respiratory symptoms have developed, oliguria and anuria usually follow rapidly. Patients with early oliguria or anuria, or those who require haemodialysis, seldom recover renal function. Treatment involves renal support, plasmapheresis, steroids and immunosuppression with cytotoxic drugs (azathioprine). Pulmonary signs and symptoms are improved by reducing anti-GBM titres with plasmapheresis and immunosuppression.

Clinical lapses during treatment are characterised by fever and reduced pulmonary and renal function.

Death is usually due to overwhelming sepsis or pulmonary haemorrhage.

PREOPERATIVE MANAGEMENT

Elective surgery should be carried out during quiescent periods (low D_{LCO}). Preoperative blood transfusion and dialysis may be necessary to optimise fluid, electrolyte and haemodynamic status.

INVESTIGATIONS:
- Full blood count – microcytic hypochromic anaemia
- Clotting – usually normal
- Urea and electrolytes – derangement reflects degree of renal impairment
- Chest radiography – small discrete shadowing; confluent densities; bilateral alveolar infiltrates
- Pulmonary function – restrictive picture; D_{LCO} raised
- ECG – electrolyte abnormalities; systemic hypertension; pulmonary hypertension.

ANAESTHESIA

PREMEDICATION:
- Avoid respiratory depression
- Steroid cover.

MONITORING:

- Routine (defined by needs of operation)
- Airway pressures and compliance.

SPECIFIC PROBLEMS:

- If employing intermittent positive-pressure ventilation (IPPV), smaller tidal volumes and increased frequency are necessary to minimise risk of alveolar capillary membrane rupture.
- Pulmonary haemorrhage leads to airway or tracheal tube obstruction. Therefore, frequent tracheal suctioning is recommended.
- Avoid renally excreted neuromuscular blocking agents.
- Aseptic techniques for immunosuppressed patients.

POSTOPERATIVE MANAGEMENT

- Physiotherapy
- Monitor renal function
- Increased steroid dosage.

BIBLIOGRAPHY

Burton AW, Mazze RI, Prough DS. Renal diseases. In: Benumof JL, ed. Anesthesia and Uncommon Diseases, 4th edn. Philadelphia: WB Saunders 1998:Ch. 5; 123–146

Prough DS, Foreman AS. Anaesthesia and the renal system. In: Barash, Cullen, Stoelting, eds. Clinical anaesthesia. 4th edn. Philadelphia: Lippincott; 2000

Stoelting RK, Dierdorf SF, eds. Renal disease in anesthesia and coexisting disease. 4th edn. Edinburgh: Churchill Livingstone; 2002

6

Haemolytic uraemic syndrome

P. R. Saunders

The haemolytic uraemic syndrome is the most important cause of renal failure in infancy and childhood. Following a prodromal illness – usually gastroenteritis – the patient may rapidly develop the typical triad of renal failure, haemolytic anaemia and thrombocytopaenia. Many viral agents have been implicated, and bacteria such as *Shigella* and *Salmonella* have been recovered from these patients.

Most patients present for anaesthesia for the creation of arteriovenous fistulae and shunts.

PATHOPHYSIOLOGY

This is a multisystem disease that involves not only the kidneys, erythrocytes and platelets, but also the gastrointestinal tract, liver, heart and CNS.

CARDIOVASCULAR SYSTEM
Myocarditis, congestive heart failure and severe systemic hypertension.

RESPIRATORY SYSTEM
Severe respiratory insufficiency may occur, unrelated to volume overload, pulmonary oedema or congestive heart failure.

CNS
Drowsiness, seizures, hemiparesis and coma.

BIOCHEMICAL:
- Evidence of acute renal failure, including acid–base and electrolyte disturbances
- Abnormal liver function associated with hepatitis.

HAEMATOLOGICAL:
- Haemolysis appears rapidly; haemoglobin level falls to as low as 4 g dl^{-1}
- Thrombocytopaenia (lasting for 7–14 days)
- Hepatosplenomegaly.

RENAL SYSTEM
Proteinuria, haematuria and oliguria, leading to anuria.

GASTROINTESTINAL TRACT
Haemorrhagic gastritis.

IMMUNOLOGICAL
Severe infections are common, for example peritonitis, meningitis and osteomyelitis.

PREOPERATIVE ASSESSMENT

EXAMINATION:
- Full neurological and cardiovascular examination
- Evidence of hepatic dysfunction
- Evidence of clotting disorders.

INVESTIGATIONS:
- Full blood count
- Urea and electrolytes, and creatinine
- Liver function tests
- Glucose
- Clotting studies
- Arterial blood gases
- Chest radiography
- ECG.

PREOPERATIVE MANAGEMENT

Premedication is unnecessary because patients in the acute phase tend to be lethargic and drowsy. Correction of acid–base status, electrolyte and coagulation disorders should be arranged before operation. Preoperative transfusion may be necessary, and any anticonvulsant therapy should be continued perioperatively.

PERIOPERATIVE MANAGEMENT

General anaesthesia is preferred because of presence of coagulation disorders in an uncooperative and severely ill child. A reduction in the dose of thiopental (less protein binding in hepatic disease) is usual. Rapid sequence induction should be performed. Isoflurane and atracurium are the ideal agents for maintenance, although the newer agents desflurane and mivacurium are attractive alternatives. In most operations, continual monitoring of acid–base and electrolyte status, temperature and urine output will be required.

POSTOPERATIVE MANAGEMENT

Postoperative ventilation may be required in patients with severe cerebral involvement. Sepsis is a common postoperative complication.

THE LATER POSTOPERATIVE PERIOD

Repeated procedures are common. Haemolytic crisis may last for more than 2 weeks, but the anaemia continues for months. Renal function may recover completely, or the child may require permanent haemodialysis.

BIBLIOGRAPHY

Johnson GD, Rosales JK. The haemolytic uraemic syndrome and anaesthesia. Canadian Journal of Anaesthesia 1987; 34:196–199

6

Nephrotic syndrome

P. R. Saunders

Although of multifactorial aetiology, 80% of cases are due to glomerulonephritis.

PRESENTING FEATURES
- Proteinuria (>3 g 24 h^{-1})
- Hypoalbuminaemia
- Hypercholesterolaemia
- Thromboembolic episodes.

Hypoalbuminaemia leads to a fall in plasma oncotic pressure, retention of sodium and water with the build-up of peripheral oedema, ascites, pleural effusions and a hypovolaemic patient (Fig. 6.1). This physiologically deranged state puts the individual at risk of thrombo-embolic episodes, commonly venous (deep venous thrombosis, renal vein thrombosis), but also arterial.

DIAGNOSIS
Renal biopsy.

TREATMENT:
- Prednisolone
- Cyclophosphamide
- Chlorambucil
- Cyclosporin.

Without treatment, most cases spontaneously remit. Renal failure is rare.

Hypertension is common with adjunctive drug therapy.

PREOPERATIVE MANAGEMENT

- Drug history – diuretics, steroids, antihypertensives
- Clinical signs of oedema
- Central venous pressure monitoring, to assess volume status (Fig. 6.2).
- Assess renal function to determine the degree of the renal lesion
- Potassium supplementation may be required; any deficiency may be due to the disease itself, or induced by diuretics or steroids.

ANAESTHETIC CONSIDERATIONS

- Precautions and care, as for any patient with renal impairment or failure

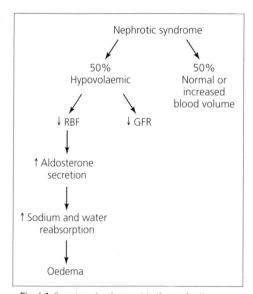

Fig. 6.1 Symptom development in the nephrotic syndrome. GFR, glomerular filtration rate; RBF, renal blood flow.

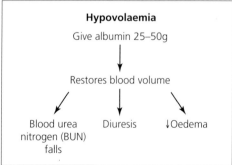

Fig. 6.2 Management of hypovolaemia in patients with the nephrotic syndrome.

- Remember: low protein levels make drugs more active. Therefore, reduce dose of induction agents, especially thiopentone. Monitor neuromuscular blockade.

POSTOPERATIVE MANAGEMENT

Thromboembolic prophylaxis.

POLYCYSTIC DISEASE

Autosomal dominant inheritance. The disease progresses slowly leading to end-stage renal failure in middle age.

PATHOPHYSIOLOGY:
- Hypertension
- Proteinuria
- Reduction in urine-concentrating ability early in the disease.

ASSOCIATED CYSTS:
- Liver
- CNS (intracranial aneurysms).

TREATMENT:
- Dialysis
- Renal transplantation.

ANAESTHETIC CONSIDERATIONS
As for end-stage renal failure, if present.

6

Patient with a transplant

P. R. Saunders

In the UK, more than 2000 cadaveric renal transplantations are performed each year. The perioperative mortality rate is less than 1%, and 80% are functioning at 1 year. These recipients may present for any operation and it is imperative that no damage occurs to the organ. Most elective procedures are well tolerated and the renal handling of drugs is good, although renal function is rarely normal.

REASONS FOR RENAL TRANSPLANTATION:
- Diabetes mellitus
- Glomerulonephritis
- Polycystic disease
- Hypertension.

PROBLEMS COMMONLY SEEN FOLLOWING RENAL TRANSPLANTATION:
- Opportunistic infection
- Hepatitis B (<5% due to vaccine)
- Cancer risk (increased 30–100 times)
- Associated medical conditions
- Large cell lymphoma (Epstein–Barr virus infection).

PREOPERATIVE PREPARATION

Discuss the patient with the renal physician. A formal assessment of renal function, coupled with a careful history and examination of any associated medical conditions, should be undertaken. Take note of any drug therapy (e.g. immunosuppressives, antihypertensives).

SPECIFIC CARDIOVASCULAR CHANGES:
- Hypertension:
  —essential
  —secondary to end-stage renal failure.
- Left ventricular failure:
  —secondary to hypertension
  —secondary to a chronic increase in cardiac output (shunts, atrioventricular fistulae and anaemia).
- Ischaemic heart disease – accelerated atherosclerosis.
- Peripheral vascular disease.
- Autonomic neuropathy – postural hypotension.

MAIN ANAESTHETIC CONSIDERATIONS

- Continue immunosuppressive regimen perioperatively – ciclosporin A reduces renal blood flow and glomerular filtration rate by preglomerular afferent arteriolar vasoconstriction, but produces less bone marrow depression (?reduced infection risk).
- Risk of aspiration.
- Infection risk.
- Avoid damage to arteries, veins and fistulae.
- Gastrointestinal bleeding:
  —steroid therapy
  —stress of operation and anaesthesia.
- Osteoporosis – care in moving and handling of patients.
- Potential for altered renal handling of drugs.

PREMEDICATION:
- Prophylactic antibiotics
- Steroid cover
- H_2 blockers, metoclopramide, proton pump inhibitors
- Benzodiazepines (avoid diazepam due to its long half-life)
- Atropine, glycopyrrolate (20–50% renal excretion)
- Opioids are not contraindicated
- Continue immunosuppression.

ANAESTHETIC TECHNIQUE
Local, general and regional techniques are well tolerated. Any general anaesthetic will reduce renal blood flow, but avoid hyperventilation, hypercapnia and high concentrations of volatile agents. Enflurane and sevoflurane are metabolised to produce fluoride ions (usually

$<15\ \mu$mol l^{-1}; nephrotoxicity at $>50\ \mu$mol l^{-1}). Isoflurane and desflurane require minimal metabolism and give good muscle relaxation, and are therefore recommended.

If the graft is functioning, all relaxants and anticholinesterases are easily dealt with, but cisatracurium and mivacurium are the relaxants of choice.

The same applies to opioids, but beware of the possible build-up of morphine-6-glucuronide and norpethidine (convulsant potential).

If a regional technique is being considered and there is a degree of doubt concerning graft function or the patient is on dialysis, coagulation studies, including bleeding time, are mandatory.

POSTOPERATIVE MANAGEMENT

Most operations are performed without any specific complications. However, renal function should be monitored closely, especially if undertaking a major procedure. Immunosuppression should be continued, with antibiotics if indicated, and any infection dealt with appropriately.

If there is any doubt regarding graft function, opioid infusions are best avoided.

CAUSES OF DEATH IN TRANSPLANT RECIPIENTS

- Sepsis
- Cardiovascular disease
- Suicide
- Gastrointestinal perforation

BIBLIOGRAPHY

Castaneda MA, Garvin PJ. General surgical procedures in renal allograft recipients. American Journal of Surgery 1986; 152:717–721

Burton AW, Mazze RI, Prough DS. Renal diseases. In: Benumof JL, eds. Anaesthesia and Uncommon Diseases, 4th edn. Philadelphia: WB Saunders 1998:Ch. 5; 123–146

Cottam S, Eason J. Renal disease. In: Kaufmann L, ed. Anaesthesia Review, vol 8. Edinburgh: Churchill Livingstone; 1991:Ch 8, 159–178

Miller RD, ed. Anesthesia and the renal and genitourinary systems. In: Miller RD, ed. Anesthesia. 5th edn. Edinburgh: Churchill Livingstone; 2000

Stoelting RK, Dierdorf SF, eds. Anesthesia and coexisting disease. 4th edn. Edinburgh: Churchill Livingstone; 2002

CROSS-REFERENCES

6

7

THE BLOOD
W. Harrop-Griffiths

Anaemia

J. Jones

Anaemia

- A common condition that rarely puts fit patients at increased risk
- There is no universally accepted minimum haemoglobin concentration
- The management of anaemia must depend on the cause, the patient's overall medical status and the operation being contemplated

DEFINITION

The World Health Organisation defines anaemia as a haemoglobin (Hb) concentration of less than:

- 13 g dl^{-1} in adult men
- 12 g dl^{-1} in adult women
- 11 g dl^{-1} in children aged 6 months to 6 years
- 12 g dl^{-1} in children aged 6–14 years.

CAUSES

The causes of anaemia may be divided into three categories:

- Defective red cell production
- Haemolysis
- Haemorrhage.

PATHOPHYSIOLOGY

The essential feature of all forms of anaemia is a decrease in the Hb content of the blood. As

> Arterial oxygen content $\propto$ Arterial oxygen saturation $\times$ Hb concentration

and

> Oxygen delivery = Arterial oxygen content $\times$ Cardiac output

it follows that a decrease in Hb concentration will, in the absence of compensatory mechanisms, be followed by a decrease in oxygen supply to the tissues.

COMPENSATORY MECHANISMS

In acute normovolaemic anaemia in otherwise healthy individuals, two mechanisms compensate for the decrease in oxygen-carrying capacity:

- An increase in cardiac output
- A decrease in blood viscosity.

In chronic anaemia a third mechanism comes into play:

- Increased 2,3-diphosphoglycerate (2,3-DPG) concentration in the red cells, which shifts the oxygen dissociation curve to the right and promotes the release of oxygen to the tissues.

CLINICAL FEATURES

The symptoms and signs of anaemia include dyspnoea on exertion, tachycardia, palpitations, angina, increased arterial pulse pressure and capillary pulsation. However, in mild chronic anaemia which is well compensated, there may be no symptoms or signs. Anaemia is poorly tolerated by patients with coronary artery disease or pre-existing myocardial dysfunction. Such patients, who are often elderly, may present with cardiac failure.

PREOPERATIVE ASSESSMENT

In some patients, anaemia is to be anticipated as a feature of the disease for which surgery is indicated. In other surgical patients, anaemia is an unexpected and unrelated finding revealed only by routine preoperative haematological testing.

Routine blood count and blood film examination will disclose:

- The severity of the anaemia
- The type of anaemia, thus suggesting its cause (Table 7.1).

TABLE 7.1

Classification of causes of anaemia according to red cell morphology

Type	Cause
Hypochromic microcytic (decreased MCV and MCHC)	Iron deficiency, thalassaemia
Normochromic macrocytic (increased MCV)	Vitamin B_{12} or folate deficiency, alcohol
Polychromatic macrocytic (increased MCV)	Haemolysis
Normocytic normochromic	Chronic disease; renal failure; haemorrhage; hypothyroidism; hypopituitarism; marrow aplasia or infiltration
Leukoerythroblastic	Marrow infiltration

MCV, mean corpuscular volume; MCHC, mean corpuscular haemoglobin concentration

FURTHER INVESTIGATIONS

It is always desirable to know the exact cause of any patient's anaemia. If surgery cannot be postponed, blood should be taken before the operation so that investigations may be performed on a specimen that is undiluted by transfused blood. Renal failure is a common and often unsuspected cause of anaemia. The serum creatinine level should always be checked.

CORRECTION OF ANAEMIA

WHAT PREOPERATIVE HB LEVEL IS ACCEPTABLE?

There is no Hb concentration that must be met by all patients in all circumstances. Although the value of 10 g dl^{-1} was generally accepted for many years, it has been shown that acute normovolaemic haemodilution to a Hb level of 5 g dl^{-1} is tolerated in healthy, resting volunteers, and there is evidence suggesting that Hb levels of the order of 8 g dl^{-1} are safe for many patients undergoing orthopaedic surgery or treatment in the ICU. The degree of anaemia

that is acceptable depends on the cardiac reserves of the patient. A frail elderly patient with severe coronary artery disease may develop cardiac failure even at a Hb concentration of 10 g dl^{-1}.

HOW MAY THE PATIENT'S HB LEVEL BE INCREASED?

By treating the cause of anaemia
This is obviously the ideal solution, but most cases of anaemia are not amenable to treatment or the treatment is surgery.

By giving specific haematinics
This is appropriate in specific deficiency states (iron, vitamin B_{12} or folic acid) only. Blind, blunderbuss haematinic treatment is useless and expensive.

By red cell transfusion
Transfusion has only a limited place because:
• A moderate degree of anaemia is well tolerated in otherwise fit patients (see above)
• Transfusion has many hazards; in particular, it is easy to overload the circulation of a normovolaemic anaemic patient

The only patients in whom preoperative transfusion is certainly indicated are some patients with sickle cell anaemia and severely anaemic patients with cardiac decompensation in whom surgery is urgent. To minimise the risks of circulatory overload, red cell concentrates should be transfused and a diuretic administered at the same time.

PERIOPERATIVE AND POSTOPERATIVE MANAGEMENT

The anaesthetist's aim is to maintain oxygen delivery. To this end:
• An adequate supply of blood must be cross-matched, and blood that is lost at operation should be replaced promptly
• Particular care should be taken to ensure that:
—hypoxaemia never develops
—cardiac output is not decreased.

Within this framework, there is a wide choice of anaesthetic techniques at the anaesthetist's disposal. There is virtually no evidence to suggest that anaemia is associated with increased morbidity or mortality at elective surgery.

7

BIBLIOGRAPHY

American Society of Anesthesiologists Task Force on Blood Component Therapy. Practice guidelines for blood component therapy. Anesthesiology 1996; 84:732–747

Carson JL, Duff A, Berlin JA et al. Perioperative blood transfusion and postoperative mortality. Journal of the American Medical Association 1998; 279:199–205

Hébert PC, Wells G, Blajchman MA et al. A multicenter randomized, controlled clinical trial of transfusion requirements in critical care. New England Journal of Medicine 1999; 360:409–417

Messmer K, Lewis DH, Sunder-Plassman L et al. Acute normovolemic haemodilution. Changes of central hemodynamics and microcirculatory flow in skeletal muscle. European Surgical Research 1972; 4:55–70

Nunn JF, Freeman J. Problems of oxygenation and oxygen transport during anaesthesia. Anaesthesia 1964; 19:206

Weiskopf RB, Viele MK, Feiner J et al. Human cardiovascular and metabolic response to acute, severe isovolemic anemia. Journal of the American Medical Association 1998; 279:217–221

7

Disseminated intravascular coagulation (DIC)

N. Watson

Disseminated intravascular coagulation (DIC):

- Associated with life-threatening conditions
- Variable presentation, with bleeding and/or thrombosis
- Aim to correct both the underlying cause and coagulopathy
- Involve a haematologist early

DEFINITION

DIC involves widespread activation of the haemostatic mechanisms that normally operate locally to halt bleeding from injured vessels. The diagnosis of DIC requires the identification of a bleeding disorder with evidence of fibrinolysis and consumption of platelets and clotting factors. Microvascular thrombosis occurs and may be associated with multiple organ failure.

PATHOPHYSIOLOGY

The normal physiological response to vascular endothelial damage involves generation of a fibrin clot at the site of injury. Thrombus formation is controlled by physiological anticoagulants such as protein C and antithrombin III, and by the fibrinolytic system. DIC involves widespread activation of coagulation with microvascular thrombosis and depletion of coagulation factors. The fibrinolytic system is activated, resulting in generation of fibrin degradation products (FDPs), which themselves have anticoagulant properties. Thus, a diagnosis of DIC requires the demonstration of a consumptive coagulopathy (thrombocytopenia, hypofibrinogenaemia, disordered clotting function tests) with evidence of excessive fibrinolysis (increased levels of FDPs such as D-dimer).

Coagulation and inflammatory pathways are closely linked. In cases of systemic sepsis, release of cytokines from monocytes and macrophages results in a generalised inflammatory response and upregulation of the host's immune responses. Cytokines also produce widespread activation of coagulation and suppression of fibrinolysis, partly by stimulating expression of tissue factor on monocytes and endothelial cells. Formation of multiple fibrin clots in the microvasculature contributes to the organ dysfunction characteristic of severe sepsis. Antithrombin III and protein C, which act as inhibitors of both coagulation and inflammation, are depleted in severe sepsis and DIC, raising the possibility that they might have a therapeutic role.

The trigger for DIC may be vascular damage, resulting in exposure of the blood to subendothelial collagen, and activation of factor XII. The process of coagulation may also be initiated by tissue damage, releasing thromboplastins into the circulation. Box 7.1 lists the common causes of DIC.

CLINICAL FEATURES

Typically, acute DIC involves depletion of clotting factors and platelets. Laboratory findings include thrombocytopenia, anaemia, prolonged prothrombin time (PT) and activated partial thromboplastin time (APTT), hypofibrinogenaemia and raised concentration of FDPs (D-dimer).

In many cases, features of the condition are limited to laboratory abnormalities. In others, there may be widespread bruising or bleeding from the gastrointestinal tract, genitourinary tract, sites of vascular access and surgical incisions. Microvascular thrombosis may cause tissue ischaemia and necrosis, resulting in organ dysfunction that typically affects the kidneys, lungs and liver. The clinical presentation of DIC varies depending upon the aetiology, so that retained products of conception typically cause uterine haemorrhage, whereas carcinoma is associated with chronic vascular thrombosis.

7

BOX 7.1

Causes of DIC

Infection

- Septicaemia
- Viraemia
- Fungaemia
- Protozoal (e.g. malaria)

Obstetric

- Pre-eclampsia
- Placental abruption
- Amniotic fluid embolism
- Retained products of conception
- Placenta praevia

Malignancy

- Acute promyelocytic leukaemia
- Metastatic carcinoma

Traumatic

- Multiple trauma, especially with shock
- Surgery – cardiopulmonary bypass, neurosurgery
- Burns
- Fat embolism

Intravascular haemolysis

- ABO transfusion reaction
- Snake venom

Other

- Shock of any cause
- Aortic dissection
- Extensive haemangioma
- Severe liver disease

PREOPERATIVE PREPARATION

The underlying cause is often of greater clinical significance than the DIC itself. Antibiotics should be given for infection, and hypovolaemia must be corrected. Fluids and blood products should be warmed, as hypothermia will further impair clotting.

Surgery intended to remove the cause of the DIC, such as evacuation of retained products of conception, should be delayed no longer than is necessary to correct the coagulopathy to an acceptable level and to ensure cardiovascular stability.

Administration of blood products should be guided by the clinical condition of the patient and the results of laboratory investigations; it is important that a haematologist is involved. Correction of coagulopathy may require platelet concentrate and fresh frozen plasma (FFP) infusion. Severe depletion of fibrinogen (blood level < 1 g l^{-1}) is an indication for giving cryoprecipitate. Anaemia, due to haemorrhage or microangiopathic haemolysis, will require blood transfusion. An adequate supply of blood and blood components must be available before surgery starts.

Low-dose heparin has been used to interrupt the vicious cycle of intravascular coagulation and consumption coagulopathy, particularly in conditions such as acute promyelocytic leukaemia. However, control is difficult, bleeding may be exacerbated, and heparin is best avoided before surgery.

Antithrombin III therapy has shown promise in animal studies of sepsis and DIC, but the results of human studies have been inconclusive. A large phase III trial of recombinant protein C administration to patients with severe sepsis showed a decrease in the procoagulant state, a decrease in inflammatory markers and a significant decrease in mortality rate. The precise role of this novel agent in the management of DIC and sepsis has yet to be established.

Premedication is usually unnecessary or inadvisable in the critically ill patient. Intramuscular injections are best avoided.

PERIOPERATIVE MANAGEMENT

Coagulopathy is a contraindication to regional anaesthesia, so general anaesthesia is usually used. The choice of anaesthetic agents and monitoring is dictated by the patient's clinical condition and the nature of the operation. DIC is usually a disease of the critically ill, so controlled ventilation and invasive cardiovascular monitoring are usually appropriate. Large-bore intravenous lines are necessary to allow the rapid transfusion of blood and blood products, and all intravenous fluids should be warmed. Nasotracheal intubation should be avoided if coagulopathy is significant and care should be exercised during the insertion of nasogastric tubes.

Blood loss should be measured and promptly replaced. Platelet concentrate, FFP and cryoprecipitate are given according to clinical need and laboratory results. When blood loss is excessive, platelet count and clotting function (including plasma fibrinogen) should be measured regularly.

7

POSTOPERATIVE MANAGEMENT

Patients with clinically significant DIC are best managed in an ICU; they often require continued mechanical ventilation and intensive cardiovascular monitoring and support. Frequent measurement of haematological parameters should continue, with judicious administration of blood and blood products after consultation with a haematologist. Surgery, particularly in obstetric cases, may remove the cause of DIC and result in rapid resolution.

BIBLIOGRAPHY

Bernard GR, Vincent JL, Laterre PF et al. Efficacy and safety of recombinant human activated protein C for severe sepsis. New England Journal of Medicine 2001; 344:699–709

Isbister JP. Haemostatic failure. In: Oh TE, ed. Intensive care medicine. 4th edn. Oxford: Butterworth Heinemann; 1997:773

Parmet JC, Horrow JC. Hematologic diseases. In: Benumof JL, ed. Anesthesia and uncommon diseases. 4th edn. Philadelphia: WB Saunders, Philadelphia; p 302

ten Cate H, Schoenmakers S, Franco R et al. Microvascular coagulopathy and disseminated intravascular coagulation. Critical Care Medicine 2001; 29:S95–S97

7

Glucose 6-phosphate dehydrogenase deficiency

N. Denny

Glucose 6-phosphate dehydrogenase deficiency:

- An inherited condition
- Haemolysis, which may be severe, can be triggered by certain agents
- Few triggering agents are in routine anaesthetic usage

BOX 7.2

Some oxidant drugs capable of triggering haemolysis in patients with G6PD deficiency

- Analgesics
  - —aspirin in high dose
  - —phenacetin
  - —acetanilide
- Sulfonamides
- Antibiotics
  - —ciprofloxacin
  - —chloramphenicol
- Antimalarials
  - —primaquine
  - —chloroquine
  - —quinine
- Miscellaneous drugs
  - —methylene blue
  - —vitamin K
  - —nalidixic acid
  - —naphthalene
  - —quinidine
  - —probenecid
  - —phenylhydrazine
  - —nitrates
  - —nitrofurantoin
  - —ascorbic acid in high dosage

Glucose 6-phosphate dehydrogenase (G6PD) deficiency is the most common inherited metabolic disorder of red blood cells (RBCs), affecting over 100 million people worldwide with varying degrees of severity. The enzyme G6PD governs the rate at which RBCs consume, utilise and detoxify oxygen. Its deficiency makes RBCs vulnerable to haemolysis. G6PD deficiency does not usually result in complications during or after anaesthesia, provided oxidant agents known to trigger haemolysis are avoided.

PATHOPHYSIOLOGY

Low levels of G6PD result in failure to generate NADPH, which is needed to maintain red cell glutathione in a reduced state. Low levels of reduced glutathione render red cell proteins susceptible to oxygenation, resulting in the formation of masses of denatured globin (Heinz bodies), which are attached to the red cell membrane. Heinz bodies are extracted from the red cells by macrophages during passage through the spleen. The inclusion-free red cells have damaged membranes and are haemolysed. Box 7.2 lists oxidant drugs that may cause haemolysis in patients with G6PD deficiency, although the response is somewhat idiosyncratic.

CLINICAL MANIFESTATIONS

The structural gene for G6PD resides on the X chromosome and is therefore inherited as a sex-linked characteristic. G6PD deficiency is most common in hemizygous males but is also seen in homozygous females. Heterozygous females may occasionally show clinical manifestations. There are more than 200 variants of G6PD; the clinical manifestations range from negligible to severe, depending on the activity of the abnormal G6PD and whether the patient is a heterozygote or a homozygote–hemizygote. Two distinct clinical syndromes may result:
- In the African variant (the gene in this variant is termed A⁻) the patient is asymptomatic until exposed to oxidant drugs or a severe infection. Some 11% of African Americans have the A⁻ gene.

- In the Mediterranean and Oriental groups of variants, the G6PD deficiency is generally more severe and may be a cause of neonatal jaundice. Nevertheless, the patient is usually asymptomatic until a drug or infection precipitates haemolysis. Some individuals can also develop a fulminant haemolytic anaemia after exposure to the fava bean (favism).

ANAESTHETIC MANAGEMENT

Elective surgery should not be performed during a haemolytic crisis. The classical features of such a crisis include abdominal pain, jaundice, a decrease in haemoglobin concentration, an increasing reticulocyte count and the presence of Heinz bodies in the peripheral blood film.

When providing anaesthetic care for patients with G6PD deficiency, it is important to avoid oxidant agents associated with the triggering of haemolysis. These are listed in Box 7.2. In addition to these, it has been recommended that nitroprusside, and prilocaine in large amounts, be avoided.

BIBLIOGRAPHY

Cuthbert RJG, Ludlam CA, MacRae WR. Blood disorders. In: Vickers MD, Jones RM, eds. Medicine for anaesthetists. 3rd edn. Oxford: Blackwell Scientific; 1989:384–386

Handl J. Heinz body hemolytic anemias. In: 'Blood'. Textbook of Hematology. 1st edn. Boston: Little, Brown; 1987:338–341

Mehta A, Mason PJ, Vulliamy TJ. Glucose-6-phospahte dehydrogenase deficiency. Baillieres Clinical Haematology 2000; 13:21–38

Smith CL, Snowdon SL. Anaesthesia and glucose-6-phosphate dehydrogenase deficiency. Anaesthesia 1987; 42:281–288

7

Idiopathic thrombocytopenic purpura

T. Ainley

Idiopathic thrombocytopenic purpura (ITP):

- Thrombocytopenia can lead to severe haemorrhage
- Platelet count should be increased to above 100×10^9 l^{-1}, if possible
- Patients may be taking drugs (e.g. steroids) with significant side-effects
- Platelet transfusions may increase the platelet count for no more than 1 h

PATHOPHYSIOLOGY

ITP is a destructive thrombocytopenia caused by the presence of an antibody (usually IgG) against platelet membrane glycoproteins IIb/IIIa. The binding of antibody to platelets leads to their phagocytosis by cells of the reticuloendothelial system (mainly in the spleen but also in the liver) and, therefore, to a decreased platelet lifespan.

ITP may be acute or chronic. The acute form occurs most commonly in children (of both sexes). It is usually preceded by a viral infection and leads to spontaneous remission in the vast majority of patients. The chronic form of the disease affects mainly young women and is a relatively common haematological disorder.

CLINICAL FEATURES

- Petechial haemorrhage
- Easy bruising
- Skin purpura
- Menorrhagia
- Mucosal bleeding
- Rarely, intracranial haemorrhage.

DIAGNOSIS

- Decreased platelet count (usually $10-50 \times 10^9$ l^{-1})

- Increased megakaryocytes in an otherwise normal marrow
- Splenomegaly is unusual and suggests another diagnosis
- Increased platelet-associated IgG (PAIgG) in most patients – this test is not sufficiently sensitive or specific to justify its routine use in uncomplicated ITP.

The diagnosis of ITP is made after the exclusion of other causes of thrombocytopenia based on the history, physical examination, blood count and blood film. Many feel that additional investigations such as bone marrow and platelet antibodies are unnecessary except in patients aged over 65 years, those with atypical findings or those who are refractory to treatment.

TREATMENT

There is a lack of randomised clinical trials comparing the different treatment options, and treatment should therefore be tailored to the individual patient.

High-dose corticosteroids can lead to a rapid increase in platelet numbers and long-term remission, but continued low-dose therapy is often required to produce adequate platelet counts. As the side-effects of long-term steroid therapy are not inconsiderable, the aim of therapy should be to provide adequate platelet numbers for haemostasis rather than to achieve a normal platelet count.

In general, patients with a platelet count above 30×10^9 l^{-1} do not need treatment unless they require surgery, dental procedures or are shortly to give birth.

Recommendations for 'safe' platelet counts in adults:
- Minor surgery: $= 50 \times 10^9$l^{-1}
- Major surgery: $= 80 \times 10^9$ l^{-1}
- Pregnancy: see below.

Splenectomy is often recommended if steroid therapy fails. The operation carries a low mortality rate in experienced hands and the response, if it occurs, is usually rapid, with normalisation of platelet count within 2 weeks. Unfortunately, relapse is common. Patients should be given prophylactic polyvalent pneumococcal vaccine, haemophilus influenza B (Hib) vaccine and meningococcal C conjugate vaccination at least 2 weeks before splenectomy. The efficacy of lifelong antibiotics is unproven.

Around 70–85% of patients achieve remission with steroid therapy and/or splenectomy. For patients refractory to these treatments, the options are many, but, even if therapy is successful, relapse is common. The treatment options include vinca alkaloids, cyclophosphamide, azathioprine, danazol, colchicines, intravenous anti-D, dapsone and intravenous γ globulins.

ITP IN PREGNANCY

ITP may occur *de novo* in a pregnant patient or pregnancy may occur in a patient with pre-existing ITP. ITP must be distinguished from gestational thrombocytopenia (platelet count rarely less than 80×10^9 l^{-1}), which is a benign self-limiting condition not associated with a bleeding risk to mother or child.

Intrapartum and postpartum haemorrhage may prove life-threatening to the mother. As PAIgG can cross the placenta, the fetus may become thrombocytopenic and is at risk of haemorrhage, particularly in the CNS. There has been debate on whether vaginal delivery or caesarean section is the safer option for the baby. It is now generally agreed that the mode of delivery should be determined by obstetric considerations alone. In the neonate, the platelet count may be low and continue to decrease in the first week of life.

The asymptomatic mother with ITP does not need therapy until delivery is imminent if the platelet count is above 20×10^9 l^{-1}, but should be monitored closely both clinically and haematologically. If the platelet count falls below this level, low-dose steroid therapy or immunoglobulin may be given. The neonate may also receive steroids and immunoglobulin if necessary.

- A platelet count above 50×10^9 l^{-1} should be considered safe for vaginal delivery in patients with otherwise normal coagulation.
- A platelet count above 80×10^9 l^{-1} should be considered safe for caesarean section, spinal or epidural anaesthesia in patients with otherwise normal coagulation.

ANAESTHETIC MANAGEMENT

Advice should be sought from a haematologist. If the procedure is elective, steroid and immunoglobulin administration may increase platelet count sufficiently for surgery to be undertaken safely. A platelet count of 80×10^9 l^{-1} is an acceptable target. Platelet transfusion is rarely indicated, as platelet survival is usually less than 1 h. However, it may be the only option in acute life-threatening haemorrhage.

The side-effects of drug therapy should be looked for and managed appropriately if present. For steroids, these include hyperglycaemia, hypokalaemia and hypertension.

During splenectomy, platelets should be given once the splenic artery has been clamped. This is logical but is based only on relatively poor published evidence. Regional anaesthetic techniques should usually be avoided if the platelet count is less than 100×10^9 l^{-1}. The trend in recent years has been to lower this threshold to 80×10^9 l^{-1}. Each case should be considered individually and both the benefits and risks of regional anaesthesia considered.

BIBLIOGRAPHY

Andersen JC. Response of resistant idiopathic thrombocytopenic purpura to pulse high dose dexamethasone therapy. New England Journal of Medicine 1994; 330:1560–1564

British Committee for Standards in Haematology. Guidelines for the investigation and management of idiopathic thrombocytopenic purpura in adults, children and in pregnancy. British Journal of Haematology 2003; 120:574–596

McVerry BA. Management of ITP in adults. British Journal of Haematology 1985; 59:203–208

7

Inherited coagulopathies

M. Price

Inherited coagulopathies:

- Rare
- Most patients presenting for anaesthesia are already aware of their disease
- Specific concentrates are available for all the commoner types

---

Inherited coagulopathies are rare, but the anaesthetist may encounter the following more common conditions:

- Factor VIII deficiency – haemophilia A or classical haemophilia
- Factor IX deficiency – haemophilia B or Christmas disease
- Von Willebrand's disease
- Factor XI deficiency
- Factor VII deficiency.

HAEMOPHILIA

There are about 5500 patients with haemophilia A in the UK, of whom 34% are human immuno-deficiency virus (HIV) positive. There are about 1100 patients with haemophilia B in the UK, of whom 5% are HIV positive.

The genes for factor VIII and factor IX production are carried on the X chromosome, and consequently haemophiliacs are usually male. The severity of haemophilia A is determined by the level of functional factor VIII (Table 7.2).

CLINICAL MANIFESTATION

The mild form (factor VIII level 25–50 units 100 ml^{-1}) is asymptomatic, and the diagnosis may not be made until the patient has surgery. Any family history of abnormal bleeding, however vague, should be taken seriously and the patient's haemostatic mechanisms thoroughly investigated. In the severe form, spontaneous bleeding into joints, muscles and other organs occurs, and may give rise to long-term dysfunction of the sites of bleeding. The

TABLE 7.2

Relationship between plasma factor VIIIc levels and severity of bleeding in classical haemophilia

Factor VIIIc level (units 100 ml^{-1})	Bleeding symptoms
50	None
25–50	Excess bleeding after major surgery or accident
5–25	Excess bleeding after minor surgery
1–5	Severe bleeding after minor surgery and some spontaneous haemorrhage

clinical manifestations of haemophilia B are similar and depend on the level of factor IX.

The APTT is prolonged in haemophilia and can be corrected by the addition of normal plasma. Quantitative assays of factor VIII or IX will identify the type and severity of the disease.

MANAGEMENT

A haematological opinion should be sought if possible. For minor surgery, factor VIII or IX levels should be $\geq$ 50% of normal. For major surgery, the levels should be as near normal as possible before the operation, and should be maintained above 50% of normal for several days after surgery.

Cryoprecipitate and FFP should be given to patients with haemophilia only in extreme emergencies, as the possibility of viral transmission has given rise to medical and medicolegal concern. Most hospitals now have adequate supplies of factor VIII and factor IX concentrates, all of which have been subject to some form of virucidal treatment. Hospitals that do not stock these concentrates can usually obtain supplies within 24 h.

Older patients who received factor concentrates before 1985, when heat treatment was introduced, may be infected with some or all of the following viruses:

- Hepatitis B
- Hepatitis C
- HIV.

VON WILLEBRAND'S DISEASE

Von Willebrand's disease (vWD) is an autosomal dominant disease and is therefore seen in both sexes. Severe forms of the disease are probably about as common as factor IX deficiency. It is caused by a deficiency of von Willebrand factor (vWF), which has a complex molecular biology. It can be associated with gene deletion, point mutations or intragenic replications. Although the frequency of abnormal genes may be as high as 1 in 2000 in the UK population, relatively few affected people have a haemostatic abnormality.

vWF is a multifunctional plasma glycoprotein that is secreted by endothelial cells and binds to factor VIII, collagen and heparin, and to platelet membrane glycoproteins. In severe vWD, platelets do not adhere to endothelium, and the factor VIII level is low due to lack of carrier protein.

CLINICAL MANIFESTATIONS

The severity of the disease depends upon the vWF level. Problems range from frequent nose bleeds, heavy periods and marked bleeding after dental extraction to more serious problems such as mucosal bleeds and haemarthroses. Diagnosis is by the demonstration of a prolonged bleeding time, the ristocetin-induced platelet agglutination test and by a quantitative vWF radioimmunoassay.

MANAGEMENT

DDAVP treatment can increase vWF levels for a few days, but does so at the expense of body stores. For severe forms of the disease, replacement therapy can be given using intermediate-purity factor VIII concentrate, which contains some vWF (high-purity factor VIII concentrate is unsuitable as it contains no vWF).

FACTOR XI DEFICIENCY

There are about 250 patients with factor XI deficiency in the UK, of whom around half are Ashkenazi Jews. It is an autosomally inherited condition. A heat-treated factor XI concentrate is available on a named-patient basis.

FACTOR VII DEFICIENCY

Factor VII deficiency is very rare and, in the UK, is usually seen in Muslims of Indian origin, probably as a result of consanguinity. It is autosomally inherited. A specific heat-treated concentrate for treatment of factor VII deficiency is available on a named-patient basis.

BIBLIOGRAPHY

Rizza CR. Clinical management of haemophilia. British Medical Bulletin 1977; 33:225–230

7

Massive transfusion, microvascular haemorrhage and thrombocytopenia

K. Ashpole

Massive transfusion

- Restore and maintain adequate circulating blood volume
- Maintain sufficient oxygen-carrying capacity
- Transfusion related coagulopathy is unlikely to occur until at least one blood volume has been transfused
- Secure haemostasis:
  - Give FFP if prothrombin time ratio and activated partial thromboplastin time ratio (PTR, APTTR) > 1.5
  - Give platelet concentrate if platelet count < 50 × 10^9 l^{-1}, or < 100 × 10^9 l^{-1} if there is a risk of intracranial haemorrhage
  - Give cryoprecipitate if fibrinogen level < 80–100 mg dl^{-1}

DEFINITION

A massive transfusion is required at times of major haemorrhage. Major haemorrhage can be defined as the loss of one circulating blood volume in a 24-h period. This equates to a blood loss of 5 litres in a 70-kg man, and represents the transfusion of 10–12 units of stored blood to an adult patient. More practical definitions have been developed to allow earlier recognition of major haemorrhage, and because the rate of blood loss has important haemostatic consequences. Massive transfusion can therefore also be defined as a greater than 50% loss of circulating blood volume in 3 h, or a rate of blood loss greater than 150 ml min^{-1}.

PATHOPHYSIOLOGY

Major haemorrhage leads to a decrease in circulating blood volume, and the effects of hypovolaemia must be separated from those of anaemia. The clinical manifestations of hypovolaemic shock related to percentage blood loss are given in Table 7.3.

Massive transfusion is associated with microvascular haemorrhage in 30% of patients.

TABLE 7.3

Classification of hypovolaemic shock according to blood loss in a 70kg man

	Class I	Class II	Class III	Class IV
Blood loss				
Percentage	< 15	15–30	30–40	> 40
Volume (ml)	750	800–1500	1500	> 2000
Blood pressure				
Systolic	Unchanged	Normal	Reduced	Very low
Diastolic	Unchanged	Raised	Reduced	Very low, Unrecordable
Pulse (beats min^{-1})	Slight tachycardia	100–120	120 (thready)	> 120 (very thready)
Capillary refill	Normal	Slow (> 2 s)	Slow (> 2 s)	Undetectable
Respiratory rate	Normal	Normal	Tachypnoea	Tachypnoea
Urinary flow rate (ml h^{-1})	> 30	20–30	10–20	0–10
Extremities	Normal colour	Pale	Pale	Pale and cold
Complexion	Normal	Pale	Pale	Ashen
Mental state	Alert	Anxious or aggressive	Anxious, aggressive or drowsy	Drowsy, confused or unconscious

In the absence of inherited disorders of haemostasis, the main causes are a dilutional deficiency of clotting factors and disseminated intravascular coagulation (DIC). The development of component therapy and the use of plasma-poor red cells (SAGM blood; see Box 7.3) means that a clotting factor deficiency is now more of a problem than thrombocytopenia. DIC is a feared complication of major haemorrhage and is more likely to develop in conjunction with prolonged shock, hypothermia, and extensive muscle or cerebral damage. It causes bleeding, tissue necrosis and microthrombosis, which can lead to irreversible organ damage. The coagulation defect occurs as a result of consumption of coagulation factors and platelets, and increased fibrinolytic activity.

BOX 7.3

Contents of blood components

Red cells in additive: stored at 4 ± 2°C; use within 4 h at room temperature
- SAGM (saline, adenine, glucose, mannitol) units = 350 ± 70 ml

Platelet concentrates: stored at 22 ± 2°C, continuously agitated; use within 2 h
- Single unit = 50 ± 10 ml fresh plasma; contains 55×10^9 platelets
- Pooled platelet pack = 320 ± 26 ml fresh plasma; contains 250×10^9 platelets

Fresh frozen plasma: 30 min to thaw; use within 2 h
- Single unit = 150 – 200 ml; dose is 12–15 ml kg^{-1}

MANAGEMENT

The mortality and morbidity rates associated with major haemorrhage are high, and the institution of a locally agreed major haemorrhage protocol is recommended to ensure effective management (Fig. 7.1). Initial management of the patient requires a full clinical assessment, insertion of large-bore intravenous lines and invasive monitoring. The clinical priority is rapid restoration of circulating blood volume with simultaneous surgical, medical or radiological intervention to stop the bleeding. It is important to prevent prolonged hypotension, as this leads to a progressive acidosis, and tissue and organ damage, which predisposes to the development of DIC. The mortality rate increases with the duration and severity of shock.

Debate continues as to the preferred choice of initial resuscitation fluid: crystalloid or colloid. About 50–75% less colloid than crystalloid is needed to achieve the same volume expansion, but at increased cost, risk of allergic reactions and, in large volumes, altered haemostasis. Pragmatically, it seems reasonable to use a combination of both crystalloids and colloids.

The critical level of oxygen delivery (D_{O_2}) as a generic value is unknown. Recent evidence suggests that a Hb concentration of 7–8 g dl^{-1} may be sufficient for the majority of patients. The Association of Anaesthetists of Great Britain and Ireland has recommended that when the Hb level is 7 g dl^{-1} a blood transfusion is strongly advised, and that when Hb concentration is 5 g dl^{-1} it becomes essential. A blood transfusion is likely to be required when 30–40% of total blood volume is lost. This decision should always be guided by laboratory investigations and the clinical picture, including an evaluation of the patient's cardiorespiratory reserve and the rate of blood loss, together with the extent of anticipated further blood loss.

Formulaic replacement therapy, i.e. the automatic administration of a unit of FFP and/or platelets for each set number of units of blood transfused, has not been shown to be effective in preventing microvascular haemorrhage. The results of regular haemostatic tests should be monitored and transfusions of platelets and FFP should be given when appropriate. A moderate deficiency of coagulation factors is common in massively transfused patients, but does not contribute to microvascular haemorrhage until levels fall to less than 20% of normal. These levels are reliably reflected by the prolongation of the PTR and APTTR to above 1.5. The APTT and PT should be monitored regularly, but interpretation must always be related to the clinical picture. Stress stimulates the synthesis and release of factor VIII and fibrinogen, so a deficiency is rare and cryoprecipitate is not usually needed unless the situation is complicated by DIC.

A dilutional thrombocytopenia is unlikely unless more than two blood volumes are lost or the patient's platelets are functionally abnormal. Extracorporeal circulatory techniques used in cardiac surgery, the administration of aspirin, uraemia and the intake of large amounts of alcohol can cause an acquired functional defect causing a prolongation of the bleeding time.

DIC can be caused by a variety of triggers, including shock. The coagulation defect occurs as a result of consumption of coagulation factors and platelets, and increased fibrinolytic activity. Laboratory investigations show a mixed picture of low platelets, low fibrinogen, prolonged PT

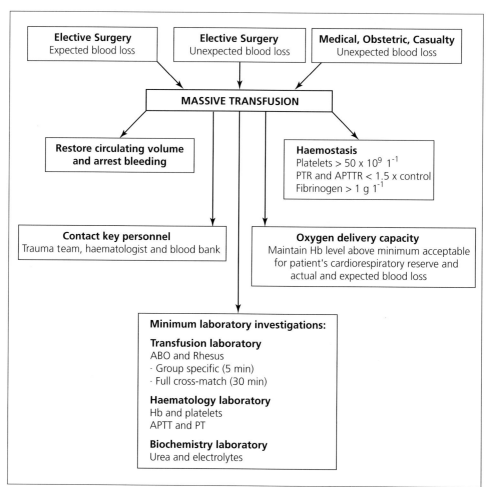

Fig. 7.1 Key issues in massive blood loss and transfusion. PTR, prothrombin time ratio; APTTR, activated partial thromboplastin time ratio; APTT, activated partial thromboplastin time; PT, prothrombin time.

and APTT, and increased FDPs or D-dimer. Senior haematological advice, platelets, FFP dimers and cryoprecipitate will all be required.

The Serious Hazards of Transfusion (SHOT) annual report 2000–2001 highlighted a 6% increase in the number of incorrect blood com-ponent transfusions. Protocols for accurate iden-tification of transfusion specimens and of desig-nated units of blood, platelets and FFP must be adhered to, even in the stress of an emergency situation, as clinical errors at this time account for most transfusion-related error morbidity.

BIBLIOGRAPHY

American Society of Anesthesiologists Task Force on Blood Component Therapy. Practice guidelines for blood component therapy. Anesthesiology 1996; 84:732–747

British Committee for Standardisation in Haematology Blood Transfusion Task Force. Guidelines for transfusion for massive blood loss. Clinical and Laboratory Haematology 1988; 10:265–273

Donaldson MDJ, Seaman MJ, Park GR. Massive blood transfusion. British Journal of Anaesthesia 1992; 69:621–630

Hiippala S. Replacement of massive blood loss. Vox Sanguinis 1998; 74 (Suppl 2):399–407

Murphy MF, Wallington TB, Kelsey P et al, British Committee for Standardisation in Haematology Blood Transfusion Task Force. Guidelines for the clinical use of red cell transfusions. British Journal of Haematology 2001; 113:24–31

Stainsby D, MacLennan S, Hamilton PJ. Management of massive blood loss: a template guide. British Journal of Anaesthesia 2000; 85:487–491

7

Mastocytosis

J. Handy

Mastocytosis

- Rare but potentially fatal
- Premedicate with antihistamines and cromoglycate
- Avoid histamine-releasing agents
- Be prepared for cardiovascular instability

DEFINITION

Mastocytosis is a rare disorder (1–4 per 10 000 population) of mast cell proliferation that occurs in both cutaneous (urticaria pigmentosa) and systemic (in about 10% of cases, particularly affecting the reticuloendothelial system) forms. Two-thirds of patients develop the disease in childhood, with an equal distribution between the sexes, and the condition has been reported in all races. Familial cases have been documented, although most patients have no familial association. Symptoms and signs result from immune and non-immune stimulation of mast cells resulting in the local and systemic release of a variety of biologically active mediators.

PATHOPHYSIOLOGY

Currently, the only established pathological mechanism appears to be the presence of a somatic mutation in codon 816 of the c-*kit* proto-oncogene, leading to constitutive activation of the KIT receptor (a type III tyrosine kinase receptor), which drives mast cell proliferation and survival.

Stimulation of the mast cells results in the release of preformed mediators (including histamine, heparin, chemotactic factors and cytokines) and newly formed mediators (including prostaglandin D, leukotrienes and platelet-activating factor). Clinically, the most important of these are histamine and prostaglandin D_2 (PGD_2), their physiological effects being widespread:

- *Cardiovascular*:
  —Venous dilatation resulting in increased vascular capacity
  —Arteriolar dilatation resulting in decreased arterial pressure
  —Increased capillary permeability with rapid loss of fluid into the tissue spaces.
- *Respiratory* – bronchospasm and increased production of airway secretions.
- *Cutaneous*:
  —Increased blood flow to the skin with erythema and flushing
  —Pruritus.
- *Gastrointestinal*:
  —Increased gastric secretions
  —Increased gut motility.
- *Other* – increased uterine contraction.

SYMPTOMS

The diverse nature of the disease, with both acute 'attacks' and chronic organ involvement, results in symptoms that are variable in terms of severity and duration. Symptoms range from pruritus and flushing to dyspnoea, abdominal pain and even syncope, and are attributable to the wide-ranging physiological effects of the secreted mast cell mediators (Box 7.4). Episodes of syncope and hypotension are rare, as are deaths associated with mast cell mediator release.

PRECIPITATING FACTORS

Mast cell stimulation results from both immune and non-immune mechanisms. In the perioperative period, the latter are of greater significance and may be classified into non-pharmacological or pharmacological triggers.

NON-PHARMACOLOGICAL TRIGGERS
Mechanical irritation of the lesions, temperature changes, exercise, vomiting, pain and psychological stress.

BOX 7.4

Symptoms and signs of mastocytosis

Cardiopulmonary	Gastrointestinal
Chest pain	Abdominal cramps
Dizziness	Diarrhoea
Dyspnoea	Epigastric pain
Palpitations	Nausea and vomiting
Syncope	Hepatosplenomegaly
Skin	Neurological
Bullae	Cognitive
Urticaria and	disorganisation
oedema	Headaches
Flushing and	Constitutional
pruritus	Fatigue
Skeletal	Fever
Bone pain	Malaise
Pathological	Weight loss
fractures	
Haematological	
Anaemia and	
thrombocytopenia	
Bleeding diathesis	

PHARMACOLOGICAL TRIGGERS

A multitude of drugs have been implicated including alcohol, opiates, curare, non-steroidal anti-inflammatory drugs, vancomycin, suxamethonium, aspirin, radiocontrast media, β-receptor antagonists, α-receptor agonists and drug preservatives, including sodium metabisulphate and parabens.

PREOPERATIVE ASSESSMENT

A detailed history may suggest organ involvement and may highlight any known trigger agents. All patients with suspected systemic involvement should have a full blood count and a peripheral smear to exclude an associated haematological disorder. Abnormal findings should prompt a bone marrow biopsy. Although liver function tests are usually normal, abdominal ultrasonography should be performed to rule out hepatic or splenic involvement.

Serum α-tryptase concentration is increased in patients with systemic mastocytosis regardless of whether or not they are experiencing acute symptoms, and this can be used to assess the total-body mast cell burden. Urinary methylimidazole acetic acid (a histamine metabolite) levels have been shown to correlate closely to the extent of mast cell disease, being highest in patients with widespread systemic involvement. Beyond these tests, any additional investigation should be tailored to individual specific symptoms and may include gastrointestinal tract endoscopy, bone scans and lymph node biopsy.

PREOPERATIVE PREPARATION

Adrenaline (epinephrine) and other resuscitation drugs and equipment must be immediately available. Premedication with H_1 and H_2 histamine receptor antagonists and non-steroidal anti-inflammatory agents is recommended, although the latter can act as trigger agents. Sodium cromoglycate may help stabilise mast cells, although prophylactic steroids have not been shown to be of any benefit. There are several reports of preoperative intradermal skin tests being used to identify drugs that may be safely administered during anaesthesia. However, the specificity of these tests is uncertain.

PERIOPERATIVE MANAGEMENT

PREMEDICATION

Anxiolysis and sedation may be achieved using benzodiazepines. Anticholinergic drugs such as hyoscine should be avoided.

MONITORING

In addition to standard monitoring, invasive blood pressure, temperature and urine output should be measured. Central venous access and pressure measurement should be considered, depending on the type of operation.

INDUCTION AND MAINTENANCE OF ANAESTHESIA

Haemodynamic instability should be anticipated, and resuscitation drugs and equipment must be immediately available at all times. Large-bore intravenous cannulae should be inserted and monitoring instituted before induction of anaesthesia. Drugs known to cause histamine release should be avoided. Drugs that have been safely administered include propofol, etomidate, fentanyl, vecuronium, volatile anaesthetic agents (ether-linked anaesthetic agents inhibit mast cell degranulation), benzodiazepines and preservative-free amide local anaesthetics. If an anticholinergic drug is required, glycopyrrolate is preferred. The number of pharmacological agents used should be kept to a minimum. Regional anaesthetic techniques may be used, although these have been associated with acute reactions.

7

ENVIRONMENT

A warm, calm environment should be maintained throughout the perioperative period. Hypothermia should be prevented by both active and passive means. Local tissue trauma should be minimised by careful patient handling, positioning and padding of all pressure points. Tourniquets should be used with caution if they are deemed necessary.

POSTOPERATIVE MANAGEMENT

A calm environment, adequate analgesia and normothermia should be maintained after surgery. Skin irritation and trauma should continue to be minimised, and resuscitation drugs and equipment should remain immediately available.

BIBLIOGRAPHY

Hartmann K, Bruns SB, Henz BM. Mastocytosis: review of clinical and experimental aspects. Journal of Investigative Dermatology Symposium Proceedings 2001; 6:143–147

Lerno G, Slaats G, Coenen E, Herregods L, Rolly G. Anaesthetic management of systemic mastocytosis. British Journal of Anaesthesia 1990; 65:254–257

Parris WCV, Scott HW, Smith BE. Anesthetic management of systemic mastocytosis: experience with 42 cases. Anesthesia and Analgesia 1986; 65:S117

Rosenbaum KJ, Strobel GE. Anaesthetic considerations in mastocytosis. Anesthesiology 1973; 38:398–401

Tharp MD, Longley BJ Jr. Mastocytosis. Dermatologic Clinics 2001; 19:679–696

7

Multiple myeloma

C. Gomersall

Myeloma can cause:

- Severe bone pain and spontaneous fractures
- Renal failure
- Hypercalcaemia

DEFINITION

Multiple myeloma is a diffuse proliferation of B lymphocytes and plasma cells largely confined to bone marrow. It is characterised by the production of a paraprotein and the occurrence of osteolytic bone lesions. The diagnosis is made by the coexistence of at least two of the following:

- Excess plasma cells in the marrow
- Paraprotein concentration greater than 1 g dl^{-1} (IgG or IgA) or excess light chains in the urine
- Radiographic evidence of lytic lesions.

It is a disease of the elderly, with a mean age at diagnosis of 60 years.

PATHOPHYSIOLOGY

BONE LESIONS

Lytic lesions, through which pathological fractures occur, result from the secretion of an osteoclast-stimulating cytokine by the abnormal plasma cells. Bones fracture either spontaneously or after trivial injuries; vertebral collapse is particularly common. Patients often suffer from severe bone pain.

HYPERCALCAEMIA

In general, this occurs only in patients with extensive osteolysis. It is exacerbated by dehydration secondary to vomiting and the inability to retain salt and water due to renal involvement. It may also be precipitated by bedrest and infection. Hypercalcaemia can cause vomiting, constipation, anorexia, depression, confusion, drowsiness and even coma.

RENAL IMPAIRMENT

Renal impairment is due to a combination of dehydration, hypercalcaemia, pyelonephritis, deposition of myeloma protein in the kidney and, in some cases, renal amyloidosis. In acute renal failure secondary to myeloma, the most important measure is correction of dehydration and treatment of any precipitating renal infection.

HAEMATOLOGICAL ABNORMALITIES

Normochromic, normocytic anaemia is common and may be severe due to marrow failure or renal failure. Haemostatic abnormalities may be due to interference with clotting and platelet function by paraprotein, hyperviscosity, renal failure or, rarely, thrombocytopenia as a result of marrow infiltration or chemotherapy.

HYPERVISCOSITY

This is a rare complication associated with high plasma levels of paraprotein. It is more likely to occur in IgA myelomatosis where there is polymerisation of paraprotein molecules. It can cause a variety of neurological, ocular, haematological and cardiac problems, including cardiac failure. It may also result in spurious hyponatraemia and predispose to venous thrombosis.

IMMUNE SYSTEM

Synthesis of all immunoglobulins apart from the paraprotein is depressed, leading to increased susceptibility to infection, especially by staphylococci and Gram-negative organisms.

NERVOUS SYSTEM

The most important neurological manifestations are peripheral neuropathy, paraplegia secondary to an epidural plasmacytoma, and spinal root compression due to paravertebral masses or collapsed vertebrae.

ANAESTHETIC MANAGEMENT

There has been little research into the anaesthetic management of patients with multiple

7

myeloma; no papers have been published in the English literature on this subject in the last 13 years and, therefore, all recommendations have to be based purely on an understanding of the abnormalities associated with the disease.

PREOPERATIVE

Management should be directed towards the detection and correction of abnormalities associated with myeloma, with particular attention to fluid balance, hypercalcaemia, haemostatic abnormalities and renal impairment. Patients with symptomatic hyperviscosity should be treated with plasmapheresis before surgery.

INTRAOPERATIVE
Regional anaesthesia
This may be absolutely contraindicated for medical reasons (haemostatic abnormalities) or relatively contraindicated for medicolegal reasons (active neurological disease).

General anaesthesia
Attention to the positioning of the patient is essential in view of the increased susceptibility to fractures. Strict asepsis is important because of the impairment of immune function, which may be further impaired by general anaesthesia. In theory, adjustment of doses of intravenous agents may be necessary in view of changes in plasma proteins.

POSTOPERATIVE
Duration of immobility should be minimised to decrease the risk of precipitating hypercalcaemia and of developing venous thrombosis.

BIBLIOGRAPHY

Dewhirst WE, Glass DD. Haematological diseases. In: Katz J, Benumof JL, Kadis LB, eds. Anaesthesia and uncommon diseases. Philadelphia: WB Saunders; 1990:406–408

7

Polycythaemia

R. Balon

Polycythaemia

- Is often secondary to clinically significant conditions
- Can be associated with abnormal bleeding during and after surgery
- Postoperative thromboembolic events are common
- Poses a greater risk to the patient than anaemia

DEFINITION

Polycythaemia may be defined as an increase in red blood cell mass such that Hb concentration and packed cell volume (PCV) exceed the following values:

	Male	Female
Hb (g dl^{-1})	17.5	15.0
PCV	0.51	0.48

CAUSES:

- Primary polycythaemia – increased red cell mass
- Secondary polycythaemia – increased red call mass
- Apparent polycythaemia – normal red cell mass.

A red cell mass more than 25% above the predicted value signifies real or absolute polycythaemia.

PRIMARY POLYCYTHAEMIA

Also known as polycythaemia rubra vera, this is a non-malignant stem cell disease of clonal origin; it gives rise to an increase in granulocyte and platelet count in addition to an increase in red cell mass. Hb can exceed 20 g dl^{-1}, platelet count is often in the range 450–800 $\times$ 10^9 l^{-1} and can exceed 1000 $\times$ 10^9 l^{-1}. It is a disease of older adults (median age 55–60 years) and of both sexes. Less than 5% of cases present before the age of 40 years.

Splenomegaly and hepatomegaly are common. High blood viscosity resulting from the high haematocrit can lead to episodes of thrombosis with resulting ischaemic damage. Primary polycythaemia may be an incidental finding but is classically associated with digital ischaemia, stroke, headache, mental clouding, facial plethora, myocardial infarction, pruritus, bleeding and gout. Although thrombosis is more common in patients with a high platelet count, it can also occur with normal platelet numbers. Paradoxically, patients with primary polycythaemia may also suffer from abnormal bleeding, as platelet function is sometimes abnormal. Rarely, patients with primary polycythaemia may present with anaemia as a result of chronic gastrointestinal haemorrhage.

Without treatment, the median survival of patients with primary polycythaemia is about 2 years after diagnosis. The mainstay of treatment is repeated venesection to maintain the PCV below 0.45. Hydroxyurea is given to control the platelet count. Phophorus-32 and busulfan are now used only in elderly patients because these drugs are associated with an increased risk of the development of leukaemia.

SECONDARY POLYCYTHAEMIA

The majority of secondary polycythaemias are caused by a compensatory increase in erythropoietin production in response to hypoxia. Common causes include chronic obstructive pulmonary disease, high altitude and congenital cyanotic heart disease. A smaller number of patients have abnormal excess secretion of erythropoietin. Causes include hypernephroma, hepatoma, cerebellar haemangioblastoma and phaeochromocytoma. Polycystic and transplanted kidneys can secrete inappropriately large amounts of erythropoietin.

7

APPARENT POLYCYTHAEMIA

This term is applied to patients who have an increased PCV but normal red cell mass. The mechanism is unclear but smoking, hypertension, obesity, diuretics and high alcohol intake have all been associated with apparent polycythaemia. Management is aimed at reversing any potential cause (e.g. stopping smoking), and treatment by venesection is recommended in patients with a PCV above 0.54 or in those with an increased risk of vascular occlusion. In addition, there are clinical situations in which the normal ranges for Hb and haematocrit are exceeded with a normal red cell mass if the plasma volume is substantially reduced, for example plasma loss in burns and severe fluid loss suffered as a result of gross dehydration or prolonged bowel obstruction.

ANAESTHESIA AND POLYCYTHAEMIA

Polycythaemia probably presents a much greater risk to the patient undergoing surgery than anaemia. It is not surprising that controlled randomised studies of patients who have undergone surgery with or without treatment of their polycythaemia are not available. A retrospective uncontrolled and non-randomised study reported more than 30 years ago suggested some important points about the anaesthetic and surgical management of patients with primary polycythaemia:

- Patients with untreated primary polycythaemia experience substantially greater morbidity and mortality rates after surgery than those who are adequately treated.
- Patients with adequately treated primary polycythaemia may have a similar morbidity and mortality rate to unaffected patients.
- The commonest complications in patients with untreated primary polycythaemia are haemorrhage and thrombosis.
- The decrease in postoperative morbidity and mortality rates seen in patients whose primary polycythaemia has been treated is proportional to the duration of haematological control.

PREOPERATIVE MANAGEMENT

Polycythaemia most often comes to light during the investigation of some other disorder or at routine preoperative testing. It should be considered when small vessel occlusive disease is the indication for surgery, or when the patient has plethoric facies, a history of ischaemic heart disease or abnormal bleeding.

If a high Hb concentration or haematocrit is identified before surgery, acute plasma volume reduction as a cause can usually be excluded on history and clinical grounds. If true polycythaemia is identified, hypoxaemia as a cause can be readily excluded by performing arterial blood gas measurement. If the surgical procedure is elective, the patient should be referred to a haematologist for investigation and treat-

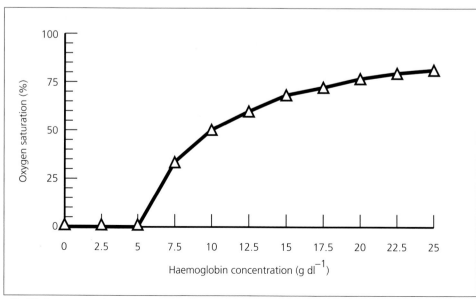

Fig. 7.2 Oxygen saturation at which cyanosis may occur over a range of haemoglobin concentrations.

ment. It has been suggested that the peripheral blood count and the blood volume should be normalised before surgery.

If the operation is urgent and blood volume is clinically normal, isovolaemic haemodilution can be performed by venesecting the patient and replacing the withdrawn volume with colloid. It is logical to retain the withdrawn blood for administration to the patient should surgical blood loss be excessive. Subcutaneous low molecular weight heparin administration should be considered.

PERIOPERATIVE MANAGEMENT

If the polycythaemia is secondary, steps must be taken to account for the primary disease process, for instance chronic obstructive pulmonary disease, congenital cyanotic heart disease. Venous stasis and hypotension, both of which can cause thrombosis, should be avoided. Regional anaesthesia offers advantages to the polycythaemic patient in that the incidence of postoperative thromboembolic events may be decreased. The anaesthetist should take care to ensure that the results of clotting and platelet function tests are normal before embarking on neuraxial blocks.

Cyanosis occurs when the concentration of reduced (deoxygenated) haemoglobin exceeds a value of about 5 g dl^{-1}. This will occur at higher oxygen saturations in patients with a high Hb concentration. If the Hb concentration exceeds 20 g dl^{-1}, cyanosis may occur at saturations equal to the normal mixed venous oxygen saturation (i.e. 75%). Figure 7.2 shows the oxygen saturation at which cyanosis may occur for a range of Hb concentrations.

BIBLIOGRAPHY

Barabas AP. Surgical problems associated with polycythaemia. British Journal of Hospital Medicine 1980; 23:289–290

Messinezy M, Pearson TC. ABC of clinical haematology. Polycythaemia, primary (essential) thrombocythaemia and myelofibrosis. British Medical Journal 1997; 314:587–590

Provan D, Weatherall D. Red cells II: acquired anaemias and polycythaemia. Lancet 2000; 355:1260–1268

Wasserman LR, Gilbert HS. Surgical bleeding in polycythaemic patients. Annals of the New York Academy of Sciences 1964; 113:122

7

Sickle cell syndrome

I. Munday

Sickle cell syndromes:

- Include HbSS, HbSC and HbSThal
- Life-threatening sickle crises can occur
- Finding compatible blood can be difficult as a result of red cell antibodies

---

DEFINITION

Sickle cell syndromes are inherited haemoglobinopathies in which the dominant haemoglobin (Hb) is the unstable haemoglobin S. They include sickle cell anaemia (HbSS) and the double heterozygote conditions sickle C (HbSC) and sickle thalassaemia (HbSThal).

PATHOPHYSIOLOGY

The sickle gene causes a single amino acid substitution on the ß chain of the Hb molecule. There is some evidence that haemoglobin S confers a limited resistance to infection with malaria, a fact that may explain the greater incidence of the sickle gene in equatorial Africa.

When HbS is deoxygenated, the molecules polymerise into long chains called 'tactoids' and become insoluble. This results in deformation of the red cell membrane into the characteristic sickle shape. Although the process is often reversible with oxygenation, haemolysis will occur if the cell membrane is damaged. During prolonged periods of deoxygenation, irreversible sickling may occur. In this situation, the cells aggregate and occlude small blood vessels, which leads to tissue infarction and further hypoxia. Hypoxia is aggravated by lung infarction, which is a common cause of death. The major features of sickle cell disease are therefore chronic anaemia and the occurrence of sickle cell 'crises' in which multiple episodes of tissue infarction occur.

Sickling occurs in individuals who are homozygous for the sickle gene (HbSS) and also in those in whom the sickle gene is inherited along with another variant such as HbC or β-thalassaemia. Tactoid formation is enhanced in the presence of HbC compared with the normal HbA. Patients with HbSC may have a Hb concentration towards the lower end of the normal range, but are liable to sickle and have a high incidence of venous thrombosis. Inheritance of the ß-thalassaemia gene results in greatly reduced ß-chain synthesis.

Individuals with sickle cell trait (HbAS) are usually asymptomatic, although sickling may occur under conditions of severe hypoxaemia. Patients with sickle cell trait are not at increased risk during a properly conducted anaesthetic, although the use of a tourniquet may be hazardous.

PREOPERATIVE ASSESSMENT

Patients from susceptible populations should be screened for HbS with a quick solubility test (e.g. Sickledex). This will not distinguish between HbAS and the more dangerous phenotypes, but other abnormalities in the full blood count and examination of the blood film should alert the laboratory to the presence of an important haemoglobinopathy. Haemoglobin electrophoresis is necessary to confirm the diagnosis.

Patients with HbSS are usually well adapted to their low haemoglobin concentration, and increases in the haematocrit will increase the risk of a vaso-occlusive crisis. Patients who have received multiple transfusions in the past may have many red cell antibodies. Consequently, compatible blood may be difficult to find and transfusion reactions are relatively common. The optimum Hb concentration and the acceptable proportion of HbS are both debatable, and are determined in part by the proposed surgical procedure. In general, blood transfusion is usually unnecessary for patients undergoing minor operations. For major surgery, simple red cell transfusion to increase the haemoglobin concentration to 10 g dl^{-1} seems to be as effective in preventing complications as more complex transfusion regimens to reduce the HbS concentration. However, a haematologist must be involved in this aspect of the patient's management.

See also Box 7.5.

PERIOPERATIVE MANAGEMENT

No specific anaesthetic technique is recommended. The principal objectives are to avoid any factors that may promote sickling. In partic-

ular, care should be taken to maintain good oxygenation, hydration, normothermia and normal acid–base balance. Limb tourniquets are best avoided, although there have been reports of their uncomplicated use. If a tourniquet is essential, it should be applied as distally as possible, the limb should be thoroughly exsanguinated and the ischaemic time should be minimised.

The high standard of care delivered in the operating theatre must continue in the postoperative period. This may require advance planning to ensure that a bed on a HDU is available.

Pain management presents a number of problems. Opioids may cause respiratory depression with consequent acidosis and hypoxia. Some patients may have developed a tolerance to opioids if they have required frequent treatment for sickle cell crises. In theory, regional pain techniques seem preferable, but there is little evidence to support this. Careful patient monitoring is essential.

Painful sickle crises may present in the postoperative period; these need to be distinguished from the surgical pain and treated appropriately. The acute chest syndrome is an acute pain crisis presenting as pleuritic chest pain, fever, hypoxaemia, and lung infiltration on the chest radiograph. It has a high mortality rate and requires urgent treatment with oxygen therapy and exchange transfusion to decrease the HbS concentration.

BIBLIOGRAPHY

Vijay V, Cavenagh JD, Yate P. The anaesthetist's role in acute sickle cell crisis. British Journal of Anaesthesia 1998; 80:820–828

Stenberg MH. Management of sickle cell disease. New England Journal of Medicine 1999; 340:1021

7

Thalassaemia

M. Weisz

> **Thalassaemia:**
>
> - β Thalassaemia major, a transfusion-dependent anaemia, is the form most likely to present problems
> - The major problems are:
>   —cardiomyopathy and liver disease as a result of haemosiderosis
>   —difficult airway management
>   —difficulty in finding compatible blood

DEFINITION

The thalassaemias are an inherited group of haematological diseases in which there is deficient synthesis of α or β globin chains. They are the most common monogenic blood diseases and are more frequently found in people originating in the Mediterranean, Central Africa, China and South-East Asia.

In normal adults, the majority of haemoglobin is HbA, which has two α and two β chains, i.e. α2β2. There are four genes controlling α-chain production (two on each chromosome 16) and two controlling β-chain production (one on each chromosome 11).

α THALASSAEMIA

The classification of α thalassaemia into α0 and α+ has replaced the older nomenclature of type 1 (severe) and type 2 (mild).

α0 Thalassaemia results from elimination of α1 and α2 genes and/or regulatory sequences. α+ Thalassaemia results from a single gene deletion or point mutation that prevents normal α-chain production. Deletion of only one gene controlling α-chain production produces haematological indices that overlap with those of the normal population. α Thalassaemia trait is caused by the interaction of the normal haplotype with α0 or α+ thalassaemia determinant or homozygosity for two α+ haplotypes.

The resulting anaemia is mild and of little anaesthetic significance.

HbH disease is caused by the interaction of α0 and α+ determinants (loss of three genes). The clinical picture is of chronic haemolytic anaemia with Hb levels of 8–10 g dl^{-1}. This stimulates erythropoietin production and results in excess production of large amounts of β chains that form insoluble tetramers (HbH). The anaemia is characterised by jaundice, hepatosplenomegaly, leg ulcers, gallstones and folic acid deficiency. Haemolysis may be increased by oxidant drugs. Inability to produce any α chains results in hydrops fetalis, in which death occurs *in utero* or soon after birth.

β THALASSAEMIA

Usually inherited as a recessive disorder (some cases in which unstable β chains are produced are dominantly inherited), β thalassaemias present as a quantitative reduction in β-chain production. Underproduction of β chains results in an excess of α chains, which are unstable and precipitate in red cell precursors, which are destroyed in the bone marrow.

β Thalassaemia trait results from the inheritance of a single abnormal gene (β0 or β+) and is associated with mild iron-resistant hypochromic anaemia but with little or no other disability.

β Thalassaemia major results from the presence of two abnormal genes, and sufferers are unable to produce any β chains. Production of fetal haemoglobin (α2γ2) leads to a Hb concentration of 30–50% of the normal adult levels. This condition is associated with a severe anaemia that requires blood transfusion from the first year of life. Patients almost invariably develop antibodies, making cross-matching of blood difficult. Patients must be treated with desferrioxamine (an iron-chelating agent) to decrease iron overload and haemosiderosis. Patients may be treated with bone marrow transplantation early in life before iron overload occurs.

CLINICAL FEATURES OF THALASSAEMIA

Clinically significant forms of thalassaemia are associated with bone marrow hyperplasia because of excessive erythropoietin production. This can lead to skeletal abnormalities including head bossing, prominent maxillae and a sunken nose, which may make tracheal intubation difficult.

There may be gross hepatosplenomegaly with hypersplenism. Repeated transfusion puts the patients at risk of bloodborne infections and haemosiderosis. The latter may give rise to cardiomyopathy, left ventricular dysfunction and clinically significant heart failure. In addition, haemosiderosis can cause hepatic failure, diabetes, hypothyroidism, hypoparathyroidism and adrenal insufficiency. Individuals who have undergone bone marrow transplantation may be taking immunosuppressant drugs.

PREOPERATIVE ASSESSMENT

Careful assessment of the patient's airway is essential. Ease of venous access should be assessed as repeated transfusions may have damaged peripheral veins. Skeletal abnormalities should be assessed as the patient may be kyphoscoliotic, which may have implications for lung function and positioning on the operating table. Symptoms and signs of cardiac, hepatic or endocrine disorders should be sought.

Investigations should include a full blood count, urea and electrolytes, blood glucose estimation, liver function tests and ECG (and echocardiography if cardiac dysfunction is suspected). Allow extra time for blood cross-matching.

PERIOPERATIVE MANAGEMENT

Appropriate steps should be taken for any abnormalities identified before surgery. Transfusion to normal Hb levels is not indicated unless it is necessary to improve cardiorespiratory function. If the patient has an associated cardiomyopathy, intensive preoperative chelation therapy may improve cardiac function. Individuals who have had a splenectomy (for hypersplenism) should have had pneumococcal vaccine and should receive antibiotic prophylaxis.

BIBLIOGRAPHY

Aldouri MA , Wonke B, Hoffbrand AU. High incidence of cardiomyopathy in β thalassaemia patients receiving regular transfusion and iron chelation. Acta Haematologica 1990; 84:113–117

Modell B, Letskey EA, Flynn DM. Survival and desferrioxamine in thalassaemia major. British Medical Journal 1986 ; 284:2031–2039

Orr B. Difficult intubation: a hazard in thalassaemia. British Journal of Anaesthesia 1967; 39:585

Rodgers GP. Pharmacological therapy. Ballieres Clinical Haematology 1998; II(1):239–255

Schrier SL. Pathophysiology of thalassaemia. Current Opinion in Haematology 2002; 9:123–126

Weatherall DJ. Fortnightly review: the thalassaemias. British Medical Journal 1997; 314:1675–1678

Zurlos MG, de Stefans P, Borgna-Pignatti C et al. Survival and causes of death in thalassaemia major. Lancet 1989; ii:27–30

7

8

BONES AND JOINTS
A. Campbell
C. Hamilton-Davies

Ankylosing spondylitis

A. Campbell and C. Hamilton-Davies

Ankylosing spondylitis is an inflammatory arthropathy affecting 1.6% of the population, although most cases are likely to be relatively mild. The condition commonly begins at between 16 and 35 years of age. Four times as many males as females are diagnosed with the disease, but this may be because females tend to have much milder symptoms and may never be diagnosed. Despite primarily affecting the joints it is a systemic disorder, and 50% will experience extraspinal involvement at some time. There is a known association between development of the disease and presence of the genetic marker HLA-B27 (96% of patients with ankylosing spondylitis compared with 4% of controls).

PATHOPHYSIOLOGY

MUSCULOSKELETAL DISEASE

The disease usually starts in the sacroiliac joints and spreads up to involve the spine and the costovertebral joints. Decreased movement of the lumbar spine results, with a proportion progressing to ankylosis and complete rigidity with a classical radiographic picture of 'bamboo spine'.

Cervical spine disease ranges from mild limitation of flexion and extension to complete ankylosis. These patients also have an increased incidence of cervical fracture (often undiagnosed) and may have associated neurological deficit.

Thoracic spinal disease may lead to restrictive lung disease as a result of reduced rib-cage movement. Involvement of the lumbar spine leads to calcification of the intraspinous ligaments of the vertebral column.

The incidence of temporomandibular joint involvement varies between 10% and 40%. Cricoarytenoid disease may present as dyspnoea or hoarseness.

RESPIRATORY SYSTEM

Upper lobe pulmonary fibrosis is a recognised complication of long-standing ankylosing spondylitis. Along with the costovertebral involvement this may significantly impair the respiratory reserve of the patient.

CARDIOVASCULAR SYSTEM

Disease of the connective tissue of the aorta and aortic valve cusps may give rise to aortitis and aortic incompetence. As in rheumatoid arthritis, disease of the conduction tissue of the heart may lead to conduction defects. Rarely, mitral valve disease occurs. Cardiovascular involvement is found in up to 10% of patients with severe spondylitis. Long-term disease is associated with a greatly increased cardiovascular mortality rate.

NEUROLOGICAL SYSTEM

In long-standing spondylitis, one study found that 22% of patients had neurological symptoms and signs. Spinal cord compression, cauda equina syndrome, vertebrobasilar insufficiency and peripheral nerve lesions have all been described. There is a greater than normal incidence of vertebral fractures, which may lead to neurological symptoms.

OTHER

Uveitis is found in up to 40% of sufferers and, rarely, there may be evidence of renal impairment secondary to an IgA nephropathy. Uraemia from amyloidosis may occur.

Non-steroidal anti-inflammatory drugs (NSAIDs) and phenylbutasone are often used for pain relief, with the usual associated gastrointestinal morbidity. One study demonstrated death from peptic ulcer to be four times greater in spondylitics than in controls. Phenylbutasone may rarely cause severe blood dyscrasias, and monitoring is essential. Steroid therapy is reserved for eye involvement.

PREOPERATIVE ASSESSMENT

MORPHOLOGICAL:
- Neck movement, mouth opening, dentition
- Suitability for regional techniques
- Joint limitations.

HISTORY:

- Previous anaesthetic problems
- Complete respiratory and cardiovascular history
- Drug history.

INVESTIGATIONS

See Table 8.1.

TABLE 8.1

Investigations and results in patients with ankylosing spondylitis

Investigation	Result
Full blood count	Anaemia (?iatrogenic gastrointestinal bleed) Pancytopenia (?iatrogenic – NSAIDs)
Urea and electrolytes	Abnormal Iatrogenic from NSAIDs
ECG	Left ventricular hypertrophy Valvular disease
Chest radiography	Upper lobe fibrosis
Spirometry	Restrictive flow pattern

PERIOPERATIVE MANAGEMENT

Regional techniques are frequently not possible in these patients owing to ankylosis of the intervertebral joints, or are ill advised because of neurological complications of the disease. Ankylosing spondylitis has been reported as an independent risk factor for spinal haematoma after epidural anaesthesia. This may be due to technical difficulties and repeated trauma, or perhaps to NSAID therapy. Careful airway management of the patient with this condition is paramount.

PREMEDICATION

If fibreoptic intubation is to be performed or difficulty with intubation is anticipated, an antisialogogue should be prescribed with or without an antacid.

AIRWAY

In this group of patients it is prudent to ensure a secure airway before embarking on a surgical procedure where there is a risk of having to convert to an emergency intubation due to either loss of airway control or failure of regional technique. In severe spondylitics early consideration should be given to awake fibreoptic intubation methods. Inhalational induction with sevoflurane followed by intubation through an intubating laryngeal mask is a reasonable option for patients who refuse awake intubation. Advantages of this method are that intubation can be achieved without head or neck movement, and ventilation can continue during intubation. However, insertion of the intubating laryngeal mask may not be possible if mouth opening is limited (<2 cm for intubating laryngeal mask, <1.2 cm for laryngeal mask). Excessive force to overcome a fixed flexion cervical spine deformity whilst trying to intubate under general anaesthesia may result in vertebral fractures.

The 'intubate at all costs' approach is not appropriate for elective surgery, and if maintaining the airway is reasonably easy a laryngeal mask is useful. If airway maintenance is extremely difficult or impossible, then allowing the patient to wake up and postponing the operation is prudent.

In the emergency situation there may be insufficient skill or equipment available to perform fibreoptic intubation, and emergency tracheostomy or cricothyrotomy may be necessary (However, with a severe flexion deformity these may be impossible.)

RESPIRATORY SYSTEM

Preoperative assessment should indicate whether any degree of respiratory compromise exists and whether consideration should be given to postoperative ventilation.

CARDIOVASCULAR SYSTEM

Aortic or mitral incompetence should be treated as in primary cardiac disease, with caution in the use of vasodilating drugs. Antibiotic cover may be appropriate and preoperative pacing may be necessary.

CONDUCT OF ANAESTHESIA

There are no specific contraindications to the use of any anaesthetic agent. Care should be taken with regard to patient transfer and positioning for the operation in order to avoid vertebral or neurological damage and to minimise backache after operation.

Ensuring that the patient has full control of their airway prior to extubation is essential, as reintubation may prove impossible.

POSTOPERATIVE MANAGEMENT

Analgesia often proves to be difficult in these patients, as regional techniques are rarely available even for the most major procedures and high doses of opioids must be balanced against the risk of oversedation and compromising the airway. Patient-controlled analgesia (PCA) may be very useful in these circumstances.

Re-establishment of regular NSAID therapy will help to relieve pain due to ankylosing spondylitis, which may be greater than the surgical pain.

LONG-TERM MANAGEMENT

Patients with ankylosing spondylitis may present for any type of operation, but as the duration of the disease lengthens so does the likelihood of the operation being relating to the disease or to the complications of its treatment.

Previous anaesthetic notes are essential, with particular reference to intubation or airway difficulties.

BIBLIOGRAPHY

Calin A. Seronegative spondarthritides. Medicine International 1984; 22:146–149

Sinclair JR, Mason RA. Ankylosing spondylitis – the case for awake intubation. Anaesthesia 1984; 39:3–11

Lu PP, Brimacombe J, Ho AC, Shyr MH, Liu HP. The intubating laryngeal mask airway in severe ankylosing spondylitis. Canadian Journal of Anaesthesia 2001; 48:1015–1019

CROSS-REFERENCES

Restrictive lung disease
    Patient Conditions 3: 101
Aortic valve disease
    Patient Conditions 4: 115
Conduction defects
    Patient Conditions 4: 126
Mitral valve disease
    Patient Conditions 4: 133
Difficult airway
    Anaesthetic Factors 28: 660

8

Dwarfism

A. Campbell and A. T. Lovell

People with short stature conventionally are divided into two categories: those with proportionate growth and those with disproportionate growth. It is people in the latter group who are classified as dwarfs. Patients with dwarfism are often considered to have a single disease entity, but this is an oversimplification. There are more than 100 different types of dwarfism, many of which pose specific anaesthetic problems.

INCIDENCE

Although each type of dwarfism is relatively rare, the large number of types means that any practising anaesthetist is likely to meet dwarfs. Achondroplasia, the commonest cause of dwarfism, has an incidence of 1 in 10 000. There is a defect of the fibroblast growth factor receptor. This affects endochondral bone formation (i.e. long bone growth), while membranous and periosteal bones are unaffected.

ANAESTHETIC PROBLEMS

These patients may have multiple problems. Monitoring and anaesthetic techniques need to be considered in relation to both the underlying diagnosis as well as the planned surgical procedure.

Traditionally, general anaesthesia has been the technique of choice – despite the risks of airway obstruction with some syndromes. This is in part due to the difficulties encountered in performance of spinal and epidural blockade: poor landmarks, spinal deformities including lumbar lordosis, spinal stenosis with a narrow epidural space. Nevertheless, there are numerous reports of successful spinal and epidural anaesthesia for caesarean section. Decreased volumes of local anaesthetic are needed and epidural administration may be preferable to spinal as the dose can be titrated according to the height of the block.

PREOPERATIVE ASSESSMENT

RESPIRATORY SYSTEM:
- Clinical assessment of airway
- Obstructive airway lesions, especially in patients with mucopolysaccharidosis
- Previous problems with airway maintenance or intubation
- Restrictive defects secondary to rib hypoplasia and kyphoscoliosis
- Sleep apnoea.

CARDIOVASCULAR SYSTEM:
- Pulmonary hypertension
- Congenital heart disease
- Coronary artery disease
- Valvular heart disease
- Cardiomyopathy.

NEUROLOGICAL SYSTEM:
- Macrocephaly and hydrocephaly
- Cervical spine instability
- Spinal cord compression
- Nerve root compression
- Temperature regulation problems.

OTHER:
- Endocrinopathy
- Bleeding problems
- Renal function.

PREMEDICATION

Anticholinergic agents are used widely in patients with marked secretions and in patients in whom problems with the airway or intubation are anticipated. Avoid sedatives in patients with potential upper airway obstruction.

VENOUS ACCESS

Peripheral and central access are often difficult. These patients are frequently obese and, in addition, may possess subcutaneous infiltrates

8

with lax skin. Cervical abnormalities, including very short necks and, frequently, stabilisation devices, may make access to the jugular vein extremely difficult. In these circumstances there may be no option but to use either a femoral or subclavian approach.

INDUCTION

Awake intubation and an inhalational induction with the maintenance of spontaneous respiration are thought to be relatively safe techniques in patients in whom difficulties with airway maintenance or intubation are predicted. Restrictive lung disease, if present, will prolong an inhalational induction. It is vital that muscle relaxants are avoided until it is certain that the patient can be ventilated by mask.

INTUBATION

This can prove to be extremely difficult and exposure of the larynx may prove impossible with a conventional laryngoscope in some dwarfs with very short necks. In these circumstances a short-handled laryngoscope may enable visualisation of the glottis, but, if this fails, fibreoptic guided intubation either awake or under general anaesthesia will be required. In patients with foramen magnum stenosis or atlantoaxial instability it is important to avoid neck movements during attempts at intubation, and under these circumstances fibreoptic control of the airway may be preferable.

There is some controversy as to the selection of correct size of tracheal tube. For achondroplastics the formula (Age/4) + 4 usually give a correct prediction of the internal diameter. In extreme circumstances a tracheostomy may be necessary, but in patients with mucopolysaccharidoses this may not relieve the tracheal obstruction completely because of distal tracheal distortion.

RESPIRATORY SUPPORT

The low functional residual capacity (FRC) and high closing volume frequently found in dwarfs with respiratory involvement predisposes these patients to atelectasis and V/Q mismatching. This may cause severe problems with oxygenation. For all but the shortest and simplest surgical procedures, arterial cannulation for intraoperative and postoperative blood gas estimation is strongly recommended for any dwarf with respiratory dysfunction. Postoperative ventilation, which can be prolonged, may be required, especially in patients with thoracic dystrophy.

CARDIOVASCULAR PROBLEMS

Cardiology opinion may be required to delineate the extent of cardiac compromise. Pulmonary hypertension is the most frequent cardiovascular complication seen in dwarfs. Clinical suspicion may be raised by the presence of a parasternal heave, a loud, widely split, second heart sound and a pulmonary systolic ejection murmur. Right ventricular enlargement may be confirmed by either electrocardiography or echocardiography. In patients with pulmonary hypertension the anaesthesia has to be planned to avoid pulmonary arterial vasoconstriction whilst still maintaining an adequate cardiac output. Care must be taken to avoid hypoxia, hypercapnia, and respiratory or metabolic acidosis, which can cause profound rises in pulmonary artery pressures. In mildly affected individuals, oxygen and inhalational anaesthetics are often used. In patients with right ventricular failure, high-dose narcotic techniques are preferred. In children, ketamine has been used safely, even in those with right ventricular failure, although this is not recommended in adults. In patients with congenital heart lesions, or corrected lesions, endocarditis prophylaxis is mandatory.

NEUROLOGICAL PROBLEMS

Most of these problems revolve around the stability of the cervical spine, especially at the atlantoaxial and craniocervical junctions, and problems with raised intracranial pressure (ICP). In patients with spinal cord compression an autonomic hyperreflexic state may develop. Document any pre-existing neurological deficit if central blockade is being considered.

The problems of anaesthetising a dwarf with raised ICP are formidable: an inhalational induction can be associated with hypercapnia and a rise in ICP, whilst an intravenous induction can be associated with apnoea in a patient who cannot be intubated or ventilated. These patients thus require consideration on a case-by-case basis.

Rarely, hyperthermia, usually without the clinical features of malignant hyperthermia,

8

develops. Therapy consists of simple cooling measures alone. A few cases that are clinically indistinguishable from malignant hyperthermia have been observed in patients with osteogenesis imperfecta. It was only by muscle biopsy that the diagnosis was able to be refuted. Thus potential trigger agents do not need to be avoided unless malignant hyperthermia is suspected clinically.

BLEEDING PROBLEMS

Osteogenesis imperfecta is the only chondrodystrophy associated with a coagulopathy. These patients require formal evaluation with a bleeding time before operation. Platelets and fresh frozen plasma should be available.

BIBLIOGRAPHY

Berkowitz ID, Raja SN, Bender KS, Kopits SE. Dwarfs: pathophysiology and anesthetic implications. Anesthesiology 1990; 73:739–759

Borland LM. Anesthesia for children with Jeunne's syndrome (asphyxiating thoracic dystrophy). Anesthesiology 1987; 66:86–88

Walts LF, Finerman G, Wyatt GM. Anaesthesia for dwarfs and other patients of small stature. Canadian Journal of Anaesthesia 1975; 22:703–709

8

Marfan's syndrome

A. Campbell and V. Taylor

Marfan's syndrome is a generalised connective tissue disorder caused by abnormal formation of fibrillin – a glycoprotein in elastic fibres. The defect decreases the tensile strength and elasticity of connective tissue. It is inherited as an autosomal dominant trait, with variable expression. Its incidence is 1 per 10 000 births. The mean age of death is early in the fourth decade, often from cardiovascular causes.

PATHOPHYSIOLOGY

CARDIOVASCULAR MANIFESTATIONS

There is degeneration of the media of the pulmonary artery, aorta and distal arteries, leading to 'cystic medial necrosis' and weakness. This causes aneurysm formation, especially in the aortic root and the ascending aorta. The dilatation of the aortic root leads to aortic regurgitation, ventricular hypertrophy, ventricular dilatation, mitral valve regurgitation or prolapse, heart failure and angina. Conduction abnormalities are seen (especially bundle branch block).

Dissection of an aneurysm may cause aortic regurgitation or it may extend into the pericardium with cardiac tamponade. Intimal tears with dissection may occur in the absence of an aneurysm. Beta-blockers seem to slow the progress of aortic dissection or dilatation. Aortic arch replacement is considered when aortic root diameter is more than 55 mm.

SKELETAL MANIFESTATIONS

There is disproportionate growth of long bones, leading to arachnodactyly with hyperextensible joints, which are prone to dislocation. Patients have high arched palates. Kyphoscoliosis (40–70%), pectus excavatum and pectus carinatum may be present.

RESPIRATORY MANIFESTATIONS

Patients with Marfan's syndrome are prone to develop emphysema, accentuating the lung defect secondary to kyphoscoliosis. There is a higher than normal incidence of spontaneous pneumothorax. Sleep apnoea occurs due to maxillary abnormalities, producing high nasal airway resistance and also increased upper airway collapsibility. Diaphragmatic herniae occur.

OCULAR MANIFESTATIONS

These include lens dislocation, myopia, retinal detachment, glaucoma and cataracts.

PREOPERATIVE ASSESSMENT

Particular attention should be paid to cardiopulmonary investigations. These should include chest radiography, ECG, echocardiography, lung function tests and arterial blood gas estimation.

Vital capacity and forced expiratory volume in 1 s (FEV_1) may appear to be lower than expected when compared with predicted values, owing to greater height or arm span.

PERIOPERATIVE MANAGEMENT

Prophylactic antibiotics must be given due to the high risk of bacterial endocarditis.

Careful handling and positioning are essential to avoid joint trauma and dislocation.

Intubation may be difficult because of the long high-arched palate. Gentle laryngoscopy should be performed to avoid cervical spine and temporomandibular joint damage.

Surges of blood pressure should be avoided, for example on laryngoscopy or in response to surgical stimulation. Beta-blockade will reduce aortic wall tension. Blood pressure should be maintained with the diastolic pressure high enough to ensure good coronary flow, but not too high so as to risk dissection. There may be little cardiac reserve, and volatile agents may be very depressant.

Spontaneous pneumothorax may become a tension pneumothorax in a patient on positive-pressure ventilation. Maintain low airway pressures and avoid overinflation of the lungs.

The risk of malignant hyperthermia may be increased.

MONITORING:

- ECG
- Pulse oximetry
- Capnography
- Airway pressures
- Arterial cannulation (but increased risk of morbidity because of weak arterial wall)
- Temperature.

CHOICE OF ANAESTHETIC

The choice of anaesthetic technique is broad and no one agent or technique is suggested. After careful induction with thiopental, propofol or etomidate while monitoring blood pressure, anaesthesia may be maintained with nitrous oxide, oxygen, narcotic, muscle relaxant and volatile agent. Blood pressure may be further controlled by beta-blockade, if needed. Care must be taken to maintain intravascular volumes and filling pressure.

BIBLIOGRAPHY

Dean JCS. Management of Marfan syndrome. Heart 2002: 88(1):97–103

Katz J, Benumof JL, Kadis LB, eds. Anaesthesia and uncommon diseases. 3rd edn. Philadelphia: WB Saunders; 1990:144–145, 294–295

Steolting RK, Dierdors SF, McCammon RL, eds. Anaesthesia and co-existing disease. 2nd edn. Edinburgh: Churchill Livingstone; 1988:640–641

CROSS-REFERENCES

Restrictive lung disease
    Patient Conditions 3: 101
Aortic valve disease
    Patient Conditions 4: 115
Cardiac conduction defects
    Patient Conditions 4: 120
Mitral valve disease
    Patient Conditions 4: 133
Cataract surgery
    Surgical Procedures 11: 332
Abdominal aortic reconstruction – elective
    Surgical Procedures 20: 497

8

Metabolic and degenerative bone disease

A. Campbell and A. T. Lovell

OSTEOMALACIA

Osteomalacia is a metabolic disease of bone in which normal bone is replaced by unmineralised osteoid. When this condition occurs in children the disease is called rickets. Clinically it can be extremely difficult to differentiate osteomalacia and osteoporosis. The finding of a low serum level of phosphate suggests osteomalacia, but the only certain diagnostic method is to take a bone biopsy.

Osteomalacia is caused by an inadequate level of 1,25-dihydrocholecalciferol (1,25-DHCC); this is an active metabolite of vitamin D. The commonest cause of osteomalacia is deficiency of vitamin D due to diet or inadequate exposure to sunlight. Rarely, malabsorption can interfere with the absorption of vitamin D, leading to osteomalacia. Severe renal disease is a potent cause of osteomalacia because 25-hydroxycholecalciferol is converted to the active 1,25-DHCC only in the kidney. Osteomalacia may develop in patients on long-term therapy with drugs that induce the hepatic mixed-function oxidase, because this interferes with vitamin D metabolism.

Clinical features include bone pain, pathological fractures and proximal myopathy.

Treatment of the underlying cause involves the replacement of vitamin D. This may be administered either as calciferol or as the active metabolite 1-α-cholecalciferol. Replacement therapy must be closely monitored because there is a risk of hypercalcaemia developing. Calcium supplements are used only if the patient is hypocalcaemic.

ANAESTHETIC PROBLEMS OF OSTEOMALACIA:
- Abnormal drug metabolism of mixed-function oxidase induced
- Potential for hypercalcaemia if on therapy with vitamin D supplements
- Great care with positioning (fractures can occur easily)
- Deformity, if occurs before epiphyseal fusion
- Hypocalcaemia – may increase the duration of action of non-depolarising muscle relaxant
- Aetiology may be chronic renal failure

OSTEOPOROSIS

In osteoporosis the overall quantity of bone is reduced, whilst its shape, composition and morphology remain normal. Osteoporosis generally occurs in the elderly, especially women. The commonest precipitating factor is the menopausal withdrawal of oestrogens. However, endocrinopathies, long-term corticosteroid therapy, smoking, alcohol, poor nutrition or malabsorption, and immobilisation can also result in osteoporosis. The net effect appears to be a relative overactivity of the osteoclasts, leading to bone loss. Because of the bone loss, fractures occur far more readily, frequently after minimal trauma.

COMMON SITES OF FRACTURES IN OSTEOPOROSIS:
- Vertebrae (usually crush or wedge fractures)
- Neck of femur
- Distal radius
- Proximal humerus
- Pelvis.

Multiple vertebral fractures leading to a kyphosis are not uncommon. This may be associated with marked respiratory impairment. Despite their frequency, it is unusual for vertebral fractures to be associated with serious neurological sequelae, although sciatica is common.

Patients may require surgical stabilisation, but any immobilisation tends to worsen the conditions. Current attempts are directed at prevention by increasing the bone mass before the menopause with the aid of calcium supplementation and physical activity, and reducing the rate of bone resorption by using hormone replacement therapy, bisphosphonates and vitamin D.

PAGET'S DISEASE

Paget's disease is a metabolic disease of unknown aetiology, although a viral aetiology has been suggested. It is characterised by excessively rapid remodelling of bone. There is intense resorption of bone by abnormal osteoclasts. The new bone formed by osteoblasts is architecturally distorted and its mineralisation is defective. The affected bones and bone marrow are initially very vascular. Eventually, the bone may become dense and hard with a reduced vascularity. It is these sclerotic areas that are weak and lead to the common complication of fractures.

The incidence of Paget's disease is approximately 5% in people aged more than 55 years, and the condition tends to run in families. The most frequently affected sites are the pelvis, femur, tibia, skull and spine. Because of the involvement of the skull and spine, spinal cord compression, atlantoaxial instability and brain stem compression may develop.

Patients may be asymptomatic, but commonly bone pain or fractures are the presenting feature. Occasionally, patients present in high-output cardiac failure due to the increased bone vascularity. Some 1% of patients develop bone sarcoma.

Specific treatment is indicated for patients with symptoms or complications of the disease. Calcitonin, which acts primarily as an inhibitor of bone resorption, has been used in patients with bone pain and before orthopaedic procedures to reduce the vascularity of the bone. Increasingly, the bisphosphonates (e.g. alendronate) are being used to control bone pain; their effect often far outlasts the duration of treatment. They are adsorbed on to hydroxyapatite crystals, so slowing both their rate of growth and dissolution, and reducing the rate of bone turnover.

ANAESTHETIC MANAGEMENT OF PAGET'S DISEASE:

- Careful evaluation for atlantoaxial and craniocervical instability.
- Assess lung function in patients with a kyphosis.
- Cardiac failure, if present, must be treated.
- Careful moving and positioning of the patient (fractures occur easily).
- General or regional techniques may be used. Spinal and epidural placement can be difficult. Most dental cases are performed under general anaesthesia because extractions are difficult and the risk of postoperative bleeding is increased.
- Corticosteroid treatment may be required, depending on previous treatment.
- Consideration should be given to the use of calcitonin before major orthopaedic procedures.

OSTEOARTHRITIS

Osteoarthritis is a common degenerative disease of the joint surface. There is damage to hyaline cartilage, with sclerosis and osteophyte formation in underlying subchondral bone. This leads to a reduced joint space. The aetiology is unclear, but may be related to joint trauma and joint overuse. Osteoarthritis is a major cause of disability and is universally evident after the age of 60 years.

Patients usually complain of pain which is worse with movement and at the end of the day, and of stiffness that improves with use. Characteristically, the hip and knee joints are involved, but there may be involvement of the distal interphalangeal joints and degeneration of the spine. The middle and lower cervical spine and lower lumbar spine are the areas most likely to be involved. Spinal cord compression or nerve root compression can occur due to degenerative discs. Spinal fusion is rare.

Treatment of osteoarthritis is symptomatic, using physiotherapy and NSAIDs. Corticosteroids are not used because they are associated with a worsening of the degenerative process. Reconstructive joint surgery has much to offer these patients, but can be associated with considerable blood loss and carries a high risk of thromboembolic phenomena. The use of regional anaesthesia for these procedures, either alone or in combination with general anaesthesia, has been shown to reduce the blood loss and to decrease the incidence of deep venous thrombosis from 33% to 9%. Graduated compression stockings and heparin prophylaxis are also used in an attempt to reduce the incidence of thromboembolism further.

8

CROSS-REFERENCES

Repair of fractured neck of femur
Surgical Procedures 22: 544
Epidural and spinal anaesthesia
Anaesthetic Factors 30: 696

Rheumatoid disease

A. Campbell and C. Hamilton-Davies

Rheumatoid disease is a common systemic chronic inflammatory disease affecting up to 3% of women and 1% of men in the UK, with an onset typically between 30 and 50 years of age. It is HLA-DR4 linked, and is thought to be an autoimmune condition perhaps triggered by an infectious agent. Rheumatoid disease may involve every organ system in the body, but of particular relevance to the anaesthetist are disorders of the musculoskeletal and respiratory systems. These patients present for surgery commonly because of the degenerative nature of the condition.

PATHOPHYSIOLOGY

MUSCULOSKELETAL

The destructive synovitis associated with rheumatoid disease attacks the small joints of the hands, ankles, knees, temporomandibular joints, wrists, elbows and joints of the spinal column. The disease progresses until the inflammation eventually moves into a fibrotic phase, leaving characteristic fixed deformities in the joints of the hands. The cervical spine is involved in the disease process in up to 80% of affected individuals, with 30% showing clinical signs of cervical spine instability. Involvement of the temporomandibular and cricoarytenoid joints is also commonly seen.

RESPIRATORY

Pleural disease occurs in 3–12.5% of patients, more commonly in men. Rib cage stiffness and interstitial lung fibrosis combine to produce a restrictive picture. Other pulmonary manifestations include the presence of rheumatoid nodules in the lungs that may rupture or cavitate and become sites of infection, pleural effusions (typically unilateral) and rarely fibrosing alveolitis. Pulmonary vasculitis should be considered as a potential cause of pulmonary hypertension. Iatrogenic pulmonary disease occurs in up to 5% of patients treated with methotrexate, and appears as a progressive interstitial fibrosis. Sulfasalazine therapy may lead to the development of eosinophilic pneumonitis.

CARDIOVASCULAR

The prevalence of cardiovascular disorders has been estimated to be up to 40%, with pericardial disease being the most common. Of rheumatoid patients, 1–5% have mitral valve disease, with other valves being less commonly involved. Direct myocardial involvement rarely causes symptoms, although involvement of the conduction pathways may lead to heart block. Systemic vasculitis is rare, but is more common in patients with high titres of rheumatoid factor. Symptoms of mononeuritis multiplex indicate neurovascular involvement and extensive, severe, vasculitic disease.

HAEMATOPOIETIC

A mild normocytic anaemia is common in rheumatoid patients and tends to correlate with disease activity. It is important that other causes of anaemia are excluded, in particular bleeding from the gastrointestinal tract secondary to either steroid or NSAID therapy. The normal responses to infection may not be present due to concomitant immunosuppressive therapy. Methotrexate, sulfasalazine, gold, azathioprine and penicillamine may induce bone marrow suppression.

OTHER

Gastrointestinal symptoms are generally secondary to drug therapy: NSAIDs and steroids produce ulceration, azathioprine leads to nausea and vomiting – and possibly even pancreatitis – and oral gold therapy causes irritation of the gut.

Renal impairment may occur secondary to gold, penicillamine, ciclosporin or NSAID administration, or rarely, amyloidosis.

Methotrexate, sulfasalazine, azathioprine, gold and ciclosporin can all cause hepatotoxicity.

Neurological complications include peripheral neuropathy (usually mainly sensory), mononeuritis multiplex, entrapment neuropathy (e.g. carpal tunnel syndrome) and spinal cord lesions secondary to cervical disease.

Infections of all kinds are more common in rheumatoid disease, especially joint infections.

8

PREOPERATIVE ASSESSMENT

MORPHOLOGICAL:
- Neck movement, mouth opening and dentition
- Veins, arteries and bruising
- Presence of painful joints and limitations
- Suitability for regional technique.

HISTORY:
- Complete neurological, respiratory and cardiovascular history
- Drug history
- Previous anaesthetic problems.

INVESTIGATIONS
See Table 8.2.

PERIOPERATIVE MANAGEMENT

Consideration should be given to performing the procedure under local or regional blockade if feasible, as this will avoid the need for airway manipulation. However, the involvement of the spine may make epidural or spinal anaesthesia difficult, if not impossible. Blocks should be established gradually in these patients with difficult airways. Maintenance of awkward positions for surgery may not be feasible in the rheumatoid patient, because of discomfort.

TABLE 8.2

Investigations and results for patients with rheumatoid disease

Investigation	Result
Full blood count	Anaemia – normochromic, normocytic (severe hypochromic – ?gastrointestinal bleed)
Urea and electrolytes	Abnormal (iatrogenic – gold, ciclosporin)
ECG	Heart block
	Ischaemic (arteritis)
	Left ventricular hypertrophy (valvular heart disease)
Chest radiography	Rheumatoid nodules
Cervical spine radiography (?lateral and odontoid views)	Atlantoaxial subluxation; subatlantoaxial subluxation
Spirometry	Restrictive flow pattern
Indirect laryngoscopy	Degree of cricoarytenoid involvement

If general anaesthesia is to be used, the cervical spine and airway are the areas likely to cause most concern.

PREMEDICATION
If fibreoptic intubation is to be performed, or difficulty with intubation is anticipated, an antisialogogue should be prescribed.

CERVICAL SPINE
On induction of anaesthesia the cervical spine will lose any protective tone around the unstable neck, and thus it is important to determine the range of comfortable neck movement before induction and limit it to this with the use of sandbags, etc. If tracheal intubation is necessary in a patient with severe cervical spine involvement, early consideration may need to be given to awake fibreoptic intubation, especially if there is posterior atlanto-axial subluxation (neck extension potentially hazardous).

Where intubation is not required, oropharyngeal or nasopharyngeal airways may reduce the amount of cervical manipulation required. The laryngeal mask is useful in longer procedures, although the larynx can be displaced in cervical spine disease, making placement difficult. Manual-in-line stabilisation should be used during airway manipulation in unconscious patients, unless there is certainty that the cervical spine is stable.

AIRWAY
Temporomandibular joint involvement may lead to difficulty in mouth opening and forward jaw protrusion, thus leading to difficulty in inserting a laryngoscope as well as viewing the larynx. Rarely, cricoarytenoid involvement can result in acute airway obstruction. Anticipated problems or previous difficulty should lead to early consideration of the fibreoptic laryngoscope.

CONDUCT OF ANAESTHESIA
There are no restrictions on anaesthetic agents used in rheumatoid disease, although iatrogenic, hepatic or renal disease may alter the amount of free drug available and increments should be administered with care.

Great care should be taken to protect the joints during anaesthesia, with careful handling and positioning of the patient and protection of pressure points.

Mechanical ventilation may be necessary in patients with severe pulmonary disease.

8

POSTOPERATIVE MANAGEMENT

Analgesia is the main problem in the postoperative period, as these patients tend to be more sensitive to opioids. Patient-controlled analgesia may be difficult for the rheumatoid patient because of hand deformities, although special modifications are available. Regional blockade may provide the optimal form of analgesia in this group of patients, if appropriate.

Early physiotherapy is indicated, both to prevent chest infections in a patient who has a restrictive lung defect, and thus a propensity to develop atelectasis, and for a patient who is more difficult to mobilise because of musculoskeletal dysfunction.

Steroid cover should be continued where indicated, and there should be close monitoring of renal function, especially if preoperative dysfunction was present.

LONG-TERM MANAGEMENT

These patients tend to require multiple surgical procedures due to the relentless progression of their disease. Careful attention should be paid to previous anaesthetic notes and any problems with intubation, analgesia, etc., noted.

BIBLIOGRAPHY

Helmers R, Galvin J, Hunninghake GW. Pulmonary manifestations associated with rheumatoid arthritis. Chest 1991; 100:235–238

Macarthur A, Kleiman S. Rheumatoid cervical joint disease – a challenge to the anaesthetist. Canadian Journal of Anaesthesia 1993; 40:154–159

Skues MA, Welchew EA. Anaesthesia and rheumatoid arthritis. Anaesthesia 1993; 48:989–997

8

Scoliosis

A. Campbell

Scoliosis is a complex deformity of growth of the vertebral column resulting in lateral curvature and rotation of the vertebrae. The spinous processes rotate toward the concavity of the curve. In the thoracic spine, scoliosis results in abnormal development of the thoracic cage and, consequently, abnormalities of respiratory and cardiovascular function.

AETIOLOGY

Scoliosis is a sign, not a disease. It may arise from several different causes; although presentation, complications and management may be similar, the prognosis may differ greatly for different aetiologies.

CLASSIFICATION OF SCOLIOSIS

FUNCTIONAL SCOLIOSIS
Secondary to discordant leg length, etc. Curve disappears when patient lies down.

STRUCTURAL SCOLIOSIS
There are three main groups:
- *Congenital* – associated with vertebral anomalies. May have abnormalities of the heart and genitourinary tract.
- *Idiopathic* – accounts for 60–80% of cases and has the best prognosis of all aetiologies. This is a diagnosis of exclusion.
- *Neuromuscular* – scoliosis occurring secondary to a neuropathy (upper or lower motor neurone or other neuropathy) such as cerebral palsy, poliomyelitis or Friedreich ataxia, or to a myopathy (e.g. Duchenne muscular dystrophy). This group includes many of the syndromes associated with scoliosis, such as Prader–Willi syndrome.

In addition:
- *Mesenchymal* – abnormalities of the tissues (e.g. Marfan syndrome, Ehlers–Danlos syndrome).

- *Trauma*.
- *Tumours* – intraspinal or skeletal.
- *Metabolic* – this category includes several miscellaneous causes (e.g. rickets, hyperphosphataemia).

The severity of scoliosis can be defined by the Cobb angle (Fig. 8.1), which is measured from an anteroposterior radiograph of the spine. The first line is taken from the most tilted vertebral body above the scoliosis and extended laterally. The second line is taken from the most tilted vertebra below the scoliosis. The measured angle is at the intersection of these two lines. Although occasional patients may have a scoliosis that is largely in the lumbar region, it is more often the case that the thoracic vertebrae are involved. In these circumstances, the larger the angle, the more severe is the scoliosis and the greater the likelihood of compromised respiratory and cardiovascular function. Patients with neuromuscular-type scoliosis may have significant impairment despite lesser abnormalities.

PATHOPHYSIOLOGY

RESPIRATORY SYSTEM
Respiratory impairment usually shows a restrictive pattern, with lung volumes being

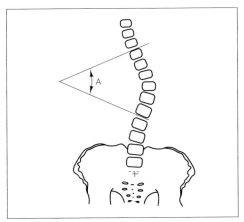

Fig. 8.1 The Cobb angle (A).

related inversely to the angle of curvature. Vital capacity is the most severely affected, but total lung capacity and FRC are also reduced. The abnormalities of rib cage development cause abnormal development of the underlying lung, with alveolar volume being compressed to, or below, the FRC. Rib abnormalities result in mechanical disadvantage of muscles of respiration and reduced chest wall compliance. This results in alveolar hypoventilation. The commonest arterial blood gas abnormality is a reduced PaO_2.

Associated with the compressed alveoli is restricted development of the pulmonary vascular bed and diversion of blood into high-resistance extra-alveolar vessels. The resulting ventilation–perfusion mismatch causes an increased alveolar to arterial oxygen gradient and exacerbates the alveolar hypoventilation. An increase in $PaCO_2$ occurs late and is a poor prognostic indicator. In addition, patients with more severe scoliosis have a decreased respiratory sensitivity to increased $PaCO_2$.

CARDIOVASCULAR SYSTEM

There is a relatively high incidence of congenital heart disease in patients with scoliosis.

Thoracic scoliosis of any aetiology may result in right-sided cardiac problems. The ventilation–perfusion mismatch causes an increased pulmonary vascular resistance.

Low lung volumes, chronic hypoxia and abnormal development of the pulmonary vascular bed all contribute to these changes. Right atrial dilatation and right ventricular hypertrophy are late in appearance.

PREOPERATIVE ASSESSMENT

Assessment involves determining the aetiology of the scoliosis and associated problems.

RESPIRATORY FUNCTION:

- Clinical assessment of airway – intubation may be difficult in, for example, patients with fixed flexion deformities, large meningomyelocele with or without encephalocele, 'halo' or other neck-immobilising traction.
- Exercise tolerance.
- Chest expansion and ability to cough.
- Formal lung function tests – if the scoliosis is <65° or lung function tests are >30% of the predicted value, ventilation problems are rare. If vital capacity is <30%, the patient is more likely to need postoperative mechanical ventilation.

- Arterial blood gas measurements – if the patient is unable to perform lung function tests or has scoliosis >65°.

CARDIAC FUNCTION:

- Clinical examination – right ventricular enlargement, loud pulmonic second sound, murmur of pulmonary insufficiency.
- ECG – P wave >2.5 mm, and R > S in V_1 and V_2. These changes are rare and occur late.
- Echocardiography – a more sensitive detector of cardiac abnormalities secondary to pulmonary hypertension.

PERIOPERATIVE MANAGEMENT

PREMEDICATION

Narcotics should be avoided if there is significant respiratory impairment (curve >60° or lung function <30% predicted). Consider an anticholinergic agent if cough is inadequate or there are problems clearing secretions. Consider preoperative physiotherapy in those with poor respiratory function.

MONITORING

Monitoring should be started in the anaesthetic room.
- ECG
- SaO_2
- Blood pressure – arterial cannulation is useful both for measuring blood pressure and for postoperative determination of arterial blood gases.
- Core temperature – there is a higher incidence of malignant hyperthermia in patients with scoliosis.
- Nasogastric tube – decompression of the stomach assists ventilation, and distraction of the spine may be associated with the development of paralytic ileus.
- Consider central venous pressure and urine output monitoring, particularly for operations associated with high blood loss.

ANAESTHESIA

- Hyperkalaemia may occur following the use of suxamethonium in patients with neuromuscular problems.
- Rhabdomyolysis and myoglobinuria may occur following the use of suxamethonium and halothane in patients with myopathy.

SURGERY – GENERAL

Evidence of pulmonary hypertension or right ventricular hypertrophy carries a poor progno-

8

sis. Right ventricular failure must be treated before operation.

There is no specific contraindication to local or regional anaesthesia. However, central neural blockade may be difficult in scoliotic patients.

SURGERY – FOR SCOLIOSIS

Most patients who undergo scoliosis surgery are children or young adults. The aims are:
- Correction of curve
- Prevention of progression of curve
- Relief or prevention of back pain
- Prevention of neurological compromise
- Prevention of respiratory compromise
- Cosmetic.

Patients usually present for corrective surgery before the onset of pulmonary hypertension. Surgery may be via an anterior approach, posterior approach, or both (carried out as two separate procedures several days apart or during a single session). The anterior approach requires access to the vertebrae on the convex side of the curve. This is achieved via thoracotomy and costectomy, and usually precedes posterior fusion. The posterior approach requires the patient to be placed prone.

ANAESTHETIC – SPECIFIC CONSIDERATIONS:
- Blood loss may be considerable and rapid. Hypotensive techniques have been associated with spinal cord ischaemia and paresis. Consider methods of blood preservation: cell salvage, haemodilution, etc. Attempt to maintain temperature with fluid warmers, warming blanket. Patients with Duchenne muscular dystrophy appear to bleed more.
- Postoperative pain, hypoventilation and atelectasis are severe following thoracotomy. Thoracic epidural analgesia provides good operating conditions and excellent pain relief, and may be continued for several days after operation.
- Anaesthesia must facilitate spinal cord monitoring ('wake-up' test, sensory or motor evoked potentials). Total intravenous anaesthesia using an infusion of propofol is a suitable technique.
- The prone position is used for the posterior approach. Careful positioning is required including abdominal decompression (decreases blood loss). Complications of the prone position include retinal artery thrombosis, brachial plexus injury and suprascapular nerve injury.

POSTOPERATIVE CARE

- ITU or HDU care is required following corrective scoliosis surgery, major general surgery and minor surgery under general anaesthesia if there is significant respiratory or cardiovascular compromise.
- Postoperative intermittent positive-pressure ventilation (IPPV) may be required.
- Continuous oxygen therapy.
- Regular physiotherapy.
- Analgesia.

BIBLIOGRAPHY

Kafer ER. Respiratory and cardiovascular functions in scoliosis and the principles of anaesthetic management. Anesthesiology 1980; 52:339–351

Porter SS. Anesthesia for surgery of the spine. New York: McGraw-Hill; 1995

Sharrad WJW. Congenital and developmental abnormalities of the spine. In: Paediatric orthopaedics and fractures, vol. 1. 3rd edn. Oxford: Blackwell Scientific; 1993:556–659

CROSS-REFERENCES

Muscular dystrophies
    Patient Conditions 2: 78
Restrictive lung disease
    Patient Conditions 3: 101
Marfan's syndrome
    Patient Conditions 8: 238

9

CONNECTIVE TISSUE
B. J. Pollard

Bullous and vesicular skin disorders

B. J. Pollard

This section considers bullous and vesicular skin disorders with the exception of epidermolysis bullosa, which is the subject of a separate entry.

PEMPHIGUS AND PEMPHIGOID

These rare autoimmune conditions are characterised by a bullous eruption of the skin and mucous membranes. There are several variants of each disease. In pemphigus, blisters form intradermally; in pemphigoid, lesions occur at the dermal–epidermal junction.

PATHOPHYSIOLOGY

Pemphigus vulgaris is the most common form of pemphigus and occurs predominantly in patients of Mediterranean or Jewish origin, with a peak incidence between 30 and 50 years of age. It was uniformly fatal before the advent of steroid therapy. There is a familial tendency and an increased incidence of HLA-13 amongst affected individuals. There may be an association with other autoimmune diseases such as thymoma, myasthenia gravis and systemic lupus erythematosus (SLE). The large (> 1 cm), superficial, flaccid blisters may occur spontaneously or in response to trauma, and are found in the groin, axilla and over the trunk. Oral lesions may predate the cutaneous bullae by several months. Pressure with torsion may result in blister formation in normal-looking skin (Nikolsky's sign). The bullae are fragile, rupturing easily with coincident loss of large areas of skin; healing occurs without scarring. Lesions may occur on the lips and in the mouth, nose, pharynx and larynx, causing difficulty in eating and hoarseness. Pemphigus vegetans has a course similar to that of pemphigus vulgaris.

In some variants of pemphigus, such as pemphigus erythematosus and pemphigus foliaceus, bulla formation occurs more superficially within the epidermis. These forms tend to be less severe.

There are two forms of pemphigoid: bullous pemphigoid and cicatricial pemphigoid. Bullous pemphigoid is clinically similar to pemphigus, but occurs predominantly in patients over 50 years of age. If untreated, it follows a chronic relapsing course and the mortality rate is low. It tends to be self-limiting and the patient's health remains good. The characteristic feature of the condition is large tense bullae, often occurring on the inner aspects of the thighs, on the flexor surfaces of the forearms, axillae and groins, and over the lower abdomen. The oral cavity may be affected but, unlike pemphigus, is rarely the site of initial manifestation. Blister formation is thought to result from the activation of complement in association with neutrophil and eosinophil migration. Cicatricial pemphigoid is rare and primarily affects the mucous membranes. Skin is involved in 10–30% of cases, but rarely in the absence of mucosal lesions. It is a chronic condition and the lesions usually heal with scarring. This may lead to nasal obstruction, dysphagia and laryngeal stenosis. Blindness may complicate ocular involvement.

TREATMENT

Treatment of both pemphigus and pemphigoid is with steroids and, occasionally, other immunosuppressant drugs (e.g. methotrexate, azathioprine and cyclophosphamide). Lower doses of corticosteroids are used in pemphigoid. Gold injections and plasmapheresis may also be used in pemphigus.

ERYTHEMA MULTIFORME

Erythema multiforme is more common and is an acute, self-limiting eruption of the skin and mucous membranes. Stevens–Johnson syndrome (SJS) is a more severe form of erythema multiforme, with involvement of mucosal surfaces and viscera in association with marked constitutional symptoms.

Erythema multiforme is characterised by the distinctive target or iris lesions. Some 50% of cases have no identifiable cause but, for the rest, a wide variety of triggers, including infective agents, drugs and neoplasms, has been described. Those of particular importance to the anaesthetist include barbiturates, antibiotics, anticonvulsants, antipyretics and cimetidine. The pathogenesis of erythema multiforme is not fully understood, but there is evidence that it may be a hypersensitivity reaction. It may present in various forms (hence its name), ranging from a mild self-limiting skin eruption through to SJS with its systemic involvement and high mortality rate (5–15%) if untreated. Erythema multiforme may present as symmetrical target lesions (dull red macules up to 2 cm in diameter with a clear centre) on the extensor surfaces of the extremities, as a series of urticarial plaques or with vesicle or bulla formation.

SJS has a prodrome lasting for up to 14 days, consisting of fever, malaise, myalgia, arthralgia, respiratory and gastrointestinal symptoms. It is followed by the explosive eruption of bullous lesions of the mouth, lips and conjunctiva, and variable skin involvement. In severe cases the oesophagus and respiratory tract are involved. Pneumonitis, pleural effusions and bullae of the visceral pleura are seen, the latter occasionally leading to pneumothorax or even bronchopleural fistula. Myocarditis, atrial fibrillation and renal failure are recognised complications. There may also be anaemia and fluid and electrolyte imbalance. Treatment of SJS is supportive, although steroids have also been used, as for severe cases of EM.

PREOPERATIVE ASSESSMENT
History and examination:
- Fully assess the disease together with its extent and the duration of the illness. In particular, assess the distribution and severity of lesions, especially those involving the airway.
- Assess nutritional state.
- Note drug therapy and dose, especially systemic corticosteroids and immunosuppressants.
- Consider the effects of plasmapheresis on cholinesterase levels in pemphigus.

Investigations:
- Full blood count:
  —anaemia may occur in SJS
  —leukopaenia and thrombocytopaenia may result from immunosuppressant therapy
- Urea and electrolytes – abnormalities may exist in SJS or as a result of steroid therapy
- Assess renal function, especially in SJS
- Blood glucose – level may be raised due to steroid therapy

- Flow–volume loops may be of use where upper respiratory tract stenosis is suspected
- Consider cholinesterase activity following plasmapheresis.

Premedication:
- Ensure that premedication is sufficient to prevent struggling during induction. Struggling may risk new bulla formation.
- The intramuscular route might appear unsuitable for fear of inducing new lesions; however, when intramuscular premedication has been used in pemphigus and SJS, new bulla formation has not been reported.

PERIOPERATIVE MANAGEMENT
Induction:
- Intramuscular ketamine has been used successfully in pemphigus and SJS.
- Suture intravenous cannulae in place or secure with vaseline gauze and ties.
- Avoid barbiturates in patients with erythema multiforme or SJS.
- For children, encourage the presence of parents in the anaesthetic room in order to reduce the chances of struggling and restlessness on induction, thereby reducing likelihood of blister formation.

Airway considerations
A major concern in all the blistering diseases must be the potential to cause the formation of new bullae during airway manipulation or intubation. It is wise to use manoeuvres that avoid unnecessary airway manipulation:
- Use face-masks with a soft air cushion.
- Pad face-masks with vaseline gauze.
- Place vaseline gauze under chin to protect skin from anaesthetist's fingers.
- If possible, avoid the use of airway adjuncts, such as Guedel airways.
- An inhalational induction may be required when laryngeal stenosis is present. Helium–oxygen mixtures may help.
- Consider the use of an 'anaesthetic hood' for inhalational induction.
- Protect front of neck with vaseline gauze if cricoid pressure must be employed.
- Laryngoscopy and oral intubation may be difficult in all of the blistering diseases due to pre-existing airway bullae.
- Laryngeal stenosis has been reported in SJS and cicatricial pemphigoid. The use of small uncuffed tracheal tubes may be necessary.
- The use of nasotracheal tubes has not been reported in pemphigus, pemphigoid, erythema multiforme or SJS.

9

- Secure tracheal tubes with simple loose ties rather than with adhesive tape.

Maintenance:
- Intermittent positive-pressure ventilation (IPPV) may be hazardous in SJS because of the risk of pneumothoraces and bronchopleural fistulae.
- Drug disposition will be affected by hypoalbuminaemia and renal disease in SJS.
- Intravenous ketamine and diazepam infusions, in the absence of intubation, have proven useful in SJS.

Regional techniques:
- Intrathecal and epidural anaesthetic techniques appear safe in pemphigus and pemphigoid. No new lesions have occurred at the sites of spinal needle insertion.
- Modifications should be made to the skin cleansing routine, for example:
  —soak skin with povidone–iodine (Betadine) swabs or pour Betadine over skin
  —avoid rubbing the skin
  —avoid subcutaneous injections of local anaesthetic solutions.
- Use EMLA cream for skin anaesthesia.

Monitoring:
- Well padded non-invasive blood pressure cuffs do not appear to cause bullae, probably because direct pressure is less harmful than frictional or shearing forces.
- The pulse oximeter should be attached using a simple clip rather than adhesive or tape.
- Use ECG pads without adhesive; needle ECG electrodes may be an alternative.
- A weighted untaped precordial stethoscope may be useful.
- Secure intravenous lines with sutures, not tape.
- Arterial lines may be of considerable use – secure with sutures.
- Do not use self-adhesive electrodes for monitoring neuromuscular function.

Positioning:
- Keep sheets and other linen free from creases.
- Pad heels, elbows and bony prominences using foam.

- Allow patients to move themselves on to trolleys or the operating table in order to minimise skin trauma.
- Inform operating-room staff of the need for special care during patient positioning.
- Take care with the positioning of a diathermy pad and do not use a self-adhesive type.

Emergence and recovery:
- If pharyngeal suction is required, use a soft flexible catheter.
- Use protective vaseline gauze under oxygen masks.
- For children, encourage the presence of parents in the recovery room in order to reduce the chances of struggling and restlessness on emergence.
- Regional techniques may allow the provision of high-quality continuous postoperative analgesia.

POSTOPERATIVE MANAGEMENT:
- New skin lesions are a common complication.
- Continue steroid supplements.

BIBLIOGRAPHY

Cucchiara RF, Dawson B. Anesthesia in Stevens–Johnson syndrome: report of a case. Anesthesiology 1971; 35:537–539

Drenger B, Zidenbaum M, Reifen E, Leitersdorf E. Severe upper airway obstruction and difficult intubation in cicatricial pemphigoid. Anaesthesia 1986; 41:1029–1031

Prasad KK, Chen L. Anesthetic management of a patient with bullous pemphigoid. Anesthesia and Analgesia 1989; 69:537–540

Vatashsky E, Aronson HB. Pemphigus vulgaris: anaesthesia in the traumatised patient. Anaesthesia 1982; 37:1195–1197

CROSS-REFERENCES

Disorders of epidermal cell kinetics and differentiation

B. J. Pollard and G. B. Smith

PSORIASIS

Psoriasis is a chronic skin disorder characterised by an accelerated epidermal turnover and epidermal hyperplasia. These are caused by an increased rate of epidermal protein synthesis, rapid epidermal cell growth, shortened epidermal cell cycle and an increase in the proliferative cell population. The exact aetiology of psoriasis is unknown, although both genetic and environmental factors are thought to play a part. The lesions, which tend to involve the extensor surfaces (elbows and knees), sacral area and scalp, consist of loosely adherent, thickened, noncoherent, silver skin scales which have an increased vascularity. Mechanical trauma leading to removal of skin causes small blood droplets to appear on the skin (Auspitz's sign). Psoriatic lesions often follow trauma of the skin (Köbner's phenomenon). Psoriatic arthropathy occurs in 5–10% of patients and resembles seronegative rheumatoid arthritis. Psoriasis is also associated with ulcerative colitis and Crohn's disease. Psoriatic lesions have a tendency to increased colonisation by bacteria, especially *Staphylococcus aureus*, compared with normal skin. Severe psoriasis may be associated with hyperuricaemia, anaemia (chronic illness, folate or vitamin B_{12} deficiency), negative nitrogen balance, iron loss and hypoalbuminaemia.

Two forms of psoriasis produce marked systemic effects on the body: psoriatic erythroderma (see below) and generalised pustular psoriasis. The latter is characterised by waves of sterile pustules over the skin of the trunk and extremities, together with fever of up to 40°C lasting for several days. There may be associated weight loss, muscle weakness, congestive cardiac failure and hypocalcaemia.

The treatment of psoriasis involves the use of topical steroids, coal tar or dithranol, ultraviolet light (with or without a psoralen), retinoids (vitamin A derivatives), cytotoxic agents (e.g. methotrexate, azathioprine) and ciclosporin A.

ERYTHRODERMA

Eyrthroderma (or exfoliative dermatitis) describes a generalised inflammatory disorder in which there is widespread scaling and erythema of the skin. The skin is hot and oedematous, and the disorder is associated with systemic effects including disturbances of the cardiovascular, thermoregulatory and metabolic systems. In the acute stages of the disorder there may be marked hypothermia, pyrexia-related hypovolaemia and heart failure. The more common causes are psoriasis, eczema, drug reactions and the reticuloses. Normally, total skin blood flow is approximately $1 \ l \ min^{-1}$ at 37°C; however, in erythroderma, this may increase to $5 \ l \ min^{-1}$, reaching as much as $10 \ l \ min^{-1}$ in the presence of pyrexia. As a result, high-output cardiac failure is a risk and may be exacerbated by hypoalbuminaemia, hypercatabolism and an iron- or folate-deficiency anaemia. Treatment of erythroderma relies on treating the cause of the disorder.

ICHTHYOSIS

Ichthyosis describes a group of conditions that are characterised by the accumulation of large amounts of dry scales on the skin. It is a disorder of keratinisation. The most common form is ichthyosis vulgaris, an autosomal dominant disease. Other common forms include X-linked ichthyosis, lamellar ichthyosis (autosomal recessive) and epidermolytic hyperkeratosis (autosomal dominant). Ichthyosis is also seen in association with neoplasia such as lymphoma, multiple myeloma and carcinomas of the lung and breast. Treatment of ichthyosis is directed at increasing the water content of the skin (urea-containing creams), causing separation of the cells using keratolytic agents (salicylic acid ointment), or by affecting epidermal metabolism (lactic acid ointment). Occasionally, methotrexate and the retinoids are used.

9

PREOPERATIVE ASSESSMENT
History and examination:
- Fully assess the disease together with its extent and the duration of the illness. In particular, assess the distribution and severity of lesions.
- Assess nutritional state.
- Assess any cardiovascular dysfunction, for example congestive cardiac failure in erythroderma or generalised pustular psoriasis.
- Exclude hypovolaemia (due to increased transepidermal water loss or pyrexia) in erythroderma.
- Check core temperature in erythroderma and pustular psoriasis.
- Note drug therapy and dose, especially immunosuppressants and steroids.

Investigations:
- Full blood count:
  —anaemia may be due to chronic illness or deficiencies of iron, vitamin B_{12} or folate
  —leukopaenia and thrombocytopaenia may result from immunosuppressant therapy.
- Urea and electrolytes:
  —abnormalities may exist in erythroderma
  —measure calcium levels if hypoalbuminaemia exists.
- Assess renal function in erythroderma.
- ECG and chest radiography if there is clinical evidence of heart failure.
- Cross-match blood in erythroderma (risk of blood loss).

Premedication
Do not inject intramuscular premedication into areas of psoriasis (risk of Auspitz's phenomenon and infection due to skin colonisation).

PERIOPERATIVE MANAGEMENT
Induction:
- Avoid using psoriatic sites for intravenous access (risk of Auspitz's phenomenon and infection due to skin colonisation).
- Suture intravenous cannulae in place or secure with vaseline gauze and ties. Adhesive tape is likely to denude skin (ichthyosis or psoriasis), cause bleeding (psoriasis) or the Koebner phenomenon (psoriasis).
- The hyperdynamic circulation in erythroderma may alter the speed of onset of intravenous and inhalational anaesthetic agents.
- Hypervolaemia, hypovolaemia, congestive cardiac failure, hypoalbuminaemia and a reduction in renal blood flow may affect the kinetics of drug distribution and excretion.

Maintenance:
- Hypervolaemia, hypovolaemia, congestive cardiac failure, hypoalbuminaemia and a reduction in renal blood flow may affect the kinetics of drug distribution and excretion.
- The increased skin blood flow and high cardiac output in erythroderma may lead to excessive bleeding during surgery.
- Use space blanket or warm air blankets with care in erythroderma because of the risk of hyperthermia. These patients have difficulty in regulating their body temperature, have an increased metabolic rate, and may not be able to sweat.

Regional techniques:
- Avoid using psoriatic sites for regional techniques (risk of Auspitz's phenomenon and infection due to skin colonisation).
- Modifications should be made to the skin-cleansing routine, for example:
  —soak skin using swabs soaked in an aqueous solution of antiseptic or pour solution over skin in ichthyosis (alcohol-based solutions may cause intense pain)
  —avoid skin scrubbing.
- Secure extradural catheters using bandage, as adhesive tape may cause skin loss.

Monitoring:
- Attach ECG electrodes and pulse oximeter to unaffected skin areas.
- Central venous pressure monitoring will be of use in erythroderma where fluid replacement must be undertaken with care.
- Use ECG pads without adhesive in patients with ichthyosis or erythroderma.
- A weighted, untaped, precordial stethoscope may be useful in ichthyosis and erythroderma.
- Monitor core temperature in erythroderma.
- Blood pressure cuffs may cause the Koebner phenomenon, so pad them underneath.

BIBLIOGRAPHY

Greaves MW, Weinstein GD. Treatment of psoriasis. New England Journal of Medicine 1995; 332:581–588

Love JB, Wright CA, Hooke DH et al. Exfoliative dermatitis as a risk factor for epidemic spread of methicillin resistant Staphylococcus aureus. Intensive Care Medicine 1992; 18:189

Smart G, Bradshaw EG. Extradural analgesia and ichthyosis. Anaesthesia 1984; 39:161–162

9

CROSS-REFERENCES

Assessment of renal function
    Patient Conditions 6: 186
Anaemia
    Patient Conditions 7: 202

9

Ehlers–Danlos syndrome

B. J. Pollard

Ehlers–Danlos syndrome (EDS) consists of a group of hereditary disorders of connective tissue characterised by hypermobile joints, extensibility and fragility of skin, and easy bruising. There are nine distinct types (I–IX) depending on the severity of joint and skin manifestations and the degree of involvement of other tissues and organs.

PATHOPHYSIOLOGY

In most forms of EDS, the condition is inherited as an autosomal trait. Specific mutations of genes for collagen (*COL1*, *COL3*, *COL5*), collagen-modifying enzymes and tenascin have been described in most of the different types of EDS. Variations in the specific types of collagen involved and their distribution in different tissues result in diverse clinical manifestations (Table 9.1). Type IV, the vascular–ecchymotic form, is the most severe form (and the only one with an increased risk of death) and results from mutations that cause deficiency of type III procollagen, resulting in marked weakness of blood vessels and the possibility of spontaneous rupture.

Other features of EDS include cardiac conduction defects, mitral valve prolapse, pes planus, scoliosis, herniae, bladder diverticuli, pulmonary emphysema, spontaneous pneumothorax, periodontitis and loose teeth. Clotting is usually normal, but severe bruising, due to friable vessels, is common. Type IV EDS is diagnosed by the presence of two of the following:
• Thin, translucent skin
• Arterial, intestinal or uterine rupture
• Easy bruising
• Characteristic facial appearance.

PREOPERATIVE ASSESSMENT

HISTORY AND EXAMINATION:
• Determine the exact form of EDS and manifestations present in the patient.
• Assess pre-existing cardiovascular and arterial disease with emphasis on valvular abnormalities, aneurysms and arrhythmias.
• Assess jaw opening.
• Assess cervical spine mobility (prone to atlantoaxial dislocation).
• Check for loose teeth and periodontitis.

INVESTIGATIONS:
• Coagulation studies, especially bleeding time
• Cross-match blood – large volumes may be required
• ECG to exclude dysrhythmias and conduction defects.

PERIOPERATIVE MANAGEMENT

PREMEDICATION:
• The patient should be warned of the risks of specific modes of anaesthesia.

TABLE 9.1

Clinical manifestations of different forms of EDS

Form	Effects
I, III, V, VI, VII, X	Hyperextensible joints resulting in recurrent dislocations
IV	Thin skin with prominent veins
Spontaneous rupture of major vessels, uterus, bowel
Aneurysmal dilatation
VI	Blue sclera
Rupture of eye
Most types	Laxity of skin
I, IV, VIII	Easily torn skin that heals with 'cigarette paper' scars
V	Mitral and tricuspid valve prolapse

- Avoid intramuscular premedication – risk of haematoma formation.
- Ensure prophylaxis for subacute bacterial endocarditis if mitral valve disease is present.
- Consider cardiac pacing in the presence of conduction defects.

INDUCTION:
- Cannulation of vessels may be difficult:
- Lax mobile skin makes vessel fixation difficult.
- There may be loss of the normal sensation when a vessel wall is pierced.
- Vessels may be fragile.
- There is a risk of haematoma formation with all vessel punctures, especially of arteries and central veins.
- Securing cannulae may be difficult due to mobile skin.
- Subcutaneous extravasation may be marked and undetected due to skin laxity.

MAINTENANCE:
- Care with insertion of nasogastric tubes – risk of haemorrhage.
- Avoid systemic hypertension – risk of haemorrhage and aneurysmal rupture.

Airway considerations:
- Avoid tracheal intubation if possible, because of potential for local haemorrhage.
- Modify the hypertensive response to intubation to reduce the risk of aneurysm rupture.
- Special care should be taken during intubation owing to the risk of cervical spine damage.
- Use oral route for intubation in preference to nasal.
- Avoid IPPV if possible as there is a risk of pneumothorax if high inflation pressures are required.

Regional techniques
Regional techniques are said to be inadvisable in patients with easy bruising because of risk of haematoma formation. However, intradural and epidural techniques have been employed without complication. Epidural ropivacaine and fentanyl has been found to be safe in obstetric anaesthesia.

Positioning
Lax and fragile skin demands that extra care be taken when moving and positioning the patient for surgery. Also take care with movements of joints.

Other considerations
- During operation, meticulous attention should be paid to haemostasis.
- Risk of major blood loss is significant.
- Ligaments and skin may not hold sutures – risk of wound dehiscence.

POSTOPERATIVE CARE

- Intramuscular injections are best avoided in case of haematoma formation.
- Intravenous opiate infusions or continuous regional techniques appear to be most suitable.

BIBLIOGRAPHY

Abouleish E. Obstetric anaesthesia and Ehlers–Danlos syndrome. British Journal of Anaesthesia 1980; 62:1283–1286

Brighouse D, Guard B. Anaesthesia for caesarean section in a patient with Ehlers–Danlos syndrome type IV. British Journal of Anaesthesia 1992; 69:517–519

Campbell N, Rosaeg OP. Anesthetic management of a parturient with Ehlers–Danlos syndrome type IV. 2002 Canadian Journal of Anesthesia 49:493-496

Dolan P, Sisko F, Riley E. Anaesthetic considerations for Ehlers–Danlos syndrome. Anesthesiology 1980; 52:266–269

Prockop DJ, Kuivaniemi H, Tromp G, Ala-Kokko L. Inherited disorders of connective tissue. In: Harrison's principles of internal medicine. 15th edn. New York: McGraw-Hill; 2001:2295–2297

Pyeritz RE. Ehlers–Danlos syndrome. New England Journal of Medicine 2000; 342:730–732

Schalkwijk J, Zweers MC, Steijlen PM, et al. A recessive form of the Ehlers-Danlos syndrome caused by tenascin-X deficiency. New England Journal of Medicine 2001; 345:1167–1175

9

Epidermolysis bullosa

B. J. Pollard and G. B. Smith

Epidermolysis bullosa (EB) encompasses a group of hereditary diseases characterised by blistering of the skin, either spontaneously or following minimal mechanical trauma. Direct pressure to the skin seems less likely to cause damage than frictional or shearing forces. Separation of the outer layer of the epidermis with accumulation of fluid within the space occurs, forming a large blister. Mucous membranes, particularly those of the mouth, pharynx and oesophagus, may also be affected. More than 20 different subtypes of EB exist, and they can be classified into three major groups – dystrophic (EBD), junctional (EBJ) and simplex (EBS) – depending on the plane within the skin where separation occurs. EBD has the greatest anaesthetic significance.

PATHOPHYSIOLOGY

DYSTROPHIC EPIDERMOLYSIS BULLOSA

EBD may be transmitted as either an autosomal dominant or a recessive disorder, with an incidence ranging from 1 in 50 000 to 1 in 300 000 births. An abnormality of type VII collagen, possibly due to excessive collagenase activity, is implicated in some forms. Blister formation occurs beneath the lamina densa of the epidermal basement membrane. The disease may start at birth or in early infancy, and is characterised by extensive skin bullae, scarring and dystrophic nail lesions. The bullae are large and flaccid, and may become infected or haemorrhagic. In the hand, scar formation eventually results in digital fusion with the formation of 'mitten-like' hands. Flexural contractures also occur. Involvement of the mucous membranes of the mouth, pharynx and oesophagus may lead to feeding difficulties, microstomia, fixation of the tongue to the floor of the mouth, and oesophageal stricture. Anaemia is common and poor nutrition leads to growth retardation in severe cases. The skin lesions of EB have often been confused with those of por-

phyria cutanea tarda (PCT) and have led to the suggestion that there is a strong association between EBD and porphyria. However, these two diseases can now be distinguished on the basis of histopathological, immunofluorescence and porphyrin studies. Equally, PCT does not hold the same significance for the anaesthetist as do the hepatic porphyrias.

JUNCTIONAL EPIDERMOLYSIS BULLOSA

EBJ describes a group of autosomal recessive conditions that lead to blister formation immediately above the basal membrane in the lamina lucida. Death usually occurs in the first 2 years of life. Patients who survive infancy often develop many of the complications of EBD.

SIMPLEX EPIDERMOLYSIS BULLOSA

EBS may be generalised or localised. Some forms are inherited as autosomal dominant disorders, others as autosomal recessives. EBS is the least disabling form of EB.

TREATMENT

EB has been treated using systemic corticosteroids or drugs with collagenase activity, for example phenytoin and minocycline. Patients with EB often require repeated surgery for repair of syndactyly, oesophageal dilatation, skin grafting, dental surgery, removal of skin cancer or change of dressings. Infections of bullae are common.

PREOPERATIVE ASSESSMENT

HISTORY AND EXAMINATION:

- Fully assess the form of EB, together with the extent and duration of the illness.
- Note drug therapy, especially systemic corticosteroids and phenytoin.
- Assess venous access.

INVESTIGATIONS:

- Full blood count – anaemia and thrombocytosis are both common; anaemia may be due to iron or folate deficiency
- Urea and electrolytes – abnormalities may exist in severe EB; assess renal function
- Serum iron, folate and vitamin B_{12} levels
- Liver function tests
- Albumin level – hypoalbuminaemia is common
- Phenytoin levels – to exclude toxicity.

PREMEDICATION:

- Ensure that premedication is sufficient to keep the patient calm during induction – struggling may risk new EB lesions.
- Traditionally, the intramuscular route has been avoided for fear of inducing new EB lesions; however, it now seems unlikely that intramuscular injections cause such problems.
- Prophylaxis against gastric aspiration (ranitidine, metoclopramide, sodium citrate) may be required if oesophageal complications exist.

PERIOPERATIVE MANAGEMENT

INDUCTION:

- Venous access may be difficult – cut-down or central vein cannulation may be necessary.
- An inhalation induction may be needed if venous access is difficult.
- Intramuscular ketamine has proven extremely useful.
- Suture intravenous cannulae in place or secure with vaseline gauze and ties – do not use adhesive tape.
- Suxamethonium appears safe in EB:
  —there have been no new EB lesions reported after muscle fasciculations
  —hyperkalaemia response is not seen, despite obvious muscle atrophy.
- Thiopental appears to be safe, despite fears of associated porphyria.
- For children, encourage the presence of parents in the anaesthetic room in order to reduce the chances of struggling and restlessness on induction.

AIRWAY CONSIDERATIONS

Concern has been expressed over the possibility of causing new EB lesions during airway manipulation or intubation. Although pharyngeal lesions do occur, the hazards of intubation appear to have been overstated, as there are no reports of laryngeal or tracheal lesions following tracheal intubation or tracheostomy. However, spontaneous EB lesions are possible in all of these sites.

- Use face-masks with a soft air cushion.
- Pad face-masks with vaseline gauze.
- Place vaseline gauze under chin to protect skin from anaesthetist's fingers.
- If possible, avoid the use of airway adjuncts, such as Guedel airways.
- On theoretical grounds, the laryngeal mask (LM) would seem inappropriate because of the risk of producing pharyngeal lesions; however, studies to date suggest that the use of well lubricated and carefully placed LMs may be safe.
- Consider the use of an 'anaesthetic hood' (a bag or a box) for inhalational induction.
- Use a rapid sequence induction when there are oesophageal symptoms – regurgitation is a risk.
- Protect front of neck with vaseline gauze when applying cricoid pressure.
- New head and neck lesions are often associated with difficult or failed intubation.
- Laryngoscopy and oral intubation may be difficult:
  —poor dentition
  —limited mouth opening
  —adhesion of tongue to floor of mouth
  —consider fibreoptic intubation
- Nasal airways or tubes should be avoided or well lubricated and used with great care.
- Lubricate the laryngoscope blade well.
- Hydrocortisone ointment has been recommended for lubrication but care must be taken with potential absorption of steroid through mucous membranes.
- Use small uncuffed tracheal tubes if possible, always taking into account the surgical field and the need to prevent airway soiling.
- Secure tracheal tubes with simple loose ties rather than with adhesive tape.
- Treat haemorrhage from mucous membrane lesions using sponges soaked in adrenaline (epinephrine) (1 : 200 000).
- Avoid nasogastric tube if possible – risk of oesophageal lesions.

MAINTENANCE

Drug disposition will be affected by decreased muscle bulk, hypoalbuminaemia and any renal disease.

REGIONAL TECHNIQUES

Although regional anaesthesia has traditionally been avoided, the following blocks have been used without complication:

9

- Brachial plexus blocks – use the supraclavicular approach if there are axillary contractures
- Subarachnoid blocks
- Epidural anaesthesia – lumbar and caudal
- Femoral nerve block
- Digital block
- Wrist block
- Lateral cutaneous nerve of thigh blocks.

Modifications should be made to the skin cleansing routine, for example:

- Soak skin using povidone–iodine (Betadine) swabs or pour Betadine over skin.
- Avoid rubbing the skin.
- Avoid subcutaneous injections of local anaesthetic solutions.
- Use EMLA cream for surface anaesthesia. Landmarks are usually easy to locate.

Tourniquets do not appear to be hazardous if the skin is protected by sufficient padding; however, intravenous regional anaesthesia remains an unreported option.

MONITORING:

- Well padded non-invasive blood pressure cuffs do not appear to cause bullae, probably because direct pressure is less harmful in EB than frictional or shearing forces.
- The pulse oximeter should be attached using a simple clip rather than adhesive or tape.
- Use ECG pads without adhesive; needle ECG electrodes may be an alternative.
- A weighted, untaped, precordial stethoscope may be used.
- Secure the intravenous cannula with sutures, not tape.
- Arterial lines may be of considerable use; secure with sutures, not tape.

POSITIONING:

- Protect the eyes using bland ointment and vaseline gauze pads – bullae may lead to corneal ulceration and globe perforation.
- Keep sheets and other linen free from creases.
- Pad heels, elbows and bony prominences using foam.
- Allow patients to move themselves on to trolleys or the operating table to minimise skin trauma.
- Inform operating-room staff of the need for special care during patient positioning.
- Take care with the positioning of a diathermy pad and do not use the self-adhesive type.

EMERGENCE AND RECOVERY:

- Pharyngeal suction must be performed extremely carefully using a soft flexible catheter.
- Use protective vaseline gauze under oxygen masks.
- For children, encourage the presence of parents in the recovery room in order to reduce the chances of struggling and restlessness on emergence.

POSTOPERATIVE CARE

Common problems and complications include:
- New skin lesions
- Regurgitation during anaesthetic induction, perhaps leading to aspiration pneumonia
- Need to continue preoperative drug treatment, including steroid supplements.

BIBLIOGRAPHY

Boughton R, Crawford MR, Vonwiller JB. Epidermolysis bullosa – a review of 15 years' experience, including experience with combined general and regional anaesthetic techniques. Anaesthesia and Intensive Care 1988; 16:260–264

Fine J, Bauer EA, Briggaman RA et al. Revised clinical and laboratory criteria for subtypes of inherited epidermolysis bullosa. Journal of the American Academy of Dermatology 1991; 24:119–135

Griffin RP, Mayou BJ. The anaesthetic management of patients with dystrophic epidermolysis bullosa. A review of 44 patients over a 10 year period. Anaesthesia 1993; 48:810–815

James I, Wark H. Airway management during anaesthesia in patients with epidermolysis bullosa dystrophica. Anesthesiology 1982; 56:323–326

Smith GB, Shribman AJ. Anaesthesia and severe skin disease. Anaesthesia 1984; 39:443–455

9

Mucopolysaccharidoses

B. L. Taylor

A group of rare familial disorders caused by deficiencies of enzymes required to metabolise the mucopolysaccharide (MPS) constituents of connective tissue. MPS accumulates in skin, bone, blood vessels, brain, heart, liver, spleen, cornea and the tracheobronchial tree, causing anatomical and biochemical malfunction. All sufferers exhibit progressive joint, skeletal and craniofacial abnormalities. Survival beyond the second decade is rare, the majority of childhood deaths being attributable to recurrent pneumonia or cardiac disease. In later years, death occurs from cardiac failure or related complications.

PATHOPHYSIOLOGY

MPS enzyme deficiencies are recessively inherited. All variants are autosomal, with the exception of Hunter's syndrome, which is X-linked. Urinary excretion of connective tissue substrates assists diagnosis, but skin biopsy and biochemical enzyme analysis may also be required. Anaesthesia may be required for surgical correction of anatomical abnormalities, relief of distressing symptoms, diagnostic investigation or coincidental disease. The MPSs present a wide range of potential anaesthetic problems (Table 9.2).

CARDIOVASCULAR SYSTEM

The mitral and aortic valves are distorted and thickened, causing incompetence or stenosis. Myocardial and coronary vessel involvement leads to hypertrophic cardiomyopathy, congestive cardiac failure, myocardial ischaemia and infarction. Arrhythmias and conduction block may occur. Chronic respiratory disease and airway obstruction may produce cor pulmonale.

RESPIRATORY SYSTEM

Airway obstruction may occur due to an enlarged tongue, orofacial abnormalities, adenotonsillar hypertrophy, laryngomalacia, tracheomalacia and mucosal deposition of MPS throughout the respiratory tree. Excessive secretions may cause further compromise. Age-related anterocephalad displacement of the larynx occurs in some types. Kyphoscoliosis and obstructive lung disease increase susceptibility to pulmonary sepsis. Mitral valve disease, pulmonary hypertension and chronic right ventricular failure may further affect respiratory function.

CENTRAL NERVOUS SYSTEM

Mental function ranges from normal intellect to severe intellectual impairment. Intellectual

TABLE 9.2

Anaesthetic problems associated with various syndromes

Syndrome	Type	Major anaesthetic considerations
Hurler	I	Macroglossia, kyphoscoliosis, odontoid hypoplasia, mitral incompetence, cardiomegaly
Scheie	I	Macroglossia, prognathia, short neck, aortic incompetence
Hurler–Scheie	I	Macroglossia, micrognathia, short neck, mitral and aortic incompetence
Hunter	II	Hydrocephaly, short neck, ischaemic cardiomyopathy
San Filippo	III	Macroglossia, vertebral abnormalities
Morquio	IV	Kyphoscoliosis, odontoid hypoplasia, short neck, C1–C2 instability, aortic regurgitation
Maroteaux–Lamy	VI	Macroglossia, kyphoscoliosis, odontoid hypoplasia, mitral and aortic valve lesions
Sly	VII	Contractures, thoracic gibbus, odontoid hypoplasia, mitral and aortic valve lesions, aortic dissection

9

deterioration may arise from the disease process or be secondary to hydrocephalus and raised intracranial pressure (ICP). Visual and hearing impairment may complicate assessment.

GASTROINTESTINAL TRACT
Hepatosplenomegaly is routinely present, but liver and splenic functions are usually unaffected. Umbilical and inguinal herniae are common owing to abdominal wall weakness.

SKELETAL
Macrocephaly, hypertelorism and abnormalities of the oropharynx and temporomandibular joints occur frequently. Abnormalities of the neck and cervical spine are common, including 'silent' atlanto-occipital subluxation and delayed vertebral ossification. Joint deformities may be aggravated by muscle contractures.

PREOPERATIVE ASSESSMENT

HISTORY:
- Previous operations and anaesthetic problems
- Physical and mental disability
- Respiratory or cardiovascular history
- Symptoms of obstructive sleep apnoea.

EXAMINATION
General:
- Skeletal abnormalities – craniofacial, contractures, etc.
- Skin and peripheral veins.

Respiratory:
- Upper airway and orofacial abnormalities
- Axial anomalies – cervical spine, kyphoscoliosis, etc.
- Proximal and distal airways obstruction
- Evidence of chronic lung disease
- Secretion and sputum production
- Active pulmonary infection.

Cardiovascular:
- Cardiac valve incompetence or stenosis
- Cardiomegaly, left ventricular hypertrophy
- Cor pulmonale
- Univentricular and biventricular failure
- Arrhythmias.

Central nervous system:
- Raised ICP, papilloedema
- Visual and hearing impairment.

INVESTIGATIONS
See Table 9.3.

TABLE 9.3

Investigations for mucopolysaccharidoses

Investigation	Result
Spirometry	Decreased vital capacity, FRC, TLC
Arterial blood gases	Hypoxaemia, hypercapnia
Chest radiography	Pneumonia, atelectasis, subglottic narrowing
ECG	LVH, RVH, arrhythmias, conduction block
Echocardiography	Decreased ejection fraction, valve lesions, dyskinesia
Cardiac catheterisation	Valve pressure gradients, coronary artery occlusion
Computed tomography of brain	Hydrocephaly, increased ICP
Cervical spine radiography	Decreased ossification, atlanto-occipital instability
MRI of cervical spine	Decreased ossification, atlanto-occipital instability
Haematology profile	Increased white cell count, anaemia
Urea and electrolytes	Diuretic and digoxin effects
Liver function tests	Liver dysfunction

FRC, functional residual capacity; TLC, total lung capacity; LVH, left ventricular hypertrophy; RVH, right ventricular hypertrophy; ICP, intracranial pressure.

PREOPERATIVE PREPARATION

- Treatment of active respiratory infection
- Chest physiotherapy
- Treatment of cardiac failure and arrhythmias
- Full discussion with parents and consideration of parental accompaniment to anaesthetic room.

PREMEDICATION:
- Increased sensitivity to narcotic analgesics
- Risk of respiratory depression and sleep apnoea
- Antisialagogue advisable – use glycopyrrolate if tachydysrhythmias are predicted
- Benzodiazepines effective, but unpredictable
- Ketamine useful if difficult airway anticipated
- Consider the need for prophylaxis against bacterial endocarditis

- Use of EMLA cream helps maintain cooperation of child.

PERIOPERATIVE MANAGEMENT

INDUCTION:
- Arrange a full range of airway adjuncts.
- Tracheal tube size is not predictable from age and weight, so a full range of sizes must be available.
- Oral abnormalities and temporomandibular stiffness may reduce airway access.
- There is a strong case for using fibreoptic intubation in the majority of patients with MPS. Difficulties in intubation are common and cervical spine abnormalities may cause critical spinal stenosis, which may be asymptomatic. In such patients positioning the patient for conventional laryngoscopy may produce significant cord compression. Fibreoptic intubation avoids the necessity to extend the neck and should reduce this risk. When a laryngeal mask is inserted to facilitate endoscopic intubation, neck extension should similarly be avoided.
- Nasal intubation may cause epistaxis; adenoidal tissue may obstruct nasal tube.
- Laryngeal mask is useful, but may cause excessive secretions or laryngospasm.
- Inhalational induction with oxygen–halothane is useful if difficult airway is likely.
- Small titrated doses of intravenous anaesthetic drug maintaining spontaneous ventilation may be used until the airway is secured.
- Ketamine is often used; avoid if ICP is raised.
- Intravenous induction agents should be used cautiously, as they may precipitate apnoea.
- Avoid neuromuscular blockade until trachea intubated or ventilation can be assured.

REGIONAL TECHNIQUES
These are seldom appropriate for surgery alone because of the intellectual impairment of many patients.

AIRWAY CONSIDERATIONS:
- Always consider cervical spine involvement.
- Oral airways may cause obstruction by pushing epiglottis backwards; nasal airways less so.
- Difficult intubation is common and becomes progressively more so with increasing age.

- Cartilaginous softening or airway distortion may make tracheostomy and cricothyrotomy difficult.

MAINTENANCE:
- A nitrous oxide–volatile agent mix is appropriate.
- Use caution with narcotic analgesics because of increased sensitivity.
- Spontaneous breathing techniques are generally inadvisable unless the procedure is of short duration or intubation proves impossible.

MONITORING
In addition to standard anaesthesia monitoring techniques, it is recommended that somatosensory evoked potentials should be monitored in patients with a high risk of compression of the cervical spinal cord (types I, IV, VI and VII), particularly during airway manipulations. In such patients preoperative magnetic resonance imaging (MRI) may be valuable in assessing the risk of cord compression.

POSITIONING
This may be difficult due to kyphoscoliosis.

EMERGENCE AND RECOVERY:
- Delayed awakening is a recognised problem.
- Extubate when awake to avoid airway obstruction; consider nasopharyngeal airway.

ANALGESIA:
- Titrate narcotic analgesics in reduced dosage.
- Local or regional technique is beneficial.

POSTOPERATIVE CARE

- Consider ITU admission for close monitoring
- Chest physiotherapy and antibiotics
- Common problems include:
  —restlessness or aggressive behaviour
  —arrhythmias
  —respiratory obstruction or depression
  —obstructive sleep apnoea
  —pulmonary infection
  —reduced cough and secretion clearance.

OUTCOME

With appropriate management, the perioperative morbidity and mortality rates of patients with mucopolysaccharidoses are low.

BIBLIOGRAPHY

Diaz JH, Belani KG. Perioperative management of children with mucopolysaccharidoses. Anesthesia and Analgesia 1993; 77:1261–1270

CROSS-REFERENCES

9

Polyarteritis nodosa

B. J. Pollard and G. B. Smith

Polyarteritis nodosa (PAN) is a rare systemic disease in which a necrotising arteritis affects the small- and medium-sized arteries. The consequence of this vasculitis depends on the site and number of vessels involved, and may range from localised lesions with clinically insignificant effects to life-threatening organ failure. Typically, there is aneurysm formation in the medium-sized arteries, and both haemorrhage and infarction in major organs. Prognosis in PAN is significantly influenced by the size of vessel affected and by the presence of renal involvement. Up to 40% of patients with PAN die within 1 year of diagnosis.

PATHOPHYSIOLOGY

The histological finding in classical PAN is a fibrinoid necrosis of the media of affected arteries associated with infiltration of the intima and media by polymorphs. The condition occurs more often in women, with a peak incidence in the 40–50 years age group. Presenting symptoms often include malaise, fever and weight loss. Approximately 60% have arthralgia, 50% a rash (erythematous, purpuric or vasculitic) and 40% a peripheral neuropathy. The gastrointestinal system is involved in about 45% of cases; gut or gallbladder infarction, gastrointestinal haemorrhage and pancreatitis being the common presentations. Approximately 25% have renal impairment. Myalgia may also be a presenting symptom. Classical PAN is treated with immunosuppressant drugs (e.g. cyclophosphamide) and systemic corticosteroids.

In some patients with PAN there is little evidence of major organ involvement, with the exception of severe renal disease (necrotising glomerulonephritis). This disorder, which has a mean age of onset of 50 years and a male predominance, is often termed microscopic polyarteritis. Although all of the features of classical PAN can occur in microscopic polyarteritis, they are less frequent. The patient often presents with haematuria (microscopic or macroscopic), proteinuria or oliguria. Haemoptysis, frank pulmonary haemorrhage (occasionally requiring controlled ventilation), pleurisy and asthma may also be the initial symptoms. In microscopic polyarteritis histological examination reveals a focal segmental necrotising glomerulonephritis with fibrinoid necrosis and thrombosis of the glomerular tufts. Treatment of microscopic polyarteritis is as for PAN; azathioprine is occasionally added. Plasmapheresis may be used when cytotoxics and steroids appear to have no benefit.

PREOPERATIVE ASSESSMENT

HISTORY AND EXAMINATION:

- Assess the extent and duration of the illness. Discover whether the patient has an acute arteritis or is in remission, as this will affect perioperative risk and outcome.
- Assess systemic involvement:
  —cardiovascular – angina, heart failure, cardiomegaly, pericarditis
  —respiratory – asthma, pneumonia, haemoptysis, pleurisy
  —renal – renal failure, hypertension
  —CNS – peripheral neuropathy, stroke
  —airway – acute pharyngeal oedema.
- Check drug history:
  —systemic corticosteroids
  —other immunosuppressant drugs
  —cardiac drugs.

INVESTIGATIONS
ECG:
- Cardiac ischaemia, myocardial infarction
- Dysrhythmias
- Pericarditis.

Echocardiography
Assess cardiac contractility, pericardial effusions.

Chest radiography:
- Pulmonary infection, haemorrhage
- Pulmonary infiltrates – pulmonary eosinophilia

9

- Pulmonary fibrosis
- Cardiac failure.

Arterial blood gases:
- Look for hypoxaemia.
- The critically ill patient is likely to have a metabolic acidosis.

Urea and electrolytes:
- Usually normal until disease is very severe
- Assess renal function – creatinine and potassium.

Full blood count:
- Anaemia is common.
- Leukocytosis is a frequent finding.
- Leukopaenia may result from immunosuppressant drug therapy.

Liver function tests:
- Albumin and clotting factors as indicators of liver function
- Approximately 30% of patients with PAN carry the hepatitis B surface antigen (HBsAg).

Lung function tests:
- Request if there is clinical evidence of lung disease.
- Pulmonary fibrosis will cause a restrictive defect.

Coagulation studies
May be abnormal due to hepatic involvement.

HBsAg
Approximately 30% of patients carry HBsAg.

Urinalysis
PAN may cause the nephrotic syndrome.

Plasma cholinesterase levels:
- Reduced by plasmapheresis
- Action inhibited by cyclophosphamide.

PREOPERATIVE PREPARATION

- Preoperative optimisation of cardiovascular and respiratory systems
- Chest physiotherapy
- Antibiotics
- Control of hypertension
- Treatment of angina (e.g. nitrates).
- Patients with severe cardiovascular disease may require perioperative invasive haemodynamic monitoring (e.g. central venous catheter, pulmonary artery catheter).

- If surgery is required urgently for patients with acute complications of PAN (e.g. gut ischaemia), the following may be required perioperatively:
  —invasive haemodynamic monitoring
  —controlled ventilation
  —inotropic or vasopressor agents
  —renal replacement therapy.
- Perioperative steroid cover needed for patients receiving systemic steroids.

PERIOPERATIVE MANAGEMENT

Throughout the perioperative phase there should be scrupulous anti-infection measures because of the high risk of sepsis in PAN.

PREMEDICATION:
- Use an anxiolytic to reduce the risk of tachycardia and hypertension from catecholamines.
- Avoid anticholinergic premedication – risk of tachycardia.

INDUCTION:
- Avoid drugs and techniques likely to cause tachycardia, hypertension, hypotension or reduced myocardial contractility (e.g. ketamine, thiopental).
- Use a 'cardiac' anaesthetic (e.g. high-dose opioid technique) to limit the hypertensive response to laryngoscopy.
- Preoxygenate prior to induction.
- Administer high concentrations of oxygen when there is a history of cardiac or respiratory disease.
- Maintain good tissue blood and oxygen supplies.

AIRWAY CONSIDERATIONS
Pharyngeal oedema, although rare, has been reported in PAN.

MAINTENANCE:
- Avoid drugs and techniques likely to cause tachycardia, hypertension, hypotension or reduced myocardial contractility.
- Administer high concentrations of oxygen when there is a history of cardiac or respiratory disease.
- Maintain good tissue blood and oxygen supplies.
- Avoid hypotension and maintain fluid balance, especially in patients with renal involvement.
- Drug handling is altered in renal disease. Avoid drugs that are excreted primarily by the kidneys.

9

- Hypoalbuminaemia will affect drug distribution.
- Avoid vasoconstrictor drugs, if possible, because of the risk of vascular occlusion.
- When plasmapheresis has been recent, remember that the action of ester drugs (e.g. suxamethonium) will be prolonged.
- The action of suxamethonium may be prolonged by cyclophosphamide.

REGIONAL TECHNIQUES:
- Avoid use of adrenaline (epinephrine)-containing local anaesthetic solutions because of the risk of vascular occlusion.
- Document existing sensorimotor neuropathies prior to use of regional techniques.

MONITORING:
- CM5 lead for ECG useful to detect myocardial ischaemia and arrhythmias.
- Radial artery cannulation may be inadvisable in the presence of aneurysmal disease because of the risk of vascular occlusion.

- Blood pressure measurement essential.
- Transoesophageal echocardiography may be helpful during operation if there is severe cardiac disease; it has been used during surgery in infant PAN.

POSTOPERATIVE MANAGEMENT

Common problems and complications include:
- Deterioration in cardiovascular function
- Respiratory failure resulting from pneumonia
- Risk of systemic sepsis.
- Continue systemic steroid supplements.

CROSS-REFERENCES
Chronic renal failure
    Patient Conditions 6: 189
Obstruction or perforation
    Surgical Procedures 16: 432

9

Polymyositis and dermatomyositis

B. J. Pollard and G. B. Smith

Dermatomyositis and polymyositis are members of an uncommon group of connective tissue disorders known as idiopathic inflammatory myopathies (Box 9.1). Their cause is unknown but genetic factors, toxins, drugs and infectious agents probably all play a part. The incidence of malignancy is increased. Both dermatomyositis and polymyositis present with muscle weakness, usually involving proximal muscle groups, and are associated with other multisystem connective tissue diseases such as SLE, rheumatoid arthritis, Hashimoto's thyroiditis and systemic sclerosis. In dermatomyositis there are characteristic violaceous skin lesions, often involving the upper eyelid.

BOX 9.1

Idiopathic inflammatory myopathies

- Polymyositis
- Dermatomyositis
- Cancer-associated myositis
- Connective tissue disease-associated myositis
- Childhood dermatomyositis
- Inclusion body myositis
- Eosinophilic myositis
- Other rare forms

PATHOPHYSIOLOGY

MUSCLE
Chronic inflammation leads to weakness, muscle tenderness, myalgia and, eventually, both atrophy and fibrosis of skeletal muscle. Characteristically there is a rise in the serum concentration of enzymes derived from muscle, such as creatine phosphokinase (CPK); the levels usually parallel disease activity. Myoglobin may be released from muscle, leading to myoglobinaemia and myoglobinuria. The risk of malignant hyperthermia is unknown, but recent *in vitro* studies have shown that muscle from some patients produces significant contracture to caffeine or halothane, but not both (i.e. malignant hyperthermia equivocal).

RESPIRATORY
Of patients with idiopathic inflammatory myopathies, 5–10% have associated interstitial pulmonary disease, predominantly fibrosis. Pulmonary compromise can also occur because of intercostal and diaphragmatic weakness or aspiration pneumonia. Patients with myositis who have no pulmonary symptoms and a normal chest radiograph may exhibit abnormal pulmonary function tests. Vocal cord dysfunction may exist.

CARDIAC
Cardiac disease is a major cause of death. The principal cardiac manifestations are dysrhythmias, conduction defects, myocarditis, cardiomyopathy and cor pulmonale. Steroid-induced hypertension may occur.

GASTROINTESTINAL
Poor coordination of swallowing, nasal regurgitation and pooling of secretions in the vallecula and cricopharyngeal spaces may predispose to pulmonary aspiration. There may also be oesophageal reflux, delayed gastric emptying and decreased intestinal motility.

TREATMENT

First-line therapy involves oral steroids. In some cases, other immunosuppressive drugs such as azathioprine, cyclophosphamide, methotrexate or ciclosporin are added. Patients may present with side-effects of therapy. Plasmapheresis has also been employed and may lower plasma cholinesterase levels.

PREOPERATIVE ASSESSMENT

From data available from the limited number of case reports of anaesthesia for these patients, the potential problems associated with these diseases do not seem to hold major implications for the anaesthetist.

HISTORY AND EXAMINATION:
- Systematic review of associated cardiovascular, respiratory and gastrointestinal disease
- Systemic assessment for other associated autoimmune disorders
- Review of drug therapy and its possible complications.

INVESTIGATIONS
See Table 9.4.

TABLE 9.4

Investigations

Investigation	Possible findings
ECG	Tachyarrhythmias
	Conduction abnormalities
	Ventricular hypertrophy
	Cor pulmonale
Chest radiography	Pulmonary fibrosis
	Ventricular dilatation
Spirometry	Decreased vital capacity
	Decreased functional residual capacity
	Decreased tidal volume
Blood gas analysis	Hypoxaemia
	Hypercapnia
Full blood count	Anaemia
	Leukopenia

PREOPERATIVE PREPARATION
Treat any chest infection.

PREMEDICATION:
- Continue systemic steroid cover
- Avoid intramuscular injections.

PERIOPERATIVE MANAGEMENT

INDUCTION AND MAINTENANCE:
- Avoid malignant hyperthermia trigger agents
- Controlled ventilation should be used in the presence of preoperative ventilatory compromise.

MUSCLE RELAXANTS
Conflicting evidence exists regarding the use of neuromuscular blocking agents. Suxa-

methonium has produced an abnormal muscle contraction prior to relaxation in a child with dermatomyositis. The use of suxamethonium has been avoided by other workers because of the potential, yet unproven, risk of malignant hyperthermia and hyperkalaemia.

The use of non-depolarising neuromuscular blocking agents has also resulted in conflicting evidence. Several workers have noted no problem, yet there are reports of prolonged neuromuscular paralysis following the use of both vecuronium in polymyositis and atracurium in eosinophilic myositis. A myasthenia-like response has been reported, but this may be related more to associated malignancy than to myositis.

- Use small doses of short-acting neuromuscular blocking agents, preferably after a test dose – remember that there is reduced muscle mass.
- Avoid suxamethonium if possible, because of the potential risk of malignant hyperthermia or, in acute myositis, of hyperkalaemia.

AIRWAY CONSIDERATIONS:
- The use of a tracheal tube is strongly recommended, especially if there is risk of aspiration.
- Rapid sequence induction should be used if pharyngeal, oesophageal or gastric symptoms are present.

INTRAOPERATIVE MONITORING:
- Neuromuscular monitoring is essential.
- Extubation and termination of assisted ventilation should follow measurement of lung volumes (e.g. tidal volume, vital capacity).

POSTOPERATIVE CARE

POSTURE
Extubate awake or in the lateral position, because of the risk of aspiration.

COMMON PROBLEMS AND COMPLICATIONS
Immediate postoperative recovery appears to be normal in most patients, yet the following complications might be expected from knowledge of the disease:
- Prolonged recovery from neuromuscular blockade, requiring IPPV
- Lung atelectasis
- Postoperative pneumonia
- Postoperative respiratory failure
- Aspiration if pharyngeal muscles are weak.

9

OTHER MEDICAL THERAPY:

- Continue systemic steroid supplementation after operation.
- Avoid intramuscular analgesics; titrate small intravenous doses of opiates to avoid respiratory depression.
- Postoperative physiotherapy, where necessary.

OUTCOME

Morbidity and mortality in these patients undergoing anaesthesia seem to be low. When they occur, it is usually because of respiratory disease.

BIBLIOGRAPHY

Flusche G, Unger-Sargon J, Lambert DH. Prolonged neuromuscular paralysis with vecuronium in a patient with polymyositis. Anesthesia and Analgesia 1987; 66:188–190

Gabta R, Campbell IT, Mostafa SM. Anaesthesia and acute dermatomyositis/polymyositis. British Journal of Anaesthesia 1988; 60:854–858

Heytens L, Martin JJ, Van de Kleft E, Bossaert LL. In vitro contracture test in patients with various neuromuscular diseases. British Journal of Anaesthesia 1992; 68:72–75

Johns RA, Finholt DA, Stirt JA. Anaesthetic management of a child with dermatomyositis. Canadian Anaesthetists Society Journal 1986; 33:71–74

Plotz PH, Dalakas M, Leff RL, Love LA, Miller FW, Cronin ME. Current concepts in the idiopathic inflammatory myopathies: polymyositis, dermatomyositis, and other related disorders. Annals of Internal Medicine 1989; 111:143–157

CROSS-REFERENCES

9

Pseudoxanthoma elasticum

B. L. Taylor

Pseudoxanthoma elasticum (PXE) is an inherited disorder of elastic and collagen tissue in which there is progressive calcification and degeneration of elastin fibres and the supportive collagen matrix in skin and mucous membranes of affected areas. Similar processes may affect the media of the arterial system, leading to arterial occlusion and ischaemia. Ocular and myocardial involvement may also occur.

PATHOPHYSIOLOGY

The underlying biochemical lesion in PXE, also known as Grönblad–Strandberg disease, is unknown, but the condition is inherited as either an autosomal dominant or a recessive disorder. Diagnosis is usually confirmed by skin biopsy. It is unclear why the areas of the body most rich in elastic tissue (e.g. aorta, lungs, palms, soles) are spared, and the pattern follows more closely the distribution of collagen. The prevalence of PXE is estimated to be between 1 in 50 000 and 1 in 200 000 adults, with women being more commonly affected. Acceleration of symptoms may occur during pregnancy, supporting the theory that some aspects of the disease may be hormonally influenced. The disease occurs at any age and, although average life expectancy is normal, premature death in childhood is a recognised risk.

SKIN

There is a variable tendency to loosening of the skin, particularly in the neck, face, axillae, abdomen and groin (including the genitalia). Most affected individuals show evidence of these changes by their second decade, but some may have minimal involvement even in later life. The loose skin becomes thickened and 'pebbled', sometimes being described as 'peu d'orange'. A characteristic skin deposition of yellowish lesions, mainly in the antecubital fossae, gives a xanthoma-like appearance and the disorder its name. Similar deposition and calcification may occur in mucous membranes, commonly the lower lip, rectum and vagina.

AIRWAY AND RESPIRATORY SYSTEM:
- Laryngeal involvement with PXE has been reported. This may cause loss of elasticity of the laryngeal structures leading to difficult tracheal intubation.
- Respiratory complications may occur secondary to cardiac involvement.

VASCULAR SYSTEM:
- Arterial involvement may lead to a reduction or absence of peripheral pulses, often with associated medial calcification. Distal ischaemic problems are uncommon, presumably because the slow process allows time for collateral circulation to develop.
- Renovascular arterial occlusion may cause severe hypertension, even in young patients.
- Vascular aneurysms also occur in PXE.

HEART:
- Calcification within the endocardium may affect conduction, and predisposes to arrhythmias.
- Mitral valve thickening and incompetence have been reported.
- Coronary arterial lesions may result in severe angina, even in the young; myocardial ischaemia and infarction may result. Coronary artery bypass grafting has been necessary in teenage sufferers and a fatal myocardial infarction has been reported in a 6-week-old infant.

EYE

PXE produces well recognised ocular manifestations in the form of retinal streaks extending radially from the optic disc over the fundus. The 'angioid streaks' are the result of reduced elasticity of Bruch's membrane, and may lead to scarring and retinal or vitreous haemorrhage.

9

GASTROINTESTINAL SYSTEM

Acute gastrointestinal haemorrhage is common, often presenting in children and young adults. The cause appears to be vascular involvement which prevents normal healing responses to minor abrasions of the mucosa. Peptic ulceration and oesophagitis also occur.

CENTRAL NERVOUS SYSTEM

Psychiatric disturbances are commonly associated with the condition. Cerebral ischaemia and haemorrhage are also recognised complications of PXE.

PREOPERATIVE ASSESSMENT

Patients with PXE may require surgery for the ocular, cardiovascular or gastrointestinal complications of the disease. Increasingly, patients present for the surgical treatment of disfiguring cutaneous manifestations.

HISTORY AND EXAMINATION:

- Assess the extent of the disease, taking note of the degree of involvement of the cardiovascular and respiratory systems:
  —angina, myocardial infarction
  —dyspnoea
  —syncopal attacks (dysrhythmias)
  —arterial pulses
  —blood pressure
  —heart murmurs.
- Assess venous access, both peripheral and central.

INVESTIGATIONS:

- ECG
- Chest radiography
- Urea and electrolytes as a baseline test of renal function.

PREOPERATIVE PREPARATION

Temporary cardiac pacing may be indicated in selected patients with conduction defects.

PERIOPERATIVE MANAGEMENT

INDUCTION:

- Venous access may be difficult due to the loose and thickened skin.
- The antecubital fossae are often unsuitable for intravenous access.
- Neck involvement may prevent use of the internal jugular veins.
- Groin involvement may prevent use of the femoral veins.

- Venous cut-down may be necessary.
- An inhalation induction may be necessary.

ANAESTHETIC TECHNIQUE

There appear to be no specific contraindications to the use of any particular anaesthetic drug during induction of anaesthesia in PXE. However, in planning the anaesthetic technique, the following points should be borne in mind:

- Risks of undiagnosed cardiac ischaemia and dysrhythmias
- Risk of major haemorrhage
- Risks of hypertension, such as subendocardial ischaemia, intracranial haemorrhage.

AIRWAY CONSIDERATIONS:

- Tracheal intubation may be difficult because involvement of the laryngeal ligaments and cartilages may cause laryngeal rigidity.
- Rigid bronchoscopy has been necessary to assist with endotracheal intubation in PXE.

MAINTENANCE

See induction (above).

Care should be taken to avoid upper gastrointestinal trauma from the use of a nasogastric tube.

REGIONAL TECHNIQUES

Thickened loose skin may make regional techniques difficult.

MONITORING:

- Blood pressure monitoring, although essential, may be difficult:
  —non-invasive oscillotonometric methods are likely to be unreliable in the presence of occlusive arterial disease
  —invasive blood pressure monitoring may be difficult because of arterial occlusion or vessel calcification.
- Central venous access for central venous pressure monitoring may be difficult (see above).
- Care should be taken to avoid upper gastrointestinal trauma from the use of an oesophageal stethoscope or oesophageal temperature probe.

OUTCOME

The majority of patients with PXE who undergo anaesthesia and surgery have an uncomplicated course and outcome. Patients with severe cardiovascular involvement are at greater risk, as are those suffering complications such as gastrointestinal haemorrhage, requiring emergency surgery.

BIBLIOGRAPHY

Levitt MWD, Collison JM. Difficult endotracheal intubation in a patient with pseudoxanthoma elasticum. Anaesthesia and Intensive Care 1982; 10:62–64

Wilson Krechel SL, Ramirez-Inawat RC, Fabian LW. Anesthetic considerations in pseudo-xanthoma elasticum. Anesthesia and Analgesia 1981; 60:344–347

CROSS-REFERENCES

Cardiac conduction defects
    Patient Conditions 4: 120
Hypertension
    Patient Conditions 4: 151
Coronary artery bypass grafting
    Surgical Procedures 25: 574

9

Scleroderma

B. J. Pollard

Scleroderma (systemic sclerosis) is a chronic multisystem disorder characterised by fibrosis of skin, vascular damage, organ involvement including the gastrointestinal tract, lungs, heart and kidneys, and evidence of an autoantibody response. There is a 4 : 1 female : male ratio, and peak age of onset is in the third to fifth decades.

PATHOPHYSIOLOGY

Scleroderma results from an excess of collagen and other extracellular matrix proteins (fibronectin, tenascin, glycosaminoglycans) in affected tissues. Sufferers often possess certain common HLA antigens and there is evidence of both disordered cell-mediated immunity and

---

BOX 9.2

Clinical features and natural history of scleroderma subtypes[a]

Diffuse cutaneous systemic sclerosis

Early onset of Raynaud's (< 1 year)
Truncal and sacral skin involved
Early systemic disease (interstitial lung fibrosis, renal failure, gastrointestinal and myocardial involvement)
Antitopoisomerase antibody in about 40%

Early (< 5 years after onset)
Rapid progression of skin thickening
Increased risk of renal, cardiac, pulmonary, articular, vascular complications and digital ulcers

Late (> 5 years after onset)
Skin involvement stable or regresses
Progression of existing visceral disease, but reduced risk of new visceral involvement

Limited cutaneous systemic sclerosis

Raynaud's phenomenon for years
Face, hands, feet and forearm skin affected
Late incidence of pulmonary hypertension, trigeminal neuralgia, skin calcification and telangiectasia
Anticentromere antibody in 70–80%

Early (< 10 years after onset)
No progression of skin lesions
Raynaud's phenomenon, digital tip ulceration, oesophageal symptoms common

Late (> 10 years after onset)
No progression of skin lesions
Raynaud's phenomenon, digital ulceration and calcification, oesophageal stricture, malabsorption and pulmonary hypertension

[a]Modified from LeRoy et al (1988) and Steen & Medsger (1990).

abnormal endothelial cell function. Additionally, some chemicals (e.g. silica) induce scleroderma-like syndromes. Most cases of scleroderma fall into one of two subsets: diffuse cutaneous systemic sclerosis or limited cutaneous systemic sclerosis (Box 9.2).

- The skin is shiny, waxen and taut with loss of skin folds in particular.
- Perioral contractures may limit mouth opening.
- Oesophageal involvement occurs in about 80% of patients, resulting in dysphagia and stricture formation.
- The heart is involved in approximately 50% of patients, leading to cardiac arrhythmias, conduction defects, cardiomyopathy, pericarditis and pericardial effusions.
- Lung involvement causes pulmonary fibrosis and pulmonary hypertension.
- Weakness of the intercostal muscles and diaphragm has been reported.
- Skin of the chest wall may be involved.
- Renal disease may lead to hypertension. Hypertensive crises may follow withdrawal of angiotensin-converting enzyme inhibitors.
- Gut involvement may cause malabsorption.
- Other findings in scleroderma include peripheral neuropathies, Sjögren's syndrome and diminished sweating.
- Autoantibodies – anti-Scl-70 (antitopoisomerase I) (specificity 100%, sensitivity 40%), anticentromere (strongly associated with CREST syndrome), anti-RNP, antinucleolar.

The CREST syndrome, a variant of scleroderma, is the combination of calcinosis, Raynaud's phenomenon, oesophageal involvement, sclerodactyly and multiple telangiectasia of the skin, lips, oral mucosa and gut.

PREOPERATIVE ASSESSMENT

HISTORY AND EXAMINATION:

- Assess the extent and duration of the illness
- Assess venous access
- Assess mouth opening
- Assess state of dentition (often poor)
- Look for mucosal telangiectasia in the mouth
- Assess neck mobility
- Assess degree of cardiac and respiratory symptoms (e.g. exertional dyspnoea or the dry cough of pulmonary fibrosis); examine for cardiac dysrhythmias, a pericardial effusion and signs of pulmonary hypertension

- Check preoperative blood pressure
- Exclude dysphagia and oesophageal reflux
- Ask about symptoms of Raynaud's phenomenon
- Check for evidence of chronic renal failure
- Examine for peripheral neuropathies
- Check drug history:
  —systemic corticosteroids
  —other immunosuppressant drugs.

INVESTIGATIONS

ECG and echocardiography:
- 24-h ECG recording (conduction defects) – the presence of a normal resting ECG does not exclude involvement of the heart in scleroderma. Up to 40% of such patients may have abnormalities on 24-h rhythm analysis.
- Diastolic dysfunction in 56% – asymmetrical septal hypertrophy, pericardial effusion.

Chest radiography:
- Look for signs of pulmonary fibrosis.
- Exclude preoperative inhalation of gastric contents.

Cervical spine radiography
Assess associated spinal disease.

Arterial blood gases
Look for hypoxaemia.

Urea and electrolytes
Baseline test of renal function.

Full blood count
Look for anaemia or leukocytosis due to treatment.

Lung function tests:
- Decreased forced vital capacity (FVC) and/or impaired carbon monoxide transfer factor ($D_L CO$) in early scleroderma is predictive of lung disease.
- Determine whether illness is of long duration or there is clinical evidence of lung disease.
- Pulmonary fibrosis may lead to decreased lung compliance and reduced total lung capacity or vital capacity.
- Impaired gas transfer may occur – $D_L CO$ is abnormal in 70% of cases of diffuse cutaneous systemic sclerosis.
- Most lung function tests are poor indicators of pulmonary hypertension in scleroderma.

Coagulation studies
These may be abnormal due to malabsorption.

9

Thyroid function tests
Hypothyroidism may occur in scleroderma.

Preoperative preparation:
- Preoperative pulmonary artery catheterisation may help to diagnose pulmonary hypertension.
- Xerostomia and poor dental hygiene may be helped by frequent preoperative mouthwashes.
- Steroid cover will be needed for patients receiving systemic corticosteroids.
- Use prophylactic H_2 blockers and prokinetic drugs (but beware of inducing arrhythmias), when oesophageal disease is present.
- Vitamin K may be required where malabsorption has led to a bleeding tendency.
- Temporary cardiac pacing may be indicated in selected patients with conduction defects.

PERIOPERATIVE MANAGEMENT

INDUCTION:
- Venous access may be difficult due to vasoconstriction; cut-down or central vein cannulation may be necessary.
- An inhalation induction or fibreoptic intubation technique may be necessary.

AIRWAY CONSIDERATIONS:
- A rapid sequence induction may not be practicable if intubation difficulties are anticipated.
- Cricoid pressure may be ineffective if the oesophagus is fibrosed.
- Consider induction of anaesthesia in the head-up position.
- Consider awake fibreoptic intubation.
- Intubation should be performed very gently to avoid injury to the mouth.
- Use oral intubation in preference to the nasal route as telangiectasia may lead to bleeding.
- In very severe cases, consider tracheostomy.

MAINTENANCE:
- Maintain patient's temperature at 37°C – risk of Raynaud's phenomenon.
- Warm all intravenous fluids.
- Reduced lung and chest wall compliance may make ventilation difficult.
- Dry eyes (Sjögren's syndrome) make eye care especially important – eyelids should be taped shut; use bland ointments or artificial tears.

- Use heat and moisture exchanger in Sjögren's syndrome.
- Avoid hypotension and maintain fluid balance, especially in patients with renal involvement.
- Drug metabolism is altered in renal failure.
- Avoid vasoconstrictor drugs, if possible.
- Increased concentrations of oxygen may be required.

REGIONAL TECHNIQUES:
- Ischaemic effects of tourniquets make the use of intravenous regional anaesthesia unwise.
- Nerve blocks, including brachial plexus and sciatic nerve, have been used successfully, but may be associated with prolonged neural blockade (this may be beneficial).
- Raynaud's phenomenon may follow wrist blocks.
- Avoid use of adrenaline (epinephrine)-containing local anaesthetic solutions.
- Unilateral local anaesthetic stellate ganglion blocks have worsened Raynaud's phenomenon on the contralateral side.

MONITORING:
- Limb contractures may make blood pressure measurement difficult.
- Radial artery cannulation may cause reflex spasm and should be avoided if possible.
- ECG monitoring to detect arrhythmias and conduction defects.

POSITIONING
Consider the risks of pressure effects on fibrotic skin during prolonged operations.

EMERGENCE AND RECOVERY:
- The maintenance of a head-down position is advisable until the patient is fully conscious.
- Patients should be nursed upright once awake, in order to prevent regurgitation.
- Increased oxygen requirements may result from a diffusion block in cases of lung fibrosis.

POSTOPERATIVE MANAGEMENT

Common problems and complications are:
- Postoperative chest infection
- Respiratory failure resulting from respiratory muscle weakness or pneumonia
- Postoperative analgesic requirements may be increased – possibly due to increased numbers of sensory nerve fibres in skin. Continue systemic steroid supplements.

BIBLIOGRAPHY

Black CM, Stephens C. Systemic sclerosis (scleroderma) and related disorders. In: Maddison PJ, Isenberg DA, Woo P, Glass DN, eds. Oxford textbook of rheumatology. Oxford: Oxford University Press; 1993:771–794

LeRoy EC, Black S, Fleischmajer R et al. Scleroderma (systemic sclerosis): classification, subsets and pathogenesis. Journal of Rheumatology 1988; 15:202–205

Neill RS. Progressive systemic sclerosis. Prolonged sensory blockade following regional anaesthesia in association with a reduced response to systemic analgesics. British Journal of Anaesthesia 1980; 52:623–625

Omote K, Kawamata M, Namiki A. Adverse effects of stellate ganglion block on Raynaud's phenomenon associated with progressive systemic sclerosis. Anesthesia and Analgesia 1993; 77:1057–1060

Roberts JG, Sabar R, Gianoli JA, Kaye AD. Progressive systemic sclerosis: clinical manifestations and anesthetic considerations. Journal of Clinical Anesthesia 2002;14(6):474–477

Smoak LR. Anesthesia considerations for the patient with progressive systemic sclerosis (scleroderma). Journal of the American Association of Nurse Anesthetists 1982; 50:548–554

Steen VD, Medsger TA. Epidemiology and natural history of systemic sclerosis. Rheumatic Diseases Clinics of North America 1990; 16:1–10

Wigley FM. When is scleroderma really scleroderma? Journal of Rheumatology 2001; 28:1471

Younker D, Harrison B. Scleroderma and pregnancy. Anaesthetic considerations. British Journal of Anaesthesia 1985; 57:1136–1139

CROSS-REFERENCES

Disorders of the oesophagus and of swallowing
    Patient Conditions 5: 162
Difficult airway – difficult mask anaesthesia and ventilation
    Anaesthetic Factors 28: 661

9

Systemic lupus erythematosus

B. J. Pollard and G. B. Smith

Systemic lupus erythematosus (SLE) is a chronic inflammatory disease affecting most body systems and characterised by abnormal immune function. Increased numbers of hyperactive B lymphocytes, together with impaired T-cell regulation, lead to the production of IgG antibodies which are specific for exogenous and endogenous antigens. The serum in SLE contains a variety of autoantibodies directed against nuclear material (anti-DNA antibodies in particular), and histological examination of affected tissue shows evidence of immune complex deposition. The origin of SLE appears to be multifactorial: diet, drugs, toxins, infection, stress, pregnancy, environment, hormones, genetics, etc. all seem to play a part. Drug-induced SLE may occur with isoniazid, hydralazine, anticonvulsants, procainamide, methyldopa and chlorpromazine.

SLE is more common in females than males (9 : 1) and the usual onset is in the third and fourth decades. It is an episodic disease with periods of prolonged remission punctuated by life-threatening exacerbations. Usually the

---

BOX 9.3

Clinical features of SLE

Bones and joints

Flitting arthralgia
Polyarthritis (wrists, elbows, knees)
Aseptic necrosis of large joints

Skin

'Butterfly' rash in malar region
Photosensitivity
Raynaud's phenomenon

Cardiovascular system

Pericarditis or pericardial effusion
Myocarditis
Endocarditis
Leg ulcers
Limb gangrene
Necrotic finger pulp lesions

Respiratory system

Pleurisy or pleural effusions
Pulmonary infiltration
Diffusion block

Renal system

Proteinuria
Nephrotic syndrome
Hypertension
Acute and chronic renal failure

Muscular system

Myalgia
Myositis
Wasting or weakness

Nervous system

Seizures
Psychosis
Peripheral sensorimotor neuropathy
Hemiplegia
Cranial nerve palsies

Gastrointestinal system

Peritonitis
Gastrointestinal haemorrhage
Vasculitic ischaemia

Haematological system

Anaemia
Leukopenia
Thrombocytopenia
Bleeding diathesis (circulating anticoagulants)

onset involves arthralgia, fever, weight loss, rash, anaemia and leukopaenia; involvement of other organs produces a wide clinical spectrum of disease (Box 9.3). The presence of hypertension and/or nephritis indicates a poor long-term prognosis.

Of particular note to the anaesthetist is involvement of the cardiovascular, respiratory and renal systems by SLE. Myocarditis occurs in approximately 15% of cases, pericarditis in up to 60% and valvular lesions (Libman–Sacks endocarditis) in almost 25%. Pleuritic pain is found in about 50% of cases of SLE, pleural effusions in 25%, and interstitial fibrosis, pulmonary vasculitis and interstitial pneumonitis in 20%. Renal disease is the most common cause of death in SLE. Of patients with renal disease, 50% have hypertension.

Up to 30% of patients with SLE have a circulating anticoagulant (lupus anticoagulant), which may prolong the activated partial thromboplastin time (APTT), but also risks the formation of arterial and venous thromboses and predisposes to recurrent abortion. The presence of the anticardiolipin antibody is also associated with these problems.

Treatment of SLE is with a combination of non-steroidal anti-inflammatory drugs (NSAIDs), antimalarial agents, corticosteroids and immunosuppressant drugs (e.g. cyclophosphamide, azathioprine). Some centres use plasmapheresis for patients who are resistant to conventional therapy.

PREOPERATIVE ASSESSMENT

HISTORY AND EXAMINATION:
- Assess the extent and duration of the illness. Discover whether the patient has acute disease or is in remission, as this will affect perioperative risk and outcome.
- Assess systemic involvement:
  —cardiovascular – tachycardia, heart failure, cardiomegaly, pericardial effusion, valve lesions
  —respiratory – pleurisy, dyspnoea
  —renal – renal failure, hypertension
  —CNS – peripheral neuropathy, stroke
  —Raynaud's phenomenon.
- Check drug history:
  —NSAIDs
  —antimalarials
  —systemic corticosteroids
  —other immunosuppressant drugs
  —cardiac drugs
  —use of plasmapheresis.

INVESTIGATIONS
ECG:
- Myocarditis
- Dysrhythmias
- Pericarditis.

Echocardiography
Assess cardiac contractility, pericardial effusions.

Chest radiography:
- Pulmonary effusion
- Pulmonary fibrosis
- Pericardial effusion
- Cardiac failure.

Arterial blood gases
Look for hypoxaemia, usually with a normal or low $Pa\text{CO}_2$.

Urea and electrolytes
Baseline test of renal function – creatinine and potassium.

Full blood count:
- Anaemia is common
- Leukopaenia may result from immunosuppressant drug therapy or from SLE itself
- Thrombocytopaenia may occur occasionally.

Lung function tests:
- Clinical signs, symptoms and chest radiograph do not reflect degree of pulmonary involvement.
- Pulmonary fibrosis will cause a restrictive defect.
- Diffusing capacity may be reduced.

Coagulation studies:
- Look for anticardiolipin antibody and lupus anticoagulant. Their presence may be associated with a prolonged APTT, although prothrombin time (PT) may be normal.
- Clotting factor assays.

Urinalysis
SLE may cause the nephrotic syndrome.

Plasma cholinesterase levels:
- Reduced by plasmapheresis
- Action inhibited by cyclophosphamide.

PREOPERATIVE PREPARATION

- Preoperative optimisation of cardiovascular and respiratory systems; in particular:
  —control of hypertension

9

—treatment of angina (e.g. nitrates)
—treatment of dysrhythmias
—treatment of heart failure
—drainage of pericardial or pleural effusions
—treatment of intercurrent pneumonia.
• Patients with severe cardiovascular disease may require perioperative invasive haemodynamic monitoring (e.g. central venous and pulmonary artery pressures).
• Perioperative steroid cover will be needed for patients receiving corticosteriods.
• Take antithrombotic measures perioperatively in patients with anticardiolipin antibody:
—antiembolic stockings
—avoid dehydration
—subcutaneous heparin.
• Patients with the anticardiolipin antibody and a history of thrombotic events require permanent anticoagulation with either warfarin or aspirin. They should receive heparin as an infusion perioperatively.

PERIOPERATIVE MANAGEMENT

Blood transfusions can exacerbate SLE.

INDUCTION:
• Avoid drugs and techniques likely to cause tachycardia, hypertension, hypotension or reduced myocardial contractility (e.g. ketamine, thiopental).
• Use a 'cardiac' anaesthetic, for example opiate induction ± intravenous lidocaine (lignocaine), to limit the hypertensive response to laryngoscopy.
• Preoxygenate prior to induction.
• Administer high concentrations of oxygen when there is cardiorespiratory disease.

AIRWAY CONSIDERATIONS
There are rare reports of a narrowed airway due to cricoarytenoid arthritis in SLE.

MAINTENANCE:
• Avoid drugs and techniques likely to cause tachycardia, hypertension, hypotension or reduced myocardial contractility.
• When plasmapheresis has been recent, the action of ester drugs (e.g. suxamethonium) may be prolonged.
• The action of suxamethonium may be prolonged by cyclophosphamide.
• Administer high concentrations of oxygen when there is cardiorespiratory disease.
• Avoid hypotension and maintain fluid balance, especially in the patient with renal involvement.

• Drug metabolism is altered in renal disease; avoid drugs that are metabolised or excreted by the kidney.
• Hypoalbuminaemia in nephrotic syndrome will affect drug distribution.
• Avoid vasoconstrictors in Raynaud's disease.

REGIONAL TECHNIQUES:
• Be absolutely sure of the patient's coagulation status before embarking upon regional anaesthetic techniques.
• Document existing sensorimotor neuropathies prior to use of regional techniques.

MONITORING:
• CM5 ECG is useful to detect myocardial ischaemia and arrhythmias.
• Radial artery cannulation may be inadvisable in the presence of Raynaud's phenomenon.
• Transoesophageal echocardiography is helpful intraoperatively in severe cardiac disease.
• Neuromuscular junction monitoring is essential if cyclophosphamide or plasmapheresis is used.

POSTOPERATIVE MANAGEMENT

Common problems and complications are:
• Deterioration in cardiovascular function
• Deterioration in renal failure
• Risk of arterial or venous thrombosis. Continue systemic steroid supplements.

BIBLIOGRAPHY

Davies SR. Systemic lupus erythematosus and the obstetrical patient – implications for the anaesthetist. Canadian Journal of Anaesthesia 1991; 38:790–796

Malinow AM, Rickford WJK, Mokkiski BLK, Saller DN, McGuinn WJ. Lupus anticoagulant. Implications for the obstetric anaesthetist. Anaesthesia 1987; 42:1291–1293

Menon G, Allt-Graham J. Anaesthetic implications of the anticardiolipin antibody syndrome. British Journal of Anaesthesia 1993; 70:587–590

9

Urticaria and angio-oedema

B. J. Pollard and P. McQuillan

Urticaria is a well demarcated, usually pruritic, skin reaction characterised by erythematous, raised, palpable lesions, often with pale centres, that blanch on pressure. Urticarial lesions result from a transient increase in capillary permeability causing focal oedema of the superficial part of the dermis. *Angio-oedema* describes a condition in which there is circumscribed, non-pitting subepithelial oedema, sometimes with erythema. It may involve the eyelids, lips, tongue, larynx, pharynx, respiratory tract, gastrointestinal tract, renal system and, occasionally, the central nervous system. This may result in airway obstruction, pleural effusions, abdominal pain, vomiting, diarrhoea, hemiplegia and seizures.

Urticaria and angio-oedema often accompany each other; however, in patients with angio-oedema due to a deficiency of C_1 esterase inhibitor (see below), urticaria does not occur. Individual attacks of urticaria and angio-oedema usually last no longer than 48 h. If episodes of urticaria or angio-oedema occur for more than 2 months, the condition is termed 'chronic'.

PATHOPHYSIOLOGY

Many common forms of urticaria and angio-oedema (Box 9.4) result from the antigen-induced release of biologically active substances from mast cells, which are found in organs rich in connective tissue (e.g. skin, respiratory tract). Urticaria and angio-oedema may also be due to drugs that cause direct mast cell degranulation or that activate the arachidonic acid or complement pathways. In all of these cases, release or activation of mediators (e.g. histamine, heparin, tryptase, chymase, chemotactic factors, prostaglandins, leukotrienes, platelet-activating factor (PAF), adenosine, oxygen radicals) causes altered vascular permeability, smooth muscle contraction and chemotaxis of leukocytes. This results in a spectrum of signs and symptoms ranging from simple urticaria or angio-oedema to fulminant anaphylaxis.

BOX 9.4

Aetiology of urticaria and angio-oedema

- Idiopathic
- Foodstuffs and additives
- Drugs:
  - antibiotics
  - muscle relaxants (e.g. tubocurarine)
  - opiates (e.g. morphine)
  - heparin
  - protamine
  - antihypertensives (e.g. angiotensin-converting enzyme (ACE) inhibitors)
  - NSAIDs
  - psychotropic drugs.
- Insect bites and stings
- Physical:
  - dermatographism
  - cold or heat
  - vibration
  - exercise
  - delayed pressure urticaria
- Infections
- Collagen vascular disease
- Endocrine disease
- Vasculitis
- Malignancy
- Hereditary and acquired angio-oedema
- Miscellaneous

Some forms of angio-oedema result from a functional deficiency of the inhibitor of the first component of the complement cascade (C_1); this is known as C_1 esterase inhibitor (C_1EI). Hereditary angio-oedema (HAO) is an autosomal dominant disorder characterised by recurrent spontaneous episodes of oedema of the skin and the mucous membranes of the respiratory tract and gut. Minor trauma, concomitant illness or perioral surgery (e.g. dentistry or tonsillectomy) may precipitate an attack. Attacks may increase during pregnancy (when C_1EI levels are low) or during menstrual bleeding. The major serious complication of an acute attack of HAO is upper airway

9

BOX 9.5

C_1 esterase inhibitor (C_1EI) deficiency

Hereditary C_1EI deficiency

- Type 1 (85%)
  - —impaired synthesis
  - —mostly autosomal dominant
- Type 2 (15%)
  - —dysfunctional protein
  - —heterogeneous genetic groups, mostly autosomal dominant

Acquired C_1EI deficiency

- Associated with:
  - —B-cell lymphoproliferative disorders
  - —connective tissue diseases
  - —monoclonal gammopathies
  - —antibodies to C_1EI

obstruction, although oedema of the bowel wall may be mistaken for an acute abdomen and result in unnecessary – and risky – surgery. Low levels of C_1EI also occur as an acquired disorder (Box 9.5). Acquired C_1EI deficiency can be distinguished from HAO by the absence of complement abnormalities in other family members, late age of onset, and the reduced level of C_1 seen in the acquired form.

LONG-TERM TREATMENT

CHRONIC URTICARIA AND ANGIO-OEDEMA:

- Identify and avoid precipitating factors.
- Avoid drugs that may aggravate disease (e.g. salicylates, NSAIDs, opiates).
- Treat with H_1-receptor antagonists (e.g. chlorpheniramine).
- Add a β-adrenergic agonist (e.g. terbutaline).
- Add an H_2-receptor antagonist (e.g. ranitidine).
- Consider use of a tricyclic antidepressant such as doxepin, which acts against both H_1 and H_2 receptors.
- Corticosteroids are used only in very severe disease.
- Adrenaline (epinephrine) is used for severe attacks of anaphylaxis.

C_1EI DEFICIENCY (HEREDITARY AND ACQUIRED):

- Androgens (e.g. stanozolol) – stimulate hepatic synthesis of C_1EI
- Antifibrinolytic agents (e.g. tranexamic acid, ε-aminocaproic acid) – these inhibit plasmin

activation.(plasmin is a potent catalyst for complement activation)
- Purified C_1EI concentrate.

PREOPERATIVE ASSESSMENT

HISTORY AND EXAMINATION

Take a careful history. Specifically ask about:
- Atopy
- Hypersensitivity
- Drug reactions
- Family history
- Previous episodes of urticaria or angio-oedema, including frequency, duration and effect
- Drug therapy (see above).

INVESTIGATIONS:

- C_1EI function in HAO
- Radioallergosorbent (RAST) tests.

PREOPERATIVE PREPARATION:

- Skin testing may be useful, but results are often unreliable and there is a small risk of severe anaphylaxis during the test.
- Avoid precipitating drugs or factors in patients with chronic urticaria or angio-oedema.

PREMEDICATION:

- Avoid precipitating drugs or factors in chronic urticaria or angio-oedema.
- In all patients with urticaria or angio-oedema, suitable premedication should be used to allay anxiety.

In those with chronic urticaria or angio-oedema, the following agents may be useful as a part of the premedication:
- H_1 antagonist (antihistamine)
- H_2 antagonist
- β-Adrenergic agonist
- Corticosteroid.

In HAO, attempts should be made to increase C_1EI levels before operation with:
- Androgens
- Antifibrinolytics
- Two units of fresh frozen plasma (FFP)
- Purified C_1EI concentrate.

If the patient is not receiving long-term therapy with androgens or antifibrinolytics, these should be administered for several days prior to surgery. Although they start to act within 24 h, 1–2 weeks is required to reach maximum effect. Alternatively, the administration of 2 units FFP given in the immediate pre-operative period will restore the C_1EI to a safe level (40% of normal) for between 1 and 4 days.

These measures also seem appropriate for the acquired form of C_1EI deficiency, although there is little documentation of their use.

PERIOPERATIVE MANAGEMENT

INDUCTION AND MAINTENANCE:
- Venepuncture has precipitated forearm angio-oedema in a patient with HAO.
- Use the most 'immunologically benign' agents, particularly in atopic patients. Avoid histamine-releasing drugs, where possible.
- Avoid airway manipulation and intubation, where possible.

In patients with cold urticaria:
- Warm intravenous fluids.
- Warm the laryngoscope blade.
- Use a warming blanket and warm air-circulating cover.
- Humidify respiratory gases.

MONITORING
Monitor core temperature, especially in cold and cholinergic (heat) urticaria.

POSITIONING
In pressure urticaria use extra protection for bony prominences, tourniquets, etc.

REGIONAL TECHNIQUES
These may allow the avoidance of tracheal intubation.

CARDIOPULMONARY BYPASS
Cardiopulmonary bypass (CPB) has been undertaken successfully in patients with certain forms of urticaria and angio-oedema.

Management of acute attacks

- Always have facilities available to treat anaphylaxis or airway obstruction (e.g. intubation equipment and tracheostomy facilities).
- Treat acute attacks of chronic urticaria or angio-oedema with adrenaline (epinephrine), steroids and antihistamines.
- Treat attacks of angio-oedema due to C1EI deficiency with FFP or purified C1EI concentrate (1000–1500 plasma units).
- There is unlikely to be any response during an acute attack of HAO to adrenaline (epinephrine), steroids or antihistamines.
- Monitor coagulation status in patients with HAO.
- Remember that C1EI levels will fall due to haemodilution in patients with C1EI deficiency undergoing CPB.
- CPB in a patient with cold urticaria has led to a rise in arterial histamine levels during rewarming.

BIBLIOGRAPHY

Johnston WE, Moss J, Philbin DM et al. Management of cold urticaria during cardiopulmonary bypass. New England Journal of Medicine 1982; 306:220–221

Kharasch ED. Angiotensin-converting enzyme inhibitor-induced angioedema associated with endotracheal intubation. Anesthesia and Analgesia 1992; 74:602–604

Razis PA, Coulson IH, Gould TR et al. Aquired C_1 esterase inhibitor deficiency. Anaesthesia 1986; 41:838–840

Wall RT, Frank M, Hahn M. A review of 25 patients with hereditary angioedema requiring surgery. Anesthesiology 1989; 71:309–311

CROSS-REFERENCES

Allergic reactions
    Anaesthetic Factors 31: 721
Intraoperative bronchospasm
    Anaesthetic Factors 31: 750
Intraoperative hypotension
    Anaesthetic Factors 31: 758

9

Glycogen storage disease

I. T. Campbell

Glycogen is a polysaccharide made up of glucose units and found in virtually every tissue in the body.

Principal storage sites of glycogen are the liver and muscle:

- Liver glycogen is concerned with maintenance of blood glucose concentrations.
- Muscle glycogen comprises the energy store for muscle itself; it does not contribute to blood glucose homeostasis.

GLYCOGEN STRUCTURE

Chains of 6–12 glucose units are joined at carbon atoms 1 and 4. The chains are joined by 1 : 6 linkages to form branching structures.

GLYCOGEN METABOLISM

- Under the control of a variety of enzymes (glucagon, adrenaline and sympathetic (noradrenaline) activation) that synthesise and break glycogen down to its constituent glucose units (liver glycogen) or to pyruvate and lactate in muscle.
- Muscle glycogen is used by muscle in aerobic exercise when the oxygen supply (cardiac output) is sufficient to meet metabolic demand.
- In high-intensity exercise, or with sudden bursts of activity, energy demand outstrips oxygen supply; lactate accumulates, diffuses into the general circulation and a metabolic acidosis develops.
- Muscle and blood lactate levels also rise in 'shock' – adrenaline stimulates glycolysis without a corresponding increase in oxygen supply.
- When lactate diffuses into general circulation, it is resynthesised to glucose by the liver and kidney.

Numerous enzymes are required in the synthesis and breakdown of glycogen. In 1952 the defi-ciency of glucose-6-phosphatase was described in Von Gierke's disease; the enzyme hydrolyses glucose 6-phosphate to glucose and phosphate immediately prior to release of glucose into the general circulation. Since then, 13 types of glycogen storage disease have been described.

TYPE I GLYCOGENOSIS: VON GIERKE'S DISEASE

Diagnosis is by liver or muscle biopsy and enzyme studies:

- Deficiency of glucose-6-phosphatase in the liver, kidney and intestine, with an inability to immobilise liver glycogen to maintain blood glucose concentration
- Autosomal recessive disorder
- Short stature; prominent rounded abdomen due to liver enlargement; kidneys also enlarge; fat deposits in cheeks and buttocks
- Hypoglycaemic, hyperlipidaemic and a tendency to acidosis (ketoacidosis and lactic acidosis)
- Prolonged bleeding time due to platelet glucose-6-phosphatase deficiency.

TREATMENT:

- Frequent or nasogastric feeding to maintain blood glucose
- A portacaval shunt enables absorbed glucose to bypass the liver
- Diazoxide, which inhibits insulin release and raises blood glucose.

TYPE II GLYCOGENOSIS: POMPE'S DISEASE

- Deficiency of 1 : 4-α-glucocidase (acid maltase)
- Deficiency of lysosomal enzyme – normally breaks 1 : 4 linkage in glucose chains
- Glycogen present in excessive quantities in:
  —liver
  —heart

—muscle
—tongue
—central nervous system
—anterior horn cells.

Blood sugar, lipid and ketone concentrations and response to glucagon and adrenaline are normal, but the prognosis is poor because of muscle weakness and heart failure.

TYPE III GLYCOGENOSIS: CORI'S DISEASE

• Deficiency of amylo 1,6-glucosidase (debranching enzyme)
• Features similar to type I but milder; able to mobilise glucose from outer chains of glycogen molecule
• Liver enlarged, growth retardation, hypoglycaemia, raised blood lipid concentrations and increased hepatic glycogen; cirrhosis later in life.
• Treatment consists of frequent feeds with a high protein diet (gluconeogenic pathway intact); hypoglycaemia can cause intellectual impairment.

TYPE IV GLYCOGENOSIS: ANDERSEN'S DISEASE

• Deficiency of 1,4-glucose-6-glucosyl transferase (brancher) enzyme
• Normal at birth, but fails to thrive
• Enlarged liver and spleen, muscles hypotonic
• Problems are those of liver disease; death in the second year of life.

TYPE V GLYCOGENOSIS: McARDLE'S SYNDROME

• Lack of muscle phosphorylase, which normally removes glucose units from glycogen as glucose 1-phosphate for metabolism to pyruvate and lactate; therefore unable to maintain glucose supply
• Symptoms usually develop in second decade of life
• Muscle glycogen concentration moderately increased; severe pain and muscle cramps at start of exercise due to lack of glucose

availability, but passes off (second wind) if exercise persists because of increased cardiac output, vasodilatation and availability of circulating glucose and fatty acids; advised to start exercise gradually.

TYPE VI GLYCOGENOSIS: HERS' DISEASE

• Reduced hepatic phosphorylase
• Clinically mild form of type I – enlarged liver and mild hypoglycaemia.

TYPES VII–XII GLYCOGENOSES

Extremely rare.

ANAESTHESIA IN GLYCOGEN STORAGE DISEASE

Experience is limited. With hepatic glycogenosis (types I and III) problems are hypoglycaemia and acidosis. Both lactic acidosis in type I and ketoacidosis in type IX have been described along with hyperthermia. It is thus important to provide enteral or parenteral nutrition before and after operation, and to monitor acid–base status and blood glucose levels, particularly during surgery.

With type II disease, problems are of myocardial involvement with congestive or obstructive cardiomyopathy and skeletal muscle weakness. A large tongue may cause airway problems. Successful surgery has been done with ketamine and vecuronium, with obsessional attention to detailed monitoring, particularly oxygenation. Also, an enlarged heart has caused bronchial obstruction.

Anaesthetic experience with type V disease is also limited. On theoretical grounds suxamethonium should be avoided because of the potential myoglobin release and renal damage. Atracurium and alcuronium have been used uneventfully, as has extradural spinal anaesthesia with bupivacaine. Any increased metabolic demand on, or diminution in, the blood supply to skeletal muscle is a potential problem (e.g. hypotension, hypothermia and shivering). Also, the use of a tourniquet should be avoided.

9

BIBLIOGRAPHY

Casson H. Anaesthesia for portocaval bypass in patients with metabolic disease. British Journal of Anaesthesia 1975; 47:969–975

Coleman P. McArdle's disease. Problem of anaesthetic management of caesarian section. Anaesthesia 1984; 39:784–787

Cox JM. Anesthesia and glycogen storage disease. Anesthesiology 1968; 29:1221–1225

Edelstein G, Hershman CA. Hyperthermia and ketoacidosis during anaesthesia in a child with glycogen storage disease. Anesthesiology 1980; 52:90–92

McFarlane HJ, Soni N. Pompe's disease and anaesthesia. Anaesthesia 1986; 41:1219–1224

Mohart D, Russo P, Tobias JD. Perioperative management of a child with glycogen storage disease type III undergoing cardiopulmonary bypass and repair of an atrial septal defect. Paediatric Anaesthesia 2002; 12:649–654

Samuels TA, Coleman P. McArdle's disease and caesarian section. Anaesthesia 1988; 43:161–162

Shenkman Z, Golub Y, Meretyk S, Shir Y, Landau D, Landau EH. Anaesthetic management of a patient with glycogen storage disease type 1b. Canadian Journal of Anaesthesia 1996; 43:467–470

Rajah A, Bell CF. Atracurium and McArdle's disease. Anaesthesia 1986; 41:93

9

PART 2

SURGICAL PROCEDURES

10

NEUROSURGERY
M. Smith

General principles of neuroanaesthesia

H. Gray and M. Smith

Neuroanaesthesia broadly concerns:
- Intracranial procedures
- Neurovascular procedures
- Spinal surgery
- Peripheral nerve surgery
- Interventional and diagnostic neuroradiology.

Neuroanaesthesia has become a subspecialty of anaesthesia following a greater awareness of the anaesthetic factors that contribute to successful neurosurgical techniques. This has been achieved because of a greater understanding of intracranial pathophysiology and an improved awareness of how systemic physiology and anaesthetic techniques may be manipulated to optimise cerebral physiology.

EFFECTS OF ANAESTHETIC AGENTS ON CEREBRAL PHYSIOLOGY

No single anaesthetic technique is suitable for all procedures and, in general terms, no technique is superior to another. The choice of anaesthetic agents and adjuvant drugs is based on consideration of their effects on cerebral blood flow (CBF) and cerebral blood volume (CBV), cerebral metabolic rate (CMR_{O_2}), intracranial pressure (ICP), cerebral autoregulation and carbon dioxide reactivity.

INTRAVENOUS AGENTS

Intravenous agents such as thiopental and propofol produce cerebral vasoconstriction and a reduction in CBF secondary to a decrease in CMR_{O_2}. Their effectiveness in reducing CBF, and hence CBV and ICP, is dependent upon the presence of cerebral metabolic activity. With the onset of an isoelectric EEG there is no further potential for intravenous anaesthetic agents to reduce CBF and ICP. Thiopental and propofol are powerful cardiovascular depressants and it is important to maintain systemic blood pressure to avoid reduction in cerebral perfusion pressure (CPP). All intravenous agents preserve autoregulation in normal sub-

jects but their influence in those with impaired autoregulation is unknown. They also have minimal effects on the carbon dioxide response of cerebral vessels.

VOLATILE AGENTS

Differences exist in volatile agents in their suitability for use in brain-injured patients and during elective neurosurgery. All volatile agents, to varying degrees, cause cerebral vasodilatation and a dose-dependent rise in CBF. Flow–metabolism coupling persists during volatile anaesthesia, but the balance may be shifted to allow a higher flow for a given metabolic rate. Volatile agents also produce a fall in CMR_{O_2} and their overall cerebrovascular effect reflects a balance between the direct vasodilatory and indirect flow–metabolism-mediated vasoconstrictive effects. Halothane is the most potent cerebrovasodilator and should be avoided. Isoflurane is the most marked metabolic depressant and therefore the least cerebrovasodilating of the volatile agents. Desflurane and sevoflurane have similar cerebrovascular effects to isoflurane. Cerebral autoregulation is impaired in a dose-dependent manner by volatile agents, being preserved at 0.5 minimum alveolar concentration (MAC) but abolished at 1.5 MAC. Some volatile agents increase CSF volume by increasing formation or decreasing absorption, but this becomes important only in prolonged extracranial procedures. Enflurane should not be used during neuroanaesthesia because it is epileptogenic in at-risk patients.

NITROUS OXIDE

Nitrous oxide is a potent cerebrovasodilator and produces a rise in ICP. It has minimal effects on autoregulation and carbon dioxide reactivity. Most neuroanaesthetists now employ an anaesthetic technique that avoids the use of nitrous oxide.

OPIOIDS

Morphine has negligible effects on cerebral haemodynamics and metabolism but may cause

10

hypotension secondary to histamine release and hypoventilation in the postoperative period if given in inappropriate doses. Synthetic narcotics have been reported to have variable cerebrovascular and metabolic effects but are unlikely to have direct effects on ICP, with the exception of alfentanil, which may increase ICP under certain circumstances. However, all opioids have the potential to cause systemic hypotension, although fentanyl is least likely to produce significant reductions in blood pressure. Remifentanil is gaining popularity in neuroanaesthesia because its favourable pharmacological profile confers many advantages over more established agents. An infusion of remifentanil allows rapid titration of analgesic level for highly stimulating periods (e.g. insertion of skull pins) but, because its context-sensitive half-life remains consistent at 3–5 min, rapid wake-up is not affected. A frequently used regimen involves infusing remifentanil at 0.05–0.25 μg kg^{-1} min^{-1}.

MUSCLE RELAXANTS

Suxamethonium causes a transient rise in ICP but this effect is not long-lasting and is irrelevant under most circumstances. Non-depolarising muscle relaxants have no effect on CBF and CMR_{O_2}.

For intracranial surgery, a balanced anaesthetic technique using sevoflurane in an air : oxygen mix is a popular choice and allows rapid wake-up and early neurological assessment. Total intravenous anaesthesia (TIVA) with propofol is an acceptable alternative, but there is no evidence to suggest that this is superior to a volatile agent-based technique under most circumstances. Intraoperative analgesia may be provided with incremental bolus doses of fentanyl or, increasingly, with a remifentanil infusion. The use of continuous neuromuscular blockade is determined by the surgical procedure and individual preference of the anaesthetist.

AIRWAY MANAGEMENT

Tracheal intubation and mechanical ventilation is recommended for intracranial neurosurgical procedures to allow control of $PaCO_2$ and maintenance of adequate oxygenation. Traditionally, reinforced tracheal tubes have been used, although preformed tracheal tubes are suitable for most procedures in the supine position. The reinforced laryngeal mask or ProSeal® laryngeal mask may be a suitable alternative in short extracranial operations and during radiological procedures.

Ventilation should be adjusted to maintain $PaO_2 > 13.5$ kPa and $PaCO_2$ between 4 and 4.5 kPa during intracranial surgery.

The head may be secured using a Mayfield three-point pin fixator rendering the airway relatively inaccessible during surgery. Care should therefore be taken during fixation of the tracheal tube and during patient positioning and draping to prevent kinks in the ventilator circuits.

Neck flexion may be required, but this should not be so excessive that it prevents proper venous drainage from the head. It should always be possible to insert at least two fingers between the chin and suprasternal notch.

Haemodynamic surges and coughing during intubation or patient positioning should be prevented by judicious use of opioids (e.g. remifentanil infusion) and muscle relaxation (monitored with a nerve stimulator).

Most patients undergoing elective surgery should be extubated at the end of the operation, even after fairly lengthy procedures. Some anaesthetists favour 'deep extubation', whereas others extubate all patients awake. Intuitively it makes sense to avoid coughing and bucking during extubation, but there is no evidence that one technique is less likely to cause this than another. The cardiovascular and intracranial effects of extubation can be blunted with 1–2 mg intravenous lidocaine (lignocaine) or a beta-blocker.

FLUID MANAGEMENT

The previous practice of restricting fluids in neurosurgical patients is inappropriate because fluid restriction leads to hypovolaemia, hypotension, raised haematocrit and hypernatraemia, which are all bad for the 'at risk' brain.

Circulating volume should be normalised during neuroanaesthesia and appropriate monitoring employed to facilitate this. The choice of fluid is probably less important than the volume given, and crystalloid or colloid can both be used for fluid replacement. Fluid flux across the blood–brain barrier is determined by osmolality rather than oncotic pressure, and therefore hypotonic fluids should be avoided. Compound sodium lactate is effectively hypo-osmolar (calculated osmolality = 273 mOsm l^{-1} – effective osmolality = 250–260 mOsm l^{-1}) because of the tendency for molecular aggregation of sodium ions. For this reason, 0.9% saline has become

10

the crystalloid of choice during neuroanaesthesia, although large volumes may cause acidosis.

Unless hypoglycaemia is suspected, glucose-containing solutions should be avoided for two reasons. First, after glucose metabolism, the residual free water can worsen cerebral oedema; and second, hyperglycaemia is correlated with poor outcome after brain injury. Hyperglycaemia produces an increased glucose concentration in the ischaemic brain, resulting in worsening of lactic acidosis, hyperkalaemia, free radical formation and intracellular oedema. Hypoglycaemia should, of course, be avoided to ensure continued glucose supply to aerobically metabolising brain. Aim for a blood sugar of 4–7 mmol l^{-1} in the perioperative period.

Blood loss should be replaced with colloid and blood products to maintain a haemoglobin level >8 g dl^{-1}.

MONITORING:

- Routine monitoring should include ECG, SpO_2, capnography and arterial cannulation for direct blood pressure measurement, as well as intermittent blood gas sampling. A large-bore cannula and a temperature probe are also mandatory.
- Central venous pressure monitoring will assist in fluid management if severe blood loss is anticipated or the patient is dehydrated preoperatively. In the UK, the antecubital fossa remains a most popular route, although femoral and internal jugular veins allow more suitable placement of multilumen catheters.
- A urinary catheter should be inserted for long operations and when mannitol is likely to be used during operation.
- ICP monitoring, Doppler ultrasonography, cerebral oxygenation monitoring and electrophysiological monitoring – somatosensory evoked potentials (SSEPs), motor evoked potentials (MEPs), seventh nerve – may be indicated for specific cases.

TEMPERATURE MANAGEMENT

There has been renewed interest in the use of moderate hypothermia for cerebral protection after traumatic or ischaemic brain injury. Although moderate hypothermia (temperature approximately 35°C) reduces ICP and excitatory amino acid release (glutamate), there are no data to recommend its routine use during neuroanaesthesia. However, many neuroanaesthetists do allow mild passive hypothermia during procedures where the brain is most at

risk of ischaemia. These include neurovascular procedures and operations where prolonged brain retraction is required. Under these circumstances, forced-air rewarming is used to restore normal temperature before the end of the procedure. If this cannot be achieved, the patient should remain sedated and ventilated until normothermia is restored. The results of prospective randomised studies investigating the role of hypothermia during neuroanaesthesia are awaited.

POSITIONING

- *Supine* – reverse Trendelenburg with 15–30° head-up tilt, modest neck flexion and back elevation to help promote venous drainage is suitable for most patients.
- *Prone* – care with eyes, face, axillae, breasts. Avoid excessive venous pressure.
- *Lateral or park bench* – ensure head and body are well supported. Avoid jugular compression and pressure on nerves, particularly brachial plexus (use axillary pad).
- *Sitting* (now rarely used) – beware hypotension and venous air embolism.

THROMBOEMBOLIC PROPHYLAXIS

Neurosurgical patients fall into the high-risk category for the development of thromboembolic disease because of release of thrombogenic factors from brain tissue and prolonged intraoperative and postoperative immobilisation. The risk is greatest after supratentorial craniotomy. Although there is no evidence that preoperative low molecular weight heparin increases the risk of perioperative bleeding, many neurosurgical teams are uncomfortable with its use. Physical methods provide a useful alternative and thromboembolism deterrent (TED) stockings in association with perioperative intermittent calf compression (continue until mobilising) should be applied in all cases. When additional risk factors are present, low molecular weight heparin should be started within the first 24 h after surgery.

POSTOPERATIVE ANALGESIA

Neurosurgical procedures can be painful, and postoperative pain is often poorly controlled. The selection of postoperative analgesics has become critical with the increased intraoperative use of the ultra-short-acting opioid remifentanil. A long-acting analgesic such as morphine should always be administered before the intraoperative opioid is discontinued.

OPIOIDS

Codeine phosphate has traditionally been used after neurosurgery because it has been claimed that it causes less respiratory depression than other opioids. However, this may merely reflect inadequate dosage. Use of morphine, including by patient-controlled analgesia (PCA), is safe and effective after craniotomy. All patients receiving potent opioids should be monitored in the postoperative period to ensure that respiratory depression does not occur. Increased $Pa\text{CO}_2$ may cause brain swelling and deterioration in neurological status. However, there is no evidence to suggest that this is more likely with one opioid than another, or that this is a problem when appropriate doses are used.

TRAMADOL

Tramadol is a novel analgesic with primary effects via serotonergic and noradrenergic pathways and some opiate-like effects (1/1000th the potency of morphine at the mu receptor). It is a suitable alternative to morphine, but must be given with an antiemetic agent.

NON-STEROIDAL ANTI-INFLAMMATORY DRUGS

NSAIDs are frequently used after spinal surgery and by many neuroanaesthetists after intracranial operations. The concern about increased bleeding tendency due to their antiplatelet action is probably unjustified, but some neuroanaesthetists prefer to wait 24 h before starting conventional NSAIDs. Specific cyclo-oxygenase (COX) 2 inhibitors may have a useful role in neuroanaesthesia.

PARACETAMOL

Simple agents have a synergistic effect with other analgesics, and paracetamol should be given routinely after intracranial surgery unless there are contraindications to its use. It is unlikely to be adequate as a sole agent but is very effective when given in combination with NSAIDs.

LOCAL ANAESTHESIA

The beneficial effects of surgical infiltration along wound edges are often underestimated. A skull block (greater and lesser occipital nerves, supraorbital, supratrochlear, auriculotemporal and greater auricular nerves) will abolish sympathetic response to head-pin insertion at the beginning of the operation and contribute to postoperative analgesia.

OTHER POSTOPERATIVE CONSIDERATIONS

Electrolyte abnormalities are common in neurosurgical patients, and urine output and plasma electrolytes should be monitored closely and treatment initiated as appropriate.

Seizures should be treated aggressively in the postoperative period to minimise the risk of secondary ischaemic brain damage. Some patients, for instance those with pre-existing epilepsy or lesions in epileptogenic areas, are at particular risk for the development of seizures. Some recommend prophylactic anticonvulsant therapy for these 'at risk' patients, whereas others treat only after the first fit. Phenytoin is the first-line agent of choice.

10

BIBLIOGRAPHY

Constantini S, Kanner A, Freidman A et al. Safety of perioperative minidose heparin in patients undergoing brain tumour surgery: a prospective, randomised double blind study. Journal of Neurosurgery 2001; 94:918–921

Duffy CM, Matta BF. Sevoflurane and anaesthesia for neurosurgery: a review. Journal of Neurosurgical Anesthesiology 2000; 12:128–140

Goldsack C, Scuplak SM, Smith M. A double blind comparison of codeine and morphine for postoperative analgesia following intracranial surgery. Anaesthesia 1996; 51:1029–1032

Mils SJ, Tomlinson AA. The use of central venous catheters in neuroanaesthesia. Anaesthesia 2001; 56:465–470

Ravussin P, de Tribolet N, Wilder-Smith OHG. Total intravenous anaesthesia is best for neurological surgery. Journal of Neurosurgical Anesthesiology 1994; 6:285–289

Smith M. Post-operative neurosurgical care. Current Anaesthesia and Critical Care 1994; 5:29–35

Spiekermann BF, Stone DJ, Bogdonoff DL, Yemen TA. Airway management in neuroanaesthesia. Canadian Journal of Anaesthesia 1996; 43:820–834

Todd MM, Warner DS, Sokoll MD. A prospective, comparative trial of three anesthetics for elective supratentorial craniotomy. Propofol/fentanyl, isoflurane/nitrous oxide, and fentanyl/nitrous oxide. Anesthesiology 1993; 78:1005–1020

Van Aken H. Anaesthetic agents: total intravenous and inhalational anaesthesia. In: Van Aken H, ed. Neuro-anaesthetic practice. London: BMJ Publishing Group; 1995:91–132

Verchere E, Grenier B, Mesli A et al. Postoperative pain management after supratentorial craniotomy. Journal of Neurosurgical Anesthesiology 2002; 14:96–101

Warner DS. Neuroanesthesia 2000. Anesthesia and Analgesia 2000; 90:1238–1240

Zornow MH, Scheller MS. Intraoperative fluid balance during craniotomy. In: Cottrell JE, Smith DS, eds. Anesthesia and neurosurgery. St Louis: Mosby; 2001:237–249

10

Anaesthesia for supratentorial surgery and shunts

G. Thomas and S. R. Wilson

Anaesthesia for supratentorial surgery requires an understanding of the regulation and maintenance of cerebral blood flow, the pathophysiology of intracranial hypertension, the effects of anaesthetic drugs on cerebral perfusion, metabolism and intracranial pressure (ICP) and the importance of the avoidance of secondary systemic physiological insults.

ANATOMY AND PATHOLOGY

The supratentorial region of the brain consists predominantly of the cerebral hemispheres and their meninges. Most brain tumours in adults are supratentorial, as shown in Box 10.1. In children, only one-third of brain tumours are supratentorial and these are predominantly glioma and craniopharyngioma.

BOX 10.1

Aetiology of supratentorial brain tumours in adults

- Glioma
- Meningioma
- Metastasis
- Craniopharyngioma
- Lymphoma

BOX 10.2

Indications for supratentorial surgery

- Burr-hole biopsy for histological diagnosis of lesion
- Craniotomy for tumour excision or debulking
- Aspiration of cerebral abscess for antibiotic sensitivities

PREOPERATIVE ASSESSMENT AND INVESTIGATIONS

The indications for supratentorial surgery are shown in Box 10.2. Patients are usually otherwise well.
- All age groups may be involved.
- If cerebral metastasis is suspected, the primary tumour might be found in lung, breast, thyroid or bowel.
- Primary sites for cerebral abscesses may be middle ear, paranasal sinuses or lung.
- Raised ICP due to the peritumour oedema is treated before surgery with dexamethasone (4 mg q.d.s.).
- Prophylactic or therapeutic anticonvulsants may be required for lesions in epileptogenic areas such as the temporoparietal or subfrontal areas. A bolus of phenytoin (15 mg kg^{-1}) followed by 300 mg daily may be given.
- Investigations:
  —Plasma glucose concentration may be raised because of preoperative steroid use.
  —Electrolyte imbalance, particularly abnormalities of plasma sodium, may result from complications of the tumour or the use of mannitol.
  —Check computed tomography (CT) or magnetic resonance imaging (MRI) scan for tumour size, site and oedema.
  —Check blood transfusion availability.
- Premedication – Patients are often extremely anxious and careful explanation is essential. Short-acting benzodiazepines may be helpful for extreme anxiety, but should be avoided in the presence of raised ICP.

INTRAOPERATIVE CONCERNS AND MANAGEMENT

INDUCTION:
- Smooth induction using propofol and an opioid with no coughing, straining or large changes in blood pressure.

10

- Non-depolarising muscle relaxant (atracurium or vecuronium).
- Orotracheal intubation with armoured cuffed tracheal tube fixed securely.
- Monitoring for all cases must include ECG, Sp_{O_2}, Et_{CO_2}, direct arterial blood pressure (consider patient position before siting arterial line) and core temperature.
- Central venous catheter should be considered if there is a risk of large blood loss (meningioma or metastatic tumour), and a urinary catheter should be sited for long procedures or where there is the possibility of intraoperative use of mannitol.
- Cover and protect eyes using tape and eye pads. Do not use eye shields, which may themselves cause damage.
- Insert large-bore intravenous cannula.
- Administer prophylactic antibiotics according to local protocols. Cefuroxime 1.5 g on induction and every 3 h thereafter during the procedure is a commonly used regimen in neurosurgery. There is no evidence to recommend the continuation of antibiotics into the postoperative period.

POSITIONING THE PATIENT:

- Patient position is dictated by the surgical approach:
  —Most procedures are carried out with the patient in the supine position, often with a small degree of head rotation and a sandbag under the shoulders.
  —Lateral (park bench) for some temporoparietal approaches.
- For all patients:
  —Head-up tilt (15–25°).
  —Maintain adequate cerebral venous drainage by avoiding extreme flexion and rotation of the neck.
  —Secure head with a horseshoe headrest or three-point pin fixator. A bolus dose of fentanyl or remifentanil may be needed to prevent hypertension during application of the head pins.
  —Perioperative thromboembolic prophylaxis using TED stockings and intermittent calf compression.
  —Check for kinks in the tracheal tube and ensure that monitors and vascular cannulae are unimpeded prior to draping of the patient.

MAINTENANCE OF ANAESTHESIA:

- Adjust ventilation to maintain Pa_{CO_2} at 4.0–4.5 kPa.
- Fi_{O_2} of 0.3–0.5 in air. Nitrous oxide may have adverse effects on CBF and ICP under certain circumstances and increases the risk of postoperative pneumocephalus. It has little place in the modern practice of neuroanaesthesia.
- Sevoflurane and/or propofol infusion supplemented with remifentanil infusion.
- Maintain normothermia using warming mattress, warm air blanket, fluid warmer and fresh gas humidification.
- Control of blood pressure – normotension is maintained for most procedures. During operation for large vascular tumours, moderate hypotension may improve the surgical field, but care should be taken because cerebral autoregulation may be impaired or abolished. Moderate hypotension is achieved by deepening anaesthesia or by the use of labetalol, short-acting beta-blockers or sodium nitroprusside.
- Fluid balance – a balanced salt solution is used for fluid maintenance and blood loss is replaced with colloid and blood to maintain a haematocrit of around 30%. Dextrose-containing fluids should be avoided.

INTRAOPERATIVE MANAGEMENT OF A TIGHT BRAIN

Bulging dura on removal of the craniotomy flap indicates a 'tight' brain. Intracranial hypertension is often secondary to peritumour oedema, and various manoeuvres may be used to improve operating conditions (Box 10.3). Swelling may also occur because of bleeding into the tumour, causing resistant hypertension and tachycardia followed by bradycardia. To preserve cerebral perfusion pressure, normotension should be maintained prior to dural opening.

BOX 10.3

Anaesthetic measures to reduce intraoperative brain swelling

- Check patient position and maintain reverse Trendelenburg position
- Avoid excessive head rotation
- Reduce or remove volatile agent – consider change to TIVA
- Ensure moderate hypocarbia (4.0–4.5 kPa)
- Control blood pressure
- Discontinue nitrous oxide if used
- Dexamethasone (8–12 mg) for tumours
- Mannitol (0.25–0.5 g kg^{-1})
- Furosemide (frusemide) (0.25–0.5 mg kg^{-1})

POSTOPERATIVE MANAGEMENT

- Return blood pressure to normal as haemostasis is achieved.
- Restore normocapnia and spontaneous breathing.
- Give analgesic (morphine) and antiemetic drugs.
- Local infiltration and scalp block may reduce the severity of postoperative pain.
- Treat hypertension on emergence with labetalol, hydralazine or a small bolus of propofol.
- Extubate at a deep plane of anaesthesia
- Return to critical care environment for postoperative monitoring.

Cerebral hyperaemia occurs during emergence from general anaesthesia irrespective of ventilation and haemodynamic changes. The reasons for this are unclear but might be due to a non-specific response to stress. Postoperative sedation and ventilation should therefore be considered only in the following circumstances:

- For a patient who was severely obtunded before operation
- Massive intraoperative haemorrhage
- Acute intraoperative brain swelling

ICP monitoring is necessary if the patient is to be sedated and ventilated after surgery.

Postoperative analgesia is achieved with an adequate dose of morphine sulfate given every 3 h or morphine via PCA. Patients will take oral fluids early in the postoperative period, and regular paracetamol and non-steroidal drugs (if appropriate) should be considered. Mechanical methods for preventing deep vein thrombosis should be continued after operation because many neurosurgeons are unhappy about using low molecular weight heparin in the early postoperative period.

Most postoperative complications occur within the first 6 h after surgery (Box 10.4).

BOX 10.4

Postoperative complications

- Bleeding at the operative site
- Subdural haematoma
- Pneumocephalus
- Remote cerebellar haemorrhage
- Limited mouth opening after frontotemporal craniotomy, which may last for up to 3 months

---

BOX 10.5

Causes of hydrocephalus

Obstructive (non-communicating) hydrocephalus

- Brain tumours (particularly midline)
- Subarachnoid haemorrhage
- Spina bifida
- Arnold–Chiari syndrome
- Head injury

Communicating hydrocephalus

- Subarachnoid haemorrhage
- Meningitis
- Head injury

SHUNT PROCEDURES

Shunts are inserted for the treatment of hydrocephalus caused by accumulation of CSF in the ventricular system. Hydrocephalus may be caused by obstruction of CSF outflow (non-communicating hydrocephalus) or by failure of absorption of CSF from the arachnoid granulations (communicating hydrocephalus) (see Box 10.5).

TYPES OF SHUNT PROCEDURE

The insertion of a shunt allows drainage of CSF to occur to a distal site. There is a variety of shunt placements:

- Ventriculoperitoneal (commonest)
- Ventriculoatrial
- Lumboperitoneal
- Ventriculopleural
- External ventricular drain (temporary).

The shunt system has several components: a catheter inserted into the subarachnoid space (usually through a burr hole), a one-way valve to control the drainage pressure, and a distal catheter that is tunnelled subcutaneously. Shunts can be positioned with conventional surgical techniques, using endoscopic procedures, or with image-guided techniques.

PREOPERATIVE ASSESSMENT AND INVESTIGATIONS

- Patients presenting for shunt surgery may have signs of raised ICP.
- All ages are represented but shunt procedures are more common in children

10

who may have associated problems, including congenital abnormalities. Children may also have abnormal head enlargement, making airway management difficult. Babies may be premature.

- Shunts often block acutely and become infected. Patients then present for emergency surgery with a full stomach and may be neurologically obtunded.
- Patients are often anxious because of previous surgery, but caution is needed with premedication because of the possibility of raised ICP.
- Dehydration and electrolyte disturbance is common because of associated vomiting.
- Attention to special needs of the premature infant is needed.

PERIOPERATIVE MANAGEMENT

ANAESTHETIC TECHNIQUE:
- Monitoring for all patients includes ECG, non-invasive blood pressure determination, SpO_2 and $EtCO_2$.
- Rapid sequence induction may be required.
- Induction and maintenance as for other supratentorial surgery.
- Antibiotics are given according to local protocols.
- Patients usually lie supine with the head turned to the opposite side with a sandbag under the shoulders. The lateral position is required for insertion of a lumboperitoneal shunt.
- Burr-hole and subcutaneous tunnelling are highly stimulating and bolus doses of opioids may be necessary.

COMPLICATIONS:
- Hypotension may occur following release of CSF and sudden reduction in ICP.
- Bradycardia or other arrhythmias may occur because of shift in intracranial contents.
- Watch for signs of pneumothorax or haemothorax when trocar is placed subcutaneously.
- Chance of air embolism is high in ventriculoatrial shunt; therefore use controlled positive-pressure ventilation to minimise air embolism.
- Rarely, blood loss from burr-hole may occur if dural veins are enlarged.

POSTOPERATIVE MANAGEMENT

- Wake patient with minimal coughing and straining.

- Analgesia provided by regular administration of paracetamol and non-steroidal drugs. Morphine may be needed for the first 24 h.
- Most pain is from the abdominal incision – infiltration of local anaesthetic at the end of surgery may help.
- Give intravenous fluids until normal oral intake is resumed.
- Any new focal neurological signs should prompt an urgent CT scan to rule out intracranial haematoma.

BIBLIOGRAPHY

Barker FG. Efficacy of prophylactic antibiotics in cerebrospinal shunt surgery: Meta-analysis. Neurosurgery 1998; 43:694

Bruden N, Pellissie D. Cerebral hyperaemia during recovery from general anaesthesia in neurosurgical patients. Anesthesia and Analgesia 2002; 94:650–654

Hamid RK, Newfield P. Paediatric neuroanaesthesia. Hydrocephalus. Anesthesiology Clinics of North America 2001; 19:207–218

Holloway KL, Smith KW, Wilberger JE et al. Antibiotic prophylaxis during clean neurosurgery: a large, multicenter study using cefuroxime. Clinical Therapeutics 1998; 18:84–94

Pickard JD, Czosnyka M. Management of raised intracranial pressure. Journal of Neurology, Neurosurgery and Psychiatry 1993; 56:845–858

Rolighed LJK, Haure P. Reverse Trendelenburg position reduces intracranial pressure during craniotomy. Journal of Neurosurgical Anesthesiology 2002; 4:16–21

Thromboembolic Risk Factors Consensus Group. Risk of and prophylaxis for venous thromboembolism in hospital patients. British Medical Journal 1992; 305:567–574

Warner DS. Remote cerebellar haemorrhage after supratentorial surgery. Journal of Neurosurgical Anesthesiology 2002; 14:167

10

Anaesthesia for posterior fossa surgery

H. Gray and M. Smith

Surgery for posterior fossa lesions is challenging for surgeons, anaesthetists and the whole perioperative team. A successful outcome for the patient requires a cooperative and coordinated approach from the entire team.

ANATOMY AND PHYSIOLOGY

The posterior fossa houses the cerebellum, pons, medulla and fourth ventricle. It is bounded by the tentorium above, the foramen magnum below, the occiput behind and the clivus in front. Even a small amount of swelling and oedema can create major neurological change because:

- The pons and medulla contain the major sensory and motor pathways, the vital vascular and respiratory centres, and the lower cranial nerve nuclei. Pressure on these structures may result in decreased levels of consciousness, rising blood pressure and falling pulse, respiratory depression and impairment of the reflexes that protect the airway.
- CSF flows from the third through the fourth ventricle and out on to the surface of the brain. Obstruction of this pathway will result in hydrocephalus.

Gross swelling will cause coning, either upwards through the tentorium, or more commonly downwards through the foramen magnum. Because the respiratory centre lies in the lower medulla, the latter will result in slow irregular respiration progressing to apnoea.

PREOPERATIVE CONSIDERATIONS

- The pathology should be noted (Box 10.6) and the scans examined to assess lesion size, degree of oedema and presence of hydrocephalus. Significant hydrocephalus will require insertion of an external ventricular drain (EVD) prior to the posterior fossa craniectomy.
- Clinical assessment of ICP – conscious state, headache and vomiting, together with response to steroids.
- Fluid and electrolyte status – may be dehydrated due to vomiting and have abnormal plasma levels of electrolytes and glucose, particularly if on steroids.
- Cardiovascular system – with reference to ability to tolerate prone or sitting positions. Hypertensive patients will be particularly prone to hypotension and cerebral ischaemia in the sitting position. Echocardiogram should be done before use of the sitting position to ensure that the patient does not have a cardiac septal defect that would predispose to paradoxical air embolism (see below).
- Respiratory status including gag reflex.

BOX 10.6

Pathology of posterior fossa lesions

Malignant tumours

- Primary – particularly astrocytomas in children
- Secondary – often metastasise to cerebellum

Benign tumours

- Acoustic neuromas in cerebellopontine angle
- Meningiomas less common than supratentorial

Vascular

- Uncommon – but angiomas, arteriovenous malformations and aneurysms can occur
- Nerve decompression for hemifacial spasm and trigeminal pain
- Haematomas – spontaneous and traumatic

10

CHOICE OF POSITION

Good positioning is important to allow visualisation of the lesion without excessive retraction of the cerebellum, whilst allowing blood and CSF to drain away from the surgical site.

PRONE

Good surgical access to midline structures, but excessive bleeding may obscure surgical field. Careful positioning with avoidance of increased venous pressure is essential.

LATERAL (PARK BENCH)

Used for laterally placed lesions, especially those in cerebellopontine angle. Avoid pressure damage to peripheral nerves, jugular compression due to excessive flexion or rotation of the neck, or damage to the eyes.

SITTING

Carries the highest risk and should be used only for highly selected cases and by experienced neurosurgeons and neuroanaesthetists (Box 10.7). The sitting position is achieved by using the standard operating table, removing the head portion, placing the back part vertically and arranging for the legs to be slightly flexed to ensure the buttocks remain firm against the vertical portion. The head is then held in a three-point pin fixator mounted on a frame across the table. Excessive head flexion should be avoided because this can cause jugular compression, swelling of the tongue and face, and cervical cord ischaemia. A minimum gap of two fingers should be maintained between the chin and suprasternal notch. Care should be taken to avoid pressure damage to peripheral nerves.

BOX 10.7

Advantages and disadvantages of the sitting position for posterior fossa surgery

Advantages (all surgical)

- Spatial orientation
- Easy access
- Good venous and CSF drainage

Disadvantages (all anaesthetic)

- Postural hypotension
- Air embolism

AIR EMBOLISM

CAUSES

Venous air embolism (VAE) is not restricted to sitting cases. It is a potential risk whenever the operative site is above the level of the heart. The greater the head-up tilt, the greater the negative hydrostatic pressure between open vein and heart, and the greater the rate at which air will tend to enter. In posterior fossa surgery the danger is increased because veins in the bone may be held open by surrounding structures. There are also large veins in the neck muscles and large venous sinuses within the skull.

INCIDENCE

This lies between 25% and 40%, depending on the sensitivity of monitoring, precautions taken, height of the head above the heart and surgical skill.

PATHOPHYSIOLOGY

Morbidity and mortality rates are directly related to the amount and rate of air entry. The fatal dose of air embolus is unknown but may be of the order of 100–300 ml. Air will be drawn down through the right atrium and ventricle into the pulmonary arterioles. Large volumes (3–5 ml kg^{-1}) will cause complete obstruction of the right ventricular outflow tract. Microvascular bubbles cause activation and release of endothelial mediators. The pulmonary vascular resistance increases, the pulmonary artery pressure rises, cardiac output falls and ECG abnormalities are seen. Gas exchange is impaired as physiological deadspace increases, causing V/Q mismatch and a fall in carbon dioxide excretion.

DETECTION

Precordial Doppler ultrasonography is the most sensitive method of monitoring for VAE, but problems include positioning the probe, diathermy interference and the need for continuous monitoring by a trained person. Capnography is generally regarded as the most useful monitoring procedure, with reasonable sensitivity although non-specific for VAE. A fall in EtCO$_2$ is an indication for immediate action. End-tidal nitrogen (EtN$_2$) is one of the most specific monitors for VAE but is not sensitive enough to detect small subclinical VAE. The use of pulmonary artery catheters and transoesophageal echocardiography, both of which are sensitive monitors for VAE, has also been described but is fraught with practical problems.

10

PREVENTION

Volume loading reduces the fall in central venous pressure (CVP) as the patient is tilted head-up. CVP must be monitored in all cases with the tip of the catheter correctly placed (see below). The use of positive end-expiratory respiration (PEEP) is controversial because it may impair surgical conditions and, by causing a rise in right atrial pressure, increase the risk of paradoxical air embolus if VAE occurs. Compression of the lower limbs and/or abdomen, by the use of bandages, a G-suit or medical antishock trousers (MAST), raises venous pressure. Nitrous oxide should not be used as it will cause expansion of any air bubble that enters the circulation.

MANAGEMENT

The aims are to stop further air entry, remove air already present and correct cardiorespiratory collapse. The immediate measures that should be taken are (in order):

- Notify the surgeons.
- Occlude the wound with a wet swab.
- Give 100% oxygen.
- Raise the venous pressure – level table and neck compression.
- Aspirate CVP line – CVP catheters, as well as allowing measurement of the effectiveness of attempts to raise venous pressure and reduce the hydrostatic gradient, can be used to aspirate air that has entered the circulation. For optimal recovery of air, the tip of the catheter should be close to where the superior vena cava enters the right atrium (usually placed with ECG guidance). Catheters with multiple orifices are more effective.
- If there is cardiovascular collapse, turn the patient on to the left side with head down to limit airflow into the pulmonary circulation. Cardiopulmonary resuscitation should be commenced. Prompt diagnosis and action will limit the need for these steps, which are barely practical and are unlikely to result in a successful outcome when the posterior fossa is exposed.

PARADOXICAL AIR EMBOLISM (PAE)

Post-mortem studies show that approximately 25% of the general population has a patent foramen ovale, which is a potential route for air to pass from the right to the left atrium. Whereas the presence of small amounts of air in the venous circulation and pulmonary vascular bed may not affect the patient adversely, the presence of minimal volumes (100–150 μl kg^{-1}) in the arterial circulation can be fatal. Even a small air embolism in the circulation of the brain or heart will result in irreversible damage. If air enters the pulmonary circulation, the obstruction to flow that occurs will cause the pressure to rise on the right side of the heart and fall on the left, thus increasing the pressure gradient. A gradient of 4 mmHg is all that is required to reverse flow through a shunt. Apart from the foramen ovale, other anatomical routes such as arteriovenous shunts may allow air to pass from the right to the left side of the circulation.

OTHER INTRAOPERATIVE CONSIDERATIONS

The choice of anaesthetic agents is not critical and most well managed techniques will suffice, although nitrous oxide should not be used.

Interference with the midbrain, vital centres and cranial nerves through direct intervention, retraction or occlusion of the blood supply may result in sudden alteration of systemic physiological variables. Traditionally it was advocated that patients undergoing posterior fossa surgery should be breathing spontaneously to allow detection of changes in respiratory pattern indicating surgical interference with the respiratory centres. However, controlled ventilation is now recommended and respiratory changes will not be detected. Cardiovascular changes can be observed but they may be abrupt and dramatic. The anaesthetist should advise the surgeon of any significant cardiovascular changes, and drugs such as atropine and beta-blockers should be used only when essential because they will mask midbrain responses. Electrophysiological techniques, such as somatosensory evoked potentials (SSEPs), are increasingly used during complex posterior fossa surgery and may assist in defining what is surgically feasible.

The facial nerve (VII) is stretched across the capsule of acoustic neuromas, and monitoring of VIIth nerve function is often performed during operation. Neuromuscular blocking drugs should therefore be avoided after the initial dose used to facilitate intubation. The use of remifentanil infusion has simplified anaesthesia under such circumstances.

Blood pressure should be brought close to normal prior to closure, in order to assess the adequacy of haemostasis.

10

POSTOPERATIVE MANAGEMENT

- Following posterior fossa surgery, patients should be managed in a critical care environment by nurses experienced in the care of neurosurgical patients.
- Poor preoperative neurological status, the occurrence of an adverse intraoperative event, prolonged surgery with significant tissue retraction and a lesion >30 mm in diameter with mass effect are all indicators of a possible slow recovery from anaesthesia, and may be indications for elective postoperative ventilation.
- Postoperative swelling in the posterior fossa is a potentially life-threatening complication. The small anatomical space, the tendency of the cerebellum to swell following prolonged retraction and the risk of bleeding all add to the threat. In addition, reduced respiration may result from, and in its turn increase, swelling. Swelling can also be delayed, sometimes developing some hours after an initially good recovery. Deterioration in neurological status after posterior fossa surgery is an indication for immediate CT.
- Hydrocephalus may occur because of occlusion of the CSF pathway. Urgent CT will confirm the diagnosis and an EVD should be placed.
- The gag reflex may be obtunded because of swelling or damage to the lower cranial nerves (glossopharyngeal and vagus). A nasogastric tube and nil by mouth are indicated until the gag reflex has been formally assessed.
- Macroglossia may occur. It is likely to be caused by prolonged surgery with excessive neck flexion causing occlusion of lingual drainage. It may also be associated with the use of oropharyngeal airways.
- Postoperative nausea and vomiting is very common, especially following cerebellopontine angle surgery.

BIBLIOGRAPHY

Artru AA, Cucchiara RF, Messick JM. Cardiorespiratory and cranial nerve sequelae of surgical procedures involving the posterior fossa. Anesthesiology 1980; 52:83–86

Duffy C. Anaesthesia for posterior fossa surgery. In: Matta BF, Menon DK, Turner JM, eds. Textbook of neuroanaesthesia and critical care. London: Greenwich Medical Media; 2000:267–280

Ingram GS, Walters FJM. Anaesthesia for posterior fossa surgery. In: Walters FJM, Ingram GS, Jenkinson JL, eds. Anaesthesia and intensive care for the neurosurgical patient. London: Blackwell Scientific; 1993:212–238

Joshi S, Dash HH, Ornstein E. Anesthetic considerations for posterior fossa surgery. Current Opinion in Anaesthesiology 1997; 10:321–326

Porter J, Pidgeon C, Cunningham A. The sitting position in neurosurgery: a critical appraisal. British Journal of Anaesthesia 1999; 82:117–128

Smith DS, Osborn I. Posterior fossa: anesthetic considerations. In: Cottrell JE, Smith DS, eds. Anesthesia and neurosurgery. St Louis: Mosby; 2001:335–351

CROSS-REFERENCES

Raised ICP/CBF control
    Anaesthetic factors 31: 787
Complications of position
    Anaesthetic factors 31: 736

10

Anaesthesia for transsphenoidal hypophysectomy

N. Curry and N. P. Hirsch

ANATOMY

The pituitary gland lies within the pituitary fossa (sella turcica) of the skull base. The floor of the fossa is formed by the roof of the sphenoid air sinus, the lateral walls by the cavernous sinus (containing the carotid arteries and cranial nerves III, IV and VI) and the roof by the diaphragma sella through which passes the pituitary stalk. The anterior lobe of the gland secretes growth hormone (GH), adrenocorticotrophic hormone (ACTH), prolactin (PRL) and thyroid-stimulating hormone (TSH). The posterior lobe secretes oxytocin and vasopressin.

PATHOLOGY

Adenomas that affect the anterior lobe are common, whereas non-pituitary derived tumours (e.g. craniopharyngiomas and Rathke pouch cysts) are rare. Most pituitary operations are performed via the transsphenoidal route.

Pituitary tumours account for 10–15% of intracranial tumours and may present in a variety of ways:
- Hypersecretion of pituitary hormones:
  —GH, resulting in gigantism in prepubertal individuals and acromegaly in adults
  —ACTH , resulting in Cushing's disease
  —PRL, resulting in galactorrhoea and infertility.
- Mass effect due to the presence of large (>1 cm in diameter) tumours. These are usually non-hormone secreting and present with:
  —headache, hydrocephalus (rare)
  —visual field defect (classically bitemporal hemianopia) due to compression of the optic chiasm.
  —hypopituitarism (especially if haemorrhage into the tumour occurs)
  —cranial nerve (III, IV and VI) palsies.

PREOPERATIVE CONSIDERATIONS

In addition to normal preoperative evaluation, attention should be directed to manifestations of hormone hypersecretion syndromes.

ACROMEGALY
- Enlarged jaw and tongue, teeth malocclusion, thickened laryngeal and pharyngeal tissues, and thyroid enlargement may pose airway problems.
- Obstructive sleep apnoea is common.
- Hypertension occurs in 30% of patients and may be associated with left ventricular hypertrophy.
- Overt diabetes occurs in 25% of patients and glucose intolerance is common.

CUSHING'S DISEASE:
- Hypertension occurs in 85% of patients and is often associated with left ventricular hypertrophy and ECG changes (increased QRS voltage and T-wave changes).
- Obstructive sleep apnoea is common.
- Glucose intolerance or diabetes occurs in 60% of patients.
- Obesity and gastrointestinal reflux are common and may warrant administration of H_2 antagonists or proton pump inhibitors.
- High levels of circulating cortisol have immunosuppressant effect predisposing to infection.
- Fragile skin requires careful handling of patients. Bruising occurs easily during intravenous access.
- Steroid cover with hydrocortisone may be necessary in the preoperative and postoperative period.

PROLACTIN-SECRETING TUMOURS:
- Do not usually cause anaesthetically important endocrine disturbance.

10

PERIOPERATIVE MANAGEMENT

- Full monitoring, including direct arterial blood pressure measurement, should be established.
- Anaesthesia is induced with thiopental or with propofol and fentanyl (1–2 μg kg^{-1}).
- Following administration of a suitable non-depolarising neuromuscular blocking agent, the trachea should be intubated with a flexometallic (non-kinkable) tracheal tube. If intubation problems are anticipated, a fibreoptic intubation should be considered.
- After intubation, the patient's lungs should be moderately hyperventilated (to PaCO$_2$ 4.0–4.5 kPa) with an oxygen–air–sevoflurane mixture. This maintenance anaesthetic regimen can be supplemented with a remifentanil infusion (0.05–2 μg kg^{-1} min^{-1}).
- After placing a throat pack, a suitable vasoconstrictor (e.g. Moffett's solution or xylometazoline) should be introduced into each nostril to improve surgical conditions.
- A single dose of a prophylactic antibiotic (e.g. cefuroxime 1.5 g i.v.) should be given.
- If the pituitary tumour is large (i.e. with suprasellar extension), a lumbar drain should be inserted into the subarachnoid space (see below).
- The patient should be placed supine on the operating table with a slight head-up tilt.
- Under radiological control, the surgeon enters the sphenoid air sinus and reaches the pituitary fossa by removing the bony floor. After incising the pituitary dura, the tumour is removed and nasal packs inserted.
- If there is suprasellar extension to the tumour, the neurosurgeon may request the introduction of 10–40 ml saline via the lumbar drain. This increases intraventricular pressure and prolapses the suprasellar part of the tumour into the operative field.
- At the end of the procedure neuromuscular block is reversed, the throat pack removed and the trachea extubated following thorough suction of pharynx and return of spontaneous respiration and airway reflexes.
- The major potential perioperative complications are haemorrhage from the cavernous sinus or carotid arteries, and persistent leakage of cerebrospinal fluid (CSF).

POSTOPERATIVE MANAGEMENT

- Patients should be nursed in a high-dependency area and routine neurological observations performed.
- Airway problems may occur, especially in patients with preoperative obstructive sleep apnoea. Nasal continuous positive pressure cannot be used immediately after transsphenoidal surgery, and continued monitoring in a critical care environment may be required for at-risk patients, particularly during the first postoperative night.
- Morphine sulfate (0.1–0.2 mg kg^{-1} i.m.) is the analgesic of choice.
- Diabetes insipidus may occur if there has been damage to the posterior lobe of the pituitary. Diagnosis should be suspected if the patient passes >1 litre of dilute urine (specific gravity <1005) within 12 h, associated with a plasma sodium concentration >143 mmol l^{-1}. A plasma osmolality >295 mOsm kg^{-1} associated with a urine osmolality <300 mOsm kg^{-1} and a high urine output (>2 ml kg^{-1} h^{-1}) confirms the diagnosis. Meticulous fluid replacement and treatment with DDAVP may be necessary, although long-term hormone replacement is rarely required.
- If a CSF leak has been produced during operation, CSF drainage via the lumbar drain may be required for 24–48 h.

BIBLIOGRAPHY

Chapman M, Smith M, Hirsch NP. Pituitary disease and anaesthesia. British Journal of Anaesthesia 2000; 85:3–14

CROSS-REFERENCES

Hypertension
     Patient conditions 4: 151
Diabetes Mellitus type
     Patient conditions 2: 56
Adrenocortical insufficiency
     Patient conditions 2: 46

Anaesthesia for stereotactic surgery

S. Galton and M. Smith

There is an increasing trend in neurosurgery towards minimally invasive operations that reduce patient discomfort, postoperative complications and length of hospital stay. There is also a need to obtain biopsies from, or to make discrete lesions in, CNS tissue that is deep in the brain or so intricately associated with important functional centres that the risks of a conventional approach are unacceptable. Stereotactic surgery has now found an established place in the diagnosis and treatment of neurological disease. This has been driven by technological advances leading to improved resolution in imaging modalities and by advances in computing power resulting in relatively inexpensive three-dimensional modelling software. The indications for stereotactic neurosurgery are listed in Box 10.8.

PRINCIPLES OF STEREOTACTIC SURGERY

Imaging of the brain with CT, MRI or digital angiography provides an accurate anatomical database that can be used singly or in combination to produce a three-dimensional coordinate system to define intracranial structures and lesions accurately. The spatial relationship of intracranial structures can be registered to an extracranial reference system present during the imaging studies. Traditionally the extracranial reference system comprises a rigid stereotactic head frame firmly attached to the head. As well as being the stereotactic fiducial marker system, this frame also acts as a platform for surgical instrumentation. More recently frameless stereotaxy has been developed in which the extracranial reference system is a series of small adhesive fiducial markers attached to the scalp. A digitiser tracks special surgical instruments in relation to the fiducial system. Frameless stereotaxy has the advantage that it is more comfortable for the patient and gives better surgical access to the operating site and access to the airway for the anaesthetist. The major disadvantage is that it is less accurate than frame stereotaxy because the adhesive fiducial markers are attached to the skin and can move slightly in relation to the skull. Using traditional stereotactic methods, a biopsy needle can be placed with an accuracy of about 1 mm.

GENERAL CONSIDERATIONS

Stereotactic procedures may be carried out using local anaesthesia, with or without sedation, or under general anaesthesia. A combination of

---

BOX 10.8

Indications for stereotactic surgery

- Stereotactic biopsy
  —allows tissue samples to be obtained from tiny deep-seated lesions inaccessible by open surgery
  —the most frequently performed stereotactic procedure in the UK.
- Aspiration of haematoma, cyst or abscess
  —decompression
  —microbiological or cytological diagnosis
- Tumour surgery
  —resection of deep-seated tumours or those intimately involved with eloquent areas
  —implantation of radioactive seeds
  —planning of surgical approach prior to open operation.
- Functional surgery
  —implantation of electrodes for deep brain stimulation in movement disorders (e.g. Parkinson's disease or dystonia) or chronic pain conditions
  —lesion generation in the thalamus or basal ganglia to control intractable tremor in Parkinson's disease
  —epilepsy surgery.

10

methods may be used at different points during the procedure. The choice of technique will depend upon the systemic condition and wishes of the patient, the nature and expected duration of procedure, and the preference of the surgeon.

In frameless stereotaxy the fiducials are attached and the imaging studies performed some time before operation, with the patient awake. Such procedures have no specific implications for the anaesthetist.

External frame systems are, however, usually applied immediately before the surgical procedure. They are attached to the skull using a series of metal pins, and therefore require local or general anaesthesia for placement. Some stereotactic frames obstruct the mouth and limit access to the airway, and general anaesthesia with an endotracheal tube in place prior to application of the head frame is the preferred technique in many centres in the UK. Following application of the head frame, the patient will be transferred to the radiology department for the imaging studies and then back to the operating theatre for the operation. Tools to release the frame should be available at all times so that the airway is easily accessible in an emergency. Some procedures (e.g. movement disorder surgery) require complex computation of the imaging studies and there may be a delay of some hours before the operation can commence. Under such circumstances, it may be appropriate to apply the head frame using local anaesthesia and allow the patient to return to the ward during the computation process. The surgical procedure itself can then be carried out using local or general anaesthesia as appropriate. Airway maintenance can be a challenge during induction of general anaesthesia in patients with a head frame in position. Some frames do not obstruct the mouth and present no difficulty, whereas others severely limit airway access. Use of a laryngeal mask airway, awake fibreoptic intubation, or other intubation aids may facilitate endotracheal intubation under such circumstances.

PREMEDICATION

Premedication is often avoided but benzodiazepines may be prescribed if required. Drugs that inhibit tremor and rigidity are contraindicated in patients undergoing stereotactic procedures for Parkinson's disease or other movement disorders.

GENERAL ANAESTHESIA

General anaesthesia has many benefits for the surgeon, including the provision of optimal operating conditions by the ability to control the $Pa\text{CO}_2$ and blood pressure, and the assurance of immobility. The advantage for the patient is, of course, unawareness of the whole procedure. There are no specific requirements for stereotactic neurosurgical procedures under general anaesthesia except that a 'full brain' facilitates stereotactic biopsy. Appropriate patient positioning and maintenance of $Pa\text{CO}_2$ within the normal range can best achieve this. Techniques that allow rapid wake-up at the end of the procedure facilitate early neurological assessment. If it is necessary to transfer the patient between radiology and operating departments, total intravenous anaesthesia using propofol and/or remifentanil is convenient, as the same technique may be used for the whole procedure.

LOCAL ANAESTHESIA AND SEDATION

This is the technique of choice in many countries, and is gaining popularity in the UK. However, some stereotactic procedures must be carried out in awake patients, particularly those in whom somatotrophic localisation is required (e.g. thalamotomy and pallidotomy). Local anaesthetic techniques require good communication between all members of the operative team, as well as careful patient selection and preparation.

Careful preoperative preparation is essential to the success of the procedure and must include a full explanation of the sequence of events to the patient. Watching a video of the procedure and a visit to the theatre suite may be an additional reassurance. The atmosphere in the theatre should be calm, with all staff fully briefed of their responsibilities beforehand. A sign on the door warns staff that the patient is awake and limits unnecessary intrusions. Relaxing music chosen by the patient can be played in the background.

An intravenous infusion and arterial line (if applicable) must be inserted using local anaesthetic. 'Awake' neurosurgical techniques rely on the provision of excellent local anaesthesia. Local anaesthetic should be applied to the sites of the fixator pins prior to application of a head frame and to the areas around the surgical incision. A mixture of 1% lidocaine (lignocaine) and 0.5% bupivacaine with 1 : 200 000 adrenaline (epinephrine) allows rapid onset of action

10

and prolonged duration of action. Scalp anaesthesia of 8–12 h has been reported using this technique. A burr-hole can be drilled without pain, but the dura must be anaesthetised separately with plain lidocaine (1%) before dural incision.

There must be careful attention to patient positioning, including a foam head-rest, leg pillows and a urinary catheter for long procedures. The surgical drapes should be positioned to allow access by the anaesthetist to the patient's airway whilst minimising obstruction to the patient's line of vision.

Incremental sedation may be administered as required using small doses of midazolam and fentanyl, usually in association with an antiemetic. Infusion of a subanaesthetic dose of propofol and/or remifentanil through a dedicated separate intravenous cannula is gaining popularity for sedation during awake procedures. In patients with raised intracranial pressure, sedation without airway control and controlled ventilation must be avoided or used with extreme care. Airway control may be enhanced in sedated patients by the use of a soft nasopharyngeal airway inserted after topical anaesthesia of the nasal passages. End-tidal carbon dioxide monitoring is possible by side-stream sampling from the end of the airway or via a nasal prong inserted directly into the nostril. Oxygen should be administered to all sedated patients via a nasal cannula. Oversedation must be avoided because of the difficulty of airway access. Equipment for emergency airway control must be readily available and should include a laryngeal mask airway and intubating fibreoptic laryngoscope. Complications of awake procedures are shown in Box 10.9. For all local anaesthetic techniques, the anaesthetist should be prepared to convert to a general anaesthetic if necessary.

POSTOPERATIVE CARE

The complication rate after stereotactic surgery is lower than for open procedures, and it is often possible to observe patients for 2–4 h in a recovery or high-dependency area prior to return to a general neurosurgical ward.

BIBLIOGRAPHY

Danks RA, Rogers M, Aglio LS, Gugino LD, Black PM. Patient tolerance of craniotomy performed with a patient under local anesthesia and monitored conscious sedation. Neurosurgery 1998; 42:28–34

Herrick IA, Craen RA, Gelb AW et al. Propofol sedation during awake craniotomy for seizures: patient-controlled administration versus neurolept analgesia. Anesthesia and Analgesia 1997; 84:1285–1291

Kelly PJ. Stereotactic surgery: what is past is prologue. Neurosurgery 2000; 46:16–27

Sahjpaul RL. Awake craniotomy: controversies, indications and techniques in the surgical treatment of temporal lobe epilepsy. Canadian Journal of Neurosurgical Sciences 2000; 27(Suppl 1):S55–S63

Sarang A, Dinsmore J. Anaesthesia for awake craniotomy – evolution of a technique that facilitates awake neurological testing. British Journal of Anaesthesia 2003; 90:161–165

Smith M. Epilepsy and stereotactic surgery. In: Walters FJM, Ingram GS, Jenkinson JL, eds. Anaesthesia and intensive care for the neurosurgical patient. Oxford: Blackwell Scientific; 1994:318–344

10

CROSS-REFERENCES

BOX 10.9

Complications of awake procedures

- Oversedation and loss of airway
- Poor control of blood pressure and Pa_{CO_2}
- Breakthrough pain
- Nausea and vomiting
- Movement
- Convulsions

Anaesthesia for intracranial neurovascular surgery

S. R. Wilson

Patients may require neurosurgery for treatment of cerebral aneurysms, arteriovenous malformations and other vascular abnormalities or following intracranial haemorrhage.

ANEURYSMS

ANATOMY AND PATHOGENESIS

Intracranial saccular aneurysms result from a progressive degenerative change of the vessel wall and usually occur at the junction of vessels in the circle of Willis. Some 90% of aneurysms are found in the anterior cerebral circulation and 10% in the posterior circulation. The commonest site is on the anterior communicating artery complex. Multiple aneurysms occur in 20% of cases. The pathogenesis of aneurysms is multifactorial, but factors such as smoking, hypertension and genetics are involved. The incidence of aneurysm increases with age, and aneurysms are more common in women. Many disease states are associated with intracranial aneurysms (Box 10.10). Mycotic aneurysms may result from a septic focus.

CLINICAL FEATURES AT PRESENTATION

The majority of aneurysms present after rupture with the signs and symptoms of subarachnoid haemorrhage (SAH). The severity of

TABLE 10.1

World Federation of Neurological Surgeons (WFNS) grading of subarachnoid haemorrhage

Grade	Glasgow Coma Score	Motor deficit
I	15	Absent
II	13–14	Absent
III	13–14	Present
IV	7–12	Present or absent
V	3–6	Present or absent

the haemorrhage is classified according to a recognised scoring system (Table 10.1). The patient will describe a very sudden onset of an extremely severe headache. The most common age of presentation is in the sixth decade, but cocaine use is associated with rupture at an earlier age. Rupture of an intracranial aneurysm may result in:
- SAH
- Intracerebral haematoma
- Subdural haematoma
- Hydrocephalus
- Mass effect resulting in:
  —cranial nerve palsies
  —raised intracranial pressure
  —seizures.

NEUROSURGICAL TREATMENT

The definitive treatment for intracerebral aneurysms is obliteration of the aneurysm sac. In the past this could be achieved only by the placement of a clip across the neck of the aneurysm under direct vision using a neurosurgical approach. More recently, techniques have been developed that allow coils to be inserted endovascularly under radiological control to pack the sac and prevent rebleeding. Although a recent trial (International Subarachnoid Aneurysm Trial; ISAT) has suggested that the endovascular route will be the treatment of

BOX 10.10

Conditions associated with intracranial aneurysms

- Familial
- Adult polycystic kidney disease
- Coarctation of the aorta
- Fibromuscular dysplasia
- Marfan syndrome
- Hereditary haemorrhagic telangiectasia

10

choice for most aneurysms in the future, there will always be aneurysms that require neurosurgical treatment. These include aneurysms with a wide neck, difficult anatomy or those that are too distal for coiling. Some patients (e.g. pregnant patients or those allergic to contrast) may also be unsuitable for prolonged radiological procedures.

A ruptured aneurysm can be treated early (within 24–48 h) or late (after 10 days), when the maximum risk of vasospasm is reduced. Most neurosurgeons favour the early approach because the chance of rebleeding is reduced and any subsequent vasospasm can be treated aggressively. However, early operation may be technically more difficult as the brain is more swollen and the clot more friable.

Most intracranial aneurysm surgery is performed urgently on unstable patients with all the associated problems of SAH. Aneurysms are treated as an elective procedure if they present with mass effect or as an incidental finding. Some patients have multiple aneurysms and those on the contralateral side may be treated when recovery from the treatment to the presenting aneurysm is complete.

ANAESTHESIA FOR ANEURYSM CLIPPING FOLLOWING SAH

PREOPERATIVE ASSESSMENT:
- Consider the many medical problems associated with SAH.
- Patients with grade I and II SAH will be extremely anxious and careful explanation is essential. Premedication is not used routinely because it may impair conscious level both before and after operation.
- Anticonvulsant drugs and calcium channel blockers should be continued before operation.
- Cardiac function must be optimised and an ECG is essential because SAH may cause ECG abnormalities.
- Patients may be intravascularly depleted and need fluid resuscitation.
- Patients with poor-grade SAH may be already intubated and ventilated on the ICU.

INTRAOPERATIVE CONCERNS AND MANAGEMENT:
The anaesthetic management is similar to that for other supratentorial neurosurgical procedures but the following points must be considered:
- Careful induction of anaesthesia to maintain cardiovascular stability is essential to minimise changes in transmural pressure in the affected cerebral artery. Hypertension may precipitate rebleeding, and hypotension may increase the risk of cerebral ischaemia and infarction in those with vasospasm. Rupture during induction of anaesthesia occurs in 1% of patients and has a mortality rate of 75%.
- Standard monitoring for all patients includes ECG, SpO_2, invasive blood pressure, $EtCO_2$, core temperature, central venous pressure and measurement of urinary output.
- Further monitoring may include EEG, evoked potentials, transcranial Doppler ultrasonography and jugular bulb oximetry.
- A lumbar drain may be required for some patients.
- Artificial ventilation to maintain $EtCO_2$ at 4.0–4.5 kPa.
- Anaesthesia is maintained by any preferred technique and may include total intravenous anaesthesia using propofol or an inhalational agent such as sevoflurane with opioid supplementation. Nitrous oxide should be avoided as it may reduce intracranial compliance.
- Neuromuscular blockade is maintained with atracurium or vecuronium.
- Normotension is maintained to maximise cerebral perfusion.
- Dysrhythmias and cardiac instability are common, particularly when aneurysms are clipped early. Cardiac dysfunction is a known association of SAH.
- Oxygen requirements may be increased.
- Mannitol may be used after the dura is opened.
- Anterior circulation aneurysms and those on the basilar artery are approached via a frontal or frontoparietal craniotomy with the patient supine and the head slightly turned.
- Aneurysms on the vertebral system require a posterior fossa craniectomy in a park-bench position.

CEREBRAL PROTECTION

Previously, systemic hypotension has been used to facilitate aneurysm surgery, but the risks of precipitating cerebral ischaemia are high. It is now more common for the tension in the aneurysm sac to be reduced by the use of a temporary clip on the feeding vessel. However, there remains the risk of cerebral ischaemia, particularly if use of a temporary clip is necessary for a prolonged time. Moderate hypothermia

10

(33–35°C) or pharmacological agents may be used for cerebral protection during prolonged temporary clipping. Both have theoretical advantages and are believed to:

- Protect the brain from ischaemic damage
- Reduce cerebral electrical activity
- Reduce metabolic requirements
- Allow a longer temporary clip time.

To be effective, these measures need to be used before the ischaemic insult, and patients should be cooled prior to temporary clip application. However, controlled trials of these treatments are awaited.

INTRAOPERATIVE ANEURYSMAL RUPTURE

Aneurysm rupture most commonly occurs as its neck is dissected. At this stage a temporary clip can be used to stop haemorrhage from the main vessel and systemic hypotension is not required. However, if the aneurysm ruptures as the dura is being opened, and the circle of Willis is not dissected, the situation will be uncontrolled. Under these circumstances deliberate hypotension is essential to allow surgical access and control of haemorrhage. Blood pressure is reduced to a level that allows the surgeon to gain control under direct vision by:

- Increased remifentanil infusion
- Thiopental 3–5 mg kg^{-1}
- Labetalol in increments of 5–10 mg
- Sodium nitroprusside infusion.

Following control of the aneurysm, hypertension should be induced to restore perfusion to the compromised area.

POSTOPERATIVE MANAGEMENT

Management is as for any craniotomy, and a rapid, smooth emergence is needed. Postoperative hypertension must be monitored carefully and treated in a critical care area. Triple H therapy (see below) may be needed if vasospasm is present.

VASOSPASM

Delayed cerebral ischaemia secondary to arterial vasospasm is a major cause of morbidity and mortality after SAH. Vasospasm presents as a focal, and often fluctuant, neurological deficit and may be confirmed on angiography. The aetiology remains unclear but it is likely that oxyhaemoglobin, or its breakdown products, may be implicated in the pathogenesis of vasospasm. Other mediators, such as serotonin, histamine, catecholamines, angiotensin and lipid peroxidase, have also been implicated.

DIAGNOSIS

Cerebral angiography is the 'gold standard' for diagnosing vasospasm. Transcranial Doppler ultrasonography is useful for monitoring the progress of vasospasm at the bedside. Flow velocity >120 cm s^{-1} in the middle cerebral artery is suggestive of the presence of vasospasm.

TREATMENT:

- *Nimodipine* – the use of nimodipine, a cerebro-specific calcium antagonist, has reduced the incidence of poor outcome after SAH by 40% and the incidence of cerebral infarction by 34%.
- *Triple H therapy* – The aim of triple H therapy is to prevent cerebral ischaemia by optimisation of cerebral perfusion using hypertension, hypervolaemia and haemodilution. This treatment can lead to significant complications, including pulmonary oedema, cardiac failure, myocardial infarction and hypertensive intracranial haemorrhage. It should therefore be administered only on the ICU in the presence of invasive cardiovascular monitoring, following protection of the aneurysm.
- *Angioplasty* – Balloon angioplasty may be effective in reducing the severity of vasospasm but there is a risk of vessel dissection or rupture. The endovascular infusion of papaverine has also been described.

ANAESTHESIA FOR ELECTIVE ANEURYSM CLIPPING

Similar techniques are used to those for emergency cases. The risk of vasospasm is greatly reduced and blood pressure control is less critical.

ARTERIOVENOUS MALFORMATIONS

Arteriovenous malformations (AVMs) are developmental; they are localised structural abnormalities of the vascular network. There is an abnormal connection between arteries and veins without intervening capillaries, resulting in a direct artery-to-venous shunt and a collection of dilated and twisted vessels between. The abnormal flow may result in adjacent aneurysm formation. These lesions are diffuse and vary in size.

CLINICAL FEATURES AT PRESENTATION

AVMs usually present in the third decade and present acutely as intracerebral haemorrhage of venous origin. Non-acute presentation includes recurrent headache, seizures and progressive neurological deficit.

ANAESTHESIA FOR AVM

The ideal treatment for AVM is excision, but this is not technically straightforward as the AVM may be extensive, difficult to access and involve eloquent areas of brain. Many are now treated by staged neuroradiological embolisation and/or radiosurgery. Some AVMs are reduced in size by preoperative embolisation and are then surgically removed. Surgery may be urgent if an expanding haematoma is causing a mass effect.

ANAESTHETIC TECHNIQUE:
- Standard techniques as for intracerebral aneurysms with particular attention to maintaining cerebral perfusion and reducing brain bulk.
- Substantial blood loss may occur during open surgery.
- Hypotension may assist the surgeon to ligate any arterial feeding vessels but this may cause ischaemia in areas of the brain with compromised autoregulation. It may also precipitate venous thrombosis.

POSTOPERATIVE PROBLEMS

- Normal perfusion pressure breakthrough – blood is chronically shunted through the AVM and the surrounding brain becomes ischaemic with loss of autoregulation. Once the AVM is removed there is a return of normal cerebral perfusion to the previously ischaemic brain. This may result in diffuse swelling and microhaemorrhage, but these effects can be reduced by staged excision of the AVM.
- Haemorrhage may occur from residual AVM.
- Hyperaemia may occur if the venous outflow is removed but arterial flow persists.

- Maintenance of normotension and immediate treatment of hypertension in the postoperative period should reduce the incidence of complications.

PRIMARY CEREBRAL HAEMORRHAGE

Primary intracerebral haemorrhage has a high mortality rate and patients often deteriorate after the ictus because of significant mass effect from the haematoma.

PATHOLOGY AND AETIOLOGY

Primary intracerebral haemorrhage occurs in late middle life and is more common in men than in women. It accounts for 15% of deaths from stroke. Haematoma enlargement is more likely in patients taking anticoagulant medication. The causes of intracerebral haemorrhage are listed in Box 10.11. Some 75% of supratentorial haemorrhages occur in the basal ganglia and thalamus, but haemorrhage may also occur in cerebral white matter, pons or cerebellum.

PRESENTATION

The specific signs and symptoms of intracerebral haematoma vary with the site and size of the haematoma, but include depressed level of consciousness, nausea and vomiting, headache and seizures. The speed with which symptoms develop depends on how quickly the clot expands but is usually maximal at 30 min. Further neurological deterioration may occur from cerebral oedema.

10

BOX 10.11

Causes of primary intracerebral haemorrhage

- Chronic hypertension – possibly arising from weakened or damaged arterioles
- Acute increase in blood pressure after sympathomimetic drug intake
- Acute increase in cerebral blood flow following carotid endarterectomy or correction of congenital heart defects
- Reperfusion of ischaemic brain in the area of embolic infarcts
- Primary neoplasm
- Metastatic neoplasm
- Subarachnoid haemorrhage
- Head injury

MANAGEMENT

- The surgical treatment of intracerebral haemorrhage is controversial, although a large multicentre study is presently ongoing. Patients with a small haematoma and little neurological deficit often require no surgery, but those with a large haematoma, mass effect and raised ICP causing depressed conscious level benefit from craniotomy and decompression. Surgery should be preceded by angiography to exclude an underlying aneurysm or AVM.
- Anaesthetic considerations are the same as those for other supratentorial lesions. Most patients requiring surgery will already be intubated, sedated and ventilated on the intensive care unit.
- Blood pressure should be controlled before operation. Patients may have cardiac and other problems resulting from chronic hypertension.
- Mannitol or furosemide (frusemide) may be needed to reduce brain swelling.
- Once the haematoma is evacuated, the blood pressure may drop dramatically as the ICP is reduced.
- Patients often require postoperative sedation and ventilation, and an ICP monitor should be inserted at the end of the procedure.

BIBLIOGRAPHY

Fleetwood IG, Steinberg GK Arteriovenous malformations. Lancet 2002; 359:863–873

Hindman BJ, Todd MM, Gelb AW et al. Mild hypothermia as a protective therapy during intracranial aneurysm surgery: a randomised prospective pilot trial. Neurosurgery 1999; 44:23–32

Lam A. Cerebral aneurysms: anesthetic considerations. In: Cottrell JE, Smith DS, eds. Anesthesia and neurosurgery. St Louis: Mosby; 2001:367–397

Molyneux A, Kerr R, Stratton I et al. International Subarachnoid Aneurysm Trial (ISAT) of neurosurgical clipping versus endovascular coiling in patients with intracranial aneurysms. Lancet 2002; 360:1262–1263

Young WL. Cerebral aneurysms: current anaesthetic management and future horizons. Canadian Journal of Anaesthesia 1998; 45:R17–R24

Young WL, Lawton MT, Gupta DK, Hashimoto T. Anaesthetic management of deep hypothermic circulatory arrest for cerebral aneurysm clipping. Anesthesiology 2002; 96:497–503

CROSS-REFERENCES

Raised ICP/CBF control
    Anaesthetic factors 31: 787
Intraoperation hypotension
    Anaesthetic factors 31: 758

10

Anaesthesia and cervical spine disease

I. Calder

TERMS AND DEFINITIONS

- Radiculopathy – disease of spinal nerve root
- Myelopathy – disease of spinal cord
- Central cord syndrome – interior of cord damaged, results in weak arms with relatively strong legs
- Anterior cord syndrome – anterior of cord damaged, results in motor weakness, loss of touch, pain, temperature, but preservation of vibration sensation
- Cauda equina syndrome – disease of neuraxis below the cord. Has lower motor neurone features and sphincter involvement
- Spinal stenosis – narrowed canal, often congenital osteophytes or disc protrusions
- Instability – loss of the ability, under normal physiological loads, to maintain normal relationships between vertebrae, In addition there should be no damage to the spinal cord or nerve roots, no development of incapacitating deformity, or any severe pain.

SURGICAL APPROACHES

An anterior approach to the spine, to left or right of the trachea in the supine position, can be used for most lesions from C3 to C7. Lesions above C3 can be approached through the mouth, from the lateral aspect, or after splitting the chin, mandible and tongue. Lesions behind the spinal cord or decompression at multiple levels are approached from the posterior aspect. The prone position is generally used, but the sitting position is occasionally necessary.

DISEASES

- *Cervical spondylosis* is the commonest indication for surgery. Osteophytes pressing on nerve roots or the cord are removed microscopically through an anterior cervical approach. The joint is then fused with iliac crest, artificial bone, or an artificial disc (Cloward or Smith–Robinson operations). Disease at multiple levels is generally treated by decompressing the canal by means of laminectomy or laminoplasty (the lamina is hinged and held open with small titanium plates).
- *Cervical disc protrusions* are not common; they are approached in the same fashion as spondylosis.
- *Tumours* – primary (of bone or neural tissue – chordoma, glioma, neurofibroma) and secondary.
- *Fracture or dislocation* – neurological deterioration can occur at any time, even long after the initial injury. Almost half of patients with fractures have vertebral artery damage. Conversely, up to 50% of patients with traumatic cord injury have no fracture.
- *Rheumatoid arthritis* – cervical involvement is common, but sometimes symptomless. It is likely that much cervical pathology was due to treatment with steroids. Important features are:
—Atlantoaxial subluxation (99% on flexion) rarely causes acute cord damage. Pain in the neck and back of the head is the usual symptom. The extent of subluxation is poorly correlated with neurological signs.
—Craniocervical 'settling' – erosion of bone, cartilage and joint space leads to shortening and immobility of the cervical spine. Erosion of C1 and the lateral masses of C2 can cause impaction of the odontoid peg on the high cord or brain stem ('vertical subluxation').
—Subaxial subluxation – staircase spine; multiple joint disease can result in subluxation at several levels.
—Temporomandibular joint disease is common.
—Arytenoid arthritis is present in about one-third of patients. Patients will often admit to intermittent hoarseness or even stridor. Exacerbations are a well

10

recognised complication of tracheal intubation.

ANAESTHESIA

There are two main problems: neurological deterioration during anaesthesia and airway management.

NEUROLOGICAL DETERIORATION DURING ANAESTHESIA

Spinal cord injury (SCI) has occurred during anaesthesia in patients with normal spines, in association with abnormal positioning or severe hypotension. Abnormality, such as spinal stenosis, instability or pre-existing myelopathy, increases the risk. Studies of cervical trauma victims have shown that patients occasionally deteriorate for no apparent reason. Vertebral artery injuries are common in patients with cervical fractures and it may be that the blood supply to the cord is unstable after injury.

Instability is hard to define and the clinical significance appears to be variable. Measurements of atlantoaxial subluxation in patients with rheumatoid arthritis have not revealed a correlation with neurological damage, whilst instability after fracture is believed to be associated with increased risk of deterioration.

Reports of cervical SCI during anaesthesia have tended to be by non-anaesthetists and may have confused association with causation. The mechanism proposed has been acute cord compression during airway management. Studies of cervical movement during intubation in unstable spinal preparations do not support this concept. The injuries described in the reports (usually central and anterior cord syndromes) would be better explained by hypoperfusion. It is likely that most injuries are due to hypoperfusion as a result of minor malposition and time.

Anaesthesia results in the loss of the normal protective reflexes that deflect the consequences of minor degrees of malposition.

Avoiding SCI during anaesthesia:
- Positioning – positions that look uncomfortable should be avoided, but in practice there is no way of telling whether a particular position will be tolerated for the duration of surgery.
- Maintain spinal cord perfusion pressure (SCPP) – serious hypotension (systolic less than normal diastolic) should be treated aggressively, especially if the cord is compressed. In practice, it is usually difficult to maintain normotension without the use of inotropes, so that a degree of hypotension is usual.
- Controlling CSF pressure by insertion of a lumbar intrathecal drain has not been investigated. The risk : benefit ratio has to be considered in each patient.
- Evoked potential spinal cord monitoring – sensory potentials recorded over the cerebral cortex following stimulation of a peripheral (median) nerve are relatively easy to record and robust to volatile agents. Motor pathways are more difficult to monitor and the signals tend to be abolished by agents other than opioids and propofol. Although it is ideal to monitor both sensory and motor pathways, only sensory evoked potentials are routinely used.
- Avoiding muscle relaxant drugs – many practitioners prefer to preserve normal neuromuscular transmission so that surgical stimulation of the cord or nerve root is betrayed by movement of an arm or leg.
- The place of high-dose steroids (methylprednisolone 30 mg kg^{-1}) when an SCI is suspected remains a matter of debate. It has not achieved the status of a 'standard of care'.

AIRWAY MANAGEMENT
Difficult laryngoscopy
This is common in patients with disease of the upper three vertebrae. An alternative to direct laryngoscopy is often required. Patients with poor craniocervical extension tend to have poor mouth opening as well, because of an association with temporomandibular joint disease and a direct effect on mouth opening. If difficulty is expected, always consider whether a nasogastric tube will be needed – it is wise to get the patient to swallow it before induction.

'Unstable' spine
There is no evidence that any method of airway management has a better outcome. Some patients are in fixation devices that will make difficult laryngoscopy likely and any difficulty with direct laryngoscopy should prompt the use of an alternative technique, rather than the application of force.

Cervical haematoma
There is a small incidence of airway obstruction after anterior cervical surgery. The haematoma may be small, and the tissue oedema marked. Opening the wound is a priority, to reduce lymphatic and venous obstruction. Patients com-

plain of not being able to breathe and want to sit up. They rarely have stridor and do not desaturate until the obstruction is nearly complete. The wound should be opened and the patient transferred to theatre. An inhalational induction with sevoflurane and oxygen is the accepted technique. A tracheal tube should be left *in situ* for at least 24 h.

BIBLIOGRAPHY

Calder I, Calder J, Crockard HA. Difficult direct laryngoscopy in patients with cervical spine disease. Anaesthesia 1995, 50:756–763

Donaldson WF III, Heil BV, Donaldson VP et al. The effect of airway maneuvers on the unstable C1–C2 segment. A cadaver study. Spine 1997; 22:1215–1218

Haldeman S, Kohlbeck FJ, McGregor M. Unpredictability of cerebrovascular ischemia associated with cervical spine manipulation therapy: a review of sixty-four cases after cervical spine manipulation. Spine 2002; 27:49–55

McCleod ADM, Calder I. Spinal cord injury and direct laryngoscopy – the legend lives on. British Journal of Anaesthesia 2000; 84:705–709

Weglinski MR, Berge KH, Davis DH. New-onset neurologic deficits after general anesthesia for MRI. Mayo Clinic Proceedings 2002; 77:101–103

CROSS-REFERENCES

10

Anaesthesia for interventional neuroradiology

M. Newton

The majority of neuroradiology units have been adapted from their original use for diagnostic imaging on awake patients to areas where complex procedures are performed for serious intracranial pathology on highly dependent patients. The resulting environment is often cramped, poorly designed for general anaesthesia, and remote from other anaesthetic areas. Long periods of darkness hinder observation of the patient, who may also be relatively inaccessible. Frequent movement of imaging equipment increases the risk of accidental extubation and decannulation. The combination of caring for patients in a 'hostile' anaesthetic environment presents a challenge – even to the most experienced neuroanaesthetist.

The same standards of anaesthetic care afforded to the neurosurgical patient in the operating theatre should extend to patients presenting for interventional neuroradiological procedures. It is essential that the anaesthetist is assisted by appropriately trained personnel, and ideally there should be a dedicated anaesthetic room. Other members of the 'radiological' team must be familiar with the clinical needs of this patient population and know how to respond to emergency situations that may arise during interventional treatments.

BOX 10.12

Commonly performed neuroradiological interventions

- Embolisation of spinal vascular malformations and tumours
- Embolisation of cerebral vascular malformations and tumours
- Endovascular coiling of cerebral aneurysms
- Angioplasty for vasospasm in subarachnoid haemorrhage
- Carotid and vertebral artery stenting
- Balloon occlusion of intracerebral vessels

RADIATION SAFETY

Multiple imaging results in high doses of radiation being used during many cases, and radiation protection of the patient and personnel is essential. The dose exposure of radiation declines proportionally to the square of the distance from the radiation source (inverse square law) and, in addition to wearing protective lead coats, personnel should therefore position themselves as far as practically possible from the radiation source to limit their exposure to radiation.

RADIOLOGICAL TECHNIQUES

The spinal and cerebral circulations are accessed by fluoroscopically guided catheters inserted through a sheath, usually via the femoral artery. Microcatheters may then be passed through the catheter to inject glue, sclerosants and particles into arteriovenous malformations or to deploy electrolytically detachable coils into aneurysms. It is essential that the radiologist and anaesthetist communicate clearly before and during interventional cases so that there is mutual understanding of concerns relating to the procedure.

Most procedures (with the exception of endovascular treatment of aneurysms) are non-urgent. The anaesthetic technique should follow the general principles of neuroanaesthesia and take into account the underlying neurological pathology.

Diagnostic cerebral angiography is virtually painless and mostly performed in conscious patients. General anaesthesia may be necessary for uncooperative patients where sedation is usually contraindicated and during spinal angiography because of its long duration.

The majority of interventional procedures (for treatment of aneurysms and arteriovenous malformations) require general anaesthesia because immobility is essential at critical periods of the procedure. Commonly performed interventional procedures are listed in

Box 10.12. The International Subarachnoid Aneurysm Trial (ISAT) demonstrated significantly improved results from endovascular coiling of aneurysms compared with open surgery and clipping. Although the results of this study are valid only for specific aneurysm types, it is likely that the number of aneurysms treated by endovascular methods will increase as further studies are reported. Other interventions in 'awake' patients command the presence of an anaesthetist for cardiovascular monitoring and possible intervention (carotid artery stenting) or management of anticoagulation ('test' balloon occlusion).

MONITORING

- In addition to minimal monitoring, most patients require intra-arterial pressure monitoring. Blood pressure may have to be manipulated in emergencies and selective changes in pressure may aid catheterisation of small arteries. Arterial lines also provide useful vascular access for monitoring anticoagulation during interventional procedures.
- Central venous access may be advisable to optimise 'filling' in patients with SAH.
- Central temperature (nasopharyngeal probes do not interfere with imaging) should be measured. The majority of patients require maintenance of normothermia but patients with aneurysms may gain some cerebral protection from being cooled (34.5°C) if the aneurysm ruptures during coiling.
- A peripheral nerve stimulator should be attached to a limb that can be observed easily if neuromuscular blocking agents are used.
- Urinary catheterisation is necessary because of the osmotic dieresis caused by the radiological contrast medium and also because of the large quantities of heparinised saline flush that are used to maintain catheter patency during the procedure.
- All intravascular lines should be extended to compensate for movement of the angiography table and have easily accessible injection points.

CONDUCT OF ANAESTHESIA FOR INTERVENTIONAL NEURORADIOLOGICAL PROCEDURES

- Meticulous control of blood pressure during induction of anaesthesia and intubation is essential. Hypertension may result in aneurysmal rupture, and hypotension may exacerbate pre-existing cerebral ischaemia.
- Patients should be intubated and ventilated as many procedures are of long duration. Some neuroanaesthetists prefer the use of a laryngeal mask airway and mechanical ventilation during interventional neuroradiological procedures.
- Maintenance of anaesthesia with intravenous or volatile agents is equally acceptable. An intravenous technique is preferable in patients with raised intracranial pressure (ICP), although theoretically the catheterisation of small arteries in the treatment of some arteriovenous malformations (AVMs) may be made more difficult by the resulting vasoconstriction.
- Studies using transoesophageal echocardiography have shown the frequent occurrence of air emboli during angiography. To reduce the risk of cerebral or spinal cord infarction caused by air emboli, nitrous oxide should be omitted from the anaesthetic technique.
- Ventilation should be adjusted to maintain normocapnia as some studies have shown a decreased reactivity to carbon dioxide in the abnormal arteries of patients with AVMs.
- Most procedures cause minimal sympathetic stimulation. Consequently 'light' anaesthesia in combination with neuromuscular blockade is advisable to maintain an adequate cerebral perfusion pressure (CPP) and prevent movement.
- Patients in the ICU may have ICP monitoring in progress; this should be continued in transit to the radiology department. Furthermore, most angiography tables cannot be positioned with head-up tilt and it is imperative that ICP monitoring is continued throughout the procedure because significant rises in ICP may occur when the patient is laid flat, particularly in the presence of pre-existing intracranial hypertension.
- A target mean arterial pressure (MAP) should be set to achieve an adequate (CPP). This may require the judicious use of vasopressors.
- Similar care must be taken with patients with an external ventricular drain *in situ*. The drain should be opened when the patient has been positioned for the procedure and personnel warned not to alter the height of the angiography table before alerting the anaesthetist.

Anticoagulation regimens vary from unit to unit. Most give heparin to achieve an activated clotting time (ACT) of twice the normal value.

Heparin should be given at the radiologist's request, and protamine must be immediately available in case of vessel or aneurysm rupture in the heparinised patient. Under certain circumstances, it may be better to continue packing a re-ruptured aneurysm as quickly as possible without reversing the heparin, but this decision must be made jointly by neuroradiologist and neuroanaesthetist. If there are signs of increasing ICP (e.g. haemodynamic changes) anticoagulation must be reversed urgently following removal of the microcatheter. A post-procedure CT scan may then determine the need for immediate operation.

CONSIDERATIONS FOR SPECIFIC PROCEDURES

ANGIOPLASTY

Symptomatic vasospasm in proximal cerebral arteries is often unresponsive to medical treatment. Angioplasty may reverse the symptoms and should be considered as soon as possible after the onset of symptoms. Under general anaesthesia a balloon is guided into the stenosed section of artery and briefly inflated. Following deflation it is advanced along the narrowed section and the process is repeated throughout the area of spasm. The effect is long-lasting but there is a high risk of rebleeding in patients with unprotected aneurysms. Vasospasm distal to the anterior, middle or posterior cerebral arteries may be treated with papaverine delivered via a superselective catheter. Papaverine-induced dilatation persists for 12–48 h.

TEST BALLOON OCCLUSION

Test balloon occlusions of the internal carotid and vertebral arteries are performed on awake patients to determine whether they will tolerate permanent sacrifice of the artery during surgery or by permanent placement of the balloon. Patients should be normotensive during the procedure to test the occlusion at their normal physiological status. Consideration should also be given to inducing slight hypotension during the occlusion to reflect the patient's 'sleeping' blood pressure. Anticoagulation is essential to prevent clot development proximal to the balloon and subsequent distal embolisation when it is deflated. Urgent anaesthetic intervention may be required if the patient fails the occlusion test and loses consciousness.

CAROTID STENTING

The placement of internal carotid artery stents as a treatment of carotid artery stenosis is performed in awake patients and again requires anticoagulation. As dilatation of the artery with stent insertion may result in profound bradycardia, it is essential that venous access is secured before that procedure and that atropine is available immediately. Vertebral arteries can also be stented.

THROMBOLYSIS

Intra-arterial injection of recombinant tissue plasminogen activator (rtPA), via a superselective catheter, has been used successfully to treat thrombotic stroke. Thrombolysis should ideally occur within 3 h of the onset of symptoms, and therefore its application is presently limited. Immobility on injection of rtPA and some stages of catheter positioning is vital and may necessitate general anaesthesia in uncooperative patients.

POSTOPERATIVE CARE

- Most angiography tables do not tilt and patients should be transferred to a tilting trolley for extubation.
- There is a significant risk of femoral artery haematoma on removal of the large-calibre arterial sheath. Coughing and leg movement should be avoided to reduce this.
- Patients must be transferred to a recovery or critical care unit experienced in the care of the neurosurgical patients.
- Most procedures do not result in pain following treatment, although some interventions to treat dural lesions and tumour embolisations may require analgesia.
- Antiplatelet agents may be prescribed for 14 days after the insertion of coils, stents and balloons to prevent thrombus formation on the surface of foreign materials and damaged endothelium.

10

BIBLIOGRAPHY

Dodson B. Interventional neuroradiology. In:
Cottrell JE, Smith DE, eds. Anesthesia and
neurosurgery. 4th edn. St Louis: Mosby; 2001:399–423

Eskridge J, Newell D, Winn H. Endovascular
treatment of vasospasm. Neurosurgery Clinics of
North America 1994; 5:437–447

Molyneux A, Kerr R, Stratton I, Sandercock P,
Clarke M, Shrimpton J, Holman R. International
Subarachnoid Aneurysm Trial (ISAT) of neurosurgical
clipping versus endovascular coiling in patients with
intracranial aneurysms. Lancet 2002; 360:1262–1263

Young WL, Pile-Spellman J. Anaesthetic
considerations for interventional neuroradiology.
Anesthesiology 1994; 80:427–456

CROSS-REFERENCES

Intraoperation hypertension
  Anaesthetic factors 31: 755
Raised ICP/CBF
  Anaesthetic factors 31: 787

10

Anaesthesia for magnetic resonance imaging

S. R. Wilson

MRI is a frequently employed imaging technique that produces particularly good images of soft tissue. It is used extensively for imaging the central nervous and musculoskeletal system and, more recently, for the cardiovascular system, the pelvis and the liver. Images are produced by placing patients within a strong magnetic field and applying pulses of radiofrequency (RF) energy. This results in intermittent release of RF energy from hydrogen nuclei, which is detected by a series of close-fitting receiving antennae known as coils. The RF signals are collected and interpreted by computer to produce extremely accurate images. The strength of the magnetic fields used during MRI is measured in Tesla (T). One Tesla is equal to 10 000 Gauss (G); the magnetic field of the earth is approximately 0.5–1.5 G. The most common strengths of magnetic resonance (MR) scanners are 0.5 and 1.5 T, although magnets of 3 and 4.5 T are now in use. Patients must be placed within the continuous magnetic field, and access during scanning is greatly restricted by the narrow bore of the magnet.

MR scans are produced in sequences of up to 10 min, and any movement during that time produces profound distortion of the final images. The aim of anaesthesia for MRI is therefore to provide immobility to obtain the best possible images, whilst maintaining safety and patient comfort throughout.

SAFETY ISSUES IN MR UNITS

- Implanted ferromagnetic objects may move in the magnet. This includes foreign bodies in the eye that may be dislodged during scanning, with the associated risk of vitreous haemorrhage.
- Non-ferromagnetic metals may heat up in the scanner, causing burns. They will also cause image artefact if they are adjacent to the area to be scanned.

- Implanted pacemakers, defibrillators and other devices may be inactivated by the magnetic field.
- Pregnant patients and staff should not to enter the scanner during the first trimester.
- The noise generated by the scanner can cause potential hearing loss, and staff and patients should wear ear protection.

PRACTICAL CONSIDERATIONS

The MR unit is often isolated from the main operating theatres and must be self-sufficient in terms of anaesthesia and resuscitation equipment. Because patients are placed inside a narrow-bore tube for the duration of the scan, they are relatively inaccessible and may be difficult to observe. Furthermore, many MR units were not designed with anaesthesia in mind, and space is usually minimal. Although the anaesthetic room and recovery area should ideally be placed adjacent to the scanner, many units have these areas in distant sites. The arrangements for anaesthesia will therefore be determined by local circumstances, but the following must always apply:

- All personnel must be trained in the local rules before entering the unit.
- Ferromagnetic items such as scissors, oxygen cylinders and laryngoscopes must never be taken into the scanning room.

MONITORING AND EQUIPMENT

Two definitions are used to describe equipment used in the MR unit. Equipment may be MR safe, which indicates that it can be used in the scanning room with no additional risk to the patient or personnel. Alternatively, equipment may be MR compatible, meaning that, as well as being MR safe, it does not degrade the images produced and its function is not affected by the scanner.

Monitoring in the MR unit must always conform to the same standards as applied in the operating theatre. In addition there are specific requirements for monitors and other equipment used during MR scanning:

- Monitoring should be established to allow the anaesthetist to view the monitor and patient from outside the scanning room.
- MR-compatible monitors allow accurate monitoring within the scanning room. Previously anaesthetists used non-MR-compatible monitoring that had been modified for use in the scanner, or placed monitors outside the scanning room and passed long cables through specially shielded holes in the scanning room wall. This practice cannot be recommended now that MR-compatible equipment is readily available.
- ECG cables must be shielded and specific electrodes used. Furthermore, the magnetic field in the MR causes specific problems with ECG interpretation. Changes in the ST segment and T wave, similar to those seen with hyperkalaemia or pericarditis, may be observed.
- Pulse oximeters must use fibreoptic cables to avoid burns.
- There may be a delay in obtaining a capnograph signal because the sampling tubing will be longer than normal.
- Measurement of temperature is difficult in the MR scanner and few compatible monitors have this facility.
- The anaesthetic machine may be sited outside the scanning room and long breathing circuits passed through the wall, as described above. However, an anaesthetic machine should always be available inside the scanning room; this should ideally be MR compatible with piped anaesthetic gases. Non-MR-compatible anaesthetic machines must either be bolted on to the floor or kept outside the 50-G line. All gas cylinders must be MR compatible.

PATIENT ASSESSMENT

The types of patients who may require general anaesthesia during MRI are shown in Box 10.13.

Screening is essential to exclude those who cannot enter the magnetic field, and this is usually performed by radiographers using a standard checklist. The exact make of an implantable device is required in order to assess its safety in the MR scanner. All patients

BOX 10.13

Patients who may require general anaesthesia during MRI

- Children
- Ventilated and other ITU patients
- Patients with severe movement disorders
- Patients whose position is limited by pain
- Adults with learning difficulties
- Claustrophobic patients
- Certain patients undergoing stereotactic neurosurgical procedures

with pacemakers and internal defibrillators are excluded because these devices may be inactivated by the magnetic field. Any metallic implants must be screened because aneurysm clips, cochlear implants and prosthetic heart valves may become dislodged, heat up or cause the induction of electric currents. Patients who are metal workers or who have known intraocular foreign bodies must also be screened with plain radiography before scanning, and all female patients should have a pregnancy test. Tattoos may heat up in the magnetic field.

ANAESTHETIC MANAGEMENT

MRI is not painful, and the requirements of anaesthesia are therefore hypnosis, amnesia and immobility. Recovery will be rapid and most patients can be treated as day cases. The following are simple rules that facilitate anaesthesia in the MRI suite:

- The patient is anaesthetised on a tipping trolley in the anaesthetic room.
- Most patients can be anaesthetised with short-acting agents and a laryngeal mask airway (LMA). With a standard LMA the pilot balloon must be taped away from the site to be scanned, because the small spring inside it may cause artefact. MR-compatible LMAs are now available.
- The airway should be clear as partial airway obstruction may cause increased respiratory movement and image artefact.
- Maintenance of anaesthesia is usually easier with an inhalational agent such as sevoflurane, as this avoids the need for a MR-compatible infusion pump or the use of long extensions from a pump placed outside the 50-G line.
- Those with a poor gag or reflux, and pregnant women, may need intubation and ventilation. A preformed tracheal tube will

10

allow close-fitting head coils to be applied, but the pilot balloon must again be taped away from the site to be scanned.

- Padding should be placed between the patient's skin and monitoring cables to prevent burns, and loops in cables must be avoided.
- Patients are transferred to a docking table or are taken into the scanning room on a non-ferromagnetic trolley.
- Contrast may be needed for scans to examine tumours or for MR angiography. The MR contrast medium is gadolinium DTPA (dimeglumine gadopentetate), which is associated with an extremely low incidence of anaphylactic reactions.
- In the event of a cardiac arrest or other critical incident, the patient must be removed from the scanner for resuscitation.

SEDATION IN THE MR UNIT

ADULTS:
- Many claustrophobic patients may be managed adequately with oral benzodiazepines.
- Pulse oximetry should be used in all cases.
- Short MR sequences may improve compliance.
- Intravenous sedation must always be given by an anaesthetist and with extreme caution.
- Monitoring of $EtCO_2$ is advisable.
- Bolus doses of midazolam can be used, or low-dose propofol–remifentanil infusions.

CHILDREN:
- Young children cannot lie still without being asleep, and conscious sedation may not ensure compliance because of the noise in the scanner.
- Small infants will sleep deeply after a feed.
- Older children (above 7 years) are often compliant without sedation.
- Many anaesthetists recommend general anaesthesia, rather than sedation, for children under 7 years of age.

- Sedation techniques must always be performed by adequately trained personnel and with extreme care. In some busy MR units nurse-led sedation techniques have been developed.
- Sedation techniques described include chloral hydrate, benzodiazepines and low-dose propofol infusions.
- Supplemental oxygen should always be given and adequate monitoring established.

BIBLIOGRAPHY

Association of Anaesthetists of Great Britain and Ireland. Provision of anaesthetic services in magnetic resonance units. London: AAGBI; 2002

Keengwe IN, Hegde S, Dearlove O, Wilson B, Yates RW, Sharples A. Structured sedation programme for magnetic resonance imaging examination in children. Anaesthesia 1999; 54:1069–1072

McBrian ME, Winder J, Smyth L. Anaesthesia for magnetic resonance imaging: a survey of current practice in the UK and Ireland. Anaesthesia 2000; 55:737–743

Menon DK, Peden CJ, Hall AS, Sargentoni J, Whitwam JG. Magnetic resonance for the anaesthetist. Part I: physical principles, applications, safety aspects. Anaesthesia 1992; 47:240–255

Morton G, Gildersleve C. Noise in the MRI scanner. Anaesthesia 2000; 55:1213

Peden CJ, Menon DK, Hall AS, Sargentoni J, Whitwam JG. Magnetic resonance for the anaesthetist. Part II: anaesthesia and monitoring in MRI units. Anaesthesia 1992; 47:508–517

Sury MRJ, Hatch DJ, Deeley T, Dicks-Mireaux C, Chong WK. Development of a nurse-led sedation service for paediatric magnetic imaging. Lancet 1999; 353:1667–1671

10

Brain monitoring

K. Hunt and M. Smith

General monitoring allows maintenance of optimal systemic physiology but will not detect changes in the brain. Cerebral monitors detect changes in cerebral compliance, haemodynamics and oxygenation, and allow therapy to be targeted to specific changes in brain function and ensure a balance between cerebral metabolic supply and demand. Electrophysiological measurements can also be made.

INTRACRANIAL PRESSURE

Intracranial pressure (ICP) can be measured using different techniques.

VENTRICULAR DRAIN
Measurement of the pressure in the CSF in the lateral ventricles, via a catheter inserted during a surgical procedure, is the 'gold standard' ICP monitoring device. Ventricular drains can also be used to drain CSF to treat intracranial hypertension. This device requires surgical expertise for placement and is associated with a higher morbidity rate (e.g. infection) than other devices. There is also a small risk of haematoma or seizures related to the insertion.

SUBDURAL MONITOR
These devices can be placed during surgery or via a threaded bolt that lies in the subdural space. Because of their position, rates of infection and damage to brain parenchyma are low, but the ICP measured by these devices may be inaccurate. They have been largely replaced by intraparenchymal monitors.

INTRAPARENCHYMAL MONITOR
These devices are inserted into brain tissue via a small bolt or burr-hole. They provide a reliable measurement of ICP and are associated with fewer complications than intraventricular catheters. Most employ modern microtransducer technology.

With the use of modern devices, ICP monitoring is a safe and straightforward technique. It also allows calculation of cerebral perfusion pressure (CPP) and detection of abnormal ICP waveforms that occur due to phasic increases in ICP triggered by cerebral vasodilatation in response to a reduction in CPP.

TRANSCRANIAL DOPPLER ULTRASONOGRAPHY

Transcranial Doppler ultrasonography (TCD) was introduced in 1982 and is a useful method of examining cerebral haemodynamics non-invasively at the bedside. An ultrasound beam is directed through an 'acoustic window' in the cranium to allow insonation of a major intracranial artery, usually the middle cerebral artery. Recognition of spatial resolution, response to compression manoeuvres and direction of blood flow in relation to the probe allows different vessels to be identified. TCD measures blood flow velocity in the insonated vessel and this can be used as a surrogate for CBF, assuming vessel diameter remains unchanged during the measurement. TCD is therefore able to identify trends in CBF and to measure cerebral vascular reactivity and assess pressure autoregulation. TCD may also be used to evaluate the degree of cerebral vasospasm after subarachnoid haemorrhage. Trained and experienced clinicians are required to use and interpret TCD.

MEASUREMENT OF CEREBRAL OXYGENATION

The benefits of monitoring cerebral oxygenation in patients at risk of cerebral ischaemia are obvious. However, the ability to do this reliably at the bedside is not straightforward.

JUGULAR VENOUS BULB OXIMETRY
The jugular bulb lies at the upper end of the internal jugular vein and is the final common pathway for venous blood draining from the

10

cerebral hemispheres. The jugular bulb oxygen saturation (SjvO_2) therefore reflects the balance between cerebral oxygen supply and demand. A catheter can be inserted in a cephalad direction via the internal jugular vein so that its tip lies in the jugular venous bulb. SjvO_2 can be measured intermittently by slowing aspirating blood from the catheter and analysing the sample in a co-oximeter or, continuously, using fibreoptic oximetry. The position of the catheter tip is crucial and should lie beyond the entry of the common facial vein to minimise the chance of extracranial contamination. A lateral cervical spine radiograph should be obtained to confirm accurate catheter placement, with the tip lying at the level of the mastoid process above the lower border of C1. SjvO_2 monitoring can accurately reflect global cerebral oxygenation only when it is placed in the dominant jugular bulb. This is usually the right side, but the direction of venous drainage may be altered in patients with head trauma. The dominant drainage side can be determined by sequential compression of each internal jugular vein in turn and observation of which causes the greatest rise in ICP. The normal range for SjvO_2 is 55–75%. Reductions in SjvO_2 below 50–55% suggest cerebral hypoperfusion (oxygen demand exceeds supply) and are associated with adverse neurological outcome after head injury. Levels above 85% indicate relative hyperaemia or ateriovenous shunting. However, because jugular venous oximetry is a 'flow-weighted' global measure, normal and supranormal values cannot exclude regional ischaemia. This is one of the major disadvantages of the technique.

NEAR-INFRARED SPECTROSCOPY

Light in the near-infrared spectrum is able to penetrate human tissue and allow tissue spectroscopy. Near-infrared spectroscopy (NIRS) is able to measure changes in the concentration of cerebral oxygenated and deoxygenated haemoglobin, and has been used as a trend monitor for cerebral haemodynamics and oxygenation. Recent advances in technology have allowed the introduction of instrumentation that can make absolute measurements of cerebral saturation. NIRS is a non-invasive real-time technique that is also able to make simultaneous measurements from different areas of the brain. However, there are significant technical problems that need to be resolved before it can be introduced into routine clinical practice.

BRAIN TISSUE OXYGEN PROBES

Microprobes can be inserted into brain parenchyma to obtain measurements of brain tissue Po$_2$ in a very focal area of brain. The normal range for brain tissue Po$_2$ is likely to lie between 3.3 and 5.9 kPa, but values <2.7 kPa have been reported in the first 24 h after head injury. Reductions in brain tissue Po$_2$ <1.0 kPa correlate with critical reductions in CBF and adverse neurological outcome after brain injury. The technology is relatively invasive and changes in local brain tissue Po$_2$ may not be reflected in global measures of cerebral oxygenation.

CEREBRAL MICRODIALYSIS

Measurement of changes in local tissue chemistry can be used to assess the balance between cerebral metabolic supply and demand. Microdialysis is a technique that relies on diffusion of substances from brain extracellular fluid across a dialysis membrane into a perfusion fluid of 'artificial CSF'. Changes in local levels of glucose, glutamate and glycerol and in the lactate : pyruvate ratio can indicate ischaemia. Microdialysis is able to sample only a limited area of tissue, and debate continues about the most appropriate location of the catheter. The catheter is usually placed in the presumed 'penumbral' zone around a focal contusion, although some also place a second catheter in 'normal' brain tissue.

ELECTROPHYSIOLOGICAL MONITORING

ELECTROESCEPHALOGRAM

The EEG is the measurement of spontaneous electrical activity in the cerebral cortex. It is measured using pairs of between 10 and 20 electrodes applied to the surface of the scalp. Characteristic waveforms are obtained in the normal EEG (Table 10.2) and classical (often diagnostic) changes are described in a large variety of clinical settings. The EEG can be used to guide the depth of sedation in head-injured patients, and to diagnose and guide therapy in those suffering from seizures or status epilepticus. Measurement and interpretation of EEG requires skilled technicians and physicians, and continuous monitoring can be cumbersome. Processed EEG techniques have been developed to allow more user-friendly continuous monitoring on the neuro-ICU.

BISPECTRAL ANALYSIS (BIS)

This processed EEG technique has been used widely to measure depth of anaesthesia. The technology measures frontal EEG and interprets segments of artefact-free non-suppressed EEG to produce a proprietary score, the BIS

TABLE 10.2

Characteristic EEG waveforms

Waveform	Frequency range (Hz)	Characteristics
Alpha	8–13	Normal waveform, seen at all ages. Disappears with attention (e.g. mental arithmetic)
Beta	>13	Small amplitude, seen in all age groups. Augmented by drugs including barbiturates and benzodiazepines
Theta	3.5–7.5	Seen in sleep. Abnormal in awake adults. Known collectively with delta waves as slow waves
Delta	<3	Seen in deep sleep in adults and infants. Abnormal in the awake adult. Large-amplitude waves

number. BIS is a dimensionless number scaled from 0 to 100, where 100 represents awake EEG and 0 complete electrical silence or cortical suppression. Although BIS is a useful measure of depth of sedation, the effect of organic brain syndromes on the BIS number has yet to be quantified. Its potential use on the neuro-ICU is therefore unclear.

EVOKED POTENTIALS

Somatosensory evoked potentials (SSEPs) are the electrical response of the cerebral cortex, brain stem and spinal cord to electrical stimulation of a peripheral nerve; they are used to assess the integrity of the relevant afferent pathway. Alternatively, in motor evoked potential (MEP) monitoring, the brain and spinal cord can be stimulated electrically or magnetically and the resultant response measured in the relevant peripheral muscle. SSEPs and MEPs are often monitored during spinal surgery to confirm the integrity of the spinal cord during manipulation or instrumentation. Anaesthetic agents have a profound depressant effect on SSEPs and MEPs. Brain stem auditory evoked potentials (BAEPs) can be used to assess brain stem function.

BIBLIOGRAPHY

Bergsneider M, Becker DP. Intracranial pressure monitoring. In: JE, Smith DS, eds. Anesthesia and neurosurgery. St Louis: Mosby; 2001:101–113

Nilsson OG, Brandt L, Ungerstedt U, Saveland H. Bedside detection of brain ischaemia using intracerebral microdialysis: subarachnoid hemorrhage and delayed ischemic deterioration. Neurosurgery 1999; 45:1176–1185

Owen-Reece H, Smith M, Elwell CE, Goldstone JC. Near infrared spectroscopy. British Journal of Anaesthesia 1999; 82:418–426

Schell RM, Cole DJ. Cerebral monitoring: jugular venous oximetry. Anesthesia and Analgesia 2000; 90:559–566

van den Brink WA, van Santbrink H, Avezaat CJ et al. Monitoring brain oxygen tension in severe head injury: the Rotterdam experience. Acta Neurochirurgica. Supplementum (Wien) 1998; 71:190–194

10

CROSS-REFERENCES

Raised ICP/CBF control
    Anaesthetic factors 31: 787

Anaesthetic and ICU management of the head-injured patient

M. Smith

INTRAOPERATIVE MANAGEMENT

Head-injured patients require anaesthesia for treatment of the primary intracranial pathology or for surgery to an associated extracranial injury.

PREOPERATIVE ASSESSMENT

Most head-injured patients present on an emergency basis, and time for assessment may be limited. However, the importance of a rapid yet thorough preoperative check cannot be overemphasised.

PRINCIPLES OF OPTIMAL ANAESTHETIC MANAGEMENT:

- Continue initial resuscitation
- Maintenance of cerebral perfusion and oxygenation
  —MAP >100 mmHg
  —PaO_2 >13.5 mmHg
  —$PaCO_2$ 4.5–5.0 kPa
  —ICP <20 cmH$_2$O
- Maintenance of low venous pressure – good neck position, head-up tilt
- Prevent or treat fluid and electrolyte abnormalities
- Correct coagulation abnormalities
- Prevent or treat seizures.

MANAGEMENT CONSIDERATIONS

Head-injured patients do not have reduced anaesthetic requirements and inadequate anaesthesia allows the surgical stimulus to increase CBF, ICP and CMRO_2, all which may be detrimental to the injured brain. The choice of anaesthetic technique depends upon the preferences of the individual practitioner, bearing in mind the effects of anaesthetic agents on intracranial physiology (see General Principles of Neuroanaesthesia) as well as the clinical state of the patient. Nitrous oxide should be avoided, but a volatile technique using an air–oxygen mix with low-dose sevoflurane is acceptable. Some recommend the use of TIVA with propofol and remifentanil, particularly

in the presence of intracranial hypertension. However, there is no firm evidence that one technique is generally better than another so long as simple principles are followed:

- Smooth induction
- No swings in blood pressure
- Maintenance of cerebral perfusion
- Prevention of rises in CBF, ICP and CMRO_2
- Consideration of the requirement for postoperative ventilation
- Rapid emergence for neurological assessment if the patient will be awakened at the end of the procedure.

INTRAOPERATIVE PROBLEMS
Bleeding

Venous bleeding occurs most frequently and can be difficult to control as cerebral venous pressure rises with increasing ICP. Treatment includes reduction of ICP, prevention or correction of venous obstruction, and correction of severe hypothermia.

Brain swelling

Acute brain swelling is life threatening. Treatment includes optimal patient position, discontinuation of volatile agent, moderate hyperventilation, propofol or barbiturates, CSF drainage and decompressive craniectomy. More aggressive hyperventilation may be life saving in the acute phase, and the risk of cerebral ischaemia can be minimised by continuous monitoring of cerebral oxygenation or the temporary use of hyperoxia.

Blood pressure

Acute intracranial lesions (particularly extradural and subdural haematoma) are often associated with intense sympathetic stimulation leading to an increase in systemic vascular resistance and tachycardia. This may mask relative hypovolaemia which, if untreated, can lead to cardiovascular collapse during surgical decompression. It is important to have a high index of suspicion and initiate early and vigorous fluid therapy. Moderate hypertension (sys-

10

tolic blood pressure ~140 mmHg) should not be treated prior to decompression of an intracranial mass lesion, because the high arterial pressure may be required to maintain an adequate cerebral perfusion pressure (CPP) in the face of raised ICP.

Coagulopathy

Coagulation abnormalities may be precipitated by ischaemic brain, particularly in the posterior fossa. Hypothermia and massive blood transfusions complicate the picture.

Fluid and electrolyte imbalance

Fluid management can be complicated in head-injured patients by multisystem injury and hypovolaemia. Maintenance of normal or supranormal circulatory volume should be achieved with colloid or crystalloid. Glucose-containing solutions should be avoided unless the patient is hypoglycaemic. Blood loss should be replaced with blood products to maintain a haematocrit of around 30%. Electrolyte abnormalities are common after head injury, and urine output and plasma electrolytes should be monitored closely and treatment initiated as appropriate.

INTENSIVE CARE MANAGEMENT

The aim of the intensive care management after head-injury patients is to prevent and treat secondary physiological insults. Novel neuroprotective agents may have promise in the future but are unlikely to affect management strategies in the short and medium terms. Although it is likely that specialist neurocritical care, with ICP- and CPP-guided therapy, might benefit patients with severe head injury, it is clear there is wide variation in clinical practice, with many units not following basic recommendations for monitoring and principles of treatment.

MONITORING

Systemic and cerebral monitoring techniques have been discussed elsewhere.

TREATMENT

The management of head-injured patients has historically concentrated on a reduction in ICP to prevent secondary ischaemic insults. Although there is limited evidence to show that this improves outcome, ICP >20 mmHg is the fourth most powerful predictor of outcome after age, post-resuscitation Glasgow Coma Score and pupillary signs. It is also accepted that treatment should be initiated if the ICP is >20–25 mmHg. However, there has recently been a change in emphasis during treatment of head injury on the ICU, and attention has focused on maintenance of adequate CPP rather than on reduction in ICP *per se*.

MAINTENANCE OF CEREBRAL PERFUSION PRESSURE

CPP should be maintained between 60 and 70 mmHg, but there is debate on the means of optimising CPP. One body of opinion recommends aggressive fluid replacement and cardiovascular support with vasopressors and inotropes to increase MAP and induce secondary reductions in ICP. However, it has recently been demonstrated that, although this strategy is associated with a reduction in secondary cerebral ischaemia, the mortality and morbidity rates are similar to those of other treatment strategies because of the high incidence of systemic (particularly respiratory) complications. Another approach is to use 'optimised hyperventilation' to reduce ICP and increase CPP. Using $Sjvo_2$ guidance, ventilation can be adjusted to reduce ICP whilst minimising the risk of secondary cerebral ischaemia from overzealous hyperventilation. Both of these approaches to treatment have a role if applied appropriately, and the risk : benefit ratio of each strategy can be assessed by appropriate monitoring techniques.

CONTROL OF ICP
Mannitol

Mannitol (0.5 g kg^{-1}) effectively reduces cerebral oedema and ICP in certain circumstances. Chronic mannitol therapy is not associated with improvement in neurological outcome and its use should be discontinued when it no longer produces a significant and sustained reduction in ICP. Plasma osmolality should be monitored regularly during mannitol therapy. The use of hypertonic saline is gaining popularity for the treatment of intracranial hypertension.

Sedation

Intravenous anaesthetic agents are often used to reduce ICP in patients with severe head injury. They produce a dose-dependent reduction in cerebral metabolism, CBF and ICP whilst maintaining pressure autoregulation and carbon dioxide reactivity. The use of barbiturates has largely been replaced by propofol, which has similar cerebrovascular effects but a more favourable pharmacological profile. Propofol has become the sedative of choice on the neurointensive care unit, but care must be taken to avoid hypotension. Neuromuscular

10

blocking drugs have no direct effect on ICP, but may prevent rises produced by coughing and straining on the tracheal tube. However, such agents are not associated with improved outcome and their use is currently the subject of much debate.

Hyperventilation

Hyperventilation was once the mainstay of treatment to reduce ICP in head-injured patients. Its aim is to reduce cerebral blood volume and ICP, but it can also cause a significant reduction in CBF. Recent evidence suggests that focal reductions in CBF occur more frequently than previously realised and that focal ischaemia, undetectable by measurement of $SjvO_2$, might occur quite commonly. The role of hyperventilation in the management of severe head injury is vigorously debated and $PaCO_2$ <4.5 kPa cannot be recommended for 'blind' therapy. In cases of intractable intracranial hypertension, when a reduction of $PaCO_2$ <4.5 kPa might be beneficial, hyperventilation should be carried out only with $SjvO_2$ guidance (see above).

CSF drainage

CSF drainage via a ventriculostomy and decompressive craniectomy are increasingly utilised methods to reduce ICP.

THERAPEUTIC HYPOTHERMIA

There has been renewed interest in the use of moderate hypothermia (33–35°C) for neuroprotection in head injury following apparent benefit in early clinical studies. Suppression of release of excitatory amino acids has been postulated as the mechanism of this effect. However, a recent prospective randomised study suggests that active cooling of patients is not effective in improving outcome after head injury, although the active warming of patients who present with spontaneous hypothermia may be detrimental. The results from further clinical studies are awaited before therapeutic hypothermia can be recommended widely but, in the meantime, it remains important to prevent pyrexia in head-injured patients because increased core temperature is associated with a worsened outcome.

GENERAL ASPECTS OF CARE

Ventilatory support of patients with head injury is vital to ensure maintenance of normal arterial blood gases. Respiratory complications secondary to head injury are common and many patients require advanced ventilatory support within a short period of time. Head-injured patients have a high calorific requirement and early feeding has been associated with an improved neurological outcome. Despite delayed gastric emptying after head injury, enteral feeding is possible in most patients and is associated with a lower incidence of hyperglycaemia than parenteral nutrition. Plasma glucose levels should be maintained within the normal range using an insulin infusion. Thromboembolic prophylaxis should be considered.

SUMMARY

The management of patients on the intensive care unit is being guided by better understanding of the pathophysiology of brain injury and by new and improved monitoring techniques. The importance of maintaining cerebral oxygenation and perfusion pressure throughout the entire management period is now accepted. The development of protocols and treatment guidelines is to be welcomed but must not prevent tailored therapy. The days of nihilism in the management of severe head injury have been replaced by the beginnings of evidence-based practice.

BIBLIOGRAPHY

Clifton GL, Miller ER, Choi SC et al Lack of effect of induction of hypothermia after acute brain injury. New England Journal of Medicine 2001; 344:556–563

Cruz J. The first decade of continuous monitoring of jugular bulb oxyhemoglobin saturation: management strategies and clinical outcome. Critical Care Medicine 1998; 26:344–351

Lam AM, ed. Anesthetic management of acute head injury. New York: McGraw-Hill; 1995

Matta BF, Menon DK. Severe head injury in the United Kingdom and Ireland: a survey of practice and implications for management. Critical Care Medicine 1996; 24:1743–1748

Patel HC, Menon DK, Tebbs S, Hawker R, Hutchinson PJ, Kirkpatrick PJ. Specialist neurocritical care and outcome from head injury. Intensive Care Medicine 2002; 28:547–553

Robertson CS. Management of cerebral perfusion pressure after traumatic brain injury. Anesthesiology 2001; 95:1513–1517

Robertson CS, Valadka AB, Hannay HJ et al. Prevention of secondary ischemic insults after severe head injury. Critical Care Medicine 1999; 27:2086–2095

Rosner MJ, Rosner SD, Johnson AH. Cerebral perfusion pressure: management protocol and clinical results. Journal of Neurosurgery 1995; 83:949–962

CROSS-REFERENCES

Raised ICP/CBF control
    Anaesthetic factors 31: 787
Management of the organ donor
    Surgical procedures 21: 529

10

11

OPHTHALMIC SURGERY
C. A. Carr

Cataract surgery

C. A. Carr

A cataract is opacity of the lens secondary to changes in the lens fibres causing significant reduction in sight. There are various underlying causes (Box 11.1).

BOX 11.1

Underlying causes of cataracts

Congenital

- Idiopathic
- Chromosomal disorders
- Inborn errors of metabolism
- Intrauterine infections

Acquired

- Age related
- Systemic disease – diabetes, hypocalcaemia
- Trauma
- Radiation
- Drugs – corticosteroids

PROCEDURE

CONGENITAL CATARACT:
Early operation to maximise visual outcome
Aspiration of lens using a suction-cutting instrument

ADULT CATARACT:

- Phacoemulsification is routine – a small incision technique without sutures
- Extracapsular cataract extraction – a larger limbal incision with sutures; eye is open during operation
- Intraocular lens implant is routine
- Intracapsular cataract extraction is rarely performed.

PATIENT CHARACTERISTICS

- The elderly with coexisting medical conditions – hypertension, ischaemic heart disease, diabetes, chronic obstructive pulmonary disease
- Neonates and young children with associated congenital syndromes

PROBLEMS

- Remote airway under the operating microscope
- Immobile eye with maximally dilated pupil and uniform intraocular pressure (IOP) provide optimal surgical conditions
- Variable length of operation – from 10 min for routine cases to 90 min for complex cases.

PREOPERATIVE ASSESSMENT

- Assessment and optimisation of associated or coexisting medical conditions as required; no routine investigations
- Assess suitability for local anaesthesia
- Assess suitability for day case or fast-track surgery.

PREMEDICATION

- Anxiolysis with a benzodiazepine if required in adults or older children
- Amethocaine (Ametop) or ELMA cream in children
- Atropine 0.02 mg kg^{-1} intramuscularly in neonates
- Avoid in local anaesthesia
- Preoperative starvation not necessary for local anaesthesia.

ANAESTHETIC MANAGEMENT

MONITORING:

- SpO_2
- ECG

- Non-invasive blood pressure (general anaesthesia)
- EtCO$_2$ (general anaesthesia)
- Peripheral nerve stimulator (general anaesthesia)
- Temperature (general anaesthesia).

LOCAL ANAESTHESIA

Local anaesthesia is the anaesthetic of choice for routine cataract surgery in adults.

CONTRAINDICATIONS TO LOCAL ANAESTHESIA:
- Patient refusal
- Inability to cooperate in lying flat and still for the operation
- True allergy to local anaesthetic agent.

TECHNIQUES OF LOCAL ANAESTHESIA
A thorough knowledge of orbital anatomy is required.

Topical anaesthesia
One per cent amethocaine or 0.4% oxybuprocaine provides good surface anaesthesia of the globe without the complications of a regional block; these drugs are frequently used alone for phacoemulsification cataract surgery.

Sub-Tenon's block
Local anaesthetic solution (3–4 ml 2% lidocaine (lignocaine) or a 2% lidocaine and 0.5% bupivacaine mixture, with hyaluronidase 15 iu ml^{-1}) is introduced to the sub-Tenon's space through a small incision in the inferior nasal quadrant of the eye using a blunt cannula. Ocular compression is not routinely required with this technique. Gives excellent anaesthesia and akinesia without the complications of sharp needle techniques.

Peribulbar block
Introduced to avoid complications of retrobulbar blocks. A 25-gauge 25-mm needle is used to place 5–10 ml of anaesthetic solution outside the muscle cone with the needle tip no further back than the equator of the globe. Two injections are used, inferolateral and medial to the globe. With larger volumes of anaesthetic, ocular compression may be required to lower IOP.

Retrobulbar block
A classical technique that provides good akinesia and anaesthesia, and is usually supplemented with a facial nerve block. Two to three millilitres of anaesthetic solution is deposited in the muscle cone at the apex of the orbit using a 40-mm needle. Rare but serious complications have led to use of the alternative techniques of local anaesthesia.

Sedation
It is vital to have full cooperation from the patient under local anaesthesia. However, the use of a small dose of an intravenous benzodiazepines (e.g. 0.5–1.0 mg midazolam) in anxious patients is beneficial.

COMPLICATIONS OF LOCAL ANAESTHESIA:
- Retrobulbar haemorrhage
- Globe perforation
- Damage to the optic nerve
- Damage to the ophthalmic artery
- Spread of local anaesthetic to the brain stem along the optic nerve dural sheath.

GENERAL ANAESTHESIA

- Techniques aim to provide stable conditions avoiding any rises in IOP with an immobile central eye.
- The operation is non-stimulating apart from the subconjunctival antibiotic injection at the end,

INDUCTION:
- Intravenous administration of propofol in adults provides a low IOP.
- Intravenous administration or inhalation in children, depending on preference.

AIRWAY MANAGEMENT:
- Intubation and ventilation with atracurium or rocuronium and alfentanil 0.01 mg kg^{-1}
- A laryngeal mask is ideal unless contraindicated as it minimises coughing on emergence
- Neonates require intubation.

MAINTENANCE:
- Moderate hyperventilation with volatile agent
- Antiemetic prophylaxis if patient susceptible to postoperative nausea and vomiting.

EMERGENCE AND RECOVERY:
- Antagonise residual neuromuscular block and extubate awake.

11

- With modern techniques, some coughing is not a problem.

POSTOPERATIVE MANAGEMENT

- Little postoperative pain, especially with small incision techniques and local anaesthesia – simple oral analgesia (paracetamol) is adequate

BIBLIOGRAPHY

Fichman RA. Use of topical anesthesia alone in cataract surgery. Journal of Cataract and Refractive Surgery 1996; 22:612–614

Johnson RW. Anatomy for ophthalmic anaesthesia. British Journal of Anaesthesia 1995; 75:80–87

McGoldrick K. Anesthesia for ophthalmic and otolaryngeal surgery. Philadelphia: WB Saunders; 1992

Rubin AP. Complications of local anaesthesia for ophthalmic surgery. British Journal of Anaesthesia 1995; 75:93–96

Stevens JD. A new local anaesthesia technique for cataract extraction by one quadrant sub-Tenon's infiltration. British Journal of Ophthalmology 1992; 76:670–674

CROSS-REFERENCES

The elderly patient
    Anaesthetic Factors 27: 606
Day-case surgery
    Anaesthetic Factors 27: 613
Infants and children
    Anaesthetic Factors 27: 610
Total intravenous anaesthesia
    Anaesthetic Factors 30: 715

11

Corneal transplant

C. A. Carr

The shape and transparency of the cornea are vital for normal vision. Disruption of these may occur with infection, trauma and underlying ophthalmic conditions.

- Routine grafts may be managed as day-case procedures
- If there is a corneal perforation, surgery may be urgent to save the eye.

PROCEDURE

PENETRATING KERATOPLASTY
A full-thickness disc (6–8 mm in diameter) of cornea is cut out and replaced with donor cornea, which is sutured in place.

DEEP LAMELLAR KERATOPLASTY
The inner layers of the cornea are left intact and the donor cornea is sutured on top.

TRIPLE PROCEDURE
A penetrating keratoplasty is combined with cataract extraction and lens implant.

PATIENT CHARACTERISTICS

- Usually adult, although occasionally small children
- Atopy associated with the corneal condition of keratoconus
- Associated connective tissue disorders such as rheumatoid arthritis and amyloidosis.

PROBLEMS

- Remote airway under the operating microscope
- Open eye for most of the procedure, so control of intraocular pressure (IOP) is vital
- May be a lengthy procedure, although not surgically stimulating
- Need to avoid postoperative coughing or vomiting because of 360° corneal suturing.

PREOPERATIVE ASSESSMENT

- Identification and optimisation of associated or coexisting medical conditions

PREMEDICATION

- Anxiolysis with a benzodiazepine (e.g. temazepam 10–20 mg orally in adults) if required
- Consider antiemetic prophylaxis in susceptible patients (e.g. metoclopramide 10 mg with ranitidine 150 mg orally in adults).

ANAESTHETIC MANAGEMENT

MONITORING:
- SpO_2
- ECG
- Non-invasive blood pressure
- $EtCO_2$
- Peripheral nerve stimulator
- Temperature.

LOCAL ANAESTHESIA

- Becoming more popular for uncomplicated corneal grafts
- May be appropriate in medically compromised patients
- Technique used must provide akinesia, IOP control and last for the duration of the operation
- Paralysis of orbicularis orbis is needed to prevent squeezing of the eye

Peribulbar anaesthesia
Ten millilitres of a mixture of 2% lidocaine (lignocaine) and 0.5% bupivacaine with hyaluronidase 150 units given as an inferolateral and a medial caruncle injection. Ocular compression for 10–15 min before operation to reduce IOP.

11

Sub-Tenon's anaesthesia

Five millilitres 0.5% bupivacaine with hyaluronidase 75 units provides lasting anaesthesia and akinesia of the globe. Orbicularis orbis is blocked with a medial caruncle injection of 2–3 ml of the same anaesthetic solution. Ocular compression to reduce IOP.

Sedation

As with all intraocular surgery, patient cooperation is required, but small doses of intravenous benzodiazepine (midazolam 0.5 1.0 mg) can make the procedure more comfortable for the patient. Careful attention to comfort and warmth ensure a relaxed and still patient.

GENERAL ANAESTHESIA

INDUCTION:

- Total intravenous anaesthesia (TIVA) with target-controlled infusion (TCI) of propofol and a remifentanil infusion provides excellent operating conditions.
- TIVA also provides rapid and smooth emergence from anaesthesia, with greatly reduced postoperative nausea and vomiting.
- Alternatively a balanced technique using intravenous induction with propofol, fentanyl, muscle relaxant and volatile agent is suitable.

AIRWAY MANAGEMENT:

- A laryngeal mask provides ideal emergence conditions.
- With an open eye the airway must be secure; a tracheal tube should be used if there is any doubt.

MAINTENANCE:

- Non-depolarising relaxant (e.g. vecuronium or rocuronium) is used for intubation and ventilation, and to ensure an immobile central eye.
- Monitor carefully to avoid sudden movements.
- Moderate hyperventilation reduces IOP.
- Antiemetic prophylaxis with ondansetron 4 mg intravenously.

EMERGENCE AND RECOVERY:

- Antagonise neuromuscular block with neostigmine and glycopyrrolate.
- Extubate awake; coughing is usually minimal.

POSTOPERATIVE MANAGEMENT

- Antiemetic prescribed in case of postoperative nausea and vomiting
- Moderate postoperative pain on the first day may necessitate a non-teroidal or narcotic analgesic
- Pain may be due to raised IOP – acetazolamide is required.

BIBLIOGRAPHY

Casey TA, Mayer DJ. Corneal grafting: principles and practice. London: Saunders; 1981

Lamb K, James MF, Janicki PK. The laryngeal mask airway for intraocular surgery: effects on intraocular pressure and stress responses. British Journal of Anaesthesia 1992; 69:143–147

Steele A, Kirkness C. Manual of systematic corneal surgery. 2nd edn. Butterworth Heinemann; 1999

Sutcliffe NP, Hyde R, Martay K. Use of 'Diprifusor' in anaesthesia for ophthalmic surgery. Anaesthesia 1998; 53(suppl 1):49–52

11

Detachment and vitreous surgery

C. A. Carr

Normal vision requires transparency of the vitreous body and integrity of the retinal layers. These may become disrupted by disease processes and trauma, resulting in separation of the photosensitive layer of the retina from the pigment epithelium with visual loss. Insulin-dependent diabetes mellitus (IDDM), myopia and increasing age predispose to retinal detachment. In IDDM and sickle cell anaemia, abnormal blood vessel growth on the retina can cause vitreous haemorrhages.

PROCEDURE

- Detachment surgery is essentially extraocular.
- The aim is to reoppose the retina to the pigment epithelium with a silicon buckle encircling the sclera over the detachment site.
- This is usually secured by diathermy or cryotherapy to the site.
- Internal tamponade may be provided by intravitreal injection of a gas bubble. This is a mixture of air and a low solubility gas such as sulfur hexafluoride (SF6). Silicone oil may be used as an alternative.
- Vitrectomy is performed for complicated retinal detachments, removal of intravitreal foreign bodies, preretinal membranes and vitreous haemorrhages.
- This is an intraocular procedure.

PATIENT CHARACTERISTICS

- Children with retinopathy of prematurity, IDDM and sickle cell anaemia are susceptible to retinal detachment.
- Adult patients may have associated medical conditions, notably IDDM.

PROBLEMS

- Remote airway and limited access to patient due to vitrectomy equipment

- Operating theatre in darkness for much of the operation
- Surgery may be lengthy
- Oculocardiac reflex
- Laser frequently used and anaesthetist has to wear goggles
- Gas bubbles may be injected into eye at the end of surgery
- Macular detachments need to be operated on within 24 h for best visual result.

PREOPERATIVE ASSESSMENT

- Assessment and optimisation of associated medical conditions, notably IDDM
- For some vitrectomy surgery, aspirin should be stopped for 2 weeks and warfarin therapy controlled to an international normalised ratio (INR) ≤ 2.0 to reduce intraocular haemorrhage at operation.

PREMEDICATION

- Usual perioperative management of IDDM if present
- Anxiolysis with oral temazepam 10–20 mg if required.

ANAESTHETIC MANAGEMENT

MONITORING:
- SpO_2
- ECG
- Non-invasive blood pressure
- $EtCO_2$
- Peripheral nerve stimulator
- Core temperature
- Audio alarms especially important in a dark theatre.

LOCAL ANAESTHESIA

- Suitable in cooperative adults for simple detachment and vitreous surgery, or in the medically compromised.

- Sub-Tenon's anaesthesia or two-injection peribulbar block (as for corneal graft surgery) provides good operating conditions.
- If the procedure is lengthy, sub-Tenon's top-up can readily given by the surgeon.
- Patient comfort is important during lengthy operations, and sedation with small doses of midazolam (0.5–1.0 mg) should be considered.
- Careful monitoring still vital as limited access to patient.

GENERAL ANAESTHESIA

General anaesthesia is the preferred technique for prolonged and complicated surgery.

INDUCTION:

Total intravenous anaesthesia (TIVA) with target-controlled infusion (TCI) of propofol and a remifentanil infusion provides excellent operating conditions.

TIVA provides rapid and smooth emergence from lengthy anaesthesia, with greatly reduced postoperative nausea and vomiting.

Alternatively a balanced technique using intravenous induction with propofol, analgesia (fentanyl), muscle relaxant and volatile agent is suitable.

AIRWAY MANAGEMENT:

- A tracheal tube is needed in view of limited access to patient.
- Muscle relaxation (e.g. vecuronium or rocuronium) – monitor carefully to avoid sudden movement of patient during operation.

MAINTENANCE:

- Ventilate with oxygen in air and avoid nitrous oxide
- Careful positioning and padding of patient
- Consider active warming and intravenous fluids for prolonged procedures or in at-risk patients
- Prophylaxis against the oculocardiac reflex with glycopyrrolate 0.01 mg kg^{-1} intravenously

- Antiemetic prophylaxis with ondansetron 4 mg intravenously
- Administration of sub-Tenon's bupivacaine by surgeon provides intraoperative and postoperative analgesia.

EMERGENCE AND RECOVERY:

- Antagonise neuromuscular block with neostigmine and glycopyrrolate.
- Extubate awake; coughing is usually minimal.

POSTOPERATIVE MANAGEMENT

- Postoperative nausea and vomiting can be a problem, especially after buckling procedures.
- Moderate to severe postoperative pain may require non-steroidal and opioid analgesia.
- Rapid recovery from anaesthesia and postoperative posturing required when gas bubble instilled.

BIBLIOGRAPHY

Charles S, Small KM. Pathogenesis and repair of retinal detachment. In: Easty DL, Sparrow JM, eds. Oxford textbook of ophthalmology, vol 2. Oxford: Oxford Medical Publications; 1999:1261–1272

Mein CE, Woodcock MG. Local anesthesia for vitreoretinal surgery. Retina 1990; 10:47–49

Stinson TW, Donlon JV. Interaction of intraocular air and sulphur hexafluoride with nitrous oxide: a computer simulation. Anesthesiology 1982; 56:385–388

11

Intraocular pressure

C. A. Carr

The balance of the inward pressure exerted by the corneoscleral envelope and extraocular muscles, and the outward pressure exerted by the contents of the globe, results in the intraocular pressure (IOP). Its importance in health is in maintaining the corneal curve and refractive index of the eye.

NORMAL VALUES

- 10–20 mmHg, with up to 3 mmHg difference between the two eyes
- Diurnal variation of up to 5 mmHg – higher in the morning.

PHYSIOLOGY

- The factors that contribute to the IOP in the intact eye are the vitreous volume, the aqueous volume and the choroid plexus volume.
- The vitreous volume is usually constant.
- The aqueous volume is maintained by a balance between production and drainage.
- Aqueous is produced from the ciliary epithelium by a mixture of secretion and ultrafiltration.
- It drains through the trabecular meshwork at the iridocorneal angle into the canal of Schlemm and the episcleral veins into the orbital venous system.
- The volume of the choroid plexus is maintained by autoregulation within physiological variations of systolic pressure.

PATHOLOGY

- Patients with glaucoma may have chronically raised IOP.
- This may be open angle, when the trabecular meshwork becomes non-porous, or closed angle, when the iris obstructs the iridocorneal angle.

- Chronically raised IOP will reduce vascular perfusion of the eye and result in optic nerve ischaemia and infarction.

MEASUREMENT OF IOP

- The IOP is measured indirectly by applanation tonometry. The principle of this is that pressure on the cornea flattens a standard area, or the extent of the flattening is measured.
- A non-contact method is to use a puff of air to flatten the cornea.

FACTORS AFFECTING IOP

ARTERIAL PRESSURE:
- Autoregulation in the retinal and choroidal circulations maintains a constant blood flow over a range of perfusion pressures.
- A sudden rise in arterial pressure may cause a transient rise in IOP but an increase in aqueous outflow and decrease in production will bring the IOP back to normal.
- A reduction in arterial pressure below 90 mmHg reduces the choroidal blood volume and the IOP. IOP will drop to zero at a systolic pressure of 50–60 mmHg.

VENOUS PRESSURE:
- Changes in choroidal blood volume and IOP are more closely related to changes in venous than arterial pressure.
- Venous congestion will cause a rise in IOP due to an increase in choroidal blood volume and a decrease in episcleral vein drainage with consequent reduction in aqueous drainage.
- Venous pressure is increased by coughing, straining, vomiting, Valsalva manoeuvre, obstructed airway, positive-pressure ventilation and obstructed venous drainage of the head.
- Head-up tilt reduces venous pressure. A 15° head-up tilt reduces the IOP to the same

extent as a reduction in $PaCO_2$ to 3.4–4.0 kPa.

BLOOD GASES:

- A rise in PCO_2 due to hypoventilation results in dilatation of the choroidal blood vessels and an increase in IOP.
- A decrease in PCO_2 causes constriction of the choroidal vessels and a fall in IOP.
- Hypoxia may dilate intraocular vessels and increase IOP, whereas hyperoxia may constrict vessels, decreasing IOP. However, the changes seen during anaesthesia will have little effect on the IOP.

ANAESTHESIA:

- Physical interventions by the anaesthetist may raise the IOP.
- Pressure on the eye by the face-mask will raise IOP.
- Laryngoscopy and intubation can markedly raise IOP by increasing the systolic pressure. Various methods have been used to obtund this reflex. The use of propofol with an opiate such as fentanyl or alfentanil for induction successfully reduces this rise.
- Insertion of a laryngeal mask causes a lesser rise in IOP.
- Extubation with coughing or gagging on the tracheal tube causes a rise in IOP.
- There is minimal coughing and straining in patients recovering with a laryngeal mask *in situ*.

ANAESTHETIC AGENTS:

- All intravenous induction agents apart from ketamine will lower IOP.
- Propofol produces the most marked reduction in IOP.
- Ketamine does not lower the IOP and may increase it.
- Inhalation anaesthetics all lower the IOP if there is a normal or low PCO_2.
- Intravenous opioids and benzodiazepines will lower the IOP.
- The non-depolarising muscle relaxants will reduce the IOP by reducing extraocular muscle tone.
- Suxamethonium will cause a rise in IOP that lasts for up to 10 min. However, if it is given after a sleep dose of propofol, the IOP does not rise to above the resting value owing to the drop in IOP caused by the propofol.
- The effect of suxamethonium is due to contraction of the extraocular muscles.

SURGICAL INTERVENTIONS:

- Chronic administration of drugs topically or systemically to lower IOP in chronic glaucoma – these work by affecting aqueous production or drainage, or by constriction of the pupil (Table 11.1).
- To treat acute glaucoma or lower IOP perioperatively, systemic agents such as 20% mannitol, 30% urea solution or oral glycerol may be used. These are osmotic diuretics that shrink the vitreous volume.
- The lid speculum and traction sutures may press on the eye during surgery and may raise the IOP.
- Intraocular gas bubbles such as sulfur hexafluoride (SF6) will expand if the patient is anaesthetised using nitrous oxide. The resultant rise in IOP may compromise perfusion of the optic nerve and retina.

LOCAL ANAESTHESIA:

- Regardless of technique, if a volume greater than 4 ml is used there will be a transient rise in IOP. This falls to normal within a few minutes.
- Oculopressor devices cause an increase in IOP while they are being applied. They

TABLE 11.1

Drugs for treatment of chronic glaucoma

Drug	Mode of action
Miotics	Constrict pupil and open up trabecular meshwork to increase drainage of aqueous.
Carbachol Pilocarpine	Given topically
Beta-blockers	Reduce rate of aqueous formation. Given topically
Timolol Betaxolol	
Carbonic anhydrase inhibitors Acetazolamide (oral) Dorzolamide (topical)	Reduce rate of aqueous formation
α_2-*Adrenoreceptor stimulant* Brimonidine (topical)	Reduce rate of aqueous formation
Prostaglandin analogues Latanoprost (topical)	Increases uveoscleral outflow of aqueous

should not exceed 30 mmHg in applied pressure.

- Once the local anaesthetic is effective, the anaesthetic has spread out in the tissues and the extraocular muscles are relaxed, resulting in a lowering of IOP.

BIBLIOGRAPHY

British Medical Association. British national formulary. London: BMA & RPSGB; 2002

Johnson RW, Forrest FC. Local and general anaesthesia for ophthalmic surgery. Oxford: Butterworth Heinemann; 1994

Murphy DF. Anesthesia and intraocular pressure. Anesthesia and Analgesia 1985; 64:520–530

Saude T. Ocular anatomy and physiology. Oxford: Blackwell Scientific; 1993

CROSS-REFERENCES

Artificial airways
    Anaesthetic Factors 28: 656
Total intravenous anaesthesia
    Techniques 30: 715

11

Penetrating eye injury

C. A. Carr

Eye trauma may result in a spectrum of injury, from superficial laceration of the cornea to complete disruption of the globe with extrusion of the contents. It may be impossible to assess the extent of the injury until the time of surgery. The trauma may be associated with other injuries. There may be a foreign body present.

PROCEDURE

- Exploration and anatomical repair in the first instance
- Removal of foreign body if present.

PATIENT CHARACTERISTICS

- All age groups
- May have coexisting medical conditions
- Presents as an emergency.

PROBLEMS

Open eye with full stomach situation
Delay before surgery for penetrating eye injury may increase risk of loss of contents of globe and increase risk of infection
Associated trauma, particularly of head and neck
Danger of extrusion of globe contents at induction.

PREOPERATIVE ASSESSMENT

- Assessment of associated injuries as resuscitation and urgent operation may be required for non-ophthalmic problems
- If surgery is within 24 h of injury, treat as a full stomach
- Assess airway for rapid sequence induction
- Assess and optimise coexisting medical conditions if time allows.

PREMEDICATION

- Sedation and antiemetics may be required, especially in tearful children
- Amethocaine (Ametop) or EMLA cream over venepuncture site in children
- Do not attempt to empty stomach before operation as crying, struggling or vomiting will increase the IOP.

ANAESTHETIC MANAGEMENT

MONITORING:
- $Sp\text{CO}_2$
- ECG
- Non-invasive blood pressure
- $Et\text{CO}_2$
- Temperature
- Peripheral nerve stimulator.

LOCAL ANAESTHESIA

Regional techniques are unsuitable. They all cause an initial rise in IOP and the injury may be more extensive than initially assessed.

GENERAL ANAESTHESIA

INDUCTION:
- There is a conflict of possible full stomach and the need for rapid sequence induction with the need to protect the eye from a rise in IOP.
- Suxamethonium causes a transient rise in IOP.
- Laryngoscopy and intubation also produce a significant rise in IOP.

Modified rapid sequence technique
May be used in experienced hands. Obtain intravenous access. Preoxygenate without pressing on eye with face-mask. Give alfentanil 0.02 mg kg^{-1}, vecuronium 0.25 mg kg^{-1}, then

propofol 3 mg kg^{-1} and apply cricoid pressure. Intubation can be performed at 90 s without coughing.

Standard rapid sequence technique
Intubation with suxamethonium, if inexperienced or anticipated difficult intubation. Use of propofol as induction agent (markedly lowers IOP) will protect against rise in IOP due to suxamethonium. Administration of lidocaine (lignocaine) 1.0 mg kg^{-1} prior to induction will attenuate rise in IOP due to laryngoscopy and intubation.

MAINTENANCE:
- With balanced technique or TIVA
- Careful monitoring of relaxation to ensure immobile patient
- Antiemetic prophylaxis
- Analgesia with non-steroidal agent or opiate.

EMERGENCE AND RECOVERY:
- Antagonism of neuromuscular block
- Extubate awake.

POSTOPERATIVE MANAGEMENT

- Antiemetics prescribed for postoperative nausea and vomiting
- Moderate postoperative pain may require non-steroidal or opioid analgesia on first postoperative day.

BIBLIOGRAPHY

Lennon RL, Olson RA, Gronert GA. Atracurium or vecuronium for rapid sequence endotracheal intubation. Anesthesiology 1986; 64:510–513

MacEwan CJ. Eye injuries: a prospective survey of 5671 cases. British Journal of Ophthalmology 1989; 73:888–894

Mirakhur RK, Shepherd WFI, Darrah WC. Propofol and thiopentone: effects on intraocular pressure associated with induction of anaesthesia and tracheal intubation (facilitated with suxamethonium). British Journal of Anaesthesia 1987; 59:437–439

Smith RB, Babinski M, Leano N. The effect of lidocaine on succinylcholine induced rise in intraocular pressure. Canadian Anaesthetists Society Journal 1979; 26:482–483

CROSS-REFERENCES

Emergency surgery
    Anaesthetic Factors 27: 619
Trauma
    Anaesthetic Factors 31: 797
Infants and children
    Surgical Procedures 27: 610

11

Strabismus correction

C. A. Carr

Misalignment of the visual axes may result in double vision (diplopia), loss of visual acuity (amblyopia) or loss of binocular vision. This occurs in about 5% of children; treatment usually requires surgical correction. Adults may require strabismus surgery due to thyroid eye disease, trauma, sixth cranial nerve palsy and following strabismus surgery as a child.

PROCEDURE

Surgery takes 20–90 min and is routinely managed as a day case.
- *Recession* – weakening an extraocular muscle by moving its insertion on the globe
- *Resection* – strengthening an extraocular muscle by removing a short piece of tendon or muscle
- *Adjustable sutures* – used in some adult patients to allow final adjustments to be made with eye movements after operation.

PATIENT CHARACTERISTICS

- The most common ophthalmic operation carried out in children
- Infantile strabismus needs early operation (6–12 months) for best visual outcome
- May be associated with congenital syndromes
- Rare association with muscle disorders and malignant hyperthermia
- Adult patients may have associated medical conditions.

PROBLEMS

- Remote airway
- Suxamethonium to be avoided as it may trigger malignant hyperthermia in susceptible patients and causes tonic contracture of extraocular muscles. This interferes with the forced duction test

- Oculocardiac reflex
- Topical adrenaline (epinephrine) is often used to reduce bleeding and may be absorbed systemically – watch dose in small children
- High incidence of postoperative nausea and vomiting.

PREOPERATIVE ASSESSMENT

- Identification, investigation and optimisation of associated syndromes or coexisting medical conditions
- Assess suitability for day-case surgery.

PREMEDICATION

- Anxiolysis if required (e.g. temazepam 10–20 mg orally in adults, midazolam 0.5 mg kg^{-1} orally in children)
- Amethocaine (Ametop) or EMLA cream to venepuncture site in children
- Anticholinergic prophylaxis for oculocardiac reflex is best given intravenously at induction.

ANAESTHETIC MANAGEMENT

MONITORING:
- SpO_2
- ECG
- Non-invasive blood pressure
- $EtCO_2$
- Core temperature
- Peripheral nerve stimulator.

LOCAL ANAESTHETIC

- May be used in cooperative adult patients for uncomplicated surgery
- Topical anaesthesia with 1.0% amethocaine allows optimal adjustment of muscle

sutures at the time of surgery. The oculocardiac reflex is not blocked; ECG monitoring and possible use of anticholinergics required
- Sub-Tenon's or peribulbar blocks (as for cataract surgery) are suitable and provide protection from the oculocardiac reflex.

GENERAL ANAESTHESIA

INDUCTION:
- Intravenous or inhalation as appropriate
- Prophylaxis against oculocardiac reflex with glycopyrrolate 0.01 mg kg^{-1} intravenously at induction
- Airway management – laryngeal mask unless contraindicated by patient factors.

MAINTENANCE:
- TIVA with propofol and remifentanil infusions provides excellent conditions and reduces postoperative nausea and vomiting.
- Non-depolarising relaxant (e.g. vecuronium or rocuronium) if intubation required. A small dose (half intubating dose) required for maintenance with TIVA to ensure a central immobile eye.
- Alternatively, use a balanced technique with fentanyl, muscle relaxant and volatile agent.

MAINTENANCE:
- Ventilation to normal EtCO$_2$
- Prophylactic antiemetic – ondansetron 0.01 mg kg^{-1} intravenously
- Analgesia with diclofenac 2 mg kg^{-1} or paracetamol 30 mg kg^{-1} rectally in children
- 1–2 ml 0.5% bupivacaine sub-Tenon's at the end of surgery gives good postoperative analgesia if adjustable sutures not used
- Alternatively, codeine phosphate 1 mg kg^{-1} intramuscularly for more extensive bilateral surgery.

EMERGENCE AND RECOVERY:
- Antagonise neuromuscular block with neostigmine and glycopyrrolate
- Extubate and remove laryngeal mask when awake.

POSTOPERATIVE MANAGEMENT

- Topical amethocaine at end of surgery for immediate postoperative pain
- Moderate postoperative pain on first day – oral paracetamol usually sufficient
- Antiemetics prescribed, but postoperative nausea and vomiting may be delayed until after discharge.

BIBLIOGRAPHY

Blanc VF, Hardy JF, Milot J, Jacob JL. The oculocardiac reflex: a graphic and statistical analysis in infants and children. Canadian Anaesthetists Society Journal 1983; 30:360–369

Carroll JB. Increased incidence of masseter spasm in children with strabismus anaesthetized with halothane and succinylcholine. Anesthesiology 1987; 67:559–561

Ing MR. Early surgical alignment for congenital esotropia. Ophthalmology 1983; 90:132–135

Mirakhur RK, Jones CJ, Dundee JW, Archer DB. I.m. or i.v. atropine or glycopyrrolate for the prevention of the oculocardiac reflex in children undergoing squint surgery. British Journal of Anaesthesia 1982; 54:1059–1063

Weir PM, Munro HM, Reynolds PI, Lewis IH, Wilton NCT. Propofol infusion and the incidence of emesis in paediatric outpatient strabismus surgery. Anesthesia and Analgesia 1993; 76:760–764

11

12

ENT SURGERY
S. M. Mostafa

Laryngoscopy and microsurgery of the larynx

P. Charters

The laryngeal inlet is the narrowest part of the upper airway. For safe management, the anaesthetist and surgeon must share responsibility. The anaesthetist needs to understand the nature and types of pathologies commonly encountered and the surgical operating requirements. Surgical work-up can provide valuable information about anatomical disturbances and assist in planning airway management.

PATIENT CHARACTERISTICS

- Often older age groups with significant co-morbidity.
- Squamous carcinoma of the larynx is associated with long-standing cigarette and alcohol consumption, and disabling cardiorespiratory and hepatic disease.
- Cigarette consumption increases airway hyperreactivity.

PREOPERATIVE ASSESSMENT

- Routine assessment of associated medical conditions.
- Appropriate investigations depend on the history and examination.
- ENT assessment of the airway, by indirect laryngoscopy and/or fibreoptic nasendoscopy.
- Radiological imaging is used to determine the extent and nature of the pathology.
- Clinical assessment for respiratory distress and presence of stridor.

PREMEDICATION

- Patients should be warned of possible temporary breathing difficulty after surgery.
- Premedication is usually unnecessary and may compromise any airway narrowing.
- Antisialogogues may decrease secretions but also make what remains thicker.

- Patients with significant stridor require oxygen during transport. (A heliox mixture can mitigate their symptoms by improving gas flow.)

THEATRE PREPARATION AND MONITORING

- Monitoring should include the routine standards of ECG, non-invasive blood pressure, SaO_2, $EtCO_2$, airway pressure, disconnection alarm and, when appropriate, neuromuscular blockade.
- Difficult intubation trolley with equipment that the anaesthetist can use and tracheal airway access devices (e.g. emergency tracheostomy) may be required.
- Position is as for most head and neck surgery – head-ring ± sandbag beneath shoulders, with due care. Excessive neck extension may cause injury.

GENERAL PRINCIPLES OF ANAESTHETIC TECHNIQUE

The main problems concern sharing the airway with the surgeon to enable access. Prevention of hypoxic brain damage is more difficult when the airway is abnormal. Induction of general anaesthesia in a compromised airway may result in total obstruction. Generally, supraglottic lesions block the view of the laryngeal inlet, glottic lesions narrow it, and subglottic lesions cause narrowing beyond what can be seen with a Macintosh laryngoscope. Neoplastic lesions can be friable and prone to bleeding with instrumentation, obscuring the view further. Airway manipulations may result in laryngeal oedema and a worse airway at reversal. The surgeon may debulk a tumour to relieve airway narrowing. The anaesthetist must anticipate the likely state of the airway at recovery and any continued bleeding.

12

- Intubation is usually necessary.
- Muscle relaxants may not be needed to effect intubation but in any case should be administered only when assisted ventilation and/or intubation are certain.
- In severely narrowed airways, elective tracheostomy under local anaesthesia may be the best option but it may be difficult in a hypoxic, distressed, uncooperative patient with an adverse neck.
- General anaesthesia alternatives include inhalation induction with sevoflurane or a 'quick look' with a small dose of propofol. (In each case the aim is to avoid apnoea and to test assisted ventilation and/or intubation conditions.) Alternatively, awake intubation is indicated.
- Surgery on the vocal cords (for biopsies or cord stripping) usually requires the patient to be fully relaxed, although assessment of vocal cord movements may need to be considered at some stage.
- Teflon injection in paralysed vocal cords (to increase bulk and decrease aspiration risk) can lead to airway obstruction. Tables anaesthesia under local or general anaesthesia (see below) best monitors the effect of the volume injected.
- Manipulation of the larynx can cause a hypertensive response and cardiac arrhythmias.
- A rapid return of consciousness and protective reflexes should be achieved whether anaesthesia is of short or prolonged duration.
- Aspiration of blood and surgical debris is possible.

ANAESTHETIC TECHNIQUE

The choice of anaesthetic technique depends on the condition of the patient at the time of surgery and the individual preference and expertise of the anaesthetist.

Cardiovascular stability, avoidance of awareness and a smooth, rapid recovery are essential.

An intravenous induction is suitable for most patients followed by maintenance with a balanced type of anaesthesia using oxygen, nitrous oxide and a volatile agent plus an opioid. A total intravenous anaesthetic (TIVA) technique is a useful alternative. This can also be used to avoid the use of muscle relaxants, although hypotension may be a problem in elderly patients. Muscle relaxation using one of the shorter-acting relaxants (e.g. miva-

curium) is usual with volatile anaesthesia. Occasionally a spontaneous breathing technique is used.

AIRWAY MAINTENANCE

- *Tracheal intubation* is the standard airway management but the need for optimal access to the vocal cords has led to alternative methods. A microlaryngoscopy tube is a tube of normal length for adults but with a small diameter. Tubes with an internal diameter of 4.0–6.0 mm are available. Such tubes have high resistance and can result in difficult ventilation of obese subjects. Nevertheless, tracheal intubation should be considered the expected technique, with other methods of ventilation the domain of specialist units because of the increased risk of aspiration and less certain airway control.
- *'Tubeless anaesthesia'* describes methods in which there is no tube between the vocal cords. One method uses intubation lower down the airway, for example cricothyroid puncture (usually with jet or high-frequency ventilation). A second method uses no tube at all, with the patient breathing spontaneously.
- *Tracheal catheter* – Various types of catheter have been used (typical diameter 14 Fr) with insertion through the cords down to the carina to deliver anaesthetic gases. Apart from increased aspiration risk, catheters tend to move with the driving gas and cause soft tissue injury by a flailing effect within the trachea.
- *Venturi jet ventilation* is when an 'injected' driving gas entrains room air. Injectors typically use oxygen as the driving gas. The injector source is firmly attached to a rigid bronchoscope to limit backlash. Ventilation is most effective when the bronchoscope tip is low down in, and well aligned with, the trachea. There is a risk of barotrauma.
- *High-frequency ventilation* uses smaller tidal perturbation at higher rates (60–100 per min) and requires specialised ventilators to deliver the driving gas, usually via a catheter below the vocal cords. The risk of barotrauma is less than with Venturi ventilation.

With any of the specialised ventilation alternatives, the important considerations are a clear route for inhalation and expiration, and awareness of the inevitable loss of normal ventilation monitoring (e.g. tidal volume, airway pressure

12

and $EtCO_2$). Hypoventilation and awareness may occur, particularly in patients who are obese or have poor pulmonary compliance. Inexperience and poor technique are also risk factors. TIVA removes dependence on the breathing circuit to maintain depth of anaesthesia. When no tube is used and the patient breathes spontaneously, local anaesthesia spray to the vocal cords decreases the need for deeper planes of anaesthesia. Close cooperation between surgeon and anaesthetist is essential. Suitability for this type of airway management must be on a case-by-case assessment.

AIRWAY MAINTENANCE FOR ANAESTHESIA FOR LASER SURGERY

Lasers are used for excision of various laryngeal lesions as they allow accurate incision and minimal tissue reaction and postoperative swelling. Carbon dioxide or neodymium–yttrium–aluminium–garnet (NdYAG)-type lasers are usual. Safety considerations for theatre staff are mandatory to prevent direct and incidental burns. The eyes are at particular risk, requiring the use of special protective glasses. When more extensive surgery is employed, the usual axial direction of the laser beam down the airway indicates the tissues most at risk from ignition. The tracheal tube itself can take fire.

FIRE PRECAUTIONS AND TREATING A FIRE

Tracheal tubes will ignite under the right conditions, and oxygen and nitrous oxide both support combustion. A 30% mixture of oxygen in nitrogen is an alternative. Specially designed, laser resistant, flexo-metallic tubes are recommended. Tube cuffs are at risk of penetration by the laser beam. These tubes have double cuffs filled with saline. The surgeon applies saline-soaked gauze pads to protect the cuffs and local soft tissue further. Wet towel drapes are used around the surgical field. If 'tubeless anaesthesia' (see above) is used instead of a laser tube, there may be increased risk of inadvertent laser injury to tissue lower down the airway. Restriction of

laser beam use to short bursts rather than continuous cutting is said to reduce the risk of fire.

When fire does occur, the first priority is to extinguish it and disconnect the gas supply to avoid further injury. Saline flushing with a syringe can be used to cool the tissue and limit secondary damage. The damaged tracheal tube will normally need to be replaced, and for this reason entirely metallic tubes are available which should be readily to hand. Reactive oedema occurs rapidly. Oxygen administration is resumed as soon as this is considered safe. The patient should be treated as having an inhalational burn injury and looked after in intensive care to monitor and treat serious complications.

POSTOPERATIVE COMPLICATIONS

- *Immediate* – transient respiratory distress; sore throat; hoarseness; laryngospasm; bleeding; stridor; oedema and aspiration of blood and surgical debris.
- *On return to the ward* – any or all of the above. Early discharge is appropriate only for carefully selected patients in whom risks are considered minimal.
- *Long-term* – tissue scarring may result and the original pathology may progress if appropriate treatment is delayed. Where radiation is the treatment for malignancy there is increased risk of reactive laryngeal oedema in the early stages.

BIBLIOGRAPHY

Rees L, Mason RA. Advanced upper airway obstruction in ENT surgery. British Journal of Anaesthesia, CEPD Reviews 2002; 2:134–138

CROSS-REFERENCES

Difficult airway – difficult tracheal intubation
    Anaesthetic Factors 28: 666
Awareness
    Anaesthetic Factors 31: 727

12

Middle ear surgery

C. Parker

PROCEDURES

Middle ear surgery involves careful dissection of small structures, such as the ossicles, using an operating microscope. The operation may take 2–3 h. These patients are not usually managed as day cases.

PREOPERATIVE INVESTIGATION

Assessment and investigations are dictated by the patient's general condition. No specific preoperative considerations arise in these patients, unless controlled hypotension is contemplated. Patients may be of any age.

PRINCIPLES OF THE ANAESTHETIC

Surgery will be made impossible by bleeding. The severity of bleeding is related as much to venous as to arterial blood pressure. Attention to the following principles ensures a satisfactory operating field:
- A clear airway is essential. A partially obstructed airway impedes expiration and raises venous pressure. An armoured endotracheal tube avoids kinking.
- Anaesthesia should be conducted smoothly. The trachea is intubated only after full muscle relaxation. Topical lidocaine (lignocaine) spray to the larynx and trachea may help to prevent subsequent responses. Straining and coughing must be avoided because they increase venous pressure and hence bleeding.
- Venous pressure should be minimised. A head-up tilt of 10–15° helps to minimise bleeding. Head posture should be adjusted to avoid extremes, which would cause venous occlusion. Neck strain and arterial narrowing should also be avoided.
- Tachycardia should be avoided. Atropine should not be given. Beta-blockers are

useful. The author titrates small doses of atenolol intravenously.
- Induced hypotension has been recommended and may be requested by the surgeon. Profound hypotension is unnecessary and may be harmful. The author does not reduce systolic blood pressure below preoperative diastolic pressure.

PREMEDICATION

Premedication is with diazepam orally.

ANAESTHETIC TECHNIQUE

The particular choice of anaesthetic agents is not crucial. The author usually ventilates the patient artificially using a tracheal tube. The main anaesthetic agents are propofol, cisatracurium, fentanyl and desflurane.

The eyes should be protected.

Two other issues may arise in middle ear surgery and influence the choice of anaesthetic technique:
- If the surgeon wishes to monitor facial nerve integrity using a nerve stimulator, muscle relaxation, induced by mivacurium, is allowed to wear off. The patient can then breathe spontaneously. Lidocaine (lignocaine) spray to the trachea prior to intubation allows the tracheal tube to be tolerated without very deep anaesthesia. Some anaesthetists control ventilation, facilitated by an infusion of remifentanil.
- The middle ear is a closed air-filled cavity. Nitrous oxide is 30 times more soluble, and hence diffusible, than nitrogen. During the early part of an anaesthetic, nitrous oxide will enter a closed cavity faster than nitrogen can leave; pressure will rise. In the recovery period nitrous oxide will diffuse out more rapidly than nitrogen can enter, and converse effects occur. The position of

12

tympanoplasty grafts can be affected. If nitrous oxide is to be avoided, advanced planning and clear communication between the surgeon and anaesthetist is necessary. The ear is bandaged at the end of the procedure. To prevent displacement of the tracheal tube and trauma to the eyes, the anaesthetist should supervise this.

MONITORING

- Minimal monitoring standards apply.
- Neuromuscular transmission should be monitored continuously.
- Invasive blood pressure monitoring is essential during hypotensive anaesthesia.

RECOVERY

Nausea, vomiting and dizziness can be a particular problem following these procedures. A suitable antiemetic agent should be given. Pain is not usually severe.

BIBLIOGRAPHY

Donlon JV Jr. Anesthesia for eye, ear, nose and throat surgery. In: Miller RD, ed. Anesthesia. 5th edn. Philadelphia: Churchill Livingstone; 2000:2173–2198

CROSS-REFERENCES

Induced hypotension, anaesthesia
    Anaesthetic Factors 30: 704

12

Oesophagoscopy

C. Parker

PROCEDURE

Oesophagoscopy can be performed using a rigid or flexible oesophagoscope. General anaesthesia is required for rigid oesophagoscopy. Sedation is usual for flexible oesophagoscopy.

INDICATIONS FOR RIGID OESOPHAGOSCOPY

- Removal of a foreign body
- Assessment and biopsy of lesions of the oesophagus
- Assessment of lesions of the lower pharynx and the postcricoid region
- Intubation or dilatation of an oesophageal stricture
- Endoscopic treatment of pharyngeal pouch.

PATIENT CHARACTERISTICS

Consideration must be given to the following:
- The oesophagus may be partially or totally obstructed, with food and saliva above the obstruction. The patient may be suffering from gastro-oesophageal reflux. These factors pose a risk of aspiration.
- Prolonged oesophageal obstruction will cause weight loss, anaemia and dehydration.
- Silent aspiration of oesophageal contents, in the weeks leading up to the oesophagoscopy, can cause pneumonia, basal lung collapse or a lung abscess.
- Rarely, a patient with a neurological or neuromuscular disease presents with dysphagia.

PREOPERATIVE INVESTIGATION AND PREPARATION

Investigations are dictated by the patient's general condition and the indication for surgery. Dehydration should be corrected before operation, and chest infections treated.

PREMEDICATION

- Sedation should be avoided. Glycopyrrolate 0.2 mg i.m. can be given to reduce secretions.
- Pharmacological means can be used to raise gastric pH. If so, remember that H_2-receptor antagonists and proton pump inhibitors do not neutralise existing acid. They require several hours to be effective.
  —Acid is not the only threat. Blood and residual food are still a potential problem.
  —The use of such medication does not remove the need to protect the airway during induction.

PRINCIPLES OF THE ANAESTHETIC

The following principles apply:
- The airway is shared with the surgeon. Close cooperation and communication with the surgeon is required.
- Tracheal intubation is necessary.
- There is a risk of regurgitation of oesophageal contents. The airway is protected during induction, using cricoid pressure.
- The tracheal tube can be compressed, kinked or displaced by the surgeon. A reinforced tracheal tube prevents kinking and compression. Ventilation by hand allows immediate detection of such events. If a mechanical ventilator is used, careful attention to airway pressure alarms is required.
- Use of a tracheal tube smaller than usual, and deflation of the cuff, make it easier to pass the oesophagoscope.
- Coughing, straining and movement during oesophagoscopy make the procedure difficult, and risk oesophageal perforation.

12

The patient should be immobile during surgery.

- Insertion of an oesophagoscope is highly stimulating, and is sustained for several minutes. The result is hypertension, tachycardia and, sometimes, myocardial ischaemia and arrhythmias.
- Biopsy of oesophageal lesions and the presence of varices can cause serious bleeding.
- The operation is of relatively short duration.
- Airway reflexes should be intact at the end of surgery, so that the patient can protect the airway after extubation.

ANAESTHETIC TECHNIQUE

An intravenous drip should be sited. Suction apparatus must be checked and switched on.

Rapid sequence induction with preoxygenation, application of cricoid pressure and tracheal intubation minimise the risk of aspiration. The author has the patient supine with a small head-up tilt. Alternative positions have been proposed and may offer theoretical advantages, but they carry their own hazards and make intubation more difficult. The tracheal tube is moved to the left side of the mouth to facilitate passage of the oesophagoscope. The patient's eyes must be protected.

The author usually uses propofol for induction and suxamethonium to provide muscle relaxation, unless it is contraindicated. If muscle relaxation needs to be continued after suxamethonium has worn off, mivacurium is used. Anaesthesia is maintained with oxygen, nitrous oxide and desflurane. The use of these agents facilitates prompt recovery of airway reflexes.

Cardiovascular disturbances are common. Blood pressure may fall profoundly due to the effect of the anaesthetic drugs on a background of undiagnosed hypovolaemia in a cachectic patient. Intravenous fluid and a small dose of vasopressor deal with this problem. On the other hand, stimulation of the procedure can cause hypertension, tachycardia and myocardial ischaemia. Hypertension and tachycardia are treated with small doses of fentanyl. If tachycardia persists and is a problem, a small intravenous dose of atenolol is given.

MONITORING

Minimal monitoring standards should be followed. Neuromuscular transmission should be monitored with a nerve stimulator.

RECOVERY

The risk of aspiration continues until full recovery. Extubate only when the patient is awake with full recovery of muscle power. This can be achieved rapidly with modern agents. If there is any doubt about whether the patient's recovery satisfies these criteria, the patient should be supervised by the anaesthetist in the lateral position, with suction available. Instrumentation by either surgeon or anaesthetist may damage teeth, lips or mouth. These structures should be examined after the trachea has been intubated, and again after surgery. Complaints of pain on swallowing are taken seriously. Perforation of the oesophagus, with pneumomediastinum, surgical emphysema and pneumothorax, is the feared risk. Chest radiography should be performed if there is any suspicion of perforation. Intravenous fluids should be prescribed after operation as patients remain nil by mouth for several hours.

CROSS-REFERENCES

Disorders of the oesophagus and swallowing
    Patient Conditions 5: 162
Hiatus hernia
    Patient Conditions 5: 166

Operations on the nose

D. T. Moloney

Nasal operations make up a large amount of the ENT workload. They are often simple and straightforward, for example manipulation of nasal bones or polypectomy. Occasionally, the procedures may be more prolonged, as in septorhinoplasty and extensive functional endoscopic sinus surgery.

As is the case with many ENT procedures, the airway is 'shared'. Cooperation between surgeon and anaesthetist is essential. An unhindered operating field is required, and coughing and straining should be avoided.

COMMON PROBLEMS

- Patients with polyps often have a history of atopy or the triad of asthma, polyps and aspirin sensitivity.
- Postnasal drip and recurrent chest infections are common.
- Patients with nasal fractures may have sustained other injuries or swallowed a significant amount of blood.

PREOPERATIVE ASSESSMENT AND PREPARATION

- History and examination with particular regard to identify the above problems.
- Treat chest infections and optimise chronic medical conditions (e.g. asthma).
- Correct hypovolaemia in patients who have bled.
- Investigations are dependent on the patient's current condition.

PREMEDICATION

- Most patients do not require premedication.
- Benzodiazepines for the over-anxious.

NASAL VASOCONSTRICTORS

Because the nose is highly vascular, some vasoconstriction, in order to decrease bleeding, is advantageous. The following may be used:
- Topical cocaine 4–10% solution – this is now less popular because of adverse effects.
- Moffett's solution (a mixture of cocaine, sodium bicarbonate, 1 : 1000 adrenaline (epinephrine) and sterile water) is still used for sinus surgery.
- Direct injection of local analgesic with 1 : 100 000 or 1 : 200 000 adrenaline at the start of the procedure.
- Lidocaine (lignocaine) 5% and phenylephrine 0.5% spray.
- Less frequently used vasoconstrictors include ephedrine, xylometazoline and felypressin.

PERIOPERATIVE ANAESTHETIC MANAGEMENT

- Standard monitoring including Sao_2, ECG, non-invasive blood pressure, $Etco_2$, disconnection alarm.
- Some operations such as septoplasty may be performed under local anaesthesia with sedation in cooperative patients. However, most nasal operations require a general anaesthetic.
- Rapid sequence induction is appropriate in patients undergoing surgery who have swallowed a significant amount of blood.
- The choice of induction agent will be influenced by factors such as anaesthetist's preference and patient's condition.
- The airway may be secured with a tracheal tube, commonly a preformed tube or, if no contraindications exist, a flexible laryngeal mask. A throat pack is then inserted. All connections must be absolutely secure as once the operation is underway access to the airway will be difficult.

12

Techniques commonly used include:

- Tracheal intubation using suxamethonium and then allowing the patient to breathe spontaneously or with controlled ventilation.
- Intubation using a non-depolarising agent and then controlled ventilation.
- Spontaneous respiration through a laryngeal mask.
- Maintenance can be achieved with either inhalation agents and narcotic or a total intravenous technique (TIVA) plus muscle relaxants. Halothane is avoided because of the incidence of arrythmias associated with the use of vasoconstrictors in the nose.
- The eyes should be taped closed and covered with protective pads. However, for sinus surgery the eyes are covered only by clear sterile tape so that the surgeon can see the eyes, as surgery is in close proximity to the orbit and optic nerve.
- Nasal surgery is often performed in the head-up position to reduce bleeding. Hypotension may occur. The thighs can be flexed at the hip to improve venous return.
- Patients with polyps occasionally receive a preoperative course of steroids. Perioperative steroid cover should be considered.

SAFE USE OF A PHARYNGEAL PACK

A throat pack is used to prevent blood and debris from contaminating the airway or being swallowed. The most common form of pack is wetted gauze, but some anaesthetists use sponge packs. The pack should be inserted under direct vision with Magill forceps and the tail of gauze left to protrude from the mouth to remind the anaesthetist of its presence at the end of surgery. An adhesive label may be applied as a further reminder, and in some centres the gauze is included in the final swab count.

When the procedure is complete and the throat pack removed, direct pharyngoscopy is performed to ensure that the pack has been removed completely, and any remaining blood clots or debris are aspirated.

POSTOPERATIVE MANAGEMENT

- The patient is extubated in the lateral position, but is sat up as early as possible to decrease bleeding.
- Encourage the patient to breathe through the mouth because nose packs are often inserted at the end of the operation.
- Plasters and tape applied to the nose may make the application of a facemask difficult.
- Administer oxygen in recovery in a routine fashion.
- Leave the intravenous cannula *in situ* in case of bleeding.
- Repacking may be necessary should bleeding from the nose continue.
- Analgesia will be required. Regular paracetamol with or without a non-steroidal anti-inflammatory drug (NSAID) is often sufficient, but opioids are needed following more extensive surgery.

BIBLIOGRAPHY

Webster AC, Morley-Forster PK, Janzen V et al. Anesthesia for intranasal surgery: a comparison between tracheal intubation and the flexible reinforced laryngeal mask airway. Anesthesia and Analgesia 1999; 88:421–425

Williams PJ, Thompsett C, Bailey PM. Comparison of the reinforced laryngeal mask and tracheal intubation for nasal surgery. Anaesthesia 1995; 50:987–989

12

Tonsillectomy and adenoidectomy

J. Beattie

PROCEDURE

Adenoidectomy and/or tonsillectomy are performed through the mouth. A Boyle–Davis gag is used for tonsillectomy. Difficulties may be encountered because of:

- Shared airway
- Difficult mask ventilation or intubation in patients with enlarged lymphoid tissue
- Poorly placed surgical gag obstructing the tracheal tube or laryngeal mask airway
- Postoperative bleeding.

Some centres choose to treat these patients as day cases. Concerns about postoperative bleeding may limit the number of centres adopting this approach.

PATIENT CHARACTERISTICS

- Children and young adults are usually operated on for chronic or recurrent infections.
- Some may have obstructive sleep apnoea or congenital abnormalities (e.g. Down syndrome).
- Older adults for tonsillectomy may have malignancy and other incidental medical conditions.
- Some have cor pulmonale as a result of long-term hypoxia.

PREOPERATIVE ASSESSMENT AND INVESTIGATIONS

- A thorough airway assessment must be performed.
- History of sleep apnoea must be carefully explored.
- Bleeding disorders are important in the patient or immediate family.
- Patients presenting on the day of surgery with an acute infection should be deferred. Except in an emergency, patients should be operated on when well.

- Tests required include full blood count, group and save, clotting studies if indicated by the history.
- Specific consent should be taken for administration of rectal analgesia.

PREMEDICATION

- Local anaesthetic gels (EMLA, Ametop) should be applied to children who request an intravenous induction.
- Sedative premedication should not be given to those with airway obstruction or a history of sleep apnoea.
- An anxiolytic may be advantageous, for example benzodiazepines for adults or older children and oral trimeprazine (1.5–2 mg kg^{-1}) or midazolam (0.05 mg kg^{-1}) for children over 2 years old.

PERIOPERATIVE MANAGEMENT

- Standard monitoring should be applied to all patients and provision made to assess blood loss.
- Intravenous or inhalational induction can be used.
- Patients are usually intubated with a 'south facing' preformed tracheal tube. Some surgeons prefer a nasal tube for tonsillectomy in adult patients.
- Check the length and patency of the tracheal tube before surgery begins.
- Intubation may be difficult because of large tonsils, but can be achieved using suxamethonium or a non-depolarising muscle relaxant, depending on personal preference.
- Oral tubes must be carefully secured in the midline to lie correctly in the Boyle–Davies gag.
- With experienced senior personnel and a regular surgical–anaesthetic team, the reinforced laryngeal mask may be used for

12

tonsillectomy. Surgeons must avoid soiling of the airway with blood.

- Patients are positioned with the neck extended.
- The eyes must be protected.
- Instrumentation of the postnasal space during adenoidectomy may induce a bradycardia requiring treatment with atropine.
- Peroperative opioid analgesia is usually required with oral or rectal paracetamol and non-steroidal drugs thereafter.
- Extubation can be accomplished either deep or awake depending on preference and the skills of recovery room staff, but patients should be in the head-down lateral position.
- Infiltration of local anaesthetic into the tonsillar bed provides good postoperative analgesia.
- Blind or aggressive suctioning of the pharynx may cause bleeding from the tonsillar bed and should be avoided.

POSTOPERATIVE MANAGEMENT

- Non-steroidal analgesics have not been found to increase bleeding significantly in patients undergoing tonsillectomy.
- Intravenous fluids are not usually required as swallowing is to be encouraged.
- Intravenous cannulae should be left *in situ* in case of early postoperative bleeding.
- Bleeding may not be detected in children until vomiting occurs.

CREUTZFELDT–JAKOB DISEASE

Transmission of prion-borne diseases, including variant Creutzfeldt–Jakob disease (vCJD), is theoretically possible with contamination of equipment during surgery on lymphoid tissues. Prions have been found in tonsillar tissue of patients with no clinical signs of vCJD. Prions are not reliably destroyed by standard surgical sterilisation. Department of Health guidelines required the use of disposable surgical and anaesthetic equipment for tonsillectomy and adenoidectomy between January and December 2001. This was revised owing to an increase in morbidity due to bleeding. The theoretical risk must, however, always be borne in mind. Single-use anaesthetic equipment, such as tracheal tubes, laryngoscope blades (or disposable sheath covering it and its handle), bougies and laryngeal mask airways, must be considered.

PERIOPERATIVE MANAGEMENT OF THE BLEEDING TONSIL

These patients require the skills of senior, experienced anaesthetists.

- Blood loss is difficult to assess as much is swallowed.
- Resuscitation with intravenous fluids and/or blood must be guided by cardiovascular parameters appropriate to the patient's age.
- Patients will have a full stomach and a potentially difficult airway with blood in the pharynx and local oedema following recent intubation.
- The recent anaesthetic record should be studied for any indication of previous airway difficulties.
- Some patients may not be fully recovered following the first anaesthetic.

INTRAOPERATIVE MANAGEMENT

- Patients should be resuscitated and have full monitoring applied.
- Suction must be immediately available and head-down tilt may keep blood away from the larynx.
- A rapid sequence intravenous induction or an inhalational induction with cricoid pressure can be used, depending on the skills of the anaesthetist. *Use the technique with which you are most familiar and which will allow the airway to be safely secured.*
- Intubation may require a size smaller endotracheal tube.
- Volume resuscitation should continue throughout the operation.
- After surgery, carefully pass a large bore orogastric or nasogastric tube to empty the stomach.
- Patients should be extubated head-down on their side and fully awake.

POSTOPERATIVE MANAGEMENT

- Patients may require midazolam or opioid analgesia to tolerate postnasal space packs if bleeding has occurred after adenoidectomy. This requires observation on a high-dependency unit because of the risk of airway obstruction.
- Check the haemoglobin level and transfuse if necessary.
- Patients should be closely monitored for further bleeding.

12

BIBLIOGRAPHY

Bolger WE, Parsons DS, Potempa L. Preoperative assessment of the adenotonsillectomy patient. Otolaryngology, Head and Neck Surgery 1990; 103:396–405

Nordbladh I, Ohlander B, Bjorkman R. Analgesia in tonsillectomy: a double blind study on pre- and post-operative treatment with diclofenac. Clinics in Otolaryngology 1991; 16:554–558

Reiner SA, Sawyer WL, Clark KF, Wood MW. The safety of outpatient tonsillectomy and adenoidectomy. Otolaryngology, Head and Neck Surgery 1990; 102:161–168

Tewary AK. Day case tonsillectomy: a review of the literature. Journal of Laryngology and Otology 1993; 107:703–705

12

Tracheostomy

R. Wenstone

Surgical

Anaesthesia is usually general with tracheal intubation (occasionally laryngeal mask); sometimes local anaesthesia in emergency (e.g. laryngeal trauma).

INDICATIONS

- Airway obstruction
- Head and neck surgery
- Laryngeal trauma
- Failed tracheal intubation
- Prolonged tracheal intubation and/or intermittent positive-pressure ventilation (IPPV)
- Prevention of pulmonary aspiration.

PREOPERATIVE ASSESSMENT AND INVESTIGATION

Look for:
- Coexisting cardiopulmonary, neurological or muscular disease
- Signs of aspiration or airway obstruction (e.g. stridor)
- Difficult laryngoscopy: intubation or ventilation
- Routine investigations plus chest and possibly cervical spine radiography, pulmonary function tests and arterial blood gases.

PREPARATION AND PREMEDICATION

- Assume difficult intubation: check equipment, have a plan.
- Various sizes of tracheostomy tube, sterile catheter mount and suction catheters should be available.
- Minimal dose of anxiolytic, if essential.
- Anticholinergic.
- Routine medications normally continued.

INDUCTION, MAINTENANCE AND PROCEDURE

- Start only when surgeon scrubbed and instruments are ready.
- Use intravenous induction only if confident; otherwise consider inhalation induction versus awake intubation.
- Fix tracheal tube to permit cautious withdrawal.
- Use balanced anaesthesia for maintenance, careful neck extension, head-ring and head elevation 10–15°.
- Clear oropharyngeal secretions.
- Tracheal incision is usually at third tracheal ring, above tracheal tube cuff.
- Ventilate manually with 100% oxygen during tracheostomy tube insertion.
- Retract tracheal tube until tip is just above incision, enabling tracheostomy tube insertion.
- Check position of tube and $EtCO_2$ trace before reattaching ventilator. Once correct position of tracheostomy tube is confirmed, withdraw tracheal tube completely.
- If local anaesthesia is used, intravenous lidocaine (lignocaine) may reduce coughing.

POSTOPERATIVE MANAGEMENT

- Check chest radiograph (tube position, pneumothorax, surgical emphysema, lobar collapse).
- Nurse in sitting-up position in appropriate ward (humidified oxygen, suction).
- Immediately available selection of tracheal and tracheostomy tubes, and tracheostomy dilator.
- Tube change is usually after a week, allowing time for formation of track.

12

COMPLICATIONS

- *Early* – malposition, displacement bleeding, surgical emphysema, pneumothorax and obstruction (blood, sputum, tracheal wall)
- *Late* – displacement, obstruction, infection, erosion, bleeding, stenosis (cuff or stoma site) and voice changes.

EMERGENCY TRACHEOSTOMY

- Usually under local anaesthetic if formal and airway is obstructed.
- Needle or cricothyroidotomy (minitracheostomy).

Percutaneous

- Elective
- At bedside – quicker, less traumatic, cost-effective
- Theatre and transfer – not needed
- Possibly higher incidence of late complications

TECHNIQUES

- Serial dilatation (Ciaglia)
- Single tapered dilatation (Blue Rhino™)
- Guidewire dilating (Griggs) forceps or screw (PercuTwist™).

INDICATIONS

- Prolonged tracheal intubation
- To facilitate weaning from ventilators and nursing.

PREOPERATIVE ASSESSMENT

- Coexisting disease, ventilation
- Consider deferring if patient is PEEP dependent or coagulopathic.

PREPARATION

- Two operators and a bronchoscope are needed.
- Give general anaesthesia with 100% oxygen.
- Some advocate change to smaller tracheal tube or laryngeal mask before starting.
- Withdraw tracheal tube to above site of tracheostomy.

- Adjust ventilation or insert a throat pack to compensate for cuff deflation.

PROCEDURE

- Use a head-ring, sandbag and head-up position.
- Infiltrate incision site with lidocaine (lignocaine) plus adrenaline (epinephrine).
- Site is usually between first and second tracheal rings.
- Dissect down to trachea.
- Check position of introducer and guidewire bronchoscopically.
- Use high-volume low-pressure cuff tracheostomy tube.

POSTOPERATIVE MANAGEMENT

- Adjust ventilator settings.
- Chest radiography.

COMPLICATIONS

- *Early* – loss of airway, malposition, displacement of tube, bleeding, infection, surgical emphysema, pneumothorax, occlusion of tube, oesophageal injury and tracheal injury
- *Late* – as for surgical tracheostomy.

12

BIBLIOGRAPHY

Donlon JV. Anesthesia and eye, ear, nose and throat surgery. In: Miller RD, ed. Anesthesia. 5th edn. Philadelphia: Churchill Livingstone; 2000:2173–2198

Norwood S, Vallina VL, Short K, Saigusa M, Fernandez LG, McLarty JW. Incidence of tracheal stenosis and other late complications after percutaneous tracheostomy. Annals of Surgery 2000; 232:233–241

Porter JM, Ivatury RR. Preferred route of tracheostomy – percutaneous versus open at the bedside: a randomized, prospective study in the surgical intensive care unit. American Surgeon 1999; 65:142–146

13

HEAD AND NECK SURGERY
S. M. Mostafa

Dental abscess

M. W. Davies

Dental abscesses usually result from infected teeth. They cause localised pain and swelling, may restrict mouth opening, and can be associated with pyrexia and malaise. They typically form 'gum-boils' and discharge into the buccal sulcus, but may 'point' elsewhere, including extraorally.

The General Dental Council (GDC) and Royal College of Anaesthetists (RCA) recommend that, whenever possible, dental procedures are performed under local anaesthesia, in combination with conscious sedation if necessary. General anaesthesia may be clinically justified when local analgesia or patient co-operation are inadequate, or when the stress of surgery whilst awake would be likely to result in dental phobia.

LUDWIG'S ANGINA

Rarely, a spreading cellulitis with extensive induration and swelling of the anterior neck may occur. Trismus, an acute confusional state, and compromise of the airway may be present. This potentially life-threatening condition requires urgent and expert help.

PROCEDURES

- Periradicular surgery (e.g. apicectomy)
- Exodontia (including surgical removal)
- Skin incision and external drainage.

PATIENT CHARACTERISTICS

The condition is not limited to those with poor dental hygiene.
- Children
- Neglected adults
- Patients with 'special needs'.

SPECIFIC PROBLEMS

- May be uncooperative patients
- May present difficult consent issues

- Parents or regular care-providers present at induction
- Airway problems:
  —shared airway
  —swelling
  —contamination (pus, etc.)
  —trismus.

IN LUDWIG'S ANGINA:

- Airway problems are more serious and also include:
  —critical patency
  —secretions
  —rigidity
  —distortion.
- Muscle relaxants may not increase mouth opening.
- Potential 'can't intubate, can't ventilate' scenario exists.

PREOPERATIVE ASSESSMENT

- Full general assessment, including appropriate investigations
- Full airway assessment, including site of abscess and restrictions imposed by it
- Resolve consent issues
- Risks and options should be understood.

IN LUDWIG'S ANGINA:

- Verbal communication may be difficult (consider text display of mobile phone)
- Co-morbidity may be impossible to assess or control fully.
- Special imaging techniques – computed tomography (CT) or magnetic resonance imaging (MRI) – may be useful.

PREMEDICATION

- 'Nil by mouth'
- Consider topical anaesthetic cream (e.g. EMLA or Ametop)
- Oral sedation if needed and airway not compromised

13

- Antisialagogue if needed
- Continue usual cardiorespiratory medication (salbutamol, GTN, etc.).

THEATRE PREPARATION

- Skilled assistance
- Association of Anaesthetists monitoring standard
- 'Difficult intubation' equipment – including laryngeal mask airways and a flexible fibreoptic laryngoscope
- *For Ludwig's angina*, facilities for immediate emergency tracheostomy are essential.

PERIOPERATIVE MANAGEMENT

- Topical anaesthesia may allow preliminary drainage of a large 'pointing' abscess
- Mask anaesthesia for simple exodontia
- Laryngeal mask for periradicular surgery or external drainage
- Tracheal intubation if clinically indicated

IN LUDWIG'S ANGINA:
- Very difficult airway
- Strongly consider awake fibreoptic intubation
- Even careful inhalational induction may result in loss of the airway.

INTRAOPERATIVE MANAGEMENT

- Use propofol and/or sevoflurane for induction and maintenance of anaesthesia.
- Small laryngeal masks are best inserted under direct vision, using a Macintosh laryngoscope.
- Monitor airway patency continuously and lift chin or thrust jaw if needed.
- Advise surgeon regarding airway care.
- Use absorbent 'pack' to reduce airway contamination.
- 'Swab count' within the oral cavity.
- Consider antibiotics and watch for dysrhythmias.
- Avoid opioids unless external drainage is extensive.
- Muscle relaxants are seldom required for uncomplicated abscesses.

IN LUDWIG'S ANGINA:
- Use intravenous fluids.
- Take extreme caution with induction.
- Use extreme caution with muscle relaxants before airway control (best avoided).

POSTOPERATIVE MANAGEMENT

- Position patient to facilitate drainage from mouth (e.g. lateral)
- Oropharyngeal suction
- Spontaneous rather than stimulated 'wake-up'
- Remove airway protection device when awake (consider removing laryngeal mask with cuff inflated)
- Ensure 'swab count' is correct
- Paracetamol and non-steroidal anti-inflammatory drugs (NSAIDs), unless contraindicated
- *In Ludwig's angina*: ventilate electively until airway is safe.

OUTCOME

- *Simple abscess* – full recovery
- *Ludwig's angina* – may require follow-up surgery.

BIBLIOGRAPHY

Atkinson RS, Rushman GB, Davies NJH. Dental anaesthesia. In: Lee's synopsis of anaesthesia. 11th edn. Butterworth-Heinemann; 1996:476–487

Moore JR, Gillbe GV. Principles of oral surgery. 4th edn. Manchester: Manchester University Press; 1991:144–159

Royal College of Anaesthetists. Standards and guidelines for general anaesthesia for dentistry. London: Royal College of Anaesthetists; 1999.

CROSS-REFERENCES

Difficult airway
    Anaesthetic Factors 28: 660

13

Dental surgery

M. W. Davies

Following GDC and RCA recommendations that local anaesthesia and conscious sedation must be used more widely, and National Institute for Clinical Excellence (NICE) recommendations that asymptomatic 'wisdom teeth' should not be removed, the demand for general anaesthesia in dentistry has fallen dramatically.

General anaesthesia is now reserved for those prolonged, unpleasant or technically difficult procedures that present an unreasonable or unacceptable burden for the patient.

General anaesthesia continues to play an important role in allowing dental care for patients with 'special needs', whether these are psychological, mental or physical. As healthcare services for these patients improve, the demand for general anaesthesia is likely to increase.

PROCEDURES

- Restorative dentistry (fillings, crowns, etc.)
- Periradicular surgery (e.g. apicectomy)
- Exodontia
- Surgical exposure or removal of teeth.

PATIENT CHARACTERISTICS

- Children
- Young adults
- Patients with special needs.

SPECIFIC PROBLEMS

- Shared airway
- Airway contamination
- Day-case anaesthesia
- Parents or regular care-providers present at induction
- Dental phobia.

PATIENTS WITH SPECIAL NEEDS:

- May have an incomplete medical history
- Co-morbidity (congenital cardiac disease, spasticity, etc.)
- May present a difficult airway
- May not understand or cooperate with treatment
- May present difficult consent issues
- May behave unpredictably and aggressively.

PREOPERATIVE ASSESSMENT

- Assessment before the day of operation is useful.
- Full general assessment, including appropriate investigations
- Full airway assessment
- Day-case suitability
- Resolve consent issues
- Risks and options should be understood.

PATIENTS WITH SPECIAL NEEDS:

- Degree of understanding should be evaluated
- May be impossible to assess fully
- Require careful observation, detailed discussion with regular care-providers
- Reference to previous anaesthetic notes
- May prefer either inhalational or intravenous induction of anaesthesia
- Cross-infection risk should be considered
- Dental treatment options and goals (short and long term) should be understood
- Key role of regular care-providers during perioperative period should be emphasised.

PREMEDICATION

- 'Nil by mouth'
Consider:
- Topical anaesthetic cream (e.g. EMLA, Ametop)
- Paracetamol and NSAIDs, (unless contraindicated)

13

- Usual cardiorespiratory medication (salbutamol, GTN, etc.)
- Thromboembolism prophylaxis if indicated.

PATIENTS WITH SPECIAL NEEDS:
- Should normally continue their usual medication
- Should attend with regular care-provider(s)
- May benefit from sedative drugs (e.g. temazepam or midazolam)
- Avoid known stressors and maintain familiar 'comforts'.

THEATRE PREPARATION

- Skilled assistance
- Association of Anaesthetists monitoring standard
- 'Difficult intubation' equipment – including laryngeal mask airways and a flexible fibreoptic laryngoscope.

PATIENTS WITH SPECIAL NEEDS:
- Consider personal safety issues
- Consider 'lifting and handling' issues
- Remove known stressors.

INTRAOPERATIVE MANAGEMENT

- Inhalational (sevoflurane) or intravenous induction – caution if difficult airway
- Flexible laryngeal mask, or tracheal intubation (rarely), needed
- Sevoflurane, desflurane or propofol (total intravenous anaesthetic; TIVA) for maintenance of anaesthesia
- Monitor airway patency continuously, and lift chin or thrust jaw if needed
- Advise surgeon regarding airway care
- Use absorbent 'pack' to reduce airway contamination
- 'Swab count' within the oral cavity
- Local anaesthesia for postoperative analgesia
- Consider antibiotics
- Opioids are seldom required.

PATIENTS WITH SPECIAL NEEDS:
- Regular care-provider(s) present whilst awake
- Flexible approach to induction of anaesthesia
- Accept goal reduction if intended treatment not possible

- Try to avoid making next time more difficult.

POSTOPERATIVE MANAGEMENT

- Position patient to facilitate drainage from mouth (e.g. lateral)
- Oropharyngeal suction
- Spontaneous rather than stimulated wake-up
- Remove airway protection device when awake (consider removing laryngeal mask with cuff inflated).
- Ensure 'swab count' is correct
- Continue paracetamol and NSAIDs, unless contraindicated
- *Patients with special needs* – write detailed notes on what worked and what didn't.

OUTCOME

Patients with special needs:
- Are likely to return
- Often appreciate being treated by staff they recognise
- May be encouraged to accept minor dental procedures without general anaesthesia.

BIBLIOGRAPHY

Department of Health. Report of an expert working party on general anaesthesia, sedation and resuscitation in dentistry. Dental Division, Department of Health; 1991

Royal College of Anaesthetists. Standards and guidelines for general anaesthesia for dentistry. London: Royal College of Anaesthetists; 1999.

Royal College of Surgeons of England. Commission on the provision of surgical services. Guidelines for day case surgery. London: Royal College of Surgeons of England; 1985

13

CROSS-REFERENCES

Day-case surgery
    Anaesthetic Factors 27: 613
Infants and children
    Anaesthetic Factors 27: 610
Difficult intubation (Difficult airway)
    Anaesthetic Factors 28: 666

Face and jaw fractures

C. A. Hodgson

13

PROCEDURES

Fractures may involve the zygoma, maxilla or mandible. Simple elevation of a fractured zygoma may be followed by internal fixation if the fracture remains unstable. Maxillary fractures are classified according to the LeFort system. A LeFort I fracture involves the lower maxilla, whereas a LeFort III fracture involves the upper maxilla and may be associated with a basal skull fracture or airway obstruction. Improved internal microplating techniques have greatly decreased the need for postoperative intermaxillary fixation (IMF).

PATIENT CHARACTERISTICS

The patients are usually young males with fractures due to trauma, for example road accidents, sports injuries or assault. Alcohol or drug intoxication may be implicated. There may be a coexisting head or cervical spine injury, or disease such as epilepsy, cardiorespiratory or cerebrovascular disease, or arrhythmias. Other organs injuries must also be excluded.

Seriously injured patients with airway difficulties need early tracheal intubation. The airway may be obstructed by blood or blood clots, dislodged teeth, displaced bone fragments, a swollen tongue or generalised oedema. A full stomach must be assumed, accompanied by a risk of aspiration of foreign material.

Patients without a compromised airway are suitable for semi-elective repair of facial fractures when the facial swelling has reduced. Definitive surgical treatment may also be delayed when there is a need to treat other major injuries first, or when there is late presentation of the maxillofacial injury.

PREOPERATIVE ASSESSMENT

This is principally directed towards assessment of the degree of airway compromise and the presence of associated injuries or coexisting medical conditions.

PREMEDICATION

No premedication is given in the emergency situation. Respiratory depressants may further compromise an obstructed airway. An antisialagogue may be given if awake intubation is planned as part of an elective procedure. An intravenous dose of an H_2 blocker (e.g. ranitidine) or a proton pump inhibitor (e.g. pantoprazole) may be given to patients known to require postoperative IMF.

PERIOPERATIVE MANAGEMENT

In the acute situation with airway compromise the priority is to secure a definitive airway. The technique chosen will depend on patient factors and the experience of the anaesthetist. Possible options include:
- Inhalational induction (airway obstruction or laryngospasm may occur)
- Use intravenous agents only if lung ventilation is certain
- Awake intubation (difficult if the patient is agitated or actively bleeding)
- Tracheostomy under local anaesthesia.

Equipment for a difficult intubation must be assembled. Standard monitoring is applied, including capnography. An oral tracheal tube is usually passed acutely and may be changed later for a nasal tube. Communication with the surgeon is necessary in deciding the route of intubation. If a basal skull fracture has not been excluded, nasal intubation or insertion of a nasogastric tube must be avoided.

Isolated mandibular fractures do not usually cause airway problems or intubation difficulty. Trismus associated with a fractured mandible is usually relieved on induction of anaesthesia.

MAINTENANCE OF ANAESTHESIA:

- A throat pack and eye protection are essential.
- Anaesthetic circuit disconnection or kinking may occur underneath the sterile towels.
- Blood loss may be significant.
- Opioid analgesics should be used sparingly.
- Dexamethasone may be given to decrease tissue swelling.
- Prophylactic antiemetics are necessary if IMF has been applied.

IMMEDIATE POSTOPERATIVE PERIOD

If facial swelling is significant, the patient should remain intubated and be transferred to an ICU until the swelling has subsided. The absence of a leak around the deflated cuff of the tracheal tube indicates that extubation would be unwise.

Patients with less swelling should be extubated when good laryngeal reflexes have returned. After a lengthy operation, a nasal tube may be withdrawn, shortened and left as a temporary nasopharyngeal airway (with a safety pin positioned through it to prevent migration). If IMF has been applied, wire cutters must be immediately available at the side of the patient, and staff must be familiar with their use. Opioids are cautiously indicated for analgesia. Intravenous fluids are continued until oral intake resumes.

COMPLICATIONS

Respiratory distress and airway obstruction may follow premature extubation of the patient. Reintubation may then be much more difficult and profound hypoxia may develop. The 1991–1992 report of the National Confidential Enquiry into Perioperative Deaths (NCEPOD) found that following maxillofacial surgery more than 50% of complications causing death were associated with cardiorespiratory problems.

BIBLIOGRAPHY

Bogdanoff DL, Stone DJ. Emergency management of the airway outside the operating room. Canadian Journal of Anaesthesia 1992; 39:1069–1089

Chesshire NJ, Knight DJW. The anaesthetic management of facial trauma and fractures. British Journal of Anaesthesia CEPD Reviews 2001; 1:108–112

Campling EA, Devlin HB, Moile RW, Lunn JN. The report of the National Confidential Enquiry into Perioperative Deaths 1991/1992. London: NCEPOD; 1993

Ochs MW, Tucker M. Current concepts in management of facial trauma. Journal of Oral and Maxillofacial Surgery 1993; 51(Suppl 1):42–55

Tomlinson S, Earlam C. Management of severe upper airway trauma. Hospital Medicine 1999; 60:844

CROSS-REFERENCES

13

Difficult airway
    Anaesthetic Factors 28: 660
Trauma
    Anaesthetic Factors 31: 797

Laryngectomy and radical neck dissection

P. Charters

Laryngectomy and its variants, such as vertical hemilaryngectomy and supraglottic laryngectomy, are performed for malignant disease of the larynx. Neck dissection is similarly for secondary spread to lymph glands or when the site of the primary tumour has not been determined. When the pharynx is involved, pharyngolaryngectomy may be required plus a reconstructive tissue flap. These procedures are discussed elsewhere. Patients presenting for surgery of this nature will have had recent endoscopy under general anaesthesia to determine the extent of the tumour. A number of patients with this form of cancer refuse surgery on account of the functional and morphological changes that result. By virtue of the removal of the internal jugular vein, radical neck dissection may lead to a rise in intracranial pressure (ICP) with oedema of the head and neck. Bilateral radical neck dissection needs a covering temporary tracheostomy until the inevitable oedema subsides.

PATIENT CHARACTERISTICS

Essentially as for patients undergoing microlaryngoscopy.

PREOPERATIVE ASSESSMENT

- These subjects may have had recent anaesthetics and an ENT work-up.
- Subjects who presented with airway narrowing, with or without tumour debulking, could have deteriorated since the earlier examination.
- Previous radiation therapy may have resulted in soft tissue fibrosis, and reactive oedema may be evident. Either complication may make airway management and intubation difficult.

PREMEDICATION

This is not usually given, especially in patients with stridor.

THEATRE PREPARATION AND MONITORING

- Full access to difficult intubation and emergency tracheostomy facilities is essential.
- Monitoring should include ECG, invasive blood pressure, Sao_2, $Etco_2$, airway pressure, disconnection alarm and neuromuscular blockade.
- Central venous access is used only if remote from the surgical site.
- Position is as for most head and neck work (head-up tilt 10-15°, head-ring ± sandbag beneath shoulders, with due care as excessive neck extension may cause injury).

GENERAL PRINCIPLES OF ANAESTHETIC TECHNIQUE

When airway problems are present, the implications for management are similar to those considered under microlaryngoscopy. Because the neck contains many vulnerable structures, complications of surgery, especially in the presence of an invasive tumour, can be dramatic but are fortunately rare. Bradycardia and hypotension may occur during dissection around the carotid vessels. Vagolytics or local anaesthesia applied by the surgeon can decrease this. The major concern is to ensure cerebral blood flow integrity. This may be compromised by:

- Asymptomatic plaques at carotid bifurcation dislodged during surgical manipulations
- Inadvertent carotid compression by *en bloc* tumour dissection
- Intentional internal jugular removal during radical neck dissection impairs venous return from the head and brain, and raises ICP
- Inadvertent disruption of a major vessel where access for control is difficult.

13

ANAESTHETIC TECHNIQUE

Co-morbidity in older patients may result in cardiovascular instability. Sputum retention may be a problem in smokers with increasing upper airway obstruction due to tumour. Pharyngeal reflex suppression and tumour mass may necessitate pharyngeal clearance by suction to improve the view at laryngoscopy. Airway considerations will be predictable on the basis of recent anaesthesia for endoscopy and will influence the induction and intubation technique. Surgical requirement for muscle relaxation is limited. Maintenance can be by most conventional methods.

AIRWAY MAINTENANCE

During laryngectomy the tracheal tube is removed and the trachea is opened to fashion the eventual tracheostomy. Cooperation between the surgeon and anaesthetist must be geared to minimise risk of loss of the airway during the change-over. Separate anaesthetic circuits helps. Preoxygenate the patient prior to incision into the trachea. The tracheal tube is identified by the surgeon and then withdrawn slowly to just above the incision under direct vision. In this position, it can be reintroduced to the lower trachea in the event of any problem while introducing the tracheostomy tube. The tube used should reflect the need to fashion the stomal site, i.e. with connection beyond the immediate surgical site and good manoeuvrability. A microlaryngeal or 'laryngectomy' tube is suitable. Confirmation of proper placement of the new tube in the trachea should include capnography and bilateral auscultation of the chest. At the end of the operation this tube is replaced with a conventional tracheostomy tube and a chest radiograph is taken to confirm its position.

POSTOPERATIVE COMPLICATIONS

Early:
- Haemorrhage
- Problematic airway integrity and poor cough, especially after hemilaryngectomy
- Various nerve palsies (phrenic nerve may be injured during neck dissection)
- Chyle leak (right-sided neck dissection)
- Rebound hypertension in the recovery room, particularly after hypotensive anaesthesia
- Increased ICP – may be prevented with mannitol
- Facial and laryngeal oedema after radical neck dissection – tends to improve over a few days but may not return to normal.

BIBLIOGRAPHY

Roland NJ, McRae RDR, McCombe AW. Key topics in otolaryngology. 2nd edn. Bios Scientific; Aberystwyth, 2001

CROSS-REFERENCES

Difficult airway – difficult tracheal intubation
    Anaesthetic Factors 28: 666
Awareness
    Anaesthetic Factors 31: 727

13

Major reconstructive surgery

S. M. Mostafa

PROCEDURES

Reconstructive procedures are carried out to repair defects or to correct deformities caused by:
- Cancer surgery of the head and neck
- Congenital craniofacial and maxillofacial deformities
- Acquired facial deformities (e.g. trauma).

The operations are usually multidisciplinary procedures involving several surgical specialties. Single-stage reconstructive surgery became possible with the use of the bicoronal approach to the anterior cranial fossa, the orbits and nasoethmoid complex, pedicled myocutaneous flaps, and the microvascular free transfer of soft tissue and bone. The need for intermaxillary and complex external fixation has decreased following mandibular reconstruction with titanium plates and internal fixation with mini-bone plating systems.

Surgery and anaesthesia are notable for:
- Complexity and length
- Inaccessibility of patient, intravenous lines and cables
- Potential for disconnection of circuit and intravenous lines
- Heat and blood loss, and infection
- Potentially difficult, shared and inaccessible airway
- Intubation is likely to be difficult
- Induced hypotension may be required
- Withdrawal problems to alcohol and nicotine.

AGE RANGES OF PATIENTS

Congenital craniofacial deformities are found in infants and children who may have other congenital defects (e.g. cardiac or spinal). The upper airway may be obstructed and intracranial pressure (ICP) is raised.

Orthognathic operations for cosmetic reasons or fractures are undertaken in young healthy adults.

Cancer is found in older malnourished patients who smoke and/or abuse alcohol. They may have associated cardiopulmonary diseases and have received radiotherapy or chemotherapy before surgery.

ASSESSMENT AND PREPARATION

Thorough evaluation is imperative. The type of patient, underlying pathology, presence of related medical conditions and planned surgery will influence assessment and preparation. Requirements for sedation, antibiotic and deep vein thrombosis prophylaxis, and blood transfusion balanced against potential risks should be determined. Discuss the technique, risks, analgesia, awake intubation and tracheostomy with the patient and relatives.

Evaluate the airway, in particular, and the potential for difficult intubation to enable safe management. Identify the following:
- Mallampati grade, thyromental distance or Wilson's score
- Abnormal or altered anatomy or presence of tumours or swellings
- Facial deformities and asymmetries
- Tongue size and mobility
- Degree of mouth opening and neck movement
- Airway obstruction (e.g. stridor, hoarseness and dysphagia) and its site
- Abnormalities on plain radiography and on CT and MRI scans of the spine, head and neck
- Previous head and neck radiotherapy or surgery, which may create difficult intubation.

ROUTINE INVESTIGATIONS:
- Full blood count, clotting profile, blood group and cross-match
- Urea and electrolytes, arterial blood gases with liver function profile
- Chest radiography, ECG and pulmonary function tests as necessary.

PREMEDICATION

This should satisfy the patient's condition and operation:

- Opioids can be used cautiously for patients who are in pain.
- A short-acting benzodiazepine orally is useful for anxiolysis.
- Chlormethiazole and nicotine patches ameliorate withdrawal symptoms.
- Atropine (preferably glycopyrrolate) is necessary in an awake intubation; it reduces oropharyngeal secretions and vagotonic responses.
- Pre-emptive antiemetics (e.g. $5HT_3$ antagonists) prevent postoperative vomiting and damage to the surgical site, pain or potential risk of aspiration if the jaws are wired.
- Avoid narcotics or sedation if the airway is compromised or ICP is raised.
- Use small intravenous doses of short-acting reversible agents (midazolam, fentanyl) – only if necessary and titrated to the patient's response – during awake intubation for a compromised airway.

THEATRE FACILITIES

Routine operating theatre facilities are needed plus:

- Assistants experienced in this field
- Fibreoptic laryngoscope and difficult airway management equipment
- Operating table with suitable mattress and padding to prevent pressure sores and nerve compression
- Equipment to maintain normothermia – warm air blankets or a warming mattress, intravenous fluid warmers, inspired gas humidifiers and raising operating theatre temperature
- Blood loss and/or haemoglobin measurement equipment.

ANAESTHETIC MANAGEMENT

GENERAL ANAESTHESIA

Induction centres on establishing control and maintenance of the airway, with thorough monitoring and maintaining a safe anaesthetic technique.

INDUCTION AND THE AIRWAY

Induction with thiopental or propofol and a muscle relaxant is acceptable in patients with a normal airway. Anticipate difficult airways, but unexpected problems occur. Patients undergoing ablative surgery on the tongue, pharynx and larynx, or prolonged postoperative controlled ventilation, will require tracheostomy. The airway and tracheal intubation can be secured by one of these techniques:

- Induction with sevoflurane in 100% oxygen, followed by intubation, then intravenous and/or inhalational agents
- Awake intubation under local anaesthesia: lidocaine (lignocaine) 6 mg kg^{-1} nebulisation and cocaine 4% 1.5 mg kg^{-1} spray to the nose (produces less coughing and laryngospasm in a compromised airway), then intravenous and/or inhalational agents
- Tracheostomy under local anaesthesia, then intravenous and/or inhalational agents
- Less often, transtracheal jet ventilation plus total intravenous anaesthesia (TIVA), followed by intubation, then intravenous and/or inhalational agents.

MAINTENANCE OF THE AIRWAY AND ANAESTHESIA

A correctly placed, secured and fixed orotracheal or nasotracheal tube, which is reinforced, is essential. It can be stabilised by a throat pack, which prevents pulmonary aspiration by reducing pharyngeal soiling. Tube route, type and fixation depend on the need of the operation and necessity for intermaxillary, mandibular or external fixation. Look out for endobronchial intubation, caused by head movement or surgical manipulation, accidental extubation and disconnection. The latter is prevented by taping of connections, using a lightweight Bain or disposable circle circuit. A risk of awareness exists when the tracheal tube is exchanged for the tracheostomy tube. Deepen anaesthesia and give 100% oxygen. To maintain anaesthesia, use volatile agents, narcotics and muscle relaxants. TIVA is an alternative. Avoid nitrous oxide in prolonged procedures because of its side-effects.

MONITORING:

- Pulse oximetry, ECG and ST-segment analysis
- Invasive blood pressure (in forearm free flaps suitable arteries are dorsalis pedis, tibial or femoral)
- Central venous pressure (CVP) – not always needed. Neck veins are unsuitable. Use long lines, subclavian or femoral veins. Note pneumothorax risk and site of myocutaneous pedicled flap
- Blood loss, fluid balance and urine output

13

- Tidal volume, respiratory rate, FiO_2, Et CO_2 and disconnection alarm
- End-tidal agent concentration and depth of anaesthesia monitor if available
- Neuromuscular blockade
- Core and peripheral temperature (groin, big toe)
- pH_i catheter or microdialysis in gastric transposition or flap surgery may be used. (pH_i <7.32 or low glucose, high lactate and glycerol concentrations indicate ischaemia).

BLEEDING

Bleeding is minimised by:
- Surgical technique
- Infiltration of vasoconstrictors
- Smooth induction and recovery
- Minimal coughing and straining
- 10–15° head-up tilt (remember risk of air embolism)
- Flexion of thighs at the hips may/can improve venous return
- Good analgesia and anaesthesia
- Controlled hypotension.

To reduce brain volume and facilitate surgery involving the cranium, modest hypocapnia, osmotic diuretics or withdrawal of CSF may be necessary.

FREE-FLAP SURGERY

Good surgical technique remains a leading factor for graft survival. Optimal anaesthetic management should prevent vasoconstriction and enhance blood flow to the flap. This is achieved and maintained by:
- Satisfactory analgesia and PaO_2
- Normotension and cardiac output
- Normovolaemia or even slight hypervolaemia
- Normothermia and normocapnia
- Optimising blood viscosity

- Use of Dextran 40 (caution in renal insufficiency)
- Minimal external compression of graft vessels by haematoma or dressings.

POSTOPERATIVE CARE

These patients will need care in the HDU/ICU. Intensive care and monitoring give confidence to patients with airway difficulties, swollen face, who are unable to see, and allow good analgesia using opioid infusion, patient-controlled analgesia (PCA) or NSAIDs for use after maxillofacial surgery. Epidural analgesia plus an opioid is useful in operations involving the thoracoabdominal area. Local anaesthetic infiltration of the donor graft site or its nerves helps in postoperative pain relief.
- The patient is extubated only when awake with intact protective reflexes and when oozing or bleeding has stopped. Prolonged controlled ventilation is uncommon unless there is coexisting cardiopulmonary disease.
- Dexamethasone may be used to reduce postoperative swelling.
- Wire cutters should be readily available if IMF is used. Where there has been major surgery to the mouth or upper airway, anticipation of severe postoperative swelling or bleeding dictates the need for extreme caution with extubation or best do a tracheostomy.
- Patients may often return to theatre due to early complications such as airway difficulties, bleeding, compromised blood supply to flaps, and haematoma formation.
- Many patients require repeat procedures, especially those with severe facial deformity or malignancy.

BIBLIOGRAPHY

Barham CJ. Anaesthesia for maxillofacial surgery. In: Patel H, ed. Anaesthesia for burns, maxillofacial and plastic surgery. London: Edward Arnold; 1993:53–77

Brooks NC, Mostafa SM. Anaesthesia and pain control for head and neck surgery. In: Jones A, Phillips DE, Hligers JM, eds. Diseases of the head & neck, nose & throat. London: Edward Arnold; 1998:142–152

Donlon JV. Eye, ear, nose and throat disease. In: Benumof JL, Benumof J, eds. Anaesthesia and uncommon diseases. 4th edn. Philadelphia: WB Saunders; 1998:38–50

Goat VA. Anaesthesia for craniofacial surgery. In: Atkinson RS, Adams AP, eds. Recent advances in anaesthesia and analgesia. Edinburgh: Churchill Livingstone; 1989:139–153

Inglis M, Robbie DS, Edwards JM, Breach NM. The anaesthetic management of patients undergoing free flap reconstructive surgery following resection of head and neck neoplasms – a review of 64 patients. Annals of the Royal College of Surgeons of England 1988; 70:235–238

Rojdmark J, Blomquvist L, Malm M, Adams-Ray B, Ungerstedt U. Metabolism in myocutaneous flaps studied by in-situ microdialysis. Scandinavian Journal of Plastic and Reconstructive Surgery and Hand Surgery 1998; 32:27–34

Sweeney DB, Sainsbury DA. Anaesthesia for cranio-maxillary-facial surgery. Current Anaesthesia and Critical Care 1992; 3:11–16

CROSS-REFERENCES

Difficult airway
    Anaesthetic Factors 28: 660
Induced hypotension
    Anaesthetic Factors 30: 704
Prolonged anaesthesia
    Anaesthetic Factors 30: 713
Trauma
    Anaesthetic Factors 31: 797

13

Operations on the salivary glands

R. Kandasamy

Surgery on the salivary glands may be simple procedures, for example for a stone blocking a duct, or more complex excision, such as glandular malignancy. The major salivary glands in humans consist of the paired parotid, submandibular and sublingual glands. Most salivary gland tumours occur in the parotid gland and represent less than 3% of head and neck neoplasms. The majority of the calculi (80%) occur in the submandibular gland and its duct. The operative approach may be either through the skin or intraorally through the mucous membrane.

Parotidectomy is a complex procedure because of the relationship of the parotid gland with the facial nerve. The facial nerve divides the parotid gland into a large supraneural and a small infraneural component. The key to parotidectomy is accurate, safe localisation of the facial nerve and the avoidance of injury to the nerve. Stimulating the facial nerve with a nerve stimulator during the operation and observing the movement of the facial muscles will achieve this. Therefore, muscle relaxants are preferably avoided for maintenance of the anaesthesia.

PREOPERATIVE EVALUATION

History, examination, evaluation of the coexisting medical condition and investigation is routine.

Assessment of the airway – swelling of the parotid or submandibular gland and involvement of the temporomandibular joint by the growth may restrict mouth opening. Discuss with the surgeon or check the CT or MRI scan to ascertain the extent of the structures involved.

Examine the tonsillar fossa and soft palate for the presence of a deep-lobe parotid tumour. Prepare the patient for fibreoptic intubation if necessary.

PREMEDICATION

A benzodiazepine is suitable. An antisialogogue (e.g. glycopyrrolate) is useful if awake fibreoptic intubation is contemplated.

PERIOPERATIVE MANAGEMENT

INDUCTION OF ANAESTHESIA
Considerations should be given to:
- Difficult airway
- Facial nerve integrity monitoring and the use of muscle relaxant
- Risk of aspiration and trauma to the face and eyes.

If no difficulties are anticipated during intubation, intravenous induction is indicated. Induction with propofol and alfentanil is safe, but etomidate is preferred in cardiac patients. Tracheal intubation is facilitated by an intermediate-acting muscle relaxant such as atracurium. Respiratory depression caused by propofol and alfentanil may allow a lower dose of muscle relaxants and recovery from relaxation to enable monitoring of the facial nerve. A preformed nasal or oral tracheal tube provides surgical access for both an intraoral and an extraoral approach. Before the operation begins, check for accidental endobronchial intubation.

A reinforced laryngeal mask (LM) with spontaneous respiration can be used, in suitable patients, as an alternative to enable facial nerve monitoring and for other operations, such as submandibular gland excision, short intraoral or extraoral procedures. Remember that a LM can be easily displaced if the head is in an abnormal position or during difficult surgical manipulation. An oropharyngeal pack is recommended for all intraoral procedures, but leave its 'tail end' outside the mouth to prompt removal at the end of the operation. The eyelids are shut and taped with clear sterile tape.

13

MAINTENANCE

Maintenance is with oxygen, nitrous oxide, a volatile agent and an opioid with controlled ventilation or spontaneous breathing with LM. Maintain deep anaesthesia without further doses of relaxant in parotid surgery. Sevoflurane may induce less tachycardia than isoflurane. TIVA with propofol and remifentanil is an alternative and may enable controlled ventilation without muscle relaxants. General anaesthesia can be supplemented with skin infiltration of 0.125% bupivacaine, but this may interfere with facial nerve conduction.

Nerve integrity is monitored during the operation by a battery-powered nerve stimulator (which has a current adjustable from 0.5 to 2.0 mA). Muscle response occurs when the probe touches exposed nerve or muscle tissue. The excitability of indirectly evoked muscle responses by stimulation of the corresponding motor nerve is substantially more sensitive than that of direct electrical muscle stimulation. Peripheral nerve stimulation for monitoring the neuromuscular blockade (e.g. train of four stimuli) will indicate when the surgeon can use the nerve stimulator.

LOCAL ANAESTHESIA

Local anaesthesia is not common; it is used for submandibular gland surgery by blocking the inferior alveolar, auriculotemporal, lingual, buccal and superficial cervical plexus.

OTHER PROCEDURES

Transposition of parotid duct into the tonsillar fossa for the treatment of drooling, excessive salivation due to trauma or spastic disorder is not an uncommon operation. The patients may be intellectually impaired. General anaesthesia with nasal intubation is usual. Submandibular diagnostic and interventional sialoendoscopy is a new procedure for ductal disorders, and may be carried out under local or general anaesthesia particularly when there are multiple and bigger stones.

POSTOPERATIVE MANAGEMENT

Analgesia with oral analgesics (e.g. diclofenac or codydramol) or occasionally parenteral opiate is adequate. Parenteral fluid may be required until oral intake is adequate.

BIBLIOGRAPHY

Granick MS, Hanna DC, Solomon MP. Management of benign and malignant primary salivary gland tumors. In: Georgiade GS, Riefkohl R, Levin LS, eds. Georgiade plastic, maxillofacial and reconstructive surgery. London: Williams & Wilkins; 1997:155–165

Marchal F, Dulguerov P, Becker M, Barki G, Disant F, Lehmann W. Submandibular diagnostic and interventional sialoendoscopy: new procedure for ductal disorders. Annals of Otology, Rhinology, and Laryngology 2002; 111:27–35

Oviedo Montes A, Ramblas Angeles P, Saucedo Najera E, Sanchez de Ovando JA. The debridement of submandibular abscesses under locoregional block. Gaceta Medica de Mexico 1992; 128:275–278

13

Thyroidectomy

J. Beattie

PROCEDURE

Thyroidectomy may be unilateral, subtotal or total. Surgery is performed through a skin crease incision approximately 4 cm above the sternum.

- Surgeons should locate and preserve the recurrent laryngeal nerves.
- Parathyroid glands should be preserved.
- In the neck, haemostasis is very important.
- Suction drains are used to minimise haematoma accumulation.
- Large retrosternal goitres may require a sternal split to allow complete excision.

PATIENT CHARACTERISTICS

Most patients presenting for thyroid surgery are females; the pathological conditions are listed below. Approximately 10% of nodules will be malignant.

- Thyrotoxicosis:
  —Graves' disease (20–40 years of age)
  —multinodular goitre (older patients)
  —toxic solitary nodule.
- Carcinoma:
  —papillary (30–40 years of age)
  —follicular or medullary (older patients)
  —anaplastic.
- Bilateral compressive or cosmetically unacceptable non-toxic goitre
- Autoimmune thyroiditis.

PREOPERATIVE ASSESSMENT

After general assessment, emphasis should be placed on the following:

- *Airway assessment*:
  —Tracheal deviation may be marked.
  —Some patients may have stridor or respiratory problems when supine.
  —Vocal cords movement should be assessed by an otolaryngologist to ensure that pre-existing laryngeal nerve palsy is recognised.
- *Cardiovascular system*:
  —Hyperthyroidism can cause tachycardia, atrial fibrillation or heart failure.
  —Large goitres may obstruct venous drainage.
- *Eyes*:
  —Lid retraction and exophthalmos mean that care is needed to protect the eyes from intraoperative drying or trauma.
- *Other conditions*:
  —Thyroid disease may be part of multiple endocrine neoplasia syndromes and conditions such as diabetes mellitus, hyperparathyroidism and phaeochromocytoma must be considered.

PREOPERATIVE INVESTIGATION

Thyroid function must be assessed and patients rendered clinically euthyroid prior to surgery. Measure serum thyroxine (T4: free, 10–40 pmol l^{-1}; total, 64–160 nmol l^{-1}; and its index, 17–47), T3 and thyroid-stimulating hormone (TSH). In another test, thyroid-releasing factor (TRF) is given and the levels of TSH are measured. Failure of TSH to rise indicates hyperthyroidism.

- Other blood tests include full blood count, group and save, serum urea and electrolytes, calcium and phosphate.
- ECG is important in older or hyperthyroid patients to assess preoperative hormone suppression regimens.
- Chest radiography and thoracic inlet views are useful to assess airway compression or deviation.
- With retrosternal disease or severe stridor, CT or MRI will delineate the degree and extent of airway narrowing.
- Surgery must be deferred if the patient remains clinically hyperthyroid.
- β-Receptor blockade must be continued beyond the day of operation.

13

DRUG TREATMENT FOR HYPERTHYROIDISM

- Carbimazole – inhibits iodination of tyrosyl residues in thyroglobulin.
- Propylthiouracil – as carbimazole, but also reduces peripheral de-iodination of T4 to T3.
- Beta-blockers – used to control cardiovascular effects. Propranolol also decreases the peripheral conversion of T4 to T3.
- Iodine – potassium iodide is given for 7–10 days before operation. It decreases gland vascularity and secretion of thyroxine.

PERIOPERATIVE CARE

- Patients often need anxiolytic premedication.
- Use routine monitoring and an intravenous fluid infusion. An arterial line may be required for those with pre-existing cardiovascular disease.
- With massive goitre or airway compromise, a gas induction or awake fibreoptic intubation may be required.
- An intravenous induction and controlled ventilation technique is usually used.
- Use a carefully secured reinforced tracheal tube.
- Careful neck extension provides surgical access.
- A head-up tilt reduces venous engorgement.
- Tracheal tube position must be checked after patient positioning as neck extension may change the location of the tube tip.
- The eyes must be protected, as drapes will be placed over the head.
- For repeat surgery, surgeons may wish to use a nerve stimulator to locate the laryngeal nerves. Muscle relaxation cannot therefore be used once intubation is completed.
- Supplementation of beta-blockade may be needed as manipulation of the thyroid may release more thyroid hormone.
- Before wound closure normotension, head-down tilt, and a Valsalva manoeuvre will assist in locating bleeding points.
- Some surgeons request direct laryngoscopy to assess vocal cord movement at the end of surgery. Others prefer a smooth extubation with no hypertensive stimuli. In some centres the tracheal tube is replaced by a laryngeal mask airway at the end of the operation. A fibreoptic endoscope is used to assess vocal cord movement.
- Surgical manipulation may kink the trachea; hence, a reinforced tracheal tube is needed.

POSTOPERATIVE CARE AND COMPLICATIONS

- Thyrotoxic patients must continue on their preoperative drug regimen until T4 levels decrease.
- Serum calcium concentration should be checked to ensure normal parathyroid gland function. Tetany or low serum calcium levels require calcium supplementation by the intravenous or oral route.
- After operation recurrent laryngeal nerve palsy (temporary due to oedema, or permanent) will cause the affected vocal cord to lie in adduction. Symptoms range from hoarse voice and dyspnoea to stridor or complete airway obstruction, requiring reintubation and possibly a tracheostomy.
- Neck haematoma and surgical tracheal retraction may cause laryngeal oedema. Removal of wound clips and sutures will decompress the neck and trachea prior to urgent evacuation and haemostasis. Gas induction or cautious intravenous induction is a suitable technique. A smaller tracheal tube may be required. Surgeons should be present in case of the need for an emergency tracheostomy.

RARE COMPLICATIONS

Tracheomalacia may be seen following resection of compressive retrosternal thyroid masses. Tracheal collapse may necessitate prolonged intubation.

Pneumothorax is occasionally seen following extensive and difficult resection, requiring insertion of a intercostal chest drain.

Thyroid storm occurs due to uncontrolled release of thyroxine in a thyrotoxic patient and may be triggered by acute illness, surgery or trauma. Signs include hyperpyrexia, tachycardia, hypertension, arrhythmias, vomiting, diarrhoea and altered mental state. During operation this may mimic malignant hyperpyrexia. This condition may occur after operation if drug treatment is stopped immediately following surgery. The half-life of T4 is about 7 days. This condition may be fatal, and

13

patients must be managed on an ICU. Treatment includes:

- Propranolol intravenously, orally or via a nasogastric tube.
- Esmolol may also be used for acute management.
- Carbimazole or propylthiouracil orally or via a nasogastric tube.
- Hydrocortisone supplementation intravenously.
- Oxygen should be given and ventilation may be required.
- Temperature monitoring and active cooling may be required.
- Use of dantrolene has been reported in these patients.

BIBLIOGRAPHY

Gravenstein N. Manual of complications during anesthesia. London: JB Lippincott; 1993:596–601

Hilary Wade JS. Respiratory obstruction in thyroid surgery. Annals of the Royal College of Surgeons of England 1980; 62:15–24

Mercer EM, Eltringham RJ. Anaesthesia for thyroid surgery. Ear, Nose and Throat Journal 1985; 64:342–375

Wheeler MH. Malignant goitre/thyroidectomy. Surgery 1984; 9:200–209

13

14

PLASTIC SURGERY
B. J. Pollard

Burns

B. J. Pollard

PROCEDURE

Burns surgery is usually required for deep dermal and third-degree burns. The aim is to harvest skin, excise the burn and cover the burn site with fresh skin. As a quick assessment of burn size, the patient's palm area represents 1% of total body surface area (TBSA) (Table 14.1).

BURNS SURGERY:
- Is usually performed in the supine position, occasionally prone
- May involve repeated procedures
- May require tourniquet(s) to reduce blood loss

TABLE 14.1

Assessment of burns

Burn	Findings
First degree	Superficial blisters, painful, heals in 3–4 days
Second degree	Partial thickness, heals in 2–3 weeks, deep dermal burns may scar
Third degree	Full thickness, anaesthetic, dermis destroyed, dry, leathery, white or brown in colour

BOX 14.1

Associated injuries

- Smoke inhalational injury:
  —cyanide and carbon monoxide poisoning
  —airway involvement, swelling
- Electrical burn:
  —myocardial damage
- Chemical burn
- Renal or hepatic damage:
  —difficult access to veins because of burn injury

- Major burn is defined as:
  —adult >20% TBSA, second or third degree
  —child >10%.

PATIENT CHARACTERISTICS

PATIENTS FOR BURNS SURGERY:
- Can be any age, but extremes of ages are common
- May have associated injuries
- May have associated medical conditions such as epilepsy
- May have an alcohol-induced injury.

See Box 14.1.

PREOPERATIVE ASSESSMENT AND INVESTIGATIONS

- Has there been any history of exposure to smoke, or inhalational injury?
- Has resuscitation been completed?
- Check availability of blood for transfusion.
- Full blood count, urea and electrolytes, chest radiography, arterial blood gases, clotting screen, urine output.

THEATRE PREPARATION:
- Ideally, two surgical teams, as well as two anaesthetists
- Prewarm operating theatre
- Warming mattress; intravenous fluid warmer
- Humidifier for breathing system.

See Table 14.2.

PREMEDICATION

- Anxiolysis may be required, especially in children (e.g. midazolam); in adults an opioid analgesic may be desirable.
- Anticholinergic premedication can be useful, particularly in children, but also in anticipated cases of difficult intubation.

14

TABLE 14.2

Resuscitation of burns patients

	Regimen
Mount Vernon regimen	0.5 x weight (kg) x %TBSA (ml) of 4.5% human albumin in each of six periods over 36 h
Lactated Ringer's (USA)	4 ml kg^{-1} per %TBSA in 24 h
Hypertonic saline	0.3 ml kg^{-1} per %TSBA in first hour, then adjust to urine output

TBSA, total body surface area.

PERIOPERATIVE MANAGEMENT

MONITORING:
- ECG
- SpO_2
- $EtCO_2$
- Non-invasive blood pressure
- Central venous pressure (CVP)
- Fluid balance and blood loss
- Urine output
- Core temperature.

Access to limbs during operation may be restricted and an intra-arterial pressure line may be necessary. CVP measurement may also be useful in the management of fluid therapy.

ANAESTHETIC TECHNIQUE

General anaesthesia is almost always the chosen technique. For change of burns dressing it is quite common practice to use ketamine (i.v. or i.m.), especially for children. Pre-treatment with a benzodiazepine or equivalent is helpful.

Intravenous induction of anaesthesia (propofol or thiopental is suitable), with a muscle relaxant (atracurium or vecuronium is suitable) and an opioid with or without an inhalational agent. Harvesting split skin grafts is intensely painful and care must be taken to use a sufficient dosage of opioid. There may be a large blood loss and large volumes of fluid administered during the procedure.

- Avoid suxamethonium, except within the first 24 h postburn.
- Anticipate blood loss. Intraoperative haemoglobin measurement may be useful (e.g. HemoCue). Beware of dilutional effect on clotting factors.

POSTOPERATIVE MANAGEMENT

- Common complications – bleeding, infection.
- Return to burns unit – nurse supine on low air-loss bed.
- Patients with large TBSA burns or inhalational injury are best ventilated after surgery.
- Postoperative pain relief may be provided by intravenous infusions of opioids or by a patient-controlled analgesia (PCA) device that can be modified for use by means other than fingers if necessary.
- Feeding – basal metabolic rate is increased by up to 100%. Early nutritional supplement is essential; 3000–5000 calories per day in an adult.

OUTCOME

- Age related – decreasing survival rate with increasing age over 30 years
- Is worse in the presence of respiratory injury
- Major reconstructive surgery may be required in the future
- Prognosis for burns over 70% TBSA is very poor, with the cut-off level for survival being about 40%. Women have a worse prognostic index than men (6.3% mortality rate, compared with 5.1%).

The trend is a decline in the number of burn cases; however, cases are increasing in severity while the mortality rate is decreasing. This may be due to earlier nutritional replacement, use of topical silver sulfadiazine cream and earlier surgery.

14

BIBLIOGRAPHY

Barisone D, Peci S, Governa M, Sanna A, Furlan S. Mortality rate and prognostic indices in 2615 burned patients. Burns 1990; 16:373–376

Muir IFK, Barclay TL. Burns and their treatment. 2nd edn. London: Lloyd Luke; 1974

Rylah LTA, ed. Critical care of the burned patient. Cambridge: Cambridge University Press; 1992

Cosmetic surgery

E. M. Grundy

PROCEDURE

Cosmetic surgery is primarily surface surgery, but this is not synonymous with minor surgery. Procedures often take several hours and multiple procedures are increasingly undertaken. While some procedures are undertaken as day cases, rarely is more than one night in hospital required.

PATIENT CHARACTERISTICS

- Patients are sensitive about an aspect of their appearance (morphophobes) or the passage of time (chronophobes)
- Young or middle-aged women predominate
- Becoming increasingly popular as the public at large become aware of what is available.

PREOPERATIVE ASSESSMENT AND CONSIDERATIONS

- These patients are almost all relatively young and fit. However, standards of preoperative assessment should be maintained.
- History, examination and investigations as indicated.
- Deep venous thrombosis (DVT) prophylaxis should be utilised for prolonged cases.

PREMEDICATION

Premedication is usually not required.

THEATRE PREPARATION

- Hypothermia should be avoided, so a warming blanket is useful.
- For surgery around the head and neck, the surgeon will expect full access, and thus the anaesthetist will be at the patient's feet.

PERIOPERATIVE MANAGEMENT

Some procedures are being performed under local anaesthesia with sedation. Standards of monitoring should be maintained. Transition from heavy sedation to light general anaesthesia occurs only too easily and should be anticipated.

During the operation, the surgeon can be expected to inject local anaesthetic solution into the surgical field. This reduces the amount of surgical stimulation and allows a lighter level of anaesthesia to be employed. It will also provide good-quality postoperative analgesia.

Intraoperative bleeding can be reduced by:
- Addition of a vasoconstrictor to the local anaesthetic – usually 5 μg ml^{-1} adrenaline (epinephrine)
- Head-up tilt in the case of upper body surgery
- Induced hypotension – most anaesthetists are prepared to bring the blood pressure down to the low end of the physiological range (around 80 mmHg systolic), but in some centres much more profound hypotension is employed on a regular basis.

HEAD AND NECK SURGERY

HEAD AND NECK SURGERY – PROCEDURES

- Blepharoplasty
- Browlift
- Facelift
- Necklift
- Rhinoplasty
- Surgery for baldness

A secure airway is mandatory and disconnection during the procedure may occur. Induced hypotension will be expected as part of the control of intraoperative bleeding. At the end of the operation, the head and neck will often be moved around significantly during the application of the dressings. With rhinoplasty, or where an intraoral incision has been made, a throat pack is usually employed, which must be removed – pharyngeal suction is necessary prior to extubation. The patient should neither buck nor become hypertensive during this period. Shortly afterwards, the anaesthetist will have to extubate the patient and must ensure that the patient is left with a safe airway. This sequence requires expertise.

ABDOMINOPLASTY

This can be a treacherous operation in the grossly obese who undergo a major reduction. Postoperative retention of secretions and postoperative respiratory failure can occur. Preoperative assessment of respiratory function is important and should not be overlooked.

LIPOSUCTION

Liposuction is the commonest surgical procedure undertaken in the USA and is reported to have a mortality rate of 1 in 5000 (Grazer & de Jong 2000, Rao et al 1999). It is almost invariably to the trunk, buttocks or lower limbs. In the early days, liposuction was performed 'dry' and 'haemoliposuction' might have been a more accurate description of the technique.

Nowadays a 'tumescent' technique is employed whereby a volume of fluid containing lidocaine (lignocaine) and adrenaline (epinephrine) greater than the volume of fat to be aspirated is injected prior to the liposuction. Care must be exercised to ensure that the 'tumescent injection' is made up according to an acceptable formula. Current practice accepts doses of lidocaine and adrenaline that exceed traditional recommended maxima. The volume injected will be up to 3 litres and, while some will be removed at liposuction, most will be absorbed by hypodermatoclysis or enter the third space produced by the liposuction. Fluid balance can be challenging.

Large-volume liposuction is defined as aspirating more than 1500 ml of fat; this requires the injection of over 3 litres of 'tumescent injection'. It is currently considered unwise.

POSTOPERATIVE MANAGEMENT

Postoperative haematomas are usually obvious because of the superficial site of the surgery; they often necessitate a return to theatre for draining (Box 14.2).

Postoperative pain is usually not great because the surgery is superficial and the surgeon will have injected local anaesthetic. Elevation of the surgical site will also help to reduce swelling, and hence pain. The use of non-steroidal anti-inflammatory drugs is controversial because of interference with clotting and the risk of haematoma. Cyclo-oxygenase 2 inhibitors may well have a role to play.

OUTCOME

Almost all patients will be mobile and out of hospital within 24 h of surgery. Postoperative pain and swelling settles within a few days; however, bruising may take 7–14 days to settle. Although rare, postoperative DVTs do occur.

BIBLIOGRAPHY

Grazer FM, de Jong RH. Fatal outcomes from liposuction: census survey of cosmetic surgeons. Plastic and Reconstructive Surgery 2000; 105:436–446

Rao RB, Ely SF, Hoffman RS. Deaths related to liposuction. New England Journal of Medicine 1999; 340:1471–1475

14

BOX 14.2

Causes of postoperative haematoma

- Stormy emergence from anaesthesia
- Rebound hypertension after intraoperative hypotension
- Bucking on tracheal tube
- Obstructed airway
- Shivering from hypothermia or other cause
- Straining from postoperative vomiting

Free flap surgery

B. J. Pollard

PROCEDURES

- Repair of a large skin tissue defect
- Autotransplantation of a distant flap of tissue complete with it own arterial and venous (and possibly nerve) supply.
- Reimplantation of limbs or digits
- An operating microscope is likely to be required
- Prolonged anaesthesia (6–12 h, or even longer) is possible.

PATIENT CHARACTERISTICS

- Almost any age group and American Society of Anesthesiologists (ASA) status may be encountered.
- Patients with malignant disease may require free flap surgery to cover a defect from the resected area.

PREOPERATIVE ASSESSMENT AND CONSIDERATIONS

- Assessment of cardiac and respiratory reserves and the ability to cope safely with an induced hyperdynamic circulation
- Assessment of the airway and the likelihood of difficult intubation if operating around the head and neck area
- Possible need for elective tracheostomy
- DVT prophylaxis
- Blood transfusion availability
- Antibiotic prophylaxis
- Discussion with the surgeon regarding accessibility of arm or leg for donor site.

PREMEDICATION

- Anxiolysis with a benzodiazepine may be useful.
- Care if there is anticipated difficult intubation.

THEATRE PREPARATION

- Skilled staffing for positioning patients
- Patient supports and padding to pressure areas (potentially long operation)
- Anaesthetic room and theatre temperature at 22–24°C and relative humidity of 50%
- Maintenance of body temperature – warming blanket, warm intravenous fluids, warm air overblanket
- Equipment for difficult intubation, including tracheostomy set.

PERIOPERATIVE MANAGEMENT

MONITORING:
- ECG
- Blood pressure – invasive advisable if a prolonged procedure
- CVP
- SpO_2
- $EtCO_2$
- Core and peripheral temperature
- Neuromuscular blockade
- Urine output and blood loss.

ANAESTHETIC TECHNIQUE

General anaesthesia is preferred because of prolonged surgery and the need to keep the patient absolutely still for microsurgery. Adjuvant local anaesthetic techniques are advantageous to promote blood flow through the flap.

Hypotensive anaesthesia may be requested during preparation of donor and recipient sites to facilitate surgery and minimise blood loss.

Following arterial and venous anastomosis of the flap in its new location, blood flow through the flap should be promoted. This can be achieved by:
- The use of isoflurane with its beneficial vasodilatory effects
- Adequate hydration with crystalloid infusion

- Replacement of blood loss as it occurs
- Maintain the CVP at about 2–3 mmHg above the baseline to promote cardiac output
- Maintain haematocrit at around 30–35% by an infusion of colloid solutions.
- Meticulous attention to maintaining body temperature (*Note*: the greatest drop in body temperature occurs in the first hour of anaesthesia)
- Provision of adequate analgesia
- Maintenance of normocapnia and good oxygenation
- Vasodilating drugs – sodium nitroprusside, glyceryl trinitrate, phenoxybenzamine, phentolamine and calcium channel blockers have all been used with success. Whichever drug is used, it is desirable for its vasodilatory effect to last into the postoperative period.

POSTOPERATIVE MANAGEMENT

Transfer to the HDU is advisable for continued monitoring of circulatory control and adequate analgesia. Colloid solution is often infused at up to 7 ml kg^{-1} day^{-1} for 3 days. The flap should be observed regularly for viability and may be monitored with impedance or photoplethys-mography or laser Doppler flowmetry. Common complications are flap arterial thrombus and haematoma requiring re-exploration.

BIBLIOGRAPHY

Green D. Anaesthesia for microvascular surgery. In: Patel H, ed. Anaesthesia for burns. Maxillofacial and plastic surgery. London: Edward Arnold; 1993:93–108

Macdonald DJF. Anaesthesia for microvascular surgery: a physiological approach. British Journal of Anaesthesia 1985; 57:904–912

CROSS-REFERENCES

14

Peripheral limb surgery

B. J. Pollard

PROCEDURES

- Include operations for the repair of bones, tendons, nerves and vessels – may be elective or urgent (trauma).
- Elective surgery also includes surgery for correction of acquired abnormalities (e.g. Dupuytren's contracture, carpal tunnel syndrome, reconstructive surgery for rheumatoid disease) and excision of tumours or skin lesions.
- A tourniquet is usually used to secure a bloodless field.
- Prolonged surgery may be involved (e.g. reimplantation surgery).

PATIENT CHARACTERISTICS

- Can be any age
- May have other trauma associated (e.g. head injury or chest trauma)
- May have alcohol-related injury
- Congenital anomalies may be multiple.

PREOPERATIVE ASSESSMENT AND INVESTIGATIONS

- Exclude concomitant abnormalities or injuries
- Look for other associated medical conditions (e.g. rheumatoid arthritis)
- Haematological and biochemical investigation, as indicated
- ECG, chest radiography and other investigations, as indicated
- Remember the sickle cell screen, especially if a tourniquet is requested.

PREMEDICATION

- Give a full explanation of the procedure and warn the patient about temporary postoperative limb numbness and weakness.

- An anxiolytic drug (e.g. a benzodiazepine) is useful.

PERIOPERATIVE MANAGEMENT

MONITORING:

- ECG
- SpO_2
- Non-invasive blood pressure
- $EtCO_2$ – not necessary for regional blocks.

Additional monitoring may be necessary if surgery is prolonged.

TECHNIQUE

Regional or local block, with or without sedation, is often the most suitable technique:

- Venous access should be established prior to block
- Suitable for a wide range of procedures
- Associated sympathetic block provides optimal perfusion for reimplantation surgery
- Check suitability for block before starting (Box 14.3)
- For details on technique, the reader is referred to a suitable major text. Regular practice with regional blocks greatly increases the success rate.

General anaesthesia, with or without a local or regional block, is also suitable:

- Useful for children
- Useful for prolonged procedures
- Useful for uncooperative patients
- If a regional block is used in addition, the associated sympathetic block provides

---

BOX 14.3

Contraindications to regional block

- Sepsis
- Anticoagulation therapy
- Coagulopathy
- Physical or mental inability to cope

optimal perfusion for reimplantation surgery.

UPPER LIMB SURGERY

BRACHIAL PLEXUS BLOCK:
- The most common block for upper limb surgery
- May be performed by the interscalene, subclavian or axillary approaches (Table 14.3).

PERIPHERAL NERVE BLOCKS:
- Ulnar, median and radial nerve blocks at the elbow and wrist may be used to supplement a brachial plexus block.
- There is a small risk of nerve damage at the elbow.

PRACTICAL POINTS WHEN PERFORMING A BRACHIAL PLEXUS BLOCK

- Use a blunt needle to decrease risk of nerve damage and increase success rate
- Use of a nerve stimulator will increase success rate
- Use of adrenaline (epinephrine) with the local analgesic agent will increase the intensity and duration of block
- A catheter can be inserted for prolonged surgery and postoperative pain relief
- Speed of onset is increased by carbonation and warming the solution
- It is best to avoid peripheral nerve blocks in unconscious patients
- If planning to use both a regional block and a general anaesthetic, it is wise to insert the regional block before induction of anaesthesia

- Digital nerve blocks may be needed – avoid adrenaline (epinephrine)-containing solutions.

INTRAVENOUS REGIONAL ANAESTHESIA (IVRA):
- Easy to perform for small or closed procedures
- The principal disadvantage is the rapid loss of analgesia on cuff deflation, which prevents further surgery to secure haemostasis should this be necessary
- Tourniquet pain may be a problem.

LOWER LIMB SURGERY

Lumbar and caudal epidural blocks and also spinal blocks are ideal for unilateral or bilateral lower limb surgery.

PERIPHERAL NERVE BLOCKS
Used mainly for pain relief in knee surgery and fractures of the lower leg:
- Femoral nerve block
- Three-in-one block – femoral, obturator and lateral cutaneous nerve of the thigh
- Sciatic nerve block.

ANKLE BLOCKS:
- Useful for surgery to the foot not requiring a tourniquet
- Nerves blocked are the sural, saphenous, posterior tibial, superficial peroneal and deep peroneal nerves.

THE USE OF A TOURNIQUET

- Maximum pressure in the leg: 300 mmHg
- Maximum pressure in the arm: 200 mmHg

14

TABLE 14.3

Common approaches to the brachial plexus block

Area blocked	Advantages	Disadvantages
Axillary Hand and forearm	Minimal complications Ideal for outpatients	Radial and musculocutaneous nerves may be missed
Subclavian perivascular Whole arm	Rapid reliable block	Risk of pneumothorax
Interscalene block Shoulder and arm	Easy access	Risk of inadvertent dural puncture or vertebral artery puncture C8–T1 area may be missed

- Maximum tourniquet time: 1–2 h
- Avoid in sickle cell disease – if use is necessary, discuss with a haematologist first.

BIBLIOGRAPHY

Baxter AG, Coventry DM. Brachial plexus blockade. Current Anaesthesia and Critical Care 1999; 10:164–169

Thompson AM, Newman RJ, Semple JC. Brachial plexus anaesthesia for upper limb surgery: a review of eight years' experience. Journal of Hand Surgery [Br] 1988; 13: 195–198

Wildsmith JA, Armitage EN. Principles and practice of regional anaesthesia. Edinburgh: Churchill Livingstone; 1993

CROSS-REFERENCES

Sickle cell syndrome
    Patient Conditions 7: 226
Day-case surgery
    Anaesthetic Factors 27: 613
Prolonged anaesthesia
    Anaesthetic Factors 30: 713
Local anaesthetic toxicity
    Anaesthetic Factors 31: 761

14

Paediatric plastic surgery

S. Berg

Children of all ages present for corrective surgery, from the neonate to the adolescent. Operations range from minor day-case procedures to major reconstructive surgery.

GENERAL FEATURES

- Most operations are elective. Children with features of a recent upper respiratory tract infection should be delayed for a minimum of 2 weeks.
- Some children may present for surgery with syndromes associated with features of anaesthetic significance (e.g. difficult intubation).
- Many children require multiple surgical procedures. It is important to establish a rapport with the child and parents. Preoperative preparation is essential and oral premedication may be required (e.g. midazolam 0.5 mg kg^{-1}).
- Heat loss is a major problem, especially for smaller children undergoing major surgery. Maintain the theatre temperature at 22–24°C and avoid unnecessary exposure of the child. Consider warming mattress, convective warm air heating blanket and overhead radiant heater. Also humidification and warming of anaesthetic gases and active warming of intravenous fluids. Temperature measurement is essential.
- Operations on the skin and superficial tissues are painful. Regional techniques including local infiltration, peripheral nerve blocks, and caudal and epidural blockade will facilitate a lighter plane of anaesthesia and provide a smoother recovery to prevent a coughing, straining restless child in the postoperative phase, which could increase bleeding and jeopardise the operation.
- Local infiltration with adrenaline (epinephrine) is used routinely by many plastic surgeons – up to 10 μg kg^{-1} can be used safely. Volatile agents may potentiate dysrhythmias.

CLEFT LIP AND PALATE

PATIENT CHARACTERISTICS:

- Common condition with an incidence of 1 in 600 live births. It is an isolated defect in 90% of cases.
- Isolated cleft palate (1 in 2000 live births) is often associated with other congenital abnormalities that may be of anaesthetic significance (Table 14.4).
- Range of deformity.
- Average age of correction:
  —cleft lip: 8–12 weeks (neonatal repair decreasing in popularity)
  —cleft palate: 6–12 months (dependent upon the size of the cleft)
- These children have multiple problems and their clinical care requires a combined team approach.

TABLE 14.4

Syndromes of anaesthetic significance associated with cleft palate

Syndrome	Significant features
Klippel–Feil	15% associated with cleft palate
	Short, webbed neck
	Fused cervical vertebrae
	Congenital cardiac disease
Pierre Robin	80% associated with cleft palate
	Severe micrognathia
	Glossoptosis
	Congenital cardiac disease
	Intubation easier with age
Shprintzen (velocardiofacial)	90% associated with cleft palate
	Facial dysmorphism
	Learning difficulties
	Congenital cardiac disease
Treacher Collins	28% associated with cleft palate
	Micrognathia
	Malar and maxillary hypoplasia
	Ear malformations
	Intubation more difficult with age

14

PREOPERATIVE ASSESSMENT AND INVESTIGATIONS:

- Assess the airway – upper respiratory tract infection will increase the risk of airway complications and compromise wound healing.
- Exclude other associated conditions (e.g. cardiac disease)
- Blood should be available for transfusion.

PREMEDICATION:

- Usually unnecessary
- Avoid opioid or sedative premedication in children under 6 months or if airway is compromised
- If difficult airway is anticipated, give atropine 20 μg kg^{-1} i.m.

THEATRE PREPARATION

Maintain body temperature by warming theatre to 22–24°C, warming fluids, humidifying gases and using warming mattress or convective blanket.

PERIOPERATIVE MANAGEMENT

Monitoring:

- ECG
- Non-invasive blood pressure
- SaO_2
- Gas monitoring
- Nerve stimulator
- Core temperature probe
- Fluid balance and blood loss.

INDUCTION OF ANAESTHESIA:

- Inhalation or intravenous induction. If there is a suspected airway problem, induce with sevoflurane in 100% oxygen. Use of continuous positive airway pressure (CPAP) will assist maintenance of the airway.
- Intubate deep with child breathing spontaneously or after a muscle relaxant once a safe airway has been established.
- Care should be taken to prevent the laryngoscope blade from lodging in the cleft. A roll of gauze can fill the defect or a lateral approach with the laryngoscope can be used.
- A preformed tracheal tube may become kinked by the gag. Using a reinforced tube will resist compression but it is more difficult to secure at the correct length.
- Throat pack.

MAINTENANCE OF ANAESTHESIA:

- Controlled ventilation. Intravenous fentanyl (1–2 μg kg^{-1}) can be used to supplement anaesthesia, but should be given cautiously in neonates or in the presence of upper airway problems.
- The use of local infiltration using either lidocaine (lignocaine) or bupivacaine with adrenaline (epinephrine) 1 : 200 000 produces good analgesia, an improved operating field and reduced blood loss.
- Infraorbital nerve block for cleft lip repair or nasopalatine and palatine block for cleft palate surgery is also effective.

POSTOPERATIVE MANAGEMENT

The patient should be extubated only when fully awake, breathing adequately and in the tonsillar position. Smooth pain-free emergence reduces crying and the risk of postoperative bleeding.

Postoperative airway obstruction can be a particular problem in cleft palate repair, and a nasopharyngeal airway or stent may be required in some patients.

The insertion of a tongue stitch to allow the tongue to be pulled forward is a useful, although uncommonly used, technique.

Postoperative analgesia for cleft lip includes regular paracetamol and codeine phosphate with feeding commonly possible within a few hours of surgery. In cleft palate repair, regular paracetamol plus ibuprofen with 'rescue' codeine phosphate is usually satisfactory; most children can feed on the following day. Ketamine may be useful as a non-respiratory depressant analgesic in the early stages of postoperative management.

CRANIOFACIAL SURGERY

- This constitutes major reconstructive surgery involving the facial skeleton, facial soft tissues and cranial shape. Children with craniosynostosis often have associated syndromes.
- Problems include difficult intubation, major blood loss and hypothermia.
- Direct arterial and central venous pressure measurement (via the femoral vein) are required.

HAEMANGIOMA

- May be complicated by airway problems, major blood loss and air embolism.
- A cutaneous haemangioma around the face and neck may be associated with a subglottic haemangioma.

CYSTIC HYGROMA

- Multiloculated cystic swelling in the neck that may invade the oropharynx and tongue; can present as an upper airway obstruction in the neonate.
- Intubation may be hazardous; spontaneous ventilation must be maintained until intubation has been achieved. Severe cases will require tracheostomy.
- Postoperative problems include bleeding and respiratory obstruction.

OTOPLASTY

Correction of prominent ears is associated with a high incidence of postoperative nausea and vomiting, which may last for up to 48 h. This can be reduced by local infiltration or nerve block, but an antiemetic will be required.

HYPOSPADIAS

- Anatomical correction of male urethra, usually infant.
- Spontaneous or controlled ventilation according to length of procedure.
- Caudal block with 0.5–1 ml kg^{-1} of 0.25% bupivacaine provides excellent analgesia that can be extended by adding clonidine, diamorphine or ketamine.

BURNS

See page 382. Similar principles apply to those used in adult practice. Analgesia is often inadequate. Ketamine is useful for minor procedures, and regional techniques should be considered for more major operations.

BIBLIOGRAPHY

Bosenberg AT, Kimble FW. Infraorbital nerve block in neonates for cleft lip repair: anatomical study and clinical application. British Journal of Anaesthesia 1995; 74:506–508

Hatch DJ. Airway management in cleft lip and palate surgery. British Journal of Anaesthesia 1996; 76:755–756

Sommerlad BC. Management of cleft lip and palate. Current Paediatrics 1994; 4:189–195

Takemura H, Yasumoto K, Toi T, Hosoyamada A. Correlation of cleft type with incidence of perioperative respiratory complications in infants with cleft lip and palate. Paediatric Anaesthesia 2002; 12:585–588

CROSS-REFERENCES

Infants and children
    Anaesthetic Factors 27: 610
Difficult airway
    Anaesthetic Factors 28: 660
Paediatric airway
    Anaesthetic Factors 28: 670

14

15

THORACIC SURGERY
J. W. W. Gothard

Overview

J. W. W. Gothard

Only 20% of patients with lung cancer have resectable tumours at presentation. The vast majority of lung resections in the UK are carried out for the treatment of lung cancer (Table 15.1), but a variety of other procedures are undertaken often via a videoscopic technique. The operative mortality rate following pneumonectomy and lobectomy remains high at 5% and 2.9% respectively. This is a result of the extensive nature of the surgery involved and intercurrent disease of the patients.

Bronchoscopy, mediastinoscopy and pleurectomy (Table 15.1) are carried out in relatively large numbers of patients, with a low mortality rate. Bronchoscopy and mediastinoscopy often precede a more major procedure, which will present a greater operative risk. Pleurectomy is,

in the main, carried out in relatively fit young patients with spontaneous pneumothoraces, so the mortality rate associated within this type of operation is very low.

ANAESTHESIA FOR THORACIC SURGERY

ENDOBRONCHIAL INTUBATION

Anaesthesia for thoracic surgery has evolved steadily since the early 1930s when Gale and Waters (USA) and subsequently Magill (UK) introduced single-lumen endobronchial tubes for selective endobronchial intubation. The double-lumen endobronchial tube of Carlens, which was originally introduced for differential spirometry in 1949, was redesigned by Robertshaw in 1962 and produced in right and left forms. More recently, plastic, disposable, double-lumen endobronchial tubes have been introduced by several manufacturers.

The 'blind' placement of endobronchial tubes has always been difficult. The introduction of relatively cheap and robust (yet slim) fibreoptic bronchoscopes now enables the thoracic anaesthetist to place endobronchial tubes under direct vision, or at least to check their position following blind placement.

ONE-LUNG ANAESTHESIA

The majority of major thoracic operations are carried out with the patient in the lateral position. When ventilation to the upper lung is discontinued to aid surgery, pulmonary blood flow continues to that lung. A 'true' shunt is therefore created and hypoxia may occur.

One-lung ventilation (OLV) should be established so that it inflates the lung adequately but also minimises intra-alveolar pressure and prevents diversion of pulmonary blood flow to the upper lung.

It is reasonable to use an inspired oxygen concentration of 50% initially. When OLV is established, the concentration can be increased to 100%, if required. This cannot affect the

TABLE 15.1

Thoracic surgical results from 47 UK centres (1999–2000)

	No. of operations	No. of deaths
Lung resection for primary malignant tumours		
Pneumonectomy	779	39 (5.0%)
Lobectomy	2208	63 (2.9%)
Video-assisted thoracoscopic surgery for pulmonary or pleural disease		
Lung biopsy	506	6 (1.2%)
Lung volume reduction surgery (unilateral)	50	3 (6.0%)
Pneumothorax (various procedures)	735	6 (0.8%)
Pleural biopsy	499	5 (1.0%)
Pleural biopsy and chemical pleurodesis	932	18 (1.9%)

Values in parentheses are percentages.
Adapted from the database of the Society of Cardiothoracic Surgeons of Great Britain and Ireland.

true shunt in the upper lung but may improve oxygenation via the alveoli with low ventilation–perfusion ratios in the lower lung.

There is increasing evidence that overinflating the single lung (volutrauma) can be detrimental and lead to acute lung injury. The use of low tidal volumes improves outcome in ventilated patients with acute respiratory distress syndrome, and this may also apply to OLV. Limiting ventilation (Box 15.1) can lead to carbon dioxide retention, but permissive hypercapnia is preferable to lung trauma. General guidelines for OLV are set out in Box 15.2.

On current evidence, hypoxic pulmonary vasoconstriction (HPV) seems to play little part in reducing hypoxaemia during the time it takes to complete a pneumonectomy or lobectomy. Thus, although many inhalational agents inhibit HPV, they do not appear to impair arterial oxygenation significantly during one-lung anaesthesia.

High-frequency jet ventilation (HFJV) has been advocated for use during thoracic surgery, but is not in widespread use. HFJV may be of benefit in patients with lung cysts and bronchopleural fistulae, but even in these conditions its use remains controversial.

POSTOPERATIVE PAIN RELIEF

Operations carried out through a lateral thoracotomy incision can be extremely painful in the postoperative period. There have been a number of advances in the provision of pain relief following thoracic surgery in recent years. These include the application of extrapleural and intrapleural analgesic techniques and the use of epidural opioid drugs.

BOX 15.1

Guidelines for the management of one-lung ventilation

- Inspired oxygen concentration of 50–100% (increase if $S_{O_2} < 90\%$)
- Normal inspiratory : expiratory ratio (increase expiratory phase if gas trapping likely)
- Consider pressure-limiting ventilation
- Use small tidal volumes (e.g. 6–7 ml kg^{-1})
- Allow permissive hypercapnia
- Use positive end-expiratory pressure (PEEP) if desaturated
- Insufflate oxygen to upper lung if hypoxic (if surgical field not obscured)
- Avoid overinflation (volutrauma)

BIBLIOGRAPHY

Gosh S, Latimer RD. Thoracic anaesthesia: principles and practice. Oxford: Butterworth Heinemann; 1999

Gothard JWW, Kelleher A, Haxby E. Cardiovascular and thoracic anaesthesia. London: Elsevier Science; 2003

CROSS-REFERENCES

Preoperative assessment of cardiovascular risk in non-cardiac surgery
    Anaesthetic Factors 27: 634
Preoperative assessment of pulmonary risk
    Anaesthetic Factors 27: 638

15

Bronchopleural fistula

J. W. W. Gothard

A bronchopleural fistula (BPF) is a direct communication between the tracheobronchial tree and the pleural cavity. Causes of BPF include:

- Trauma
- Neoplasm
- Inflammatory lesion
- Dehiscence of bronchial stump.

In developed countries, dehiscence of the bronchial stump following pneumonectomy is the commonest reason for patients to present for surgical repair of BPF. The incidence of BPF following pneumonectomy is, however, extremely low in specialised surgical centres.

PROCEDURE

Minor forms of postpneumonectomy BPF can be cauterised at bronchoscopy with sodium hydroxide or, alternatively, may be sealed with fibrin glue.

Large fistulae require surgical repair (resuture of the bronchial stump) via a lateral thoracotomy through the previous incision.

PATIENT CHARACTERISTICS

- Often postpneumonectomy (3–15 days)
- American Society of Anesthesiologists (ASA) status IV or V.

PREOPERATIVE ASSESSMENT AND INVESTIGATIONS

SYMPTOMS

Symptoms relate to fluid from the infected space flowing over to the remaining lung:

- Malaise
- Low-grade fever
- Cough
- Haemoptysis
- Wheeze or dyspnoea

or, in acute onset with a large BPF:

- Severe dyspnoea

- Coughing up copious amounts of thinnish brown fluid.

INVESTIGATIONS

Chest radiography shows:

- Loss of pneumonectomy space fluid
- Consolidation or collapse of remaining lung.

Arterial blood gas analysis demonstrates:

- Hypoxia
- Hypercarbia
- Metabolic acidosis.

PREMEDICATION

None required if acute onset. Omit premedication if there is any doubt regarding the patient's condition.

THEATRE PREPARATION

- General resuscitation including oxygen by face-mask
- Sit patient up to prevent further 'spill-over'
- Insert chest drain on pneumonectomised side
- Transport patient to theatre in sitting position with drain open.

PERIOPERATIVE MANAGEMENT

MONITORING:

- ECG
- Blood pressure – preferably invasive
- SaO_2
- $EtCO_2$
- Central venous pressure or pulmonary capillary wedge pressure (PCWP)
- Core temperature
- Urine output.

ANAESTHETIC TECHNIQUE

Classically it has been advocated that a postpneumonectomy fistula should be isolated with an endobronchial tube before intermittent positive-pressure ventilation (IPPV) is employed. A double-lumen endobronchial tube (DLT) is inserted in the remaining bronchus. To secure the airway prior to the administration of a muscle relaxant, two methods were previously advocated:

- Awake endobronchial intubation using local analgesia of the upper respiratory tract
- Inhalational induction and intubation under deep inhalational anaesthesia.

The above techniques should be discussed at examinations, but in practice both are fraught with difficulty. Most experienced anaesthetists now use the following technique:

- Patient sitting upright, with drain open
- Preoxygenation
- Slow intravenous induction
- Intravenous suxamethonium (or alternative such as rocuronium)
- Insertion of DLT – use of fibreoptic bronchoscope useful
- Administer further muscle relaxant
- IPPV via endobronchial portion of tube
- Patient placed in lateral position for thoracotomy.

POSTOPERATIVE MANAGEMENT

Re-establish spontaneous respiration, in the sitting position where possible, and transfer the patient to an ITU for further management. Respiratory failure is common after this type of procedure and this should be treated conventionally where indicated, with IPPV via a tracheal tube. High-frequency jet ventilation has been advocated for the preoperative and postoperative management of bronchopleural fistulae because of the low peak airway pressures employed. The evidence that this mode of ventilation is significantly better than conventional techniques remains conflicting.

OUTCOME

The morbidity rate is high following this type of operation. The mortality rate is probably in the region of 10–20%, but national figures are not available.

BIBLIOGRAPHY

Feeley TW, Keating D, Nishimura T. Independent lung ventilation using high-frequency ventilation in the management of a bronchopleural fistula. Anesthesiology 1988; 69:420–422

Lauckner ME, Beggs I, Armstrong RF. The radiological characteristics of bronchopleural fistula following pneumonectomy. Anaesthesia 1983; 38:452–456

Ryder GH, Short DH, Zeitlin GL. The anaesthetic management of a bronchopleural fistula with the Robertshaw double-lumen tube. British Journal of Anaesthesia 1965; 37:861–865

15

Inhaled foreign body

J. W. W. Gothard

Foreign bodies can be inhaled at any age but are more common in children under 3 years of age. Foreign bodies within the tracheobronchial tree require removal at bronchoscopy. The rigid bronchoscope is by far the best instrument for this procedure, as it allows grasping forceps of an adequate size to be used.

Peanuts are of a size easily inhaled by children and they are liable to fragment in the airway, releasing an irritant oil that causes severe inflammation. Inorganic objects can also be inhaled, however, and will also require removal at bronchoscopy.

PATIENT CHARACTERISTICS

Inhalation of foreign bodies is more common in the following groups:
- Children
- The elderly
- Debilitated subjects
- Drunks.

PREOPERATIVE ASSESSMENT AND INVESTIGATIONS

SYMPTOMS
There may be a specific history of inhalation such as a bout of coughing whilst eating peanuts. Alternatively, a chronic cough with wheeze, stridor and fever may be the presenting symptoms some time after the original inhalation. A persistent chest infection in an otherwise healthy child may warrant investigation for an inhaled foreign body.

INVESTIGATIONS
A variety of chest radiographic changes may be present:
- Obstructive emphysema (seen best on expiratory film)
- Radiopaque object (e.g. pin) in tracheobronchial tree
- Non-specific changes (atelectasis, consolidation)
- Normal radiograph.

OTHER INVESTIGATIONS:
- Full blood count in children
- Standard investigations relating to age and medical condition of adult (e.g. ECG, urea and electrolytes, liver function tests).

PREMEDICATION

- Anaesthetist's preferred standard regimen in adults and children
- Anticholinergics not essential
- Omit premedication if any question of upper airway obstruction.

PERIOPERATIVE MANAGEMENT

MONITORING:
- ECG
- Non-invasive blood pressure
- SaO_2

ANAESTHETIC TECHNIQUE
General anaesthesia is preferred for rigid bronchoscopy in both adults and children.
- Preoxygenation
- Intravenous induction in adults and bigger children (use suitable local anaesthetic cream)
- Inhalational induction in smaller children
- Consider inhalational induction in all patients with upper airway obstruction.

If upper airway obstruction is present because of a foreign body lodged in the upper trachea or larynx, it may be safer to perform initial bronchoscopy under deep inhalational anaesthesia. In the majority of circumstances it will be safe to introduce the bronchoscope after the administration of suxamethonium. If the procedure is likely to be prolonged, intermittent suxamethonium can be used (NB: use an anticholinergic to prevent bradycardia), but it is preferable to use a longer-acting drug such as atracurium.

Anaesthesia can be maintained by a propofol infusion in adults, whereas a volatile agent is ideal for use with a ventilating bronchoscope in children. Ventilation in adults can be carried out satisfactorily with a Venturi system, but care must be taken not to blow fragments of foreign body further down the tracheobronchial tree. In children ventilation can be carried out via a ventilating bronchoscope and T-piece system (see section below on Rigid bronchoscopy).

POSTOPERATIVE MANAGEMENT

After a relatively short atraumatic procedure, the patient can be allowed to wake up in the usual manner, once the bronchoscope has been removed and muscular relaxation reversed. Oxygen is then administered by face-mask. If the procedure has been long and difficult, the instrumentation may cause upper airway oedema, especially in small children. It is prudent, therefore, to take the following precautions:

- Remove bronchoscope and reintubate with a small oral tracheal tube
- Allow patient to awake on side, breathing a high $F\text{iO}_2$
- Suction, as required
- Extubate when fully awake
- Be prepared for emergency reintubation.

Postextubation, children should be nursed in humidified oxygen-enriched air and monitored in a high-dependency area. In the presence of severe laryngeal oedema, a period of postoperative ventilation may be required until a gas leak appears around the tracheal tube. Steroids and nebulised adrenaline (epinephrine) may be useful at this stage.

BIBLIOGRAPHY

Gillbe C, Hillier J. Anaesthesia for bronchoscopy, tracheal and airway surgery. Anaesthesia and Intensive Care Medicine 2002; 3(11):402–404

CROSS-REFERENCES

Rigid bronchoscopy
    Surgical Procedures 15: 413
Preoperative assessment of pulmonary risk
    Anaesthetic Factors 27: 638

15

Lobectomy

J. W. W. Gothard

PROCEDURE

Lobectomy is the surgical excision of one lobe of a lung. Usual indications are:
- Malignant and benign tumours
- Bronchiectasis
- Tuberculosis and fungal infections.

PATIENT CHARACTERISTICS

LOBECTOMY FOR MALIGNANT TUMOURS:
- Elderly
- Smokers
- ASA grades II–IV.

LOBECTOMY FOR BENIGN TUMOURS:
- Younger age group.

LOBECTOMY FOR BRONCHIECTASIS:
- Children and adults
- Resection indicated if disease confined to one or two lobes
- If lung disease is generalised:
  —indicates high risk
  —patients often debilitated.

PREOPERATIVE ASSESSMENT

As for Pneumonectomy (see p. 408). Computed tomography and bronchography used to evaluate extent of any bronchiectasis.

Patients unable to tolerate pneumonectomy may withstand lobectomy.

PREMEDICATION

- Continue cardiac and respiratory medications until surgery
- Conventional benzodiazepine premedication is satisfactory
- Anticholinergic drugs not essential
- Low-molecular-weight heparin for prophylaxis of deep vein thrombosis (DVT).

Patients with bronchiectasis are admitted several days before operation for postural drainage, physiotherapy and antibiotic medication. This is intended to reduce the volume and purulence of secretions.

PERIOPERATIVE MANAGEMENT

MONITORING:
- ECG
- Blood pressure, preferably invasive
- Sao_2
- $Etco_2$
- Core temperature
- Central venous pressure
- Tidal volume and airway pressure
- Arterial blood gases
- Urine output – if epidural analgesia employed or high-risk patient.

ANAESTHETIC TECHNIQUE

General anaesthesia with muscle relaxation and mechanical ventilation is the technique of choice. Intravenous opioids can be used to supplement analgesia; alternatively, epidural techniques can be employed (see section below on Postoperative analgesia for thoracic surgery patients).

A double-lumen endobronchial tube is placed in the non-operative lung to provide one-lung ventilation and control of secretions. An unacceptable degree of hypoxaemia may occur during one-lung ventilation in patients with generalised pulmonary disease who are judged capable of withstanding lobectomy, although this is uncommon. It may be necessary to use an inspired gas concentration of 100% oxygen, possibly in combination (rarely) with oxygen insufflated at a positive pressure to the operative lung. In the presence of severe hypoxia positive end-expiratory pressure (PEEP) to the dependent lung may improve oxygenation.

In bronchiectasis, the remaining lobe or lobes on the non-operative side are unprotected from the spread of secretions if a double-lumen tube is used, and infected material may seep past the endobronchial cuff into the opposite lung. Repeated suction to both lungs limits this contamination. Spread of secretions from lobe to lobe can be reduced by using bronchial blockade (e.g. 'Arndt' blocker or the 'Univent Tube', a blocker combined with a tracheal tube) to block specific bronchi while continuing to ventilate the remaining lobes. The main drawback of blocking techniques is that if they fail (e.g. by dislodgement), all protection from the spread of secretions is lost.

PERIOPERATIVE MANAGEMENT

One-lung anaesthesia is used when requested. The integrity of bronchial suture lines is tested prior to chest closure. The bronchial stump is covered with sterile water (malignant disease) or saline (benign disease) and a pressure up to a maximum of 30 cmH$_2$O is exerted by manual compression of a rebreathing bag. Any leak is then detected. Leaks from raw lung surfaces are detected in a similar manner, but at a pressure of approximately 20 cmH$_2$O. Any significant leaks require suturing, or may be sealed with tissue glue sprayed on to the surface.

CHEST DRAINAGE

- Apical and basal drains
- Suction at 5 kPa via under water seal
- Anterior and posterior drains are occasionally used.

POSTOPERATIVE PERIOD

- Extubate patient in the sitting position, breathing spontaneously
- Administer humidified oxygen by face-mask
- Management of other complications as for pneumonectomy
- Persistent air leak can be a problem.

OUTCOME

The 30-day operative mortality rate for lobectomy in primary malignant tumours of the lung is currently 2.9% in the UK.

BIBLIOGRAPHY

Wright IG (1999) Surgery on the lungs. In: Ghosh S, Latimer RD, eds. Thoracic anaesthesia: principles and practice. Oxford: Butterworth Heinemann; 1999:73–99

CROSS-REFERENCES

Bronchiectasis
    Patient Conditions 3: 90
Pneumonectomy
    Surgical Procedures 15: 408
One-lung anaesthesia
    Anaesthetic Factors 30: 710
Preoperative assessment of respiratory risk
    Anaesthetic Factors 27: 638

15

Mediastinal operations

J. W. W. Gothard

15

PROCEDURES

Mediastinal surgery can be split into two categories:
- Diagnostic – mediastinoscopy, mediastinotomy
- Therapeutic – excision of tumours and cysts.

Mediastinoscopy and mediastinotomy are commonly carried out to assess mediastinal lymph node involvement in the staging of lung cancer. These patients are in the categories outlined for pneumonectomy and lobectomy, and are in a relatively low-risk category for the staging procedure. Patients with mediastinal tumours are in a very different category. Some are at low risk, for example those with mediastinal cysts, small intrathoracic thyroids or thymomas. Many, particularly patients with large anterior mediastinal tumours, are at high risk. These high-risk patients may present for a histological diagnosis to be determined. If this is the case, the problems outlined for major mediastinal surgery must also be taken into account for the lesser procedures.

MEDIASTINOSCOPY AND MEDIASTINOTOMY

In mediastinoscopy, a mediastinoscope is passed into the pretracheal area via a small incision above the suprasternal notch. Biopsies can then be taken and nodes palpated digitally. A mediastinotomy allows direct surgical access to the anterior mediastinum via an incision through the bed of the second costal cartilage.
- Rigid bronchoscopy is usually performed first.
- Position the patient supine with a sandbag under the shoulders, the head on a ring, and the neck extended.

PATIENT CHARACTERISTICS

As for pneumonectomy (see p. 408) and lobectomy (see p. 402).

PREOPERATIVE ASSESSMENT AND CONSIDERATIONS

As for pneumonectomy and lobectomy.

PREMEDICATION

As for pneumonectomy and lobectomy.

PERIOPERATIVE MANAGEMENT

Monitoring:
- ECG
- Non-invasive blood pressure
- SaO_2
- $EtCO_2$
- Intravenous infusion is essential – vascular structures may be biopsied in error.

ANAESTHETIC TECHNIQUE:
- Intravenous induction
- Muscular relaxation (atracurium, vecuronium, rocuronium)
  Note: different considerations apply in the presence of myasthenia gravis.
- Maintenance – volatile agent
- Low- to moderate-dose opioid.

PERIOPERATIVE MANAGEMENT

Mediastinotomy is often on the left side. Pleura may be breached surgically. This is drained via a wide-bore nasogastric tube, which is removed as the anaesthetist applies continuous positive pressure to the lungs and the surgeon completes the suture line to prevent recurrence of the pneumothorax.

POSTOPERATIVE MANAGEMENT:
- Extubate
- Sit up
- Check chest radiograph for pneumothoraces.

MEDIASTINAL TUMOURS

Mediastinal tumours are rare. The tumours that more commonly present for surgical excision are:

- Retrosternal thyroid
- Thymectomy for myasthenia gravis
- Neurogenic tumours
- Reduplication cysts
- Thymoma without myasthenia.

PROCEDURE

Most resectable mediastinal tumours are removed surgically via a median sternotomy, with the patient in a supine position. Anterior mediastinal tumours are particularly likely to cause problems during anaesthesia. The major problems encountered are:

- Airway obstruction
- Compression of intrathoracic vascular structures
- Effects of radiotherapy and chemotherapy (NB: bleomycin lung)
- Intraoperative bleeding
- Section of phrenic and recurrent laryngeal nerves at operation.

PATIENT CHARACTERISTICS

Mediastinal tumours appear more commonly in young adults.

PREOPERATIVE ASSESSMENT AND CONSIDERATIONS

As for other major thoracic surgery, such as pneumonectomy (see p. 408). Further investigations will depend on symptoms:

- Respiratory symptoms (cough, dyspnoea, orthopnoea):
  —CT or MRI of airway
  —Lung function with flow volume loop.
- Superior vena cava (SVC) obstruction:
  —CT or MRI of airway.
- Cyanosis with reasonable lung function (?pulmonary artery occlusion):
  —Pulmonary angiography may be indicated.
  —Consider echo investigation in addition to CT or MRI.

PREMEDICATION

Omit in airway obstruction.

PERIOPERATIVE MANAGEMENT

Monitoring:

- Standard monitoring as for pneumonectomy and lobectomy
- Additional venous access required in lower limb in the case of major surgical disruption of SVC.

ANAESTHETIC TECHNIQUE

General anaesthesia with muscle relaxation and mechanical ventilation. Special considerations apply if the patient has myasthenia gravis (see p. 80). Major problems with large tumours relate to external compression of airway at induction of anaesthesia. To circumvent this:

- Splint airway with bronchoscope following intravenous induction and intravenous suxamethonium
- Pass long tracheal or endobronchial tube through the compression
- Consider the use of cardiopulmonary bypass, especially in the presence of pulmonary artery compression (very rare)
- *Note*: inhalational induction is very difficult if there is gross external compression of the airway.

PERIOPERATIVE MANAGEMENT:

- IPPV
- Replace blood loss, which may be substantial (NB: lower-limb intravenous access)
- Use lowest F_{IO_2} compatible with adequate arterial oxygen saturation if patient has had recent bleomycin therapy.

POSTOPERATIVE MANAGEMENT

Consider mechanical ventilation:

- After a long operation
- If major nerves (e.g. phrenic) are sectioned
- When airway patency is still a problem.

OUTCOME

Good results if tumour resectable. Very low operative mortality rate in the UK, despite potential difficulties. Recurrence is a problem with some tumours, but these may respond to chemotherapy or radiotherapy. Some tumours (e.g. secondary teratoma) may require reoperation.

15

BIBLIOGRAPHY

Feneck RO. Mediastinal surgery. In: Ghosh S, Latimer RD, eds. Thoracic anaesthesia: principles and practice. Oxford: Butterworth Heinemann; 1999:123–143

Gothard JWW. Anaesthesia for thoracic malignancy. In: Filshie J, Robbie DS, eds. Anaesthesia and malignant disease. London: Edward Arnold; 1989:175–197

Pleurectomy

J. W. W. Gothard

PROCEDURE

- Parietal pleura is stripped over all but the diaphragmatic and mediastinal surfaces of the lung.
- This is the surgical treatment of choice for fit patients with a spontaneous pneumothorax.
- This procedure is now commonly carried out endoscopically utilising a video-assisted thoracoscopic surgical (VATS) technique, with the patient in a lateral or semilateral position. Occasionally an open surgical approach may be required via a small lateral or anterolateral thoracotomy.
- Lesser procedures (e.g. pleurodesis) are indicated in debilitated patients and those with malignant disease; these are commonly carried out endoscopically with a VATS technique.

PATIENT CHARACTERISTICS

Spontaneous pneumothorax commonly occurs in:
- Young fit adults
- Tall and thin subjects
- More frequently in males and smokers.
Secondary pneumothorax occurs in:
- Chronic bronchitis and emphysema
- Tuberculosis
- Cystic fibrosis
- Lung cancer.

PREOPERATIVE ASSESSMENT AND INVESTIGATIONS

- General medical condition – particularly with secondary pneumothorax
- Size of existing pneumothorax, presence of functioning drain, etc.
- Rarely possible to obtain meaningful lung function studies.

PREMEDICATION

- Conventional benzodiazepine premedication satisfactory
- Anticholinergic drugs not essential
- Low-molecular-weight heparin for DVT prophylaxis.

PERIOPERATIVE MANAGEMENT

MONITORING:
- ECG
- Blood pressure (preferably invasive)
- Sao_2
- $Etco_2$
- Tidal volume and airway pressure.

PROBLEMS OF PNEUMOTHORAX DURING ANAESTHESIA:
- Size of pneumothorax will increase with uptake of nitrous oxide.
- Positive-pressure ventilation may create tension pneumothorax.
- Both of the above are unlikely with a functioning chest drain.
- It is safer to drain a large pneumothorax before operation (a minor air space is usually tolerated).

ANAESTHETIC TECHNIQUE

ENDOSCOPIC AND OPEN PLEURECTOMY
General anaesthesia with muscle paralysis and mechanical ventilation is the preferred technique. Postoperative pain relief is a much greater problem after open surgery. In general:
- Safer to avoid nitrous oxide
- Minimise inflation pressures
- Potential for pneumothorax on non-operative side (bilateral disease)
- Tracheal intubation satisfactory (for open procedure only) if:
  —no pneumothorax present, or
  —functional drain present.

15

- Double-lumen endobronchial tube (in left lung) mandatory for endoscopic (VATS) technique and in presence of a large air leak for open operation
- Facility to collapse operative lung may be requested for open technique by some surgeons
- Blood loss may be significant, particularly if pleura is diseased
- Surgeon may ligate bullae or seal leaks with tissue glue
- Test for air leaks as described for lobectomy.

BILATERAL PLEURECTOMY

This is a very painful operation that is preferably avoided or carried out as a VATS procedure if essential. Pain relief may be a problem and epidural analgesia is therefore indicated. A brief period of postoperative ventilation may be beneficial.

POSTOPERATIVE MANAGEMENT

- Generally possible and desirable to establish spontaneous respiration
- Patients after bilateral pleurectomy and those with generalised lung disease may need a period of mechanical ventilation
- Sit patient up as soon as possible
- Administer humidified oxygen by face-mask

- Pleural cavity usually drained after operation, as for lobectomy
- Adequate pain relief essential.

OUTCOME

Incidence of recurrence of pneumothorax after endoscopic and open pleurectomy is very low.

CROSS-REFERENCES

Bronchogenic carcinoma
     Patient Conditions 3: 92
Chronic obstructive airway disease
     Patient Conditions 3: 95
Cystic fibrosis
     Patient Conditions 3: 98
Postoperative analgesia for thoracic surgery patients
     Surgical Procedures 15: 411
One-lung anaesthesia
     Anaesthetic Factors 30: 710

BIBLIOGRAPHY

Millar FA, Hutchinson GL, Wood RAB. Anaesthesia for thoracoscopic pleurectomy and ligation of bullae. Anaesthesia 1992; 47:1057–1060

15

Pneumonectomy

J. W. W. Gothard

PROCEDURE

- Usual indication is carcinoma of the lung
- Performed via a lateral thoracotomy.

PATIENT CHARACTERISTICS

Patients for pneumonectomy are generally:
- Elderly
- Smokers (past or present)
- ASA status II–IV.

PREOPERATIVE ASSESSMENT AND INVESTIGATIONS

ASSESSMENT OF CARDIAC AND RESPIRATORY FUNCTION:
- Clinical examination
- ECG
- Chest radiography
- CT
- Full blood count
- Urea and electrolytes
- Arterial blood gases (breathing air)
- Lung function tests
- Cross-match (4 units blood or packed cells).

EVALUATE THE RISK OF PNEUMONECTOMY:
- Cardiac dysfunction is common.
- Cardiac risk indicators (e.g. American College of Cardiology guidelines) may be valuable.
- Forced expiratory volume in 1 s (FEV_1) and forced vital capacity (FVC) are essential baseline measurements.
- Exercise testing is useful.
- Good preoperative exercise tolerance indicates patient probably in low-risk group.
- Can identify high-risk group with full lung function testing (Box 15.2).

BOX 15.2

Criteria indicating high risk for pneumonectomy

- Age over 70 years
- Abnormal ECG
- FVC < 50% of predicted value
- FEV_1 < 50% of FVC, or less than 2 litres
- Maximum breathing capacity < 50% predicted
- $T_{L}CO$ < 50% predicted
- $Paco_2$ > 6 kPa

PREMEDICATION

- Continue cardiac and respiratory medications
- Conventional benzodiazepine premedication is satisfactory
- Anticholinergic drugs not essential
- Low-molecular-weight heparin for DVT prophylaxis.

PERIOPERATIVE MANAGEMENT

MONITORING:
- ECG
- Blood pressure (preferably invasive)
- Sao_2
- $Etco_2$
- Core temperature
- Central venous pressure
- Tidal volume and airway pressure
- Arterial blood gases
- Urine output – if epidural analgesia employed.

ANAESTHETIC TECHNIQUE

General anaesthesia with muscle paralysis and mechanical ventilation is the technique of choice. Intravenous opioid drugs can be used to provide intraoperative and postoperative analgesia; alternatively, epidural analgesia can be employed. A double-lumen endobronchial tube is used to separate both lungs and provide one-lung ventilation when required.

PERIOPERATIVE MANAGEMENT

- Blood loss may be substantial, but this is unusual.
- During one-lung ventilation:
  —monitor Sao_2, $Etco_2$ and arterial blood gases
  —adjust tidal volume, respiratory rate and Fio_2, as necessary.
- Test integrity of bronchial suture line when requested by surgeon; release clamp on double-lumen tube to the operated side and slowly apply inflation pressure up to 25–30 cmH$_2$O with the bronchial stump immersed in water.

CHEST DRAINAGE FOLLOWING PNEUMONECTOMY

As air leak does not occur, chest drainage is not mandatory.

NO CHEST DRAIN SITED
Air is aspirated from the pneumonectomy space at the end of the operation via a cannula placed through the chest wall, with the patient in a supine position. Air is aspirated until there is a negative pressure within the space. The mediastinum will then be approximately central or slightly towards the side of surgery. This is confirmed on chest radiography.

CHEST DRAIN SITED
Usually a single basal chest drain is left clamped but connected to an underwater seal drain. The drain is unclamped for 1–2 min every hour to reveal excess blood loss and centralise the mediastinum by releasing trapped air. Never apply suction to a pneumonectomy drain; this will pull the mediastinum across and severely impair venous return to the heart, with disastrous consequences.

POSTOPERATIVE MANAGEMENT

Most patients are allowed to breathe spontaneously immediately after surgery.

- Sit the patient up as soon as possible to encourage expansion of remaining lung.
- Administer humidified oxygen by face-mask.
- Chest drain is usually removed 12–24 h after surgery, if there is no significant bleeding.
- Careful attention to fluid balance is essential; do not overload the patient.

COMPLICATIONS OF PNEUMONECTOMY

HAEMORRHAGE
Perioperative bleeding may be substantial if adhesions were present. Excess accumulation of fluid in the pneumonectomy space can cause hypovolaemia and respiratory distress. The latter is relieved by chest drainage, or by release of the drain clamps.

SPUTUM RETENTION, INFECTION AND RESPIRATORY FAILURE
More likely to occur in patients with poor lung function. Treat as follows:
- Physiotherapy and antibiotics
- Consider minitracheostomy if cough is poor
- Consider mechanical ventilation if there is severe deterioration in respiratory function (high mortality rate)
- Infection in pneumonectomy space:
  —requires draining
  —associated with a bronchopleural fistula in some cases.

DYSRHYTHMIAS:
- More common after operation
- Usually atrial in origin
- Treated by digitalisation (or other suitable drug therapy such as amiodarone) rather than cardioversion
- Some surgeons favour prophylactic digitalisation.

OUTCOME

- Mortality rate up to 5% (UK)
- Cardiorespiratory dysfunction is the major cause of death.

15

BIBLIOGRAPHY

Entwistle MD, Roe PG, Sapsford DJ, Berisford RG, Jones JG. Patterns of oxygenation after thoracotomy. British Journal of Anaesthesia 1991; 67:704–711

Goldman L. Assessment of the patient with known or suspected ischaemic heart disease for non-cardiac surgery. British Journal of Anaesthesia 1988; 61:38–43

Goldstraw P. Post-operative management of the thoracic surgical patient. In: Gothard JWW, ed. Thoracic anaesthesia. Clinical anaesthesiology, vol 1. London: Baillière Tindall; 1987:207–231

Wright IG. Surgery on the lungs. In: Ghosh S, Latimer RD, eds. Thoracic anaesthesia: principles and practice. Oxford: Butterworth Heinemann; 1999:73–99

15

Postoperative analgesia for thoracic surgery patients

J. W. W. Gothard

AIM OF ANALGESIA

- Reduce distress to patient
- Improve lung function
- Allow early mobilisation
- Reduce incidence of postoperative complications and length of hospital stay
- Potential to improve outcome in terms of mortality

SOURCES OF PAIN

- Chest wall and most of pleura via intercostal nerves
- Diaphragmatic pleura via phrenic nerves
- Mediastinal pleura via the vagus nerve
- Shoulder joint via spinal nerves C5–C7

ANALGESIC TECHNIQUES

REGIONAL:

- Intercostal nerve block
- Extrapleural block
- Intrapleural block
- Paravertebral block
- Epidural block.

OPIOID:

- Parenteral
- Epidural
- Intrathecal
- Patient-controlled analgesia (PCA).

OTHER:

- Cryoanalgesia
- Non-steroidal anti-inflammatory drugs (NSAIDs).

REGIONAL ANAESTHESIA

INTERCOSTAL NERVE BLOCK

Simple to perform. Main disadvantages are short duration of action (unless indwelling intercostal catheters used) and failure to ameliorate pain from diaphragmatic pleura, mediastinal structures and areas supplied by the posterior primary rami.

EXTRAPLEURAL BLOCK

Indwelling catheter is placed in a pocket of retracted pleura so that the tip lies against a costovertebral joint. Local anaesthetic spreads to paravertebral space, providing anaesthesia of both anterior and posterior primary rami. Increasingly popular due to promising analgesic results.

INTRAPLEURAL BLOCK

Local analgesic agent deposited between visceral and parietal pleura via indwelling catheter. Analgesic action due to widespread intercostal nerve block. Does not spread to paravertebral space. Analgesia unpredictable due to variable loss of drug into chest drains, binding with blood in thorax, and rapid systemic absorption.

PARAVERTEBRAL BLOCK

Percutaneously inserted catheter at one level allows considerable spread of drug between adjacent paravertebral spaces. Provides good analgesia of both anterior and posterior primary rami, with fewer side-effects than epidural. Main disadvantages are problems of accurate siting and easy displacement.

EPIDURAL

Height of required block necessitates thoracic approach if local analgesic drug alone is used. Can provide excellent analgesia and is considered the 'gold standard'. Side-effects of extensive sympathetic block and motor weakness can be minimised by using weak local anaesthetic solutions (e.g. 0.125% bupivacaine) in combination with an opioid. A urinary catheter is inserted in most patients in whom epidural analgesia is established because urinary retention is common and needs to be differentiated from oliguria.

15

OPIOID ANALGESIA

PARENTERAL

Intermittent intramuscular opioids provide inadequate pain relief. Analgesia is improved by continuous infusion, but at the expense of excessive sedation, respiratory depression, nausea and vomiting.

EPIDURAL

Improved pain relief compared with intravenous route, with decreased total opioid requirement and less sedation, nausea and vomiting. Main disadvantage is respiratory depression (may be delayed), urinary retention and pruritus. Combined local analgesic and opioid epidural provides superior analgesia with decreased side-effects and is probably achievable by the high lumbar route with drugs such as diamorphine.

INTRATHECAL

Produces profound but short-term analgesia, unless indwelling catheter used. Risk of respiratory depression greater than with epidural opioids.

PATIENT-CONTROLLED ANALGESIA

Either intravenous or epidural. Analgesia generally superior to continuous infusions with reduced sedation and respiratory depression. Requires patient and staff education to achieve optimum effect.

OTHER

CRYOANALGESIA

Application of extreme cold (from −20 to −60°C) to intercostal nerves, under direct vision. Produces disruption of impulse transmission lasting for several months. Decline in popularity due to poor analgesic results and possible association with chronic post-thoracotomy pain syndrome.

NSAIDS

Inadequate when used alone but have synergistic action when combined with opioids and regional techniques. Adverse side-effects of platelet dysfunction, gastrointestinal bleeding and renal dysfunction preclude their use in some patients. Cyclo-oxygenase (COX) 2 NSAIDs may be preferable, but evidence is not conclusive.

BIBLIOGRAPHY

Kavanagh BP, Katz J, Sandler AN. Pain control after thoracic surgery. A review of current techniques. Anesthesiology 1994; 81:737–759

CROSS-REFERENCES

Bronchopleural fistula
    Surgical Procedures 15: 398
Lobectomy
    Surgical Procedures 15: 402
Pleurectomy
    Surgical Procedures 15: 406
Pneumonectomy
    Surgical Procedures 15: 408
Local anaesthetic toxicity
    Anaesthetic Factors 31: 761

15

Rigid bronchoscopy

J. W. W. Gothard

PROCEDURE

Isolated rigid bronchoscopy has largely been superseded by flexible fibreoptic bronchoscopy for the initial diagnosis of airway and lung disease. Rigid bronchoscopy remains the procedure of choice for surgical assessment of the airway before staging procedures such as mediastinoscopy or prior to thoracotomy. The rigid bronchoscope is also the preferred instrument for therapeutic manoeuvres such as removal of a foreign body, stent insertion and diathermy resection of airway tumour.

PREOPERATIVE ASSESSMENT AND INVESTIGATIONS

Investigations similar to those described for pneumonectomy (especially if bronchoscopy is carried out immediately before thoracotomy). Cardiac and respiratory dysfunction are both common in this group of patients.
- ECG
- Chest radiography
- Full blood count, urea and electrolytes
- Arterial blood gases (breathing air)
- Lung function tests.

It is particularly important to assess the degree of upper airway obstruction (if any) when rigid bronchoscopy is carried out as an isolated procedure. Further investigations of upper airway obstruction following clinical examination may include:
- Flow–volume loop
- Lateral radiograph of the trachea
- CT or MRI to show main airways. Rigid bronchoscopy may entail a degree of neck extension.
- Check lateral neck radiograph in rheumatoid arthritis.

PREMEDICATION

- Continue all cardiac and respiratory medication
- Anticholinergic medication not essential, but may be administered if preferred
- Anxiolysis with short-acting oral benzodiazepine, if required
- Omit sedatives if there is evidence of significant airway obstruction.

PERIOPERATIVE MANAGEMENT

MONITORING:
- ECG
- Non-invasive blood pressure
- Sao_2.

15

TABLE 15.2

Maximum inflation pressure achieved with various Venturi bronchoscope injector systems (oxygen driving pressure 410 kPa)

Negus bronchoscope	Injector needle (SWG)	Approx. maximum pressure (cmH$_2$O)
Adult	14	50
Adult	16	25–30
Child	19	14–18[a]
Suckling	19	15[a]

[a]Manual ventilation technique with Storz-type bronchoscope preferred in this age group.
SWG, standard wire gauge.

VENTILATION

The airway is 'shared' with the surgeon during rigid bronchoscopy. The main methods of providing adequate gas exchange are described.

Venturi injector

A high-pressure source of oxygen is injected intermittently through a needle at the proximal end of the bronchoscope. Air is entrained and positive-pressure ventilation produced via the distal end of the bronchoscope. Using this technique it is essential that there is always an adequate opening at the proximal end of the bronchoscope to allow entrainment of air during inspiration and egress of gas during expiration. It is also essential to match the injector needle size to the type of bronchoscope and oxygen pressure used (Table 15.2). This method of ventilation is usually used in adults.

Ventilating bronchoscope

A glass slide device at the proximal end of the bronchoscope allows manual positive-pressure ventilation with a suitable anaesthetic gas mixture via a side port built into the bronchoscope. This technique is ideal for infants and children. A T-piece circuit can be attached to the side port and anaesthesia is maintained with non-cumulative gaseous agents. This method avoids the use of injector techniques, which are more likely to cause barotrauma in children.

High-frequency jet ventilation

Not used widely in the UK, but popular in some other countries.

ANAESTHETIC TECHNIQUE

- Intravenous induction
- Short-acting muscle relaxant (suxamethonium, mivacurium)
- Inhalational induction
  —children
  —upper airway obstruction.

Maintenance of anaesthesia is usually achieved intravenously in adults and with inhalational agents in children (sevoflurane or isoflurane). Awareness is a significant problem during bronchoscopy, and it is preferable to use a constant infusion for all but the shortest cases. A total intravenous anaesthesia (TIVA) technique with propofol is particularly suitable in this respect. If the bronchoscopy is prolonged or to be followed by a surgical procedure, a longer-acting muscle relaxant such as vecuronium or atracurium can be used.

POSTOPERATIVE MANAGEMENT

- Reverse the muscle relaxant
- Administer oxygen by mask
- Allow patient to awaken
- Lie patient with suppurative side down if secretions are present
- Be prepared to reintubate in the presence of airway obstruction.

BIBLIOGRAPHY

Gillbe C, Hillier J. Anaesthesia for bronchoscopy, tracheal and airway surgery. Anaesthesia and Intensive Care Medicine 2002; 3(11):402–404

CROSS-REFERENCES

Bronchogenic carcinoma
    Patient Conditions 3: 92
Inhaled foreign body
    Surgical Procedures 15: 400
Mediastinal operations
    Surgical Procedures 15: 404
Preoperative assessment of pulmonary risk
    Anaesthetic Factors 27: 638

15

16

ABDOMINAL SURGERY
M. C. Bellamy

Overview

M. C. Bellamy

Anaesthesia for abdominal surgery embraces a wide range of disciplines. In the great majority of cases, the technique of choice involves general anaesthesia, usually in combination with thoracic epidural anaesthesia for postoperative pain relief. The conduct of anaesthesia for intra-abdominal surgery can have a major bearing on the quality of recovery, including the incidence of complications. Several studies have shown that fluid management and maintenance of adequate perfusion at the level of the tissue bed have a major bearing on surgical outcome in high-risk patients. Patients undergoing intra-abdominal surgery can be considered as falling into this category.

Not all intra-abdominal procedures necessitate general anaesthesia. Those confined to the pelvis are frequently carried out under spinal anaesthesia or epidural blockade. Some body surface procedures are carried out adequately using local nerve blocks or infiltration anaesthesia. Inguinal hernia repair falls into this category. Points of specific interest include:

- Splanchnic perfusion
- Respiratory function
- Cardiovascular function
- Temperature regulation
- Fluid and electrolyte balance.

SPLANCHNIC PERFUSION

Patients undergoing major intra-abdominal surgery, especially those who are being operated on for bowel obstruction, perforation or other acute conditions, are at high risk of sepsis and multiple organ failure. Similarly, elderly patients and those having major bowel or liver surgery are at risk. Numerous studies have suggested that perioperative optimisation reduces the risk of subsequent organ failure and postoperative morbidity. Various algorithms and monitoring techniques have been proposed to achieve this. Most are based on the concept of maintaining flow. Techniques that have been shown to be effective in various patient populations include monitoring of cardiac output, stroke volume, central venous oxygen saturation, and gastric mucosal intracellular pH. Similarly, several fluid and inotrope regimens have been proposed as 'off the shelf' recipes. Which of these, if any, is appropriate in an individual patient depends on the experience of the anaesthetist and clinical judgement, as well as on the scientific evidence.

RESPIRATORY FUNCTION

Postoperative respiratory function is often impaired following intra-abdominal surgery, for a number of reasons. First, the use of the supine position, and intraoperative administration of nitrous oxide, may contribute to the development of atelectasis. Second, postoperative pain is associated with chest wall and abdominal splinting. This results in a reduction in functional residual capacity. The consequences of this include impingement of closing volume on tidal volume breathing. This results in ventilation–perfusion mismatch and increased shunting.

The administration of general anaesthesia, together with postoperative analgesic drugs, results in disorganised central control of respiration. Further, opiate analgesics have been shown to suppress rapid eye movement (REM) sleep. After the drugs are discontinued, there is a rebound in REM sleep with consequent hypoxia. There are theoretical reasons why regional blockade may avoid a number of these complications. Although relatively few studies have been able to demonstrate a reduction in the incidence of postoperative complications when epidural anaesthesia is employed, the pooled data from a number of studies support this view. Moreover, most studies comparing epidural anaesthesia with postoperative opioids have reported an increase in the quality of pain relief as perceived by the patient. Other approaches involve specific nerve blocks and the use of non-steroidal anti-inflammatory

16

drugs (NSAIDs). Again, there is a growing body of evidence that these approaches may improve the quality of pain relief as well as reducing the rate of respiratory complications.

CARDIOVASCULAR SYSTEM

A substantial fraction of the cardiac output is delivered to the splanchnic viscera. Venous drainage from the gut and spleen passes into the portal system and on to the liver. Portal venous blood flow represents two-thirds of hepatic perfusion. The remaining third is oxygenated blood derived from the hepatic artery. Liver blood flow represents 25–30% of the cardiac output at rest. This increases following the ingestion of food. Any impairment of gut blood flow may therefore result in a reduction in liver blood flow. There are compensatory mechanisms (the hepatic artery buffer response) that normally protect the liver from such effects. Under anaesthesia, the normal buffer response becomes obtunded. Anaesthetic drugs have a differential effect on liver blood flow, with halothane exhibiting the worst profile of the commonly used agents, followed by enflurane. The newer agents have a much more benign effect.

Recent work has demonstrated quite clearly that epidural anaesthesia, while protecting against the effects of the stress response, results in a reduction in splanchnic blood flow. This can be offset by restoring normal arterial pressure.

THERMOREGULATION

Thermoregulation is a major problem in patients undergoing intra-abdominal surgery. Anaesthesia renders the patient poikilothermic. Patients cool rapidly, because of increased heat and water loss across the large surface area of exposed viscera. This can potentially be compounded by the administration of large volumes of fluids. Patients with a septic illness or a reduced metabolic rate (e.g. those with liver disease) have a reduced production of heat and therefore tend to cool more quickly and may be difficult to rewarm.

Traditional approaches to maintaining patient warmth in theatre have included maintaining the temperature of the ambient environment close to an isothermic one, that is, a temperature at which there is no tendency for a transfer of heat between patient and environment. This is a temperature in excess of 24–27°C and may result in an unacceptable working environment. Warming mattresses, equally, have proved of limited value.

More recently, the advent of forced warm air over blankets has provided a solution to maintaining patient warmth in theatre. Such devices dramatically reduce thermal losses, and may also in some cases actually transfer heat to the patient. Using both upper and lower body devices simultaneously is particularly effective.

Devices to humidify gases, including HME filters and circle systems also help to minimise thermal losses. The universal use of fluid warming devices is now considered mandatory by some. Modern devices include countercurrent fluid warmers which allow delivery of body temperature fluids at very high rates.

FLUID AND ELECTROLYTE BALANCE

Patients who present for intra-abdominal surgery may have gross derangement of fluid and electrolyte balance. Those presenting for elective surgery are particularly at risk in the event of administration of bowel preparation or laxatives.

Patients presenting for acute surgery may have lost fluids from the central circulating compartment as a result of diarrhoea, vomiting or fluid sequestration into an obstructed intestine. In addition, those with an inflammatory process may have lost fluid from the circulating compartment into the so-called 'third space', as a result of altered vascular permeability and colloid oncotic pressure.

These changes can be further exacerbated by handling the gut at surgery. This can result in translocation of bacteria and endotoxin, as well as altered liver blood flow.

Patients who have effusions (including ascites) are particularly at risk of major fluid and electrolyte shifts occurring as a consequence of surgery. Such shifts can precipitate acute haemodynamic decompensation. The anaesthetist must be aware of both the nature and the severity of any preoperative derangement, together with the contribution likely to be made by surgery. Full assessment should allow correction of fluid and electrolyte abnormalities. Patients with major derangement may require invasive vascular monitoring.

SPECIFIC POINTS

OPIOIDS AND ANASTOMOSES
The debate regarding the contribution of opiates to anastomotic disruption continues. There are differences in basic pharmacology

16

between drugs of this class. While some, including pethidine, are smooth muscle relaxants, others are smooth muscle constrictors – including morphine. The significance of this in clinical practice is unclear. However, some suggest that pethidine is superior to morphine for patients with biliary spasm, and possibly for all patients undergoing biliary surgery.

ANTICHOLINESTERASE DRUGS

These drugs can increase gut motility and intraluminal pressure. Neostigmine has been used specifically as a prokinetic drug in the treatment of pseudo-obstruction. These effects are only partially blocked by concurrent treatment with vagolytic agents, such as atropine. However, there is no good clinical evidence for an increase in anastomotic failure rate as a consequence of neostigmine use.

ANTIBIOTICS

Antibiotics are known to reduce the postoperative infection rate, and in particular the incidence of wound infection. There is no good evidence that the effects of a preinduction antibiotic can be further improved by subsequent doses. The antibiotic used for prophylaxis should be given sufficiently in advance of surgery that adequate tissue levels are obtained at the time of operation. Ideally, it should be given at the time of premedication.

Common antibiotic regimens include the combination of a penicillin or cephalosporin with metronidazole. Some drugs, particularly the aminoglycosides and streptomycin, may have the additional unwanted effect of perpetuating the effects of neuromuscular blocking agents.

VENOUS THROMBOEMBOLISM

Intra-abdominal surgery, and in particular pelvic surgery, conveys a significant risk of deep vein thrombosis (DVT). This risk can be minimised by the appropriate use of anticoagulants. Many regimens have been shown to be effective. Most centres currently use a standard dose of a low-molecular-weight heparin.

The risk can be further reduced by the use of support stockings or pneumatic compression boots. Regional anaesthesia can reduce the risk of DVT.

Recent work has suggested that low-molecular-weight heparin persists in the circulation over a number of hours. Careful thought should be given when considering siting a thoracic epidural. This should not be sited in the hours immediately after the administration of a dose of low-molecular-weight heparin.

16

Anaesthesia for open and laparoscopic cholecystectomy

H. Buglass

The incidence of gallstones is approx. 12% in men and 24% in women in the UK. The standard treatment for symptomatic gallstones is now laparoscopic cholecystectomy. There are relatively few absolute contraindications, and most surgeons proceed with laparoscopic surgery even after acute cholecystitis, previous surgery and in patients with common bile duct stones.

The main indications for open cholecystectomy are:
- Patients unfit to tolerate pneumoperitoneum (although new surgical techniques using laparoscopic retractors require a lower intra-abdominal pressure)
- Intraoperative conversion to an open technique
- Previous upper abdominal surgery (relative).

TYPICAL PATIENT CHARACTERISTICS

- Age 40–50 years
- Female : male ratio 5 : 1
- History of hypercholesterolaemia and haemolytic disease
- Obesity and its complications
- Most operations are performed electively.

PREOPERATIVE ASSESSMENT AND INVESTIGATIONS

ELECTIVE CHOLECYSTECTOMY
- History and examination
- Full blood count and electrolytes
- Liver function tests (if deranged, coagulation screen)
- Chest radiography and ECG where warranted
- Any further investigations according to coexisting medical conditions.

ACUTE CHOLECYSTECTOMY
- Patients present acutely unwell, jaundiced and/or dehydrated
- Special attention should be paid to renal function
- Hypovolaemia should be fully corrected with crystalloid and colloids according to clinical need
- If coagulation is deranged, 10 mg intravenous vitamin K ± fresh frozen plasma should be considered
- Antibiotics as per hospital protocol.

ANAESTHETIC TECHNIQUE

Preinduction:
- Routine standard monitoring – ECG, blood pressure, $EtCO_2$, pulse oximetry, temperature
- Occasionally invasive monitoring as required, depending on any co-morbidity or intercurrent condition
- Rapid sequence induction may be indicated in the acute state.

OPEN CHOLECYSTECTOMY
Induction and maintenance:
- Thoracic epidural is the pain relief of choice where coagulation is satisfactory
- In the acute state, with normal coagulation but deranged liver function tests, vitamin K is advisable before operation
- Induction – standard intravenous induction, non-depolarising muscle relaxation, tracheal intubation
- Maintenance – air–oxygen mix with a volatile agent, intermittent bolus of non-depolarising muscle relaxant, controlled ventilation
- Analgesia – opioid analgesics plus a NSAID, particularly where epidural analgesia is not employed
- Morphine used to be avoided as it was thought to cause contraction of the sphincter of Oddi. This is not now thought to be the case, although many continue to use pethidine for its supposed smooth muscle relaxant properties

16

- Reversal of non-depolarising muscle relaxant at end of procedure.

Recovery – early:
- Oxygen via face mask
- Intravenous fluid until patient is drinking adequately
- Analgesia :
  —Intravenous opioid via patient-controlled analgesia (PCA)
  —Regional technique – continuous epidural infusion of low-dose local anaesthetic and opioid. Patient-controlled epidural analgesia is increasingly being used
  —Paravertebral blocks and intercostal blocks are occasionally used.

Recovery – late:
Complications may be secondary to poor pain control, obesity or immobility. They include basal atelectasis with resultant pneumonia, and DVT. Optimising pain control, physiotherapy, early mobilisation and thromboembolic prophylaxis can reduce these problems.

The operative mortality rate is substantially below 1%. Factors increasing the risk of postoperative mortality are advancing age and acute surgery.

LAPAROSCOPIC CHOLECYSTECTOMY
Induction and maintenance:
- *Induction* – standard intravenous induction, non-depolarising muscle relaxation, tracheal intubation. In some centres, controlled ventilation via the laryngeal mask airway is used. While this may be appropriate in some cases, its general applicability is not recommended.
- *Maintenance* – air–oxygen mix with volatile agent, intermittent bolus of non-depolarising muscle relaxant, controlled ventilation.
- *Analgesia* – opioid analgesic, usually fentanyl, plus a NSAID unless specifically contraindicated
- Reversal of non-depolarising muscle relaxant at end of procedure
- This can be a deceptive operation, which may be finished very quickly – watch the screens and be aware of surgical progress!

Perioperative complications
Perioperative complications of laparoscopic cholecystectomy are shown in Box 16.1.

Recovery – early:
- Oxygen via face-mask
- Intravenous fluid until patient is drinking adequately

BOX 16.1

Perioperative complications of laparoscopic cholecystectomy

- Cardiovascular collapse – raised intra-abdominal pressure leads to decreased venous return, increased systemic vascular resistance and reduced cardiac output. Further compromised by reverse Trendelenburg (head up) position
- Gas embolism – sudden fall in $EtCO_2$, cardiovascular collapse, hypoxaemia. Differential diagnosis of above. In principle, carbon dioxide is rapidly absorbed, leading to resolution
- Direct surgical trauma – vascular or visceral injury (increased risk after gas insufflation of stomach by intermittent positive-pressure ventilation (IPPV), reduced by insertion of nasogastric tube)
- Severe dysrhythmias – severe bradycardia on inflation related to vagal stimulation due to peritoneal stretch. Many anaesthetists use prophylactic anticholinergics
- Hypercarbia – ventilation can become difficult, particularly in obese patients
- Haemorrhage – difficult to access
- Pneumothorax, mediastinal emphysema – present with cardiovascular collapse
- Hypothermia – due to large volumes of gas used; monitor temperature and warm actively.

- Analgesia – regular paracetamol supplemented with codeine or a NSAID.

Recovery – late:
- Possible as day-case procedure
- Delayed owing to conversion to open technique in 4%. Incidence of bile duct injury 0.3%.
- Mortality rate < 0.4%.

BIBLIOGRAPHY

Adams JP, Murphy PG. Obesity in anaesthesia and intensive care. British Journal of Anaesthesia 2000; 85(1):91–108

Hirvonen EA, Poikolainen EO. The adverse effects of anaesthesia, head up tilt, and carbon dioxide pneumoperitoneum during laparoscopic cholecystectomy. Surgical Endoscopy 2000; 14(3):272–277

16

Anaesthesia for pancreatic surgery

H. Buglass

The pancreas is an exocrine and endocrine gland situated in the retroperitoneal space in the upper abdomen.

INDICATIONS FOR PANCREATIC SURGERY

- Necrotising acute pancreatitis
- Chronic pancreatitis
- Trauma
- Neoplasia:
  —adenocarcinoma
  —endocrine.

ACUTE PANCREATITIS

In recent years there has been a trend against surgical intervention in acute pancreatitis. Treatment now revolves around supportive management, often involving intensive care with serial radiological imaging of the pancreas. The main indication for surgery is necrotising pancreatitis. The operation of choice is necrosectomy plus lavage. This procedure has reduced the mortality rate to 24% for this condition.

Minimally invasive, radiologically assisted necrosectomy has been described with good results, but is yet to become common practice. This procedure has many advantages.

Surgery may also be required for the complications of acute pancreatitis: persistent pseudocyst, pancreatic abscess and haemorrhage.

Epidural analgesia has been shown to be an excellent method of pain control in the acute episode.

TYPICAL PATIENT CHARACTERISTICS:
- Age 40–70 years
- History of gallstones and associated risk factors
- Alcohol
- Trauma
- 40% idiopathic

- Drugs – angiotensin-converting enzyme (ACE) inhibitors, thiazide diuretics, etc.
- Lipid abnormalities
- Hypercalcaemia.

PRESENTATION:
- Patients may present acutely unwell, complaining of epigastric pain.
- They are dehydrated and often jaundiced.
- Pleural effusions and acute lung injury may develop.
- Septic shock and multiorgan failure are indicators of the development of necrotising pancreatitis.

PREOPERATIVE ASSESSMENT AND INVESTIGATIONS:
- Full history and examination (patient may be in intensive care)
- Full blood count, electrolytes, liver function tests, coagulation screen, arterial blood gases
- Chest radiography and ECG
- Any further investigations according to coexisting medical condition(s)
- If coagulation is deranged, consider giving 10 mg intravenous vitamin K ± fresh frozen plasma
- Hypovolaemia should be fully corrected.

ANAESTHETIC TECHNIQUE
Preinduction:
- Standard monitoring – ECG, pulse oximetry, blood pressure, $EtCO_2$, temperature
- Invasive monitoring – arterial blood pressure, central venous line
- Rapid sequence induction if not intubated already (gastric stasis is likely).

Induction and maintenance:
- Thoracic epidural analgesia is the pain relief of choice where coagulation permits.
- Induction – intravenous induction, muscle relaxation, tracheal intubation. A nasogastric tube should be inserted if not already present.

16

- Maintenance – air–oxygen mix with a volatile agent, intermittent bolus of non-depolarising muscle relaxant, controlled ventilation.
- Analgesia – opioid analgesic or epidural.
- Antagonism of non-depolarising muscle relaxant at end of procedure if the patient is well enough to extubate.

Recovery:
- High-dependency unit care as minimum
- Supplemental oxygen via appropriate method
- Supportive treatment as surgery causes release of inflammatory mediators which can lead to initial clinical deterioration
- Early commencement of enteral feeding via a nasojejunal feeding tube
- Postoperative surgical complications include colonic necrosis, fistula formation and bleeding
- Respiratory and renal complications are common.

CHRONIC PANCREATITIS

Increasing in incidence – 27.4 cases per million population. Indications for surgery are:
- Palliation of pain
- Exclude suspicion of carcinoma
- Bypass or remove the complications of the disease.

Endoscopic techniques are increasingly being used as an alternative to traditional pancreaticojejunostomy.

TYPICAL PATIENT CHARACTERISTICS:
- Alcohol – 60–70% of cases in Western world
- Tropical pancreatitis
- Obstructive pancreatitis
- Hypercalcaemia
- Hereditary
- Biliary tract disease
- Idiopathic.

PRESENTATION:
- Chronic abdominal pain radiating to back
- Weight loss due to endocrine and exocrine insufficiency
- Diabetes and associated complications
- Jaundice is rare
- Alcohol abuse is common.

PREOPERATIVE ASSESSMENT, INVESTIGATION AND OPTIMISATION:
- History and examination
- Full blood count, electrolytes, liver function tests, coagulation screen and blood glucose level

- Chest radiography and ECG
- Further investigations according to coexisting medical condition(s)
- Alcohol intake should be noted and treatment for withdrawal commenced
- Diabetes should be stabilised and converted to an insulin sliding scale perioperatively
- Multivitamins and vitamin K should be considered perioperatively.

PANCREATIC NEOPLASIA

Pancreatic neoplasms comprise a spectrum of exocrine and endocrine tumours, the majority being malignant. Two-thirds of cases arise in the head of the pancreas. The incidence is 10 per million population, with a 10% 1-year survival rate. Surgery is by Whipple's pancreaticoduodenectomy or a variant of this, for example the pylorus-preserving pancreaticoduodenectomy.

TYPICAL PATIENT CHARACTERISTICS:
- Male : female ratio 1.25 : 1
- Smoker
- Occupational – exposure to α-naphthalene and benzidine
- Hereditary
- Diabetes mellitus
- Chronic pancreatitis
- Gastrectomy.

PRESENTATION:
- Obstructive jaundice, weight loss and abdominal pain
- Anorexia, nausea and vomiting
- Impaired glucose tolerance.

PREOPERATIVE ASSESSMENT, INVESTIGATION AND OPTIMISATION:
- History and examination
- Full blood count, electrolytes, liver function tests and coagulation screen
- Chest radiography and ECG
- Further investigation according to coexisting medical condition(s)
- Hypovolaemia should be corrected
- Diabetes should be stabilised and treatment converted to an insulin sliding scale perioperatively
- An endocrinologist should be consulted – endocrine tumours are often part of a more complex syndrome
- Preoperative stenting to relieve jaundice is common, but consider vitamin K 10 mg where the liver function tests remain deranged even in the presence of normal coagulation.

16

ANAESTHETIC TECHNIQUE FOR WHIPPLE'S PANCREATICODUODENECTOMY

Preinduction:
- Standard monitoring – ECG, pulse oximetry, blood pressure, $EtCO_2$, temperature
- Invasive monitoring – arterial blood pressure, central venous line.

Induction and maintenance:
- Thoracic epidural is the pain relief of choice if the coagulation is satisfactory
- Induction – intravenous induction, non-depolarising muscle relaxant, tracheal intubation
- Maintenance – air–oxygen mix with volatile agent, intermittent bolus or infusion of non-depolarising muscle relaxant
- Analgesia – epidural preferable, but where this is not possible a remifentanil infusion with a loading of morphine at the end of procedure is effective
- Reversal of non-depolarising muscle relaxant at the end of procedure.

Peroperative complications
These are shown in Box 16.2.

Recovery – early:
- Oxygen via face-mask
- High-dependency unit care
- Intravenous fluid then early introduction of enteral (jejunal) feed
- Analgesia:
  —epidural – low-dose local anaesthetic with opioid
  —intravenous opioid via PCA.
- DVT prophylaxis
- Monitor blood glucose level – manipulation of insulin and dextrose.

Recovery – late:
- The morbidity rate associated with the operation is high – up to 40%.
- Common complications are basal atelectasis with resultant pneumonia, thromboembolic disease and anastomotic leak.
- Optimising pain control, physiotherapy, early mobilisation and thromboembolic prophylaxis can reduce these.

BOX 16.2

Peroperative complications of Whipple's procedure

- Hypothermia – active warming; fluid and blankets
- Hypovolaemia – large fluid loss perioperatively plus potential large blood losses; maintain central venous pressure and monitor haematocrit; transfuse as necessary
- Hyperkalaemia – surgical manipulation leading to portal vein or hepatic artery obstruction, and hepatic ischaemia and intracellular potassium leak; monitor potassium levels
- Hypoglycaemia or hyperglycaemia – monitor closely; in insulinoma, constant infusion of dextrose infusion has been shown to reduce rebound hyperglycaemia
- Hypoxia – basal atelectasis or development of acute lung injury, increase FiO_2; add PEEP; consider facial continuous positive airway pressure (CPAP) or continued ventilation after operation
- Renal dysfunction – hepatorenal syndrome; monitor renal output; maintain circulating volume and mean blood pressure; consider mannitol or a loop diuretic

- Incidence of postoperative diabetes is dependent on size of pancreatic resection but is quoted as 50%.
- Operative mortality rate is 5%.

PANCREATIC TRAUMA

Deceleration injury is the major mechanism of blunt pancreatic injury. The force required means that other organs are often involved (see Abdominal trauma below).

BIBLIOGRAPHY

Manciu N, Beebe DS. Total pancreatectomy with islet cell autotransplantation: anaesthetic implications. Journal of Clinical Anesthesia 1999; 11(7):576–582

CROSS-REFERENCES

16

Abdominal trauma

L. Milligan

Intra-abdominal injuries may carry high morbidity and mortality rates because the diagnosis may be difficult or delayed and the severity underestimated. A high index of suspicion of abdominal trauma is required in all patients who have sustained serious injury.

The principal cause of death in abdominal trauma is uncontrolled bleeding, particularly from bursting injuries of the liver or spleen.

Abdominal trauma is classified as:

- *Blunt* – common in road traffic accidents secondary to seat-belt injuries. The spleen is the most vulnerable organ. Liver, pancreas, bowel, kidneys and bladder are injured by greater forces.
- *Penetrating* – 20% of abdominal injuries in the UK. May be caused by low-velocity projectiles (e.g. knives, hand-gun bullets) or high-velocity projectiles (e.g. rifle bullets or shrapnel from bombs or blasts). Impaled objects or weapons must be removed only under controlled circumstances in the operating theatre. Some 90% of patients with gunshot wounds sustain visceral injuries.

Patients often require exploratory laparotomy and repair of the damaged viscera.

In the last 10 years, the technique of 'damage control surgery' has been gaining popularity. The least possible is done for the patient with multiple injuries at the first operation. The patient is transferred to the intensive care unit to correct hypothermia, acidosis and coagulopathy, before definitive surgery is undertaken within the next 36 h.

Some abdominal injuries (e.g. liver and spleen) do not require surgery and improved outcomes have been shown with conservative management.

INITIAL MANAGEMENT

- Injuries to the abdomen cannot be managed in isolation and require a multidisciplinary team approach.

- The victim of major trauma requires full assessment and resuscitation before definitive investigations are carried out and the decision to embark on surgery is made.
- By following a system such as Advanced Trauma Life Support (ATLS), the trauma team is able to achieve stabilisation of the injured patient in a consistent and systematic order, and life-threatening injuries are treated according to priority.

PRIMARY SURVEY:

- An *ABC* approach is followed.
- *A*irway patency is assessed and managed as appropriate, with tracheal intubation if necessary, and the cervical spine is immobilised.
- *B*reathing is assessed and, where necessary, IPPV is commenced. Life-threatening chest injuries are excluded and treated at this stage.
- Intravenous access is obtained and overt external haemorrhage is controlled by compression. Adequacy of the *C*irculation and blood volume is then assessed clinically. It should be remembered that in young patients blood pressure is often maintained until the final phase of shock, when catastrophic and sometimes irretrievable falls occur.
- Choice of fluid for resuscitation is controversial; however, ATLS recommends starting with warmed crystalloid solutions. A request for cross-matched blood must be sent immediately. With the exception of imminent exsanguination, there is little indication for the use of O-negative or group-specific blood. Cross-matched blood should be available within 20–30 min.
- Excessive fluid resuscitation in penetrating trauma prior to haemostasis may be detrimental. In patients who have sustained major vascular injuries; increasing blood pressure leads to clot disruption and increased bleeding.

SECONDARY SURVEY

Once the patient has been stabilised a full 'top-to-toe' examination is carried out to identify all injuries.

Constant reassessment and vigilance is required at this stage for ongoing life-threatening problems that require immediate treatment.

INVESTIGATIONS

ROUTINE:

- Haematology – cross-match, full blood count, clotting screen
- Biochemistry – electrolytes, creatinine, amylase
- Radiology – C-spine, chest radiography, pelvis
- ECG.

SPECIFIC TO ABDOMINAL TRAUMA:

Erect chest and abdominal radiographs; then, as indicated, proceed to:

- Deep peritoneal lavage
- CT of abdomen
- Ultrasound scan of abdomen
- Laparoscopy
- Laparotomy.

Each of these investigations has its advantages and disadvantages. The choice will depend on the nature of the injury, stability of the patient and expertise available in imaging techniques.

Great care should be exercised when deciding to move a potentially unstable patient from the emergency department to a remote environment (e.g. CT scanner), where staff and resuscitation facilities may be limited.

There are a few indications for immediate laparotomy:

- Unexplained shock
- Rigid silent abdomen
- Evisceration
- Radiological evidence of free intraperitoneal gas
- Radiological evidence of ruptured diaphragm
- All gunshot wounds.

LAPAROTOMY FOR ABDOMINAL TRAUMA

Where possible, the patient should be resuscitated and hypovolaemia corrected prior to induction of anaesthesia. Sometimes, when haemorrhage is ongoing and exceeding trans-fusion rates, it is necessary to proceed with anaesthesia in the hypovolaemic patient.

ANAESTHETIC TECHNIQUE:

- *Monitoring* – Standard ± arterial line, central venous line, pulmonary artery catheter, temperature, urine output (these may be instituted following induction and surgical control of haemorrhage in life-threatening situations).
- *Intravenous access* – *two* large-bore cannulae ± large-bore central access where feasible. Vasopressors and inotropes should be prepared in advance and intravenous fluids should be running, with a rapid infuser and blood available.
- *Induction of anaesthesia* – should take place in the operating theatre, with the surgeon scrubbed, so that the operation can commence immediately. Severe cardiovascular decompensation may occur at induction due to the vasodilatory and myocardial depressant effects of anaesthetic drugs plus the loss of a tamponading effect from the abdominal muscles at the institution of neuromuscular blockade.
- *Rapid sequence induction* with cricoid pressure is the technique of choice in the unfasted trauma patient. Care must be taken to protect the potentially unstable cervical spine.
- *Choice of anaesthetic drugs* will depend on the stability of the patient. The dose of drug used is far more important than the actual drug given. The intravascular volume is reduced in hypovolaemic patients; therefore, usual doses will result in higher than expected plasma concentrations. Etomidate ($0.1–0.3$ mg kg^{-1}) is a popular choice for its cardiovascular stability. Ketamine ($0.3–0.7$ mg kg^{-1}) may also be used; its sympathomimetic effects help to maintain blood pressure. It should be avoided in patients with head injuries because of its effects on intracranial pressure. An alternative technique is a high-dose opioid (e.g. fentanyl) combined with a benzodiazepine (e.g. midazolam). This has minimal cardiac depressive action but may result in a decrease in endogenous catecholamine output, and the patient will require postoperative ventilation. Suxamethonium ($1.0–1.5$ mg kg^{-1}) is the neuromuscular blocking drug of choice in rapid sequence induction.
- *Intubation* may be difficult in patients with facial injuries, cervical spine immobilisation and blood in the airway.

16

- *Maintenance of anaesthesia* is with cautious amounts of volatile agent in an air–oxygen mixture. Nitrous oxide is avoided in abdominal surgery to prevent bowel distension. Once haemodynamic stability has been achieved, anaesthesia may be deepened.
- *Neuromuscular blockade* is maintained with an intermediate-acting drug. Atracurium may cause histamine release, which will result in vasodilatation compounding hypotension. Cisatracurium is an alternative, with greater cardiovascular stability. Pancuronium has some intrinsic sympathomimetic activity and may be preferred for longer operations and in patients who will require postoperative ventilation.
- A nasogastric tube is inserted and gastric contents aspirated; prophylactic broad-spectrum antibiotics are given to all patients.
- Once control of bleeding has been achieved, the patient's cardiovascular status should improve. Further fluid resuscitation with crystalloid, colloid and blood should be guided by ongoing losses, central venous pressure and urine output. Blood should be taken for estimation of arterial gases, haemoglobin concentration, coagulation screen and electrolytes.
- *Warming* the patient is essential. Hypothermia will result in platelet dysfunction, reduced metabolism of citrate and lactate, increased incidence of cardiac arrhythmias, bleeding diathesis, hypocalcaemia, metabolic acidosis and cardiac arrest. In the longer term, hypothermia impairs immune function, increases the risk of septic consequences and impairs wound healing.

MASSIVE TRANSFUSION:

- Coagulopathy is common after transfusion of about one blood volume owing to dilutional thrombocytopaenia, reduced levels of coagulation factors (approximately 40% of normal), disseminated intravascular coagulation (DIC) and fibrinolysis.
- Hypothermia causes secondary alterations in platelet function, inhibition of enzyme function and increased fibrinolytic activity.
- Massive transfusion results in metabolic acidosis, hyperkalaemia and impaired oxygen-carrying capacity (reduced levels of 2,3-diphosphoglycerate; 2,3-DPG).
- Intraoperative red cell salvage (Cell Saver) provides warm blood with normal levels of 2,3-DPG. It is, however, contraindicated if

the blood is contaminated with intestinal contents.
- Coagulopathy is corrected with fresh frozen plasma, cryoprecipitate and platelet transfusions. There is often a delay in obtaining these products, so they should be requested early if their use is anticipated.
- There may be a role for antifibrinolytic and platelet-activating drugs, such as tranexamic acid, aprotinin, DDAVP.

POSTOPERATIVE MANAGEMENT:

- Patients will require close monitoring in a high-dependency or intensive care unit.
- Those who have sustained massive blood loss and undergone transfusion are often hypothermic, coagulopathic and acidotic, requiring drugs to support the cardiovascular system. They will benefit from a period of ventilation on the intensive care unit whilst being warmed and stabilised.
- Oxygen, fluids and analgesia are prescribed. A morphine PCA system is most appropriate for major abdominal trauma where a coagulopathy exists and extradural blockade is contraindicated. However, once clotting returns to normal, the patient may benefit from the insertion of an epidural.

LIVER TRAUMA

- Liver injuries range from trivial to fatal.
- They comprise 45% of abdominal trauma; 30–40% are due to penetrating injuries and 60% are associated with other injuries, especially life-threatening head injuries.
- Liver injuries are graded from I to V, from minor lacerations to avulsion from the inferior vena cava (IVC).
- Liver injuries may be treated by the insertion of packs, which are removed a day or two later following a period of stabilisation, correction of coagulopathy and hypothermia, and transfer to a specialist centre. By this stage, haemorrhage will often have stopped.
- Patients may be investigated by angiography, permitting bleeding vessels to be embolised before further surgery to remove packs; occasionally, in a stable patient, it is the sole intervention.
- In the most severe liver injuries (grade V) with simultaneous damage to the hepatic veins or vena cava, caval–atrial or caval–caval bypass may be required. The

survival rate from such injuries is less than 10%.

- Stable patients, with a liver injury detected on CT, are best managed conservatively in a specialist centre. Transfusion requirements are reduced and there are fewer abdominal complications. In total, 34–51% of adult blunt hepatic injuries can be managed conservatively, although in grade V injury only 10% are sufficiently stable.
- Conservative management of solid abdominal visceral injuries is not a passive process; continuous assessment is required. The patient may need emergency laparotomy at any time for potentially exsanguinating haemorrhage. Intensive care monitoring is mandatory.

SPLENIC INJURY

- Splenectomy is a relatively simple surgical procedure which has saved many lives. However, it is not necessary for all injuries, and splenectomy may occasionally be associated with overwhelming postsplenectomy sepsis.
- Approximately 50% of spleens can be repaired by partial resection, ligation of bleeding vessels, and packing and enveloping the spleen in an absorbable mesh bag.
- If haemostasis is obtained, the incidence of further haemorrhage is less than 2%.
- In stable patients conservative treatment is now advocated in a similar manner to that for liver trauma. Careful patient selection is required, and laparotomy is undertaken for haemodynamic instability, signs of peritonism or transfusion requirements over 2 units. Some 50–70% of splenic injuries are now managed conservatively.

- Angiography and embolisation techniques have also been employed.
- Observation on intensive care or a high-dependency unit is essential, with continual readiness for an emergency operation.
- Patients who have undergone splenectomy are protected by daily administration of oral penicillin V for 2 years and immunised against pneumococci and *Haemophilus influenzae*.

BIBLIOGRAPHY

American College of Surgeons. Advanced trauma life support manual. Chicago: American College of Surgeons; 1997

Bickell WH, Wall MJ, Pepe PE et al. Immediate versus delayed fluid resuscitation in patients with penetrating torso injury. New England Journal of Medicine 1994; 331:1105–1109

Hishberg A, Mattox KL. Damage control surgery. British Journal of Surgery 1993; 80:1501–1502

Parks RW, Chrysos E, Diamond T. Management of liver trauma. British Journal of Surgery 1999; 86(9):1121–1135

Patcher HL, Gram J. The current status of splenic preservation. Advances in Surgery 2000; 34:137–174

Paterson-Brown S. Emergency surgery and critical care. WB Saunders; 1997

Skinner D, Driscoll P, Earlam R. ABC of major trauma. 3rd edn. London: BMJ Books; 2000

16

CROSS-REFERENCES

Trauma
    Anaesthetic Factors 31: 797

Colorectal surgery

L. Milligan

PROCEDURES

A wide range of surgical procedures is carried out on the lower gastrointestinal tract for a variety of pathologies, including carcinoma, inflammatory bowel disease, diverticular disease, motility disorders, angiodysplasia and bowel obstruction (Box 16.3).

COLORECTAL SURGERY

Procedures vary in complexity; most involve laparotomy, excision of the affected section of bowel, anastomosis of the remaining segments with or without stoma formation.

Adjacent organs may be involved (e.g. bladder, uterus), requiring a multidisciplinary approach, prolonged anaesthesia and major blood loss.

Laparoscopic techniques are now being used for appendicectomy and some bowel resections. Advantages of improved diagnosis, reduced wound size and tissue trauma must be weighed against the problems associated with laparoscopic surgery (see Laparoscopic cholecystectomy, above) and increased operating time, and the anaesthetist must be prepared for conversion to laparotomy at any stage.

BOX 16.3

Common lower gastrointestinal tract surgical procedures

- Appendicectomy
- Anterior resection (left or right hemicolectomy)
- Hartmann's procedure
- Total colectomy
- Panproctocolectomy (abdominoperineal resection)
- Ileorectal pouch formation
- Stoma formation and closure
- Fistula surgery
- Haemorrhoidectomy
- Other perianal surgery (e.g. fissure, haematoma, abscess, carcinoma)

PERIANAL SURGERY

Procedures are usually short but often intensely stimulating and extremely painful after operation. They are often carried out on a day-case basis, and therefore require anaesthetic techniques that allow the patient to be pain-free and fit for discharge within a few hours of surgery.

PATIENT CHARACTERISTICS

- Physiological status depends on:
  —underlying pathology
  —concurrent medical conditions.
- Patients with malignant disease may have significant weight loss, anaemia, bowel obstruction, electrolyte imbalance and metastatic disease.
- Patients are often elderly with one or more of the medical conditions frequently associated with this population, such as ischaemic heart disease, hypertension, pulmonary disease, diabetes mellitus, arthritis.
- Patients with inflammatory bowel disease are usually younger but have frequently undergone multiple surgical procedures and may present with severe sepsis due to bowel perforation or 'toxic megacolon'. Steroid therapy may cause immunosuppression, and signs of sepsis may be masked.
- Patients of all age groups and levels of fitness present for perianal surgery. Pregnant women may present for urgent haemorrhoidectomy.

PREOPERATIVE ASSESSMENT

- Routine history and examination with special attention to concurrent disease.
- Specific to gastrointestinal pathology:
  —anaemia
  —weight loss
  —diarrhoea and vomiting

—bowel obstruction
—sepsis
—medications (including steroids)
—metastatic disease.
* Investigations:
    —routine haematology – full blood
    count ± clotting screen; group and save
    or cross-match (depending on nature of
    operation and local transfusion policy)
    —routine biochemistry – creatinine and
    electrolytes ± glucose, amylase, liver
    function tests
    —ECG
    —chest radiography, where indicated by
    history or examination findings
    —other specialised investigations (e.g.
    echocardiography, pulmonary function
    tests) as indicated by history and
    examination.

PREMEDICATION

* Oral anxiolytic if required (e.g.
  temazepam).
* Regular medication, especially cardiac
  drugs, should be continued until the day of
  surgery, with consideration given to
  postoperative intravenous regimens.
* Intravenous fluids should be prescribed for
  patients given 'bowel prep' or those with
  diarrhoea or vomiting, to correct
  hypovolaemia and electrolyte losses prior to
  surgery.
* Diabetics are commenced on an appropriate
  intravenous insulin regimen.

PERIOPERATIVE MANAGEMENT

* *Monitoring* – ECG, non-invasive blood
  pressure, SpO_2, $EtCO_2$.
* *Intravenous access* – large-bore access required
  in major cases where blood loss anticipated.
* *Arterial line* – measure direct arterial blood
  pressure in cases involving large fluid and
  blood losses, in patients with significant
  ischaemic heart disease or arrhythmias, and
  to obtain arterial blood gases and blood
  samples.
* *Central venous line* – to monitor central
  venous pressure (CVP) and guide volume
  replacement, to enable central delivery of
  drugs (e.g. inotropes, vasopressors,
  antiarrhythmics) and to allow postoperative
  intravenous feeding if necessary.
* After *induction* of anaesthesia, a nasogastric
  tube and urinary catheter are inserted.

* *Positioning* – a variety of positions is used,
  including Lloyd-Davies, lithotomy,
  Trendelenburg, prone. Eyes should be
  taped closed and pressure points protected.
* *Temperature* – every effort should be made to
  prevent hypothermia using warming
  mattresses, forced air warmers and warmed
  intravenous fluids. Core temperature should
  be monitored with a nasopharyngeal
  temperature probe.
* Broad-spectrum prophylactic *antibiotics* are
  given at induction of anaesthesia along with
  steroid cover if indicated.

ANAESTHETIC TECHNIQUE

In emergency procedures for the 'acute
abdomen' in unfasted patients, rapid sequence
induction using thiopental and suxamethonium, with the application of cricoid pressure
and tracheal intubation, is the technique of
choice (see Ch. 28).

For elective major abdominal surgery,
general anaesthesia with tracheal intubation
and controlled ventilation is a well proven technique.

INDUCTION AGENT
The choice of induction agent depends on the
physiological status of the patient and the
length of the procedure. In fit patients, propofol or thiopental may be used. Propofol may be
more suitable for shorter cases where rapid
emergence is desirable. In septic, hypovolaemic
or haemorrhaging patients, and in those with
significant cardiovascular disease, etomidate
may be preferred for its greater cardiovascular
stability.

MAINTENANCE
Maintenance of anaesthesia is usually with a
volatile anaesthetic agent; isoflurane and
desflurane are suitable choices for longer cases,
whereas sevoflurane is often reserved for day
cases. Nitrous oxide is avoided to prevent
bowel distension. Total intravenous anaesthesia
(TIVA) with propofol and a short-acting opioid
(e.g. remifentanil) has also been employed successfully in major abdominal surgery.

MUSCLE RELAXATION
Muscle relaxation is required to facilitate surgical access and IPPV. An agent of intermediate
duration of action is chosen, such as atracurium
or vecuronium. Monitoring of neuromuscular
blockade is required to ensure that reversal is
adequate at the end of the procedure. In the

16

past, there has been concern regarding the use of anticholinesterase drugs, such as neostigmine, for reversal of neuromuscular blockade because of the possibility of increased peristaltic activity and the theoretical risk of dehiscence of the bowel anastomosis. Conclusive evidence is lacking and most anaesthetists favour the use of neostigmine to ensure adequate return of respiratory muscle function at the end of the operation.

FLUID THERAPY

Intravenous infusion of a crystalloid solution (e.g. 0.9% saline, Hartmann's solution) should be commenced via fluid or blood warmer before induction. Fluid balance should be carefully monitored throughout surgery, taking into account blood loss, evaporative losses from exposed bowel, urine output, trends in central venous pressure, etc. Crystalloids, colloids and blood are given to replace losses as appropriate. Major blood losses may occur requiring blood transfusion, and coagulopathy may ensue requiring administration of other blood products such as fresh frozen plasma and platelets.

BLOOD TRANSFUSION

Blood transfusion in cancer surgery has provoked debate over recent years. Studies have shown an increase in tumour recurrence, increased infection rates and a poorer outcome in patients who had received perioperative blood transfusions. A causative link has not been established, although a likely mechanism is via immune suppression. Transfusion should therefore be avoided if at all possible, and a haemoglobin concentration of $7-9$ g dl^{-1} is considered acceptable. Despite these risks, in patients with ongoing haemorrhage it is not advisable to withhold transfusion.

ANALGESIA

Analgesia may be provided with intravenous opioids: morphine, pethidine, diamorphine and fentanyl have all been used. Doses are titrated during operation and can be continued after surgery using a PCA system. In appropriate patients opioids can be supplemented with NSAIDs, which can have an opioid-sparing effect.

Alternatively, regional anaesthetic techniques may be employed.

REGIONAL ANAESTHESIA AND ANALGESIA

Some procedures are suitable for regional anaesthesia alone, for example perianal surgery and refashioning of stomas. Major abdominal procedures are less suited to regional techniques alone, although in some high-risk patients this may be the preferred choice of anaesthetic.

A combination of light general anaesthesia and epidural blockade is now a popular technique in major abdominal surgery. As well as providing excellent analgesia both during and after surgery, epidurals have been demonstrated to confer several major benefits to the patient (Box 16.4).

There is a lack of convincing evidence to support concerns that epidural blockade may provoke the breakdown of bowel anastomoses. Epidural blockade results in a relative increase in parasympathetic tone, which may result in increased bowel activity. This, combined with hypotension, which sometimes accompanies epidural anaesthesia, may compromise mesen-

---

BOX 16.4

Benefits of epidural blockade

General

- Good operating conditions
- Good postoperative analgesia

Reduced neuroendocrine stress response:

- Reduced oxygen consumption
- Reduced catecholamine release
- Reduced postoperative negative nitrogen balance (reduced catabolism)
- Reduced hyperglycaemia
- ?Less immunosuppression

Improved gastrointestinal function

- Shorter duration of postoperative ileus (compared with opioids)
- Reduced gut mucosal perfusion by increased mesenteric blood flow
- Faster recovery of gut function
- NB: Segmental blockade of dermatomes T5–T12 is required to reduce sympathetically mediated peristaltic inhibition, preserving vagal and sacral parasympathetic outflow.

Improved respiratory function

- Increased postoperative oxygenation
- Reduced pulmonary infection rate
- Cardiovascular benefits
- Reduced cardiac morbidity in high-risk patients
- Reduced DVT rate
- Less blood loss

teric blood flow and affect anastomotic healing. The bulk of recent evidence contradicts these concerns and supports the use of epidurals in colorectal surgery, both for their beneficial effects on bowel function and reduction in the number of systemic complications.

PERIANAL SURGERY

Surgical stimulation to the anus can cause severe pain and may precipitate reflex responses, including laryngeal spasm, tachyarrhythmias and bradyarrhythmias.

Anaesthetic techniques aim to provide sufficient depth of anaesthesia and adequate analgesia to avoid these responses and yet allow rapid emergence from what is usually a short procedure, often performed as a day case.

GENERAL ANAESTHESIA

A spontaneous breathing technique using a laryngeal mask or face mask, and intravenous induction with propofol and a potent analgesic such as fentanyl (1 μg kg^{-1}) or alfentanil (5–10 μg kg^{-1}), is commonly used.

Patient positioning for these procedures dictates airway management. Lithotomy and Trendelenburg positions increase the risk of aspiration of gastric contents and ventilatory compromise, and may necessitate tracheal intubation and controlled ventilation. Patients may also be managed in the lateral position. Certain procedures require the patient to be positioned prone and 'jack-knifed', and in this position airway and ventilation may be severely compromised. Tracheal intubation is required, with positive-pressure ventilation.

REGIONAL ANAESTHESIA

Spinal and caudal extradural anaesthesia have both been used successfully in perianal surgery. The benefits include: avoidance of general anaesthesia, good postoperative analgesia and attenuation of the stress response. Regional techniques may be less suitable for day-case surgery where urinary retention may prove a concern and early mobilisation is required. A low spinal block ('saddle block') aiming to anaesthetise S2–S5 can be performed in the sitting position (difficult in the elderly and patients with severe perianal pain) using small volumes (0.5–1.5 ml) of 0.5% heavy bupivacaine. A caudal extradural block using 15–20 ml of 0.5% bupivacaine will provide perianal analgesia. It may be used alone or in combination with general anaesthesia, and has been used successfully in day-case surgery. Local blocks, such as posterior perineal nerve blockade and local infiltration, have also been used for certain procedures, as sole anaesthetic as well as in combination with general anaesthesia to provide postoperative analgesia.

POSTOPERATIVE MANAGEMENT

- Patients who have undergone major surgery or who have significant concurrent medical problems should be managed in a high-dependency environment with invasive monitoring.
- Oxygen, intravenous fluids and appropriate analgesia should be prescribed and consideration given to antithrombotic prophylaxis.
- Antibiotics are prescribed in conjunction with the surgical team, and provision made for restarting essential medication.
- Day-case patients should be assessed according to unit policy and discharged with suitable analgesia to the care of a competent adult. Clear instructions for follow-up should be given, along with contact telephone numbers should problems occur.

BIBLIOGRAPHY

Aljafri AM, Kingworth A, eds. Fundamentals of surgical practice. Greenwich Medical Media; 1998

Amato AC, Pescatori M. Effect of perioperative blood transfusions on recurrence of colorectal cancer: meta-analysis stratified on risk factors. Diseases of the Colon and Rectum 1998; 41(5):570–585

Blajchman MA. Immunomodulatory effects of allogenic blood transfusions: clinical manifestations and mechanisms. Vox Sanguinis 1998; 74(Suppl 2):315–319

Buggy DJ, Smith G. Epidural anaesthesia and analgesia: better outcome after major surgery. British Medical Journal 1999; 319:530–531

Jackson IJB. The management of pain following day surgery. British Journal of Anaesthesia Continuing Education and Professional Development Reviews 2001; 1(2)

Williams B, Wheatley R. Epidural analgesia for postoperative pain relief. Royal College of Anaesthetists Bulletin 2000; July

16

Obstruction or perforation

R. J. Harding

These two conditions have multiple aetiologies. They can represent a major anaesthetic and surgical challenge. Gastrointestinal obstruction results in major fluid loss into the bowel lumen. It may be complicated by perforation. Perforation of the gastrointestinal tract results in peritonitis and can produce severe systemic upset.

PATIENT CHARACTERISTICS

- Neonates to the elderly, but often older age groups with medical co-morbidities
- Often unwell and may have significant pain
- Invariably hypovolaemic and may have systemic sepsis
- Associated with underlying pathologies such as malignancy.

PREOPERATIVE ASSESSMENT AND INVESTIGATIONS

Particular attention should be paid to the following areas:
- Presence and severity of co-morbid conditions, particularly of the cardiorespiratory system
- State of hydration and serum electrolytes
- Evidence of septic or hypovolaemic shock.

INVESTIGATIONS:
- *Full blood count and coagulation screen, particularly if considering epidural analgesia*
- Urea, electrolytes and creatinine
- Cross-match at least 2 units of blood (or follow locally agreed blood-ordering schedule)
- Arterial blood gases – evidence of metabolic acidosis or high lactate concentration suggests poor tissue perfusion and the need for preoperative resuscitation
- ECG and chest radiography if clinically indicated.

PREOPERATIVE PREPARATION

Patients with bowel obstruction require urgent, but not emergency, surgery. They should be fully resuscitated prior to theatre, and surgery should not be performed precipitously unless the obstruction is complicated by bowel ischaemia or perforation.

Gastrointestinal perforation is a surgical emergency, but patients will still require adequate, and sometimes aggressive, resuscitation before operation.

Any patient who is significantly unwell should be optimised with the aid of invasive monitoring in a high-dependency area. All patients require a nasogastric tube and a urinary catheter. Adequate analgesia is necessary in all patients. Consider thromboembolic prophylaxis.

PERIOPERATIVE MANAGEMENT

MONITORING:
- Routine anaesthetic monitoring
- Monitoring of core temperature
- Consider invasive arterial and CVP monitoring in all but the most straightforward of cases. This is particularly important with significant cardiorespiratory disease or poor preoperative condition
- Monitoring of cardiac output in high-risk cases.

ANAESTHETIC TECHNIQUE

Such operations almost always require general anaesthesia, but this is often supplemented with an epidural to provide postoperative analgesia. Regional anaesthesia, with a continuous spinal or epidural technique, can be used in selected cases, but adequate anaesthesia may be both difficult to achieve and associated with side-effects such as significant hypotension. An epidural can provide excellent postoperative

16

analgesia, but the following points should be considered:

- There may be a coagulopathy.
- Intraoperative use may result in profound hypotension because patients are often hypovolaemic and may have severe sepsis.
- Placement of an epidural catheter in the presence of systemic sepsis – the true risk of an epidural abscess is unknown and this is a risk–benefit decision.

GENERAL ANAESTHESIA

Large-bore intravenous access and intravenous fluid administration should be established prior to induction of anaesthesia. Aspirate the nasogastric tube and leave it open to drain freely.

Rapid sequence induction is used. There is potential for cardiovascular collapse on induction of anaesthesia if the patient is inadequately resuscitated. Be prepared for this – however adequate resuscitation appears to be.

Choice of agents used is relatively unimportant, but consider drugs with a rapid recovery profile because drug kinetics may be altered in patients who are unwell, particularly the elderly. Nitrous oxide is best avoided as it can diffuse into an already dilated bowel making closure of the abdomen difficult, and may increase intra-abdominal pressure in the early postoperative period.

Patients with an obstructed or perforated viscus may require very large fluid volumes during operation, including blood transfusion. Fluid warmers and active body warming (e.g. forced warm air over-blankets) are mandatory because heat loss will be significant. Patients may require inotropic or vasopressor support.

POSTOPERATIVE MANAGEMENT

All but the most straightforward cases should be managed in a high-dependency or intensive care unit in the early postoperative period. This is particularly true when an epidural catheter has been sited. Significant fluid loss and fluid shifts are likely to continue in the postoperative period, owing to redistribution and sequestration. There is potential for deterioration, most commonly due to sepsis or respiratory complications.

Patients require good quality analgesia. Both epidurals and opioid-based regimens are suitable.

Care should be taken when using NSAIDs if upper gastrointestinal tract perforation or renal compromise is present – this includes a substantial proportion of patients suffering a perforated or obstructed viscus.

BIBLIOGRAPHY

Callum KG et al. Extremes of age. The 1999 report of the National Confidential Enquiry into Perioperative Deaths. London: NCEPOD; 1999

Paterson-Brown S. Emergency surgery and critical care: a companion to specialist surgical practice. London: WB Saunders; 1997

CROSS-REFERENCES

Water and electrolyte disturbances
Anaesthetic Factors 27: 624

16

Oesophagogastrectomy

R. J. Harding

SURGERY FOR MALIGNANT LESIONS OF THE OESOPHAGUS AND STOMACH

There are several surgical approaches for oesophageal surgery, which are determined by the anatomical position of the tumour and by surgical preference:
- 'Ivor-Lewis' oesophagectomy – upper midline laparotomy followed by right thoracotomy for tumours in the middle and lower thirds of the oesophagus
- Left thoracoabdominal oesophagectomy – for tumours of the lower third and cardia
- Three-stage oesophagectomy – upper midline laparotomy, right thoracotomy, and left or right-sided cervical incision. For tumours of the upper and middle thirds
- Pharyngolaryngo-oesophagectomy – for tumours of the hypopharynx and cervical oesophagus. Usually an ENT procedure
- Transhiatal oesophagectomy – oesophagectomy without thoracotomy; rarely used
- Thorascopic surgery is becoming more popular.

Gastric surgery is performed via an upper midline laparotomy. This section concentrates on anaesthesia for oesophagectomy.

PATIENT CHARACTERISTICS

- Elderly
- High prevalence of tobacco and alcohol consumption
- Patients frequently suffer from smoking-related conditions, particularly ischaemic heart disease and chronic obstructive pulmonary disease
- Patients are often malnourished secondary to dysphagia and the presence of a malignancy. Operations on malnourished patients carry high morbidity and mortality rates.

PREOPERATIVE ASSESSMENT AND INVESTIGATIONS

Adequate staging of the tumour is essential to ensure that proposed surgery is appropriate. Assessment of the severity of co-morbid disease, particularly of the cardiorespiratory system, and assessment of nutritional status are important as these influence choice of anaesthetic technique.
Investigations should include:
- Full blood count
- Urea, electrolytes and creatinine levels
- ECG
- Chest radiography
- Lung function tests and arterial blood gases if patient has respiratory disease or one-lung ventilation (OLV) is required
- Further cardiovascular testing such as echocardiography should be considered.

PREOPERATIVE PREPARATION

Attention should be given to the nutritional state of the patient. Both enteral and parenteral nutrition have a role and currently there is interest in the addition of immunomodulatory substances to these. Maximum medical treatment of co-morbid conditions should be implemented. Patients with poor respiratory function may benefit from admission for pre-operative physiotherapy and treatment of infection.

Thromboembolic prophylaxis and premedication are administered.

PERIOPERATIVE MANAGEMENT

MONITORING:
- Routine anaesthetic monitoring
- Urinary catheter
- Core temperature
- Invasive arterial pressure and central venous pressure monitoring

16

- Monitoring of cardiac output in high-risk cases.

Patients can be haemodynamically unstable during thoracotomy and arterial lines are also useful for assessing the adequacy of OLV. Central lines should be sited ipsilateral to the side of the thoracotomy, because of the risk of pneumothorax or vessel damage.

ANAESTHETIC TECHNIQUE

The technique chosen most commonly involves a general anaesthetic supplemented by epidural analgesia. A balanced anaesthetic technique is used. Agents with rapid recovery profiles are useful to avoid prolonged postoperative respiratory depression. Unlike the volatile agents, propofol does not inhibit hypoxic pulmonary vasoconstriction and may therefore confer a small benefit. A double-lumen endobronchial tube is inserted to allow OLV, which may be prolonged. A left-sided tube is usually employed for oesophageal surgery. Correct positioning is vital and should be checked fibreoptically. Active patient warming is required.

SPECIAL POINTS

With multilevel approaches to the oesophagus, such as the Ivor-Lewis operation, several intraoperative changes of patient position are required. This risks displacement of the double-lumen tube, loss of invasive lines and patient injury.

- Tube position needs to be checked after each change of position.
- Surgery can be prolonged and involve significant fluid and blood loss.
- Manipulation of mediastinal structures can impede cardiac filling and produce arrhythmias.

POSTOPERATIVE MANAGEMENT

In most cases the aim is early extubation and admission to a high-dependency area. However, some patients need ventilation on the intensive care unit. Adequate analgesia is vital to avoid respiratory complications. Analgesia can be provided by an epidural, paravertebral catheter, intercostal nerve blocks or an opioid-based technique. Epidural analgesia is the most popular technique in the UK. Complete analgesia can sometimes be difficult to achieve because the operation involves many dermatome levels. A multimodal approach is advisable.

Other key therapies include:

- Aggressive physiotherapy.
- Thromboembolic prophylaxis.
- Early institution of enteral nutrition, often via a surgically sited jejunostomy, reduces the incidence of postoperative complications.
- A high index of suspicion is required for surgical complications, the most important of these being anastomotic breakdown.

OUTCOME

Oesophagectomy has an operative mortality rate of approximately 10%. Outcome is improved by performing oesophagectomies in specialist centres with experienced teams.

COMPLICATIONS

Respiratory complications occur in 25% of patients after oesophagectomy.

Cardiovascular complications (including arrhythmias) occur in approximately 10%, and thromboembolic complications in less than 10%. Anastomotic leaks occur in approximately 10%, and chylothorax in 3%. These are associated with a high mortality rate if not managed aggressively.

After operation, the 1-year survival rate is approximately 50%, with a 5-year survival rate of 20%.

16

BIBLIOGRAPHY

Braga M, Gianotti L, Nespoli L, Radaelli G, Di Carlo V. Nutritional approach in malnourished surgical patients: a prospective randomized study. Archives of Surgery 2002;137(2):174–180

Gray AJG, Hoile RW, Ingram GS, Sherry KM. The report of the National Confidential Enquiry into Perioperative Deaths 1996/1997. London: NCEPOD; 1998

Griffin SM, Raimes SA. Upper gastrointestinal surgery: a companion to specialist surgical practice. London: WB Saunders; 1997

Sherry KM. How can we improve the outcome of oesophagectomy? British Journal of Anaesthesia 2001; 86(5):611–613

Vaughan RS. Pain relief after thoracotomy. British Journal of Anaesthesia 2001; 87(5):681

Hernia repair

L. Milligan

A hernia is a protrusion of the whole or part of a viscus from its normal position through an opening in the wall of its containing cavity.

Surgical repair involves excision of the hernia sac and closure of the defect with non-absorbable sutures and/or polypropylene mesh. Occasionally, bowel resection and anastomosis is required.

TYPES OF HERNIA

- Inguinal
- Femoral
- Umbilical and paraumbilical
- Epigastric
- Incisional
- Obturator
- Spigelian
- Lumbar
- Gluteal
- Sciatic
- Perineal
- Hiatus
- Diaphragmatic.

INGUINAL HERNIA

- Most common in both sexes, comprising 75–80% of abdominal wall hernias
- Occur at any age from infancy (especially premature babies) to elderly
- Repair early to reduce risk of strangulation and minimise stretching of abdominal wall musculature, hence reducing recurrence rate
- Repaired by various techniques of herniorhaphy and, in infants, herniotomy
- 3% of herniae recur and patients may present for further repair. Such procedures may be longer and more complex.

LAPAROSCOPIC REPAIR:

- Remains currently an experimental technique

- Extraperitoneal approach, so problems of pneumoperitoneum avoided. Complexity and risk of potential complications make it an operation for experienced surgeons only.
- Reduced length of hospital stay and use of analgesia have to be weighed against increased theatre costs
- Royal College of Surgeons' review failed to demonstrate advantage over conventional approach.

STRANGULATED HERNIA

Hernia contents may become constricted by the neck of the sac or by twisting. Symptoms and signs of bowel obstruction indicate the need for urgent operation. Laparotomy and bowel resection may be required.

FEMORAL HERNIA

- Protrusion of the peritoneum into the potential space of the femoral canal.
- Sac may contain abdominal viscera (small bowel) or omentum.
- More common in multiparous women; rare in children.
- Strangulates more readily than inguinal hernia because femoral canal is small and not distensible.
- Presents with symptoms and signs of small bowel obstruction.
- Repair should be undertaken at earliest opportunity even when asymptomatic.

UMBILICAL AND PARAUMBILICAL HERNIAS

True umbilical hernias occur only in infancy. The most extreme form is exomphalos, in which the midgut fails to return to the abdominal cavity in early fetal life. Surgical repair is required urgently and prognosis is generally poor. A small hernia can occur at the umbilical cicatrix in the first few days of life. Repair is

16

rarely required unless the hernia persists after the age of 18 months.

Paraumbilical hernias are acquired and associated with: middle age, obesity, multiparous women. They occur at a small defect in the linea alba and there is a high risk of strangulation. Repair is recommended, even in relatively unfit and obese patients. Mayo's operation is the usual surgical procedure.

INCISIONAL HERNIAS

- Late complication of 10–15% of abdominal wounds; occur between 1 and 5 years after operation due to breakdown of the repair to the abdominal wall muscle and fascia.
- Predisposing factors:
  —obesity
  —distension
  —poor muscle quality
  —inadequate closure technique
  —postoperative wound infection
  —multiple operations through same incision.
- Usually asymptomatic, but occasionally a narrow-necked hernia may produce pain or strangulation, in which case surgical repair is indicated.

PATIENTS

- All ages – neonates and infants to the elderly.
- May present with any number of concurrent medical problems. The demographics of hernia repair make conditions associated with the elderly particularly common.
- Problems specifically associated with hernias:
  —chronic cough (chronic obstructive pulmonary disease, asthma)
  —chronic constipation
  —obesity (and associated problems, such as ischaemic heart disease, diabetes mellitus, sleep apnoea)
  —pregnancy.
- Approximately 50% of patients in the UK undergo day-case hernia repair. Inpatient treatment is required for those with a poor level of fitness, lack of social backup and complicated hernias. In the USA, 70% of inguinal hernia repairs are performed as a day case, the majority under local anaesthesia, and discharged within 4 h of operation.
- Some patients present as an emergency with the problems associated with bowel obstruction, including:

—vomiting
—dehydration
—hypovolaemia
—electrolyte and acid–base disturbances.

PREOPERATIVE ASSESSMENT

- Routine history and examination, with particular attention to concurrent disease
- Routine investigations – haematology, biochemistry, ECG, as dictated by local policy
- Other investigations as indicated by history and examination, for example chest radiography, arterial blood gases, pulmonary function tests.

PREMEDICATION

- Sedative premedication is not indicated for day-case patients. An oral anxiolytic (e.g. temazepam) may be prescribed for elective inpatients.
- Oral analgesia may be prescribed as part of a multimodal, pre-emptive analgesic regimen.
- Emergency cases can be prescribed an H_2-receptor antagonist (e.g. ranitidine) and a pro-kinetic drug (e.g. metoclopramide) to reduce the risk of pulmonary aspiration.
- Intravenous fluids should be commenced for patients with a history of vomiting, dehydration, hypovolaemia and electrolyte imbalance.

ANAESTHETIC MANAGEMENT

- Anaesthetic technique depends largely on the type and size of hernia, and whether elective or emergency case.
- All strangulated hernias with symptoms of bowel obstruction should be treated as an 'acute abdomen'. A general anaesthetic with rapid sequence induction and application of cricoid pressure is the technique of choice.
- For other types of hernia repair there is a wide choice of anaesthetic technique:
  —general
  —regional
  —local
  —combination of above.
- In all cases, standard monitoring is required, along with intravenous access ± intravenous fluids and broad-spectrum antibiotics.

16

GENERAL ANAESTHESIA

- General anaesthesia is used in preference to regional and local techniques in:
  —anxious patients
  —children
  —obese patients
  —patients who have difficulty lying flat (arthritis, congestive cardiac failure).
- For inguinal and femoral hernia repair, where there is no risk of vomiting or regurgitation, a spontaneously breathing technique using a laryngeal mask may be appropriate.
- For abdominal wall hernias, especially large incisional hernias and those involving bowel, muscle relaxation is required and therefore tracheal intubation and positive-pressure ventilation is needed.
- Extubation should be achieved where possible with minimal coughing and bucking to protect the hernia repair. The use of drugs (e.g. propofol and sevoflurane) that allow rapid return of consciousness and upper airway reflexes is recommended. These drugs are also advantageous in day-case surgery.
- Nitrous oxide is not recommended in patients with bowel obstruction.
- Intraoperative analgesia should be multimodal and tailored to the type of hernia repair and amount of postoperative pain expected. A short-acting opioid (e.g. fentanyl), a NSAID and infiltration of the wound with local anaesthetic may be satisfactory in inguinal and femoral hernia repairs.
- General anaesthesia can be combined with a local block (e.g. inguinal field block) to reduce intraoperative anaesthetic requirements and produce good quality, non-sedative, postoperative analgesia.
- In cases where a large laparotomy wound is explored, insertion of an epidural, which can be used for postoperative analgesia, may be beneficial, especially if the patient has concurrent pulmonary disease.

REGIONAL ANAESTHESIA:

- Regional techniques (spinal or epidural) are appropriate for the elective repair of hernias, provided an intraperitoneal approach is not required.
- Avoids complications of general anaesthesia, reduces stress response, and provides good postoperative analgesia.
- Not recommended in emergency cases with bowel obstruction and hypovolaemia.

- May be the technique of choice in high-risk elderly patients.
- Patient must be able to lie flat.
- Sedation may be required, and can be achieved with judicious boluses of midazolam (1–2 mg) or an infusion of propofol (1–2 μg kg^{-1} h^{-1}). Oxygen should be administered by face-mask or nasal cannulae.

LOCAL ANAESTHESIA:

- May be used as the sole anaesthetic in day-case surgery or in patients considered unfit for other anaesthetic techniques. Intraoperative pain has been reported as a problem. May be used in combination with general anaesthesia to reduce anaesthetic requirements and provide postoperative analgesia.
- Gaining popularity as surgical expertise increases.
- Not suitable for the anxious, obese and uncooperative patients, or those with complicated hernias.
- Shown to be the most cost-effective anaesthetic technique in inguinal hernia repair.
- All patients require standard monitoring and intravenous access.

Inguinal field block:
- Aims to block:
  —subcostal nerve (T12)
  —iliohypogastric nerve (L1)
  —ilioinguinal nerve (L1).
- *Technique* – a regional block needle is inserted 2.5 cm inferomedially to the anterior superior iliac spine and advanced through the external oblique aponeurosis. A distinctive 'click' is felt as the needle penetrates the fascia. Some 10 ml local anaesthetic (e.g. 0.5% bupivacaine, 0.5–1.0% prilocaine) is infiltrated deep to the aponeurosis, down the inner surface of the ilium through the abdominal muscle layers. A further 10 ml local anaesthetic is deposited superficial to the external oblique and medial to this point, in line with the inguinal ligament. A further injection is made over and around the pubic tubercle in a 'fan' pattern.
- Blockade produces good postoperative analgesia; however, supplementary infiltration – especially around the inguinal ring and hernial sac – is usually necessary during operation if this is the only anaesthetic employed.

16

POSTOPERATIVE MANAGEMENT

- Analgesia following hernia repair is best provided by a multimodal approach. A successful regimen includes combinations of opioids, simple analgesics (paracetamol) and NSAIDs. along with local block techniques or wound infiltration with local anaesthetic.
- Patients undergoing large or bilateral hernia repair may prefer a morphine-based PCA system, rather than repeated intramuscular injections.
- Those with significant cardiovascular or respiratory disease undergoing major abdominal wall hernia repairs may benefit from insertion of an epidural for postoperative analgesia.
- Oxygen and intravenous fluids should be prescribed and thromboprophylaxis considered.
- Chest physiotherapy is recommended for all patients with respiratory disease.
- Day-case patients must be assessed carefully prior to discharge in accordance with the unit's policy; analgesia should be prescribed and information given regarding follow-up and contacts should problems arise.

BIBLIOGRAPHY

Aljafri AM, Kingsnorth A. Fundamentals of surgical practice. Greenwich Medical Media; 1998

Burkitt HG, Quick CRG, Gatt D. Essential surgery: problems, diagnosis and management. Edinburgh: Churchill Livingstone; 1990

Callesen T, Bech K, Kehlet H. One-thousand inguinal hernia repairs under unmonitored local anesthesia. Anesthesia and Analgesia 2001; 93(6):1373–1376

Cheek CM, Black NA, Devlin HB, Kingsnorth AN, Taylor RS, Watkin DF. Groin hernia surgery: a systematic review. Annals of the Royal College of Surgeons of England 1998; 80(Suppl 1):S1–S80

Jackson IJB. The management of pain following day surgery. British Journal of Anaesthesia Continuing Educationa and Professional Development Reviews 2001; 1(2)

Wildsmith JAW, Armitage EN. The principles and practice of regional anaesthesia. Edinburgh: Churchill Livingstone; 1993

CROSS-REFERENCES

Postoperation pain management
    Anaesthetic Factors 31: 778
Day case surgery
    Anaesthetic Factors 27: 613

16

17

GYNAECOLOGICAL SURGERY
B. J. Pollard

Minor gynaecological procedures

B. J. Pollard

Dilatation and curettage (D&C), evacuation of retained products of conception (ERPC) and suction termination of pregnancy (TOP) are common minor gynaecological procedures. Additional procedures, such as hysteroscopy, may occasionally be added and these will lengthen the procedure, possibly quite considerably.

PROCEDURES

- Short in duration
- Often undertaken as day cases
- Usually performed in the lithotomy position
- Involve an initial period of intense surgical stimulation for dilatation of the cervix
- May be diagnostic (e.g. D&C for postmenopausal bleeding) or therapeutic (e.g. ERPC).

PATIENT CHARACTERISTICS

- May be of any age from puberty onwards
- Are generally young and fit for TOP and ERPC
- May have significant co-morbidity (e.g. cardiac abnormalities), possibly related to the reason for the TOP
- Those for ERPC who are beyond the first trimester of pregnancy or who have symptomatic gastro-oesophageal reflux require precautions against aspiration of gastric contents
- May be elderly for D&C with various co-morbidities and perhaps malignant disease.

PREOPERATIVE ASSESSMENT AND INVESTIGATIONS

- Assess adequacy of resuscitation if patient for ERPC has vaginal bleeding as this may have been considerable and be continuing.
- If urgent, when and what was last oral intake and what analgesia has been given as

this may indicate the possibility of a full stomach.
- What is the length of gestation, if relevant, and are there any symptoms of reflux?
- Investigations as clinically indicated.
- Measure haemoglobin level if bleeding, but remember that following acute blood loss there may be no change in the haemoglobin concentration for several hours.
- Enquire about any coexisting diseases.
- Enquire about any limitation of knee and hip movement (need for lithotomy position).
- If planned as a day case, ensure that appropriate procedures are in place for subsequent care.

PREMEDICATION

- Anxiolysis is rarely required, but a short-acting benzodiazepine may be useful if necessary
- H_2 antagonists and sodium citrate if at risk of regurgitation
- Has a prostaglandin pessary been given? This may increase requirements for postoperative analgesia.

THEATRE PREPARATION

- Routine equipment and machine check
- Adequate personnel to ensure simultaneous lifting and lowering of legs to avoid injuries to hips and knees
- Remember when positioning to avoid nerve injury due to pressure on the medial or lateral lower leg from lithotomy poles.

PERIOPERATIVE MANAGEMENT

MINIMAL MONITORING:

- F_{IO_2}
- SpO_2
- ECG

17

- Non-invasive blood pressure
- $EtCO_2$.

ANAESTHETIC TECHNIQUE:

- General anaesthesia is usually the technique of choice because these operations are short and quite stimulating.
- Regional techniques are acceptable in selected patients.
- For TOP or ERPC, uterine relaxation should be avoided if possible by selecting a total intravenous anaesthetic (TIVA) technique or using a low concentration of volatile agent.
- Intravenous induction with spontaneous ventilation using nitrous oxide–oxygen–volatile agent and a short-acting opioid (e.g. alfentanil or fentanyl) to obtund response to cervical dilatation is a suitable technique.
- Rapid sequence induction and tracheal intubation are necessary if there is risk of regurgitation.
- Oxytocics may be requested by the gynaecologist. Synthetic oxytocin (e.g. Syntocinon) is preferred. Products containing ergometrine (e.g. Syntometrine) should be avoided as these may cause hypertension, bronchospasm, nausea and vomiting, especially if given intravenously. Oxytocin may cause a fall in arterial pressure, which can be minimised by giving it slowly.
- Non-steroidal anti-inflammatory drugs (NSAIDs) are useful for postoperative analgesia, especially if prostaglandin pessaries have been used as these cause painful uterine contractions. A suitable dose of an NSAID may be given with the premed or a suppository (remember the consent) during the procedure.

- Antiemetics may be needed in view of the high incidence of postoperative nausea and vomiting in patients undergoing gynaecological surgery.
- There is little evidence that concentrations of volatile agents of 0.5 minimum alveolar concentration (MAC) or less lead to a clinically significant increase in blood loss during TOP or ERPC. Any uterine relaxation will be rapidly reversed by the administration of an oxytocic.

POSTOPERATIVE MANAGEMENT

- Nurse in the lateral position with supplemental oxygen until awake.
- If the trachea was intubated, then extubate awake in the lateral position.
- Male recovery staff should have chaperones in view of the possibility of inappropriate patient behaviour during recovery.
- Simple analgesics are usually adequate. Postoperative pain is usually minimal but may be greater in those patients who normally experience painful menstruation or who have received a prostaglandin pessary.
- If patient condition allows and domestic circumstances are suitable, most patients may be allowed home on the day of surgery with appropriate day-case procedure advice.

CROSS-REFERENCES

Complications of position
    Anaesthetic Factors 31: 736
Day-case surgery
    Anaesthetic Factors 27: 613
Premedication
    Anaesthetic Factors 27: 621

17

Hysteroscopy and laser surgery

D. Phillips and B. J. Pollard

PROCEDURES

- Direct examination of the uterine cavity using a fibreoptic endoscope.
- Surgical intervention may follow.
- Uterine distension is necessary for visualisation. The use of irrigation fluid also permits removal of blood and detritus, and dissipation of heat.
- Distension is usually achieved with a fluid (saline, glycine, dextran). Carbon dioxide may occasionally be used.
- Complications
  —fluid absorption and circulatory overload
  —dilutional hyponatraemia and hypoproteinaemia
  —transurethral resection (TUR) syndrome
  —disseminated intravascular coagulation
  —anaphylaxis.
- Complications – carbon dioxide:
  —abdominal distension during long procedures (leak via fallopian tubes)
  —carbon dioxide absorption – acidosis, arrhythmias
  —carbon dioxide embolism.

THE LASER

The commonest lasers in gynaecological use are the neodymium–yttrium–aluminium–garnet (NdYAG) and carbon dioxide lasers.

All staff concerned should be familiar with the national guidelines on the safe operation of medical lasers and also local policies. Although the laser should be operated only in the surgical field, precautions must be taken to protect against injury from inadvertent operation:

- Patient eye protection
- Staff eye protection
- Designated operating theatre with locked doors and covered windows (if any)
- Removal or covering of reflective surfaces
- No casual access
- Extra eye protection outside in case of need.

Intrauterine hysteroscopic laser surgery is carried out under fluid uterine distension. Procedures include endometrial destruction and removal of benign intrauterine pathology.

Complications include uterine perforation, haemorrhage (usually controlled with the laser but may necessitate laparotomy if uterus perforated), heat transmission (not clinically important at typical power settings for intrauterine surgery).

PATIENT CHARACTERISTICS

- May be any age from mid-teens onwards
- No particular medical disorder is associated with the need for hysteroscopic laser surgery, except anaemia
- The procedure may be performed as a day case, so check suitability (medical status, home circumstances, etc.).

PREOPERATIVE ASSESSMENT AND INVESTIGATIONS

- Check for anaemia
- Other investigations as indicated by patient's medical status.

PREMEDICATION

- Not often required. Anxiolysis with a benzodiazepine may be valuable
- Consider an antiemetic
- Antibiotic prophylaxis may be given with the premedication or on induction of anaesthesia in at-risk patients.

THEATRE PREPARATION

- Familiarity with policies on the use of the laser is essential.
- Availability of patient protection – eye pads, foil, etc.
- Availability of staff eye protection – goggles.

17

PERIOPERATIVE MANAGEMENT

MONITORING:
- ECG
- Non-invasive blood pressure
- Pulse oximetry
- Fluid balance (including uterine distension fluid)
- Capnography
- Airway pressure
- Core temperature.

ANAESTHETIC TECHNIQUE:
- Resuscitation equipment should be available.
- General anaesthesia with either spontaneous or controlled respiration.
- Choice of maintenance technique depends on patient's medical condition and anaesthetist's preference.
- Regional – epidural or spinal is suitable. Light sedation may be needed (e.g. midazolam) with oxygen via face-mask.
- Local – paracervical, intracervical and intrauterine local block may be given by the surgeon. These are not favoured by all gynaecologists. Light sedation may be needed (e.g. midazolam).
- Analgesia (e.g. ketorolac or alfentanil).
- Place patient in lithotomy position.

FLUID BALANCE

- Measurement of fluid instilled and retrieved can be difficult but should be attempted because of the possible effects of fluid absorption.

SAMPLE PROTOCOL

1000 ml absorbed – continue operation
1500 ml absorbed – end operation as soon as possible
2000 ml absorbed – stop operation.

- Excessive blood loss is rarely a problem.
- Watch for signs of TUR syndrome, especially with extensive surgery and high intrauterine pressures.

POSTOPERATIVE PERIOD

- Any postoperative discomfort can usually be managed by NSAIDs.
- Gynaecological procedures are associated with an increased incidence of nausea and vomiting; an antiemetic should be prescribed.

BIBLIOGRAPHY

Department of Health and Social Security. Guidelines on the safe use of lasers in medical practice. London: DHSS; 1984

Morrison LMM, Davis J, Sumner D. Absorption of irrigating fluid during laser photocoagulation of the endometrium in the treatment of menorrhagia. British Journal of Obstetrics and Gynaecology 1989; 96:346–352

Osborne GA, Rudkin GE, Moran P. Fluid uptake in laser endometrial ablation. Anaesthesia and Intensive Care 1991; 19:217–219

Studd J, ed. Progress in obstetrics and gynaecology, vol 9. London: Churchill Livingstone; 1991

Van Boven MJ, Singelyn F, Donnez J, Gribomont BF. Dilutional hyponatraemia associated with intrauterine endoscopic laser surgery. Anesthesiology 1989; 71:449–450

17

CROSS-REFERENCES

Complications of position
    Anaesthetic Factors 31: 736
Day-case surgery
    Anaesthetic Factors 27: 613
TUR syndrome
    Anaesthetic Factors 31: 801

Laparoscopy

S. Piggott

17

PROCEDURE

- Gynaecological laparoscopy may be diagnostic (e.g. dye studies) or therapeutic (e.g. tubal ligation).
- Carbon dioxide is insufflated at pressures of 20–40 mmHg to create a pneumoperitoneum. This allows the pelvic organs to be visualised via a fibreoptic endoscope passed through a small subumbilical incision.
- Lithotomy position with Trendelenburg tilt is required.
- Instrumentation of the vagina is needed to manipulate the uterus or to inject dye.

PATIENT CHARACTERISTICS

Most patients presenting for gynaecological laparoscopy are relatively healthy. A high proportion are day cases.

PREOPERATIVE ASSESSMENT AND INVESTIGATION

All patients should have a full blood count. Other investigations need be performed only if indicated.

PREMEDICATION

Oral benzodiazepines are suitable if a premed is required.

PERIOPERATIVE MANAGEMENT

PROBLEMS ASSOCIATED WITH LAPAROSCOPY:

- Hypercapnoea – carbon dioxide is absorbed from the peritoneum. This is compounded by a reduction in functional residual capacity and compliance secondary to the pneumoperitoneum and Trendelenburg position. $EtCO_2$ reflects changes in arterial carbon dioxide tension.
- Regurgitation is a risk because of raised intragastric pressure and head-down tilt.
- Intra-abdominal pressure in excess of 40 cmH_2O compresses the inferior vena cava and restricts venous return with a consequent fall in cardiac output of up to 40%. Blood pressure and heart rate may be unaffected because total peripheral resistance increases.
- Manipulation of the pelvic organs often causes significant bradycardia.
- Perforation of abdominal viscera or major blood vessels by trocar is possible.
- Pneumothorax.
- Carbon dioxide embolism is a rare but potentially fatal complication of laparoscopy, although successful resuscitation has been reported (Box 17.1).

MONITORING:

- ECG
- Non-invasive blood pressure
- $EtCO_2$

BOX 17.1

Carbon dioxide embolism

Diagnosis

- Sudden decrease in $EtCO_2$
- ECG changes
- Hypotension
- Decrease in saturation.

Management

- Stop carbon dioxide insufflation
- 100% oxygen
- Left lateral decubitus position
- Place central line and attempt aspiration of gas from right atrium
- Cardiopulmonary resuscitation as required.

- Pulse oximetry
- Airway pressure
- Intra-abdominal pressure.

GENERAL ANAESTHESIA

General anaesthesia with muscle relaxation, tracheal intubation and controlled ventilation is the preferred technique because it guarantees airway protection and adequate ventilation. A recent report suggests that in selected patients spontaneous ventilation via a laryngeal mask may be satisfactory.

If the Bain circuit is used for intermittent positive-pressure ventilation (IPPV), higher than normal gas flows are needed to prevent rebreathing. A fresh gas flow of 110 ml kg^{-1} min^{-1} and minute ventilation of 175 ml kg^{-1} min^{-1} should be used.

Analgesia is best achieved with an opioid combined with a NSAID. The latter reduces the requirements for opioids, which exacerbate postoperative nausea and vomiting, and sedation. The choice of opioid is influenced by the duration of surgery and whether the patient is an inpatient or day case. An antiemetic should be given before reversal.

The brevity of some procedures could make reversal of non-depolarising neuromuscular block difficult. Mivacurium, or a small dose of atracurium or vecuronium, is suitable.

REGIONAL TECHNIQUES

An epidural block from T5 to S5 can provide satisfactory anaesthesia for laparoscopy. It is also possible to perform laparoscopy under local anaesthesia, with or without sedation.

POSTOPERATIVE MANAGEMENT

- Localised pain arises because of visceral trauma, particularly to the fallopian tubes after sterilisation. This is usually short-lived.
- Residual carbon dioxide causes diaphragmatic irritation and referred shoulder tip pain. The surgeon should ensure that as much gas as possible is vented from the peritoneal cavity at the end of the procedure.
- Peritoneal inflammation has been demonstrated up to 3 days after laparoscopy and is probably responsible for any persistent discomfort.
- A combination of an opioid and a NSAID provides effective analgesia. Take-home medication should be prescribed for day patients.
- Postoperative nausea and vomiting is frequently associated with laparoscopy. Varying incidences are quoted and other factors, including the administration of opioids and the phase of the menstrual cycle, are involved, but at least 50% of patients can be expected to have symptoms after gynaecological surgery.

BIBLIOGRAPHY

Gillberg LE, Harsten AS, Stahl LB. Preoperative diclofenac sodium reduces post-laparoscopy pain. Canadian Journal of Anaesthesia 1993; 40:406–408

Goodwin AP, Rowe WL, Ogg TW. Day case laparoscopy. A comparison of two anaesthetic techniques using the laryngeal mask during spontaneous breathing. Anaesthesia 1992; 47:892–895

CROSS-REFERENCES

Complications of position
    Anaesthetic Factors 31: 736
Day-case surgery
    Anaesthetic Factors 27: 613

17

Radical cancer surgery

B. J. Pollard

PROCEDURES AND INDICATIONS

- Simple vulvectomy is undertaken for local malignancy of the vulval region. Radical vulvectomy is for more advanced malignancy of the vulva; it includes excision of the femoral and inguinal lymph nodes and may include removal of parts of the urethra, vagina and bowel.
- Wertheim's and other forms of radical hysterectomy are performed for advanced cancer of the uterine cervix. Wertheim's hysterectomy includes removal of the upper half of the vagina, broad ligaments. and often the iliac and pelvic wall lymph nodes.
- Ovarian cystectomy and oophorectomy are undertaken for cancer of the ovary. An omentectomy may be done at the same time.
- Total pelvic exenteration consists of excision of all pelvic viscera, fascia and lymphatics. It is a rare 'last resort' procedure for very advanced or recurrent cancer of the uterine cervix or, more rarely, for severe radiation damage. It may very occasionally be performed for cancer of the vagina. In anterior exenteration the rectum is preserved, whereas in posterior exenteration the bladder and ureters are preserved.
- Vaginectomy, which may include excision of the bladder or rectum, may be performed for cancer of the vagina.
- Palliative surgery, such as colostomy or urinary diversion, may be required to relieve symptoms of obstruction or when the gut or urinary tract is involved in the malignant process.

PATIENT CHARACTERISTICS

- Often elderly, frail and cachectic.
- Patients with cancer of the cervix may be young.

- Cancer of the endometrium is significantly associated with diabetes and obesity, but radical surgery is rarely required.

Specific associations with cancer of the ovary include:

- Complications of the malignant process – ascites and pleural effusions
- Complications of the large intra-abdominal mass – aortocaval compression and reduced lung compliance
- Systemic effects – anaemia, hypovolaemia.

PREOPERATIVE ASSESSMENT AND INVESTIGATIONS

- Exclude associated conditions including anaemia, pleural effusions.
- Ensure blood is available for transfusion.
- Optimise chronic medical conditions.
- Consider deep vein thrombosis (DVT) prophylaxis. The incidence of DVT is 40% in operations for gynaecological malignancy.
- Assess nutritional state where appropriate (e.g. plasma proteins, albumin).

PREMEDICATION

These patients are commonly anxious, so a sedative premedication such as a benzodiazepine is usually indicated.

THEATRE PREPARATION

- Especially with more major surgery, maintenance of body temperature is important (fluid warmer, warming mattress, warm air blanket, humidification of inspired gases)
- May require admission to ITU or to HDU after operation
- Preparations for elective induced hypotension if required
- Invasive monitoring if indicated.

17

PERIOPERATIVE MANAGEMENT

- General anaesthesia is almost invariably used for these major procedures.
- Rapid sequence induction is indicated when there is raised intra-abdominal pressure, symptoms of reflux or where the malignancy may have caused intestinal adhesions leading to obstruction.
- With massive ascites or a huge ovarian cyst, induction of anaesthesia may precipitate profound hypotension or difficulty with ventilation. Under these circumstances it is wise to have a suitable pressor agent ready to hand. It may be necessary for the surgeon to perform an immediate laparotomy to relieve the pressure.
- Choice of drug depends on the patient's or anaesthetist's personal preference. A muscle relaxant–opioid–volatile agent technique is appropriate.
- An epidural (single-shot or continuous) may be added to provide intraoperative stability and postoperative analgesia, as well as a degree of induced hypotension to reduce blood loss.

MONITORING

In addition to standard monitoring the following are necessary:
- Core temperature
- Blood loss
- Urine output (catheterise the patient)
- Invasive haemodynamic monitoring – intra-arterial pressure and central venous pressure monitoring are desirable for a major procedure such as pelvic exenteration or in high-risk patients.

PATIENT POSITIONING

Prolonged operations in the lithotomy or Lloyd-Davies positions require particular attention to pressure points and traction on joints or nerves.

The anaesthetist must be alert to the possibility of massive and/or very rapid blood loss. A considerable proportion of this may be 'occult' in the sense that it remains hidden in the abdominal cavity. Appropriate arrangements should be made with the haematology department for assessment of clotting status and provision of blood, fresh frozen plasma, platelets, etc.

POSTOPERATIVE MANAGEMENT

Analgesia may be a major problem. Patient-controlled analgesia, continuous intravenous infusions and continuation of an epidural block with opioids and/or local anaesthetics all have a place.

Fluid balance is important following these extensive intra-abdominal operations; central venous pressure monitoring may need to be continued.

ITU or HDU admission, with or without elective ventilation, may be indicated.

Postoperative nausea and vomiting may be a major problem, as in any gynaecological operation.

OUTCOME

Prognosis is poor following most of these operations (Table 17.1). It must be remembered, however, that many of these operations are carried out for relief of symptoms (e.g. pressure symptoms of an ovarian mass) or in young women who often have young families (especially cancer of the cervix).

TABLE 17.1

Five-year survival after surgery for gynaecological cancer

Operation	5-year survival (%)
Radical vulvectomy	60–65
Cancer of the vagina (any treatment)	30–35
Wertheim's hysterectomy	55–60
Cancer of the ovary (any treatment)	30–35
Pelvic exenteration	25–35

17

CROSS-REFERENCES

Induced hypotension during anaesthesia
    Anaesthetic Factors 30: 704
Thrombosis and embolism
    Anaesthetic Factors 31: 789
Complications of position
    Anaesthetic Factors 31: 736
Postoperative pain management
    Anaesthetic Factors 31: 778

Fertility surgery

B. J. Pollard

17

PROCEDURE

The most common procedure for fertility surgery is probably that for egg retrieval. Very occasionally a general anaesthetic may be required for embryo replacement, but this is rare.

More extensive procedures may be necessary in the early diagnosis of infertility; these might include hysteroscopy, laparoscopy or laparotomy. These may be of a minor diagnostic nature to check for tubal patency or more extensive with tubal reconstruction or for adhesiolysis.

The procedures may form part of an *in vitro* fertilisation (IVF) programme, such as egg retrieval (transvaginally or laparoscopically) and gamete intrafallopian transfer (GIFT).

An operating microscope may be used during tubal surgery and the procedure may be lengthy.

Patients are generally young, highly motivated and knowledgeable about their treatment, and as such often request further information and an explanation of the anaesthetic procedure. Except for procedures that require a laparotomy, the patient is likely to be managed on a day-case basis.

For egg retrieval and embryo replacement, ovarian or endometrial stimulation may have been undertaken by carefully controlled hormonal therapy. The procedure may have to be performed within a specific time window.

PATIENT CHARACTERISTICS

- Patients are generally young, physically fit women, with American Society of Anesthesiologists (ASA) grade 1 or 2.
- Infertility may sometimes be associated with specific psychological problems ranging from anxiety or stress disorders to compulsive obsessive neuroses. Such women need a sympathetic and understanding approach.
- Occasionally there may be an associated endocrine disorder.
- Very occasionally a patient may appear as an urgent case following a failed attempt under local analgesia and sedation. It is essential to determine exactly what drugs have already been administered, to avoid potentially harmful interactions.

PREOPERATIVE ASSESSMENT

- There may be a history of a recent large (1 litre) oral fluid intake to fill the bladder to facilitate a preoperative pelvic ultrasound scan.
- The patient may have had many previous anaesthetics.
- The risk of postoperative nausea and vomiting is high in this patient population.

PREMEDICATION

- Usually unnecessary
- If very anxious, a short-acting benzodiazepine is suitable.

THEATRE PREPARATION

- Routine equipment and machine check.
- Lithotomy position is likely to be required, so check leg supports, personnel for lifting the two legs simultaneously, etc.
- Bulky video and ultrasound equipment may be used by the gynaecologist.
- If the laser is to be used, arrange appropriate eye protection.

ANAESTHETIC TECHNIQUE

- For diagnostic hysteroscopy, laparoscopy, etc., any appropriate technique is suitable.
- For egg retrieval, the evidence that any anaesthetic drug or technique is associated

with higher conception rates is inconclusive. Halothane should be avoided, but all other inhalational agents are equally acceptable. It has been suggested that some NSAIDs may impair embryo development and the gynaecologist may request that these be avoided. A good general rule is to keep the technique as simple as possible and to use as few drugs as possible.

- As the patient is likely to be a day case, avoid suxamethonium and use short-acting agents.
- TIVA is favoured by many.
- Nitrous oxide may increase nausea and vomiting but there is no evidence that it is detrimental to embryo development as a component of the anaesthetic. Tracheal intubation is usually necessary only for laparotomies, laparoscopies or in patients who are at risk from regurgitation. A laryngeal mask is usually suitable for airway management.
- A spinal or epidural may be used. Motivated patients may like to take an active interest in the proceedings. Careful explanation and counselling is necessary if using a central block in a day-case patient.

INTRAOPERATIVE MONITORING

Routine monitoring should be instituted to include:
- ECG and heart rate
- Non-invasive blood pressure
- Pulse oximetry
- Inspired oxygen and inhalational agent
- Expired $EtCO_2$.

COMPLICATIONS

Unexpected collapse may be due to:
- Sudden extreme bradycardia secondary to peritoneal distension or traction on pelvic structures

- Blood loss from an unrecognised laceration to a major pelvic blood vessel – such blood loss may be retroperitoneal and thus unseen
- Venous gas embolism
- Tension pneumothorax.

POSTOPERATIVE MANAGEMENT

PAIN RELIEF
Ideally oral using paracetamol with or without codeine. A NSAID may be administered if the gynaecologist has no objection. Opioids may be required in a small number of patients.

ANTIEMETIC
Any available antiemetic drug is suitable, and is recommended if the patient is a day case.

BIBLIOGRAPHY

Bokhari A, Pollard BJ. Anaesthesia for assisted conception. European Journal of Anaesthesiology 1998; 15:391–396

Bokhari A, Pollard BJ. Anaesthesia for assisted conception: a survey of UK practice. European Journal of Anaesthesiology 1999; 16:225–230

Critchlow BM, Ibrahim Z, Pollard BJ. General anaesthesia for gamete intrafallopian transfer. European Journal of Anaesthesiology 1991, 8:381–384

17

CROSS-REFERENCES

Day-case surgery
    Anaesthetic Factors 27: 613
Complications of position
    Anaesthetic Factors 31: 736
Laparoscopy
    Surgical Procedures 17: 446
Hysteroscopy and laser surgery
    Surgical Procedures 17: 444

18

OBSTETRIC ANAESTHESIA
M. Dresner

Overview

M. Dresner

Few aspects of obstetric anaesthesia are amenable to the principles of evidence-based practice, and the measurement of quality in analgesia and anaesthesia inevitably involves subjectivity. Solutions to clinical problems depend on interpretation of the literature, local experience and cultural factors amongst staff and patients. The following sections on obstetric anaesthesia provide one author's interpretations; these are not presented as a definitive guide, but hopefully will stimulate some thought and discussion.

The basic principles of obstetric anaesthesia have not changed in the past two decades, although workloads have. Epidural and caesarean section rates continue to rise, as does the complexity of the case mix. The bulk of the patient population is young and healthy, but there are important changes in physiology that can affect anaesthetic management; their clini-

cal relevance is magnified in the presence of pathological conditions. These are summarised in Table 18.1.

Although the complications of pregnancy have also not changed in this time, their contributions to maternal mortality and their clinical management have. Multidisciplinary team working between obstetricians, anaesthetists, midwives and physicians is now the established norm, and anaesthetists have an important role to play in antenatal risk assessment, intrapartum analgesia and anaesthesia, and postpartum high-dependency or intensive care. Knowledge of the important complications of pregnancy and causes of maternal death is obviously essential, and these are discussed later.

Finally, to our knowledge of the physiology and complications of pregnancy must be added increased understanding of coexisting medical conditions. More women with serious medical-

18

TABLE 18.1

Important physiological changes in pregnancy

Physiological change	Clinical relevance	Management change
Increased blood volume	Increased cardiac workload	Careful fluid management in cardiac disease
Physiological anaemia	Increased risk of severe anaemia after haemorrhage	Close monitoring of blood loss and haematocrit
Hypercoagulable state	Increased risk of thromboembolism	Use of appropriate thromboprophylaxis
Aortocaval compression	Risk of hypotension when supine, especially after regional blockade	Use of wedge or tilt in supine women
Reduced functional residual capacity	Rapid onset of hypoxia after induction of anaesthesia	Preoxygenation and rapid intubation always required
Increased tendency for oesophageal reflux	Increased risk of pulmonary aspiration	Use of fasting, antacid regimens and cricoid pressure from 16 weeks
Multifactorial changes in visualisation of larynx	10-fold increase in risk of failed intubation	Knowledge and use of failed intubation drill
Presence of fetus and transplacental transfer of drugs	Sedating anaesthetic and analgesic agents may depress neonatal respiration	Minimise use of opioids etc. and have neonatal resuscitation facilities
Increased BMI and volume of distribution	Increased risk of awareness under general anaesthesia	Don't let worries of neonatal depression make you give inadequate anaesthesia!

TABLE 18.2	
Role of the obstetric anaesthetist	
Role	Setting
To provide antenatal risk assessment, counselling and education of women and their partners. To liaise with other professionals to institute an appropriate care plan	Antenatal anaesthetic clinic
Assemble team for management of extremely high-risk patient (e.g. cardiac disease)	Tertiary referral unit. Specialist operating theatre, anaesthetist and ICU may be required
Provide intrapartum analgesia	Properly equipped and staffed delivery suite
Provide peripartum elective and emergency anaesthesia	Properly equipped and staffed delivery suite theatre
Provide routine monitoring after anaesthesia	Properly equipped and staffed delivery suite recovery
Provide higher-level monitoring and care for complications of pregnancy or serious co-morbidity	Delivery suite HDU or general ICU with input from obstetric anaesthetists
Teaching, audit, research	Obstetric anaesthetists need office facilities

conditions are surviving to reproductive age, are better managed medically to allow them to achieve fertility, and have the expectation that childbirth is safely within their grasp. Obstetric anaesthetists should provide anaesthetic and analgesic advice in the antenatal period, assist in the peripartum medical management of these patients, and provide high-dependency, intensive care and resuscitation services. Routine analgesic and anaesthetic management may need to be modified.

In summary, while the basic principles of clinical practice have changed little, the volume and complexity of the work of obstetric anaesthetists have increased in recent times. Our role is described in Table 18.2.

natural movement and posture during labour raised hope of increasing the numbers of normal deliveries, and great interest in the topic was generated in the anaesthetic literature and lay press. There is now convincing evidence that low-dose epidurals are indeed associated with fewer operative deliveries, as well as increased satisfaction scores and reduced incidence of hypotension. However, mobility itself seems to have had disappointingly little influence and, indeed, few women in advanced labour want to walk anywhere with or without an epidural. So, while low-dose epidural cocktails have been a significant advance, mobility in the form of walking has failed to have a significant impact on obstetric outcomes.

DEVELOPMENTS AND CONTROVERSIES

MOBILE EPIDURALS

The theory was that the immobility produced by epidurals using solutions such as 0.25% bupivacaine adversely affected the progress of labour by forcing the parturient to remain in bed and by paralysing her pelvic floor muscles. Conventional epidurals were thereby held responsible for causing unnecessary forceps and caesarean deliveries. In the early 1990s it began to be realised that analgesia could still be achieved with much weaker doses of local anaesthetic such as 0.1% bupivacaine, especially if an opioid such as fentanyl was added. Between top-ups and avoiding continuous infusions, periods of ambulation became possible for women with epidurals. The promise of more

COMBINED SPINAL–EPIDURAL ANALGESIA

Confusingly, combined spinal–epidural (CSE) analgesia became well known through its association with mobile epidurals. This led to the bogus belief the intrathecal route was a vital ingredient in achieving minimal motor block. Motor blockade is affected by the strength and total doses of intraspinal local anaesthetics, not by their route of administration. The advantage of the intrathecal route is the same for analgesia as it is for anaesthesia: it provides a more reliable, rapid block, with reduced likelihood of missed segments. The author's own research and understanding of the literature leads to the conclusion that the routine use of CSE analgesia is unjustified, especially given the reports of

18

meningitis following its use. CSE does have clear advantages when rapid, reliable analgesia is required, such as in severe maternal distress, rapidly progressing labour, pushing against a partially dilated cervix, or resiting a failing epidural. Given that speed of onset is the main consideration, the most rapid needle technique of performing a spinal first, followed by the epidural component when analgesia has begun, seems more logical than a needle-through-needle alternative.

COMBINED SPINAL–EPIDURAL ANAESTHESIA

The development of small-gauge, pencil-point spinal needles allowed spinal anaesthesia to return to obstetrics after unacceptable headache rates precluded its use up until the mid 1980s. Spinal anaesthesia rapidly became the first choice of anaesthesia for caesarean section in the UK because of its rapidity and reliability, especially since the addition of lipid-soluble opioids to drug regimens. However, there are several units that almost exclusively used CSE anaesthesia. Why? The epidural component can be used as a safety net for the occasional spinal that proves to be inadequate. The number of patients that needs to be treated to gain this advantage exceeds 100 in the author's unit. It seems more acceptable to site a rescue epidural now and again than to expose many women to the unnecessary risk of a dural tap. However, CSE has the obvious advantage of allowing the duration of anaesthesia to be extended when prolonged surgery is anticipated. CSE also allows a reduced spinal dose to be given, followed by incremental epidural extension. This reduces the incidence and severity of hypotension in all women, and is particularly useful in women with cardiac disease. It also takes the dangerous guesswork out of single-shot spinal anaesthesia in women at extremes of stature. In the author's unit, these indications have led to a 3% CSE rate, and the universal use of CSEs seems inexplicable when single-shot spinals remain so efficient. If a CSE technique is chosen, a combined needle-through-needle technique reduces the discomfort produced by the 'separate space, separate needle' approach, but both techniques have their advantages.

INTRATHECAL CATHETERS

In theory, an intrathecal catheter combines the reliability of intrathecal anaesthesia with the ability to extend and prolong the block incrementally. However, size matters, in that the needle and catheter combination must be small enough to maintain an acceptable spinal headache rate. This was achievable with 32-gauge catheters passed through a 24-gauge Sprotte needle, despite the technique being fiddly. After reports of cauda equina syndrome occurring in the USA, the Food and Drug Administration (FDA) banned the use of 32-gauge catheters. Although UK interpretation of these cases laid the blame not with the catheters but with excessive use of hyperbaric lidocaine (lignocaine) solutions, the shrinkage of the commercial market for 32-gauge catheters led to the end of their production. When a reliable fine-gauge catheter system becomes available, interest in this technique may return and provide an alternative to CSE anaesthesia.

ANTICOAGULANTS AND REGIONAL ANAESTHETIC TECHNIQUES

Conditions such as recurrent venous thromboembolism and recurrent fetal loss due to systemic lupus erythematosus or factor V Leiden abnormalities have led to growing numbers of parturients receiving anticoagulants during pregnancy. Anaesthetists want to know when it is safe to site and remove spinals and epidurals. There

TABLE 18.3

Guidelines for the use of regional anaesthesia with anticoagulants

Anticoagulant	Advice
Aspirin	Of concern only when combined with other anticoagulants
Heparin	Check APTT – regional anaesthesia can proceed once ratio < 1.5
Enoxaparin (Clexane) or dalteparin (Fragmin)	Wait 8–10 h after prophylactic dose, 24 h after therapeutic dose. Delay next dose for 2 h after regional anaesthesia or removal of catheter
Tinzaparin (Innohep)	Wait 24 h after any dose before performing regional blockade. This drug is potent and long acting

APTT, activated partial thromboplastin time.

is no truly evidence-based answer to this, but some suggestions are made in Table 18.3.

MANAGEMENT OF PRE-ECLAMPSIA AND ECLAMPSIA

Deaths from severe pre-eclampsia, eclampsia and HELLP (haemolysis, elevated liver enzymes and low platelets) syndrome have always involved a high incidence of substandard care as judged by the Confidential Enquiries into Maternal Deaths. This has led to great interest in formal management policies, robust clinical audit and an evidence-based approach to this condition. Areas of controversy over the past decade have included the use of magnesium in the treatment and prevention of convulsions, and fluid management. Some clarity has now emerged. Magnesium sulfate is the proven drug of choice for the prevention of reconvulsion in women who have had an eclamptic fit. It also reduces the risk of a first fit if given prophylactically to all pre-eclamptic women, but many units have shied away from taking this approach. A third of women who fit do so before the diagnosis of pre-eclampsia has been made, so would escape prophylaxis. In the remainder, the number that would need to be treated to prevent one eclamptic fit is large, and the incidence of side-effects high. Many obstetricians therefore use prophylactic magnesium only in women with extremes of hypertension, or with cerebral symptoms.

As regards fluid management, there was a vogue for invasive central venous pressure (CVP) monitoring and restoration of circulating volumes with colloid solutions. It is now recognised that pulmonary oedema or adult respiratory distress syndrome (ARDS) is a real threat in pre-eclampsia, and is often provoked by excessive fluid therapy. It is a fact that oliguria down to 80 ml per 4 h is well tolerated in pre-eclampsia, and renal failure is extremely unusual in the absence of haemorrhage or pre-exiting renal disease. Consequently, modest fluid regimens are now favoured in many units. This is an unfamiliar and counterintuitive approach to some general intensivists, so it is important that the obstetric team assists in the management of pre-eclamptic patients who are nursed in the intensive care unit.

BACKACHE

In the early 1990s it became generally accepted that epidurals increased the incidence of post-natal backache. Several careful prospective studies have now disproved this. Excepting needle trauma, epidurals do not influence the incidence of new, significant, postnatal backache, which occurs in about 7% of women. The only clear risk factor is an antenatal history of back pain.

INADVERTENT DURAL PUNCTURE AND TREATMENT OF POSTDURAL PUNCTURE HEADACHE

It has become accepted practice to manage inadvertent dural puncture with a Tuohy needle by threading the catheter and giving drugs intrathecally. Solutions such as 0.1% bupivacaine with fentanyl 2 μg ml^{-1} used for the epidural space work just as well intrathecally in boluses of 2–5 ml. Tachyphylaxis is common. This approach maintains good analgesia, reduces CSF leak during pushing, may reduce the incidence of subsequent headaches, and avoids the stress of a second epidural attempt.

In treating an established headache, the mean duration of symptoms is 8 days without treatment, but some persist for months. This is unacceptable for the new mother. The aim should be to get her home on the day she originally planned. Results with prophylactic blood patches are disappointing, and epidural infusions, caffeine, etc. all seem to delay the onset of headaches rather than prevent or cure them. Blood patch remains the only definitive cure; complications are rare apart from temporary backache, but repeat patching is needed in one-third of patients.

INFORMED CONSENT

New Department of Health guidelines on consent have provoked some anaesthetic departments to seek written consent for anaesthesia as well as surgical procedures in the UK. This has refocused the attention of obstetric anaesthetists on the difficulties of providing information to women in labour, let alone obtaining meaningful written consent for epidural analgesia and anaesthesia for emergency caesarean section. Effort must be made to provide information to women in the antenatal period using all media available, including leaflets, videos, websites and antenatal classes. This information should be provided in all required languages. Despite such efforts, obstetric anaesthetists will still encounter

18

women who have bypassed all these information sources and will remain vulnerable to complaint if complications subsequently occur. Withholding treatment in these circumstances is surely not the solution, but careful documentation of the reasons for performing procedures without formal consent is essential.

BIBLIOGRAPHY

Collis RE, Harding SA, Morgan BM. Effect of maternal ambulation on labour with low-dose combined spinal–epidural analgesia. Anaesthesia 1999; 54:535–539

Department of Health. Why mothers die. Report on confidential enquiries into maternal deaths in the United Kingdom 1994–96. London: Stationery Office, 1999. Online. Available: http://www.cemd.org.uk

Dresner M, Bamber J, Calow C, Freeman J, Charlton P. Comparison of low-dose epidural with combined spinal–epidural analgesia for labour. British Journal of Anaesthesia 1999; 83:756–760

Eclampsia Trial Collaborative Group. Which anticonvulsant for women with eclampsia? Evidence from the collaborative eclampsia trial. Lancet 1995; 345:1455–1463

Hart EM, Ahmed N, Buggy DJ. Impact study of the introduction of low-dose epidural (bupivacaine 0.1%/fentanyl 2 μg ml^{-1}) compared with bupivacaine 0.25% for labour analgesia. International Journal of Obstetric Anesthesia 2003; 12:4–6

Howell CJ, Dean T, Lucking L, Dziedzic K, Jones PW, Johanson RB. Randomised study of long term outcome after epidural versus non-epidural analgesia during labour. British Medical Journal 2002; 325:357

MAGPIE Trial Collaborative Group. Do women with preeclampsia, and their babies, benefit from magnesium sulphate? The MAGPIE trial: a randomised placebo controlled trial. Lancet 2002; 359:1877–1889

Nelson-Piercy C. Handbook of obstetric medicine. Oxford: Isis Medical Media; 1997

Walker JJ. Pre-eclampsia. Lancet 2000; 356:1260–1265

18

Medical problems and obstetric anaesthesia

M. Dresner

This topic will be approached from the view seen from the antenatal anaesthetic clinic, which gives a real perspective on the type and frequency of problems referred to the obstetric anaesthetist. The reader will notice the absence of common medical conditions such as asthma and diabetes from the following sections, as these do not significantly alter anaesthetic management. Patients are referred for advice on anaesthetic and analgesic management, not optimisation of the conditions themselves.

BACK PROBLEMS

This is the commonest cause of women (or their obstetrician and midwife) seeking antenatal advice from the anaesthetist, usually wanting to know whether regional techniques are contraindicated. This probably stems from the now disproven belief that epidurals cause backache *per se* and therefore patients with pre-existing back pain may be more vulnerable. Patients with the following diagnoses can be reassured that surveys have revealed no increased risk of exacerbations of back problems. They can be offered normal management, but warned to take care of their posture during regional analgesia and anaesthesia:
- Chronic lumbar back pain
- Sciatica
- Prolapsed intervertebral disc
- Spondylolisthesis.

Where there is an anatomical abnormality or previous spinal surgery, the epidural space might be distorted by scarring and tethering, increasing the risks of dural puncture and poor analgesia. Spinal techniques bypass these problems, except in the few women whose spine is so distorted that the fear of neurological trauma outweighs the benefits. CSE analgesia provides the advantage of providing good initial analgesia, even if the epidural component subsequently proves unreliable. If examination reveals favourable landmarks, patients with the following conditions can be offered normal management, avoiding pure epidural techniques:
- Previous laminectomy or microdiscectomy (choose scar-free interspace)
- Spina bifida occulta (chooses interspace between two palpable spines)
- Kyphoscoliosis.

There are few absolute contraindications to regional techniques, but some conditions introduce risks of implant infection or neurological damage that outweigh the benefits of regional anaesthetic techniques. These include:
- Implanted spinal rods after scoliosis surgery
- Spina bifida with extensive lumbar scarring.

CARDIAC PROBLEMS

Adult congenital cardiac abnormalities are by far the commonest cardiac problems referred antenatally. Rarer conditions include rheumatic heart disease and cardiomyopathies, and the occasional sufferer of ischaemic heart disease. Many patients have had surgery in infancy, some of which is anatomically difficult to understand. Thankfully, detailed pathophysiological and anatomical understanding is not vital for safe anaesthetic management. Before considering management of specific conditions, some *general principles* apply:
- Some conditions are associated with death in pregnancy, but death in labour or at caesarean section is rare. Reassurance can be offered.
- Maternal or fetal deterioration may necessitate rapid surgical delivery during pregnancy. An emergency plan must be in place for 24-h implementation.
- Assume everyone is at risk of bacterial endocarditis and paradoxical air embolism, and take the appropriate precautions. With this in mind, do you really need that CVP line or PA catheter?
- A unit without dedicated 24-h anaesthetic cover is no place for these patients.

18

- If the condition could conceivably deteriorate in the peripartum period, the patient must be managed in a unit with 24-h cardiology or cardiac anaesthetic cover.
- If medical deterioration is a possibility during anaesthesia for caesarean section, an obstetric anaesthetist should team up with a cardiac anaesthetist.
- If medical deterioration during caesarean section could conceivably be managed by cardiac surgical intervention, the section should be performed in cardiac theatres with cardiopulmonary bypass immediately available and surgical teams on standby.
- Avoid aortocaval compression!

Some *conditions are associated with relatively fixed cardiac output*, because of either left ventricular outflow obstruction or myocardial insufficiency. There is little compensatory reserve for a sudden loss of peripheral resistance, and coronary blood flow can be critically compromised by sudden onset regional anaesthesia. There has to be a very good reason for not choosing cardiac-style general anaesthesia for caesarean section in these patients. Opioid-only epidurals or very low-dose local anaesthetics can be considered in labour, but if pain-induced tachycardia is considered a genuine hazard the cardiologist will probably recommend a caesarean section. Examples include:

- Any severely stenotic valve, especially aortic stenosis
- Hypertrophic obstructive cardiomyopathy
- Any other type of cardiomyopathy.

The next group of conditions has usually had *complete or partial surgical correction*, often associated with residual valvular dysfunction and shunts. Surgery is sometimes responsible for dysrhythmias or heart block, so pacemakers and implantable defibrillators are sometimes *in situ*. These devices are now too complicated for simplistic use of magnets, so the anaesthetist must liaise with the cardiology team for advice on the use of diathermy and reprogramming. In the absence of a severely stenosed valve or cyanosis, and if hypovolaemia is avoided, low-dose epidural analgesia is safe without invasive monitoring. Regional anaesthesia is an appropriate choice, but an incremental technique such as CSE or spinal catheter should be used. These conditions include:

- Septal defects with left-to-right shunts
- Tetralogy of Fallot
- Transposition of the great vessels

- Marfan's syndrome
- Coarctation of the aorta.

Cyanotic heart disease, particularly Eisenmenger's syndrome, is associated with great risk to the mother. Pain or clumsy general anaesthesia can cause increased pulmonary vasospasm, thereby increasing right-to-left shunt and hypoxia. Equally, clumsy regional techniques can rapidly reduce peripheral resistance and produce the same result. No technique is known to be superior, but a gentle, incremental technique can make either general or regional anaesthesia acceptable. Paradoxical embolus is a particular hazard. Chronic hypoxia leads to polycythaemia and an increased risk of venous embolism, so anticoagulants are usually prescribed. This has to be borne in mind if regional techniques are planned.

NEUROLOGICAL DISEASE

There is a school of thought that recommends the avoidance of regional techniques in patients with neurological disease for fear that an exacerbation will be blamed on the anaesthetist. This is no way to practise medicine. There is neither an obvious mechanism, nor convincing literature to suggest that epidurals and spinals will have any influence on multiple sclerosis, peripheral neuropathies, ME, etc. Patients with cerebral vascular abnormalities or space-occupying lesions associated with raised intracranial pressure will not be allowed to labour. If their neurosurgeon believes that a CSF leak from a spinal or dural tap could cause problems, the caesarean section should be performed under a neuro-style general anaesthesia. Conditions involving denervation, such as paraplegia, are associated with dangerous hyperkalaemia after succinylcholine use. Rocuronium is a suitable alternative for rapid sequence induction in the hands of an experienced intubator.

MISCELLANEOUS CONDITIONS

IDIOPATHIC THROMBOCYTOPAENIA:
- Numbers of platelets are reduced, but they are young and of good function.
- A count above 50×10^9/litre is acceptable for regional blockade.
- Antibodies can cause fetal thrombocytopaenia.

BIBLIOGRAPHY

Cole P, Cross M, Dresner M. Incremental spinal anaesthesia for elective caesarean section in a patient with Eisenmenger's syndrome. British Journal of Anaesthesia 2001; 86:723–726

Dresner M, Freeman J, Cole P. Obstetric anaesthesia for patients with chronic back problems. British Journal of Anaesthesia 1997; 78:A349 (abstract)

Howell CJ, Dean T, Lucking L, Dziedzic K, Jones PW, Johanson RB. Randomised study of long term outcome after epidural versus non-epidural analgesia during labour. British Medical Journal 2002; 325:357

Lewis NL, Dob DP, Yentis SM. UK registry of high-risk obstetric anaesthesia: arrhythmias, cardiomyopathy, aortic stenosis, transposition of the great arteries and Marfan's syndrome. International Journal of Obstetric Anesthesia 2003; 12:28–34

Nelson-Piercy C. Handbook of obstetric medicine. Oxford: Isis Medical Media; 1997

Smith PS, Wilson RC, Robinson APC, Lyons GR. Regional blockade for delivery in women with scoliosis or previous spinal surgery. International Journal of Obstetric Anesthesia 2003; 12:17–22

Yentis S, Dob D. Anaesthesia for the obstetric patient with cardiac disease. CPD Anaesthesia 2000; 2(3):130–133

CROSS-REFERENCES

Adult congenital heart disease
    Patient Conditions 4: 112
Cardiomyopathy
    Patient Conditions 4: 124

18

Pain relief in labour

M. Dresner

Psychoprophylaxis, Entonox, pethidine and transcutaneous electrical nerve stimulation (TENS) are provided by midwives, not anaesthetists, and so are not covered in this section.

Anaesthetists provide various types of epidural analgesia and, occasionally, patient-controlled analgesia (PCA) with intravenous opioids. In explaining epidural and CSE analgesia to non-anaesthetists, it is important to clarify the fact that the title of the technique merely describes the route of drug administration. Although this has some bearing on pharmacokinetics, pharmacodynamic effects depend mostly on the drug regimen used. Generic advice given to patients about epidurals and CSEs from textbooks is therefore of limited value, because a wide variety of drug regimens is in use.

EPIDURAL ANALGESIA

On receiving a request for an epidural, *increased risks* must be identified, considered and discussed with the patient. These include:

- Coagulopathy – international normalised ratio (INR) > 1.5, platelets < 80×10^9/litre
- Bacteraemia – this does not include a simple temperature
- Local sepsis near injection site.

The patient and partner then need the procedure explained, including potential side-effects. These include:

- Some loss of mobility of the legs
- Loss of sensation to void the bladder
- Itching if opioids are used
- Transient dizziness and nausea due to hypotension.

Complications should also be discussed. How far to go with these discussions is controversial, but the anaesthetist should attempt to gauge how much information a patient wants. Withholding information about rare complications from all and alarming every patient with dire warnings are equally inappropriate. Judgement is required, and careful documenta-

tion essential. The following list is appropriate, with incidences quoted from the author's units:

- Poor analgesia (4%)
- Inadvertent dural puncture requiring blood patch (0.6%)
- Possible prolongation of labour and increased risk of operative delivery
- Neurological damage – rarer than obstetric causes.

Preparation before performing the epidural must include documentation of maternal and fetal monitoring by the midwife. Vascular access is mandatory, but fluid preloads are unnecessary with epidural cocktails using 0.1% bupivacaine or less, unless the woman has been bleeding, vomiting, or is dehydrated for any reason. Patient positioning is of fundamental practical importance. Despite some suggesting that the sitting position is uncomfortable for women, this is not the author's experience. Sitting has the advantage of easier identification of the midline in obese patients. Aseptic technique should include the use of a surgical mask, as well as the usual precautions. Equipment and drugs should be assembled with care to avoid any chance of contamination with neurotoxic cleaning agents or drug error. Recommended technique involves:

- 16- or 18-gauge Tuohy needles
- Continuous pressure, loss of resistance to saline
- Warn of paraesthesia at catheter insertion
- Leave around 4 cm of catheter in the epidural space – more increases missed segments
- Use aspiration and syphon tests to exclude intravascular and intrathecal placement.

Once the catheter has been secured, the question that has to be asked mentally is: '*Where could this catheter be?*'. There are five possibilities:

- Epidural space
- 'Gristle'
- Subdural or extra-arachnoid
- Intrathecal
- Intravascular.

18

The last three dangerous positions are still possible despite negative aspiration and syphon tests, which can produce false-negative findings. Do not be fooled into thinking an epidural test dose such as 3 ml 0.5% bupivacaine excludes these catheter positions. This dose is insufficient to produce the classical symptoms of intravenous placement (popping and ringing in the ears, and circumoral tingling), and of insufficient volume to rupture the arachnoid to reveal a subdural catheter. It will identify an intrathecal catheter, but only by producing an unnecessarily high and dense block. A reduced dose of local anaesthetic, in a high volume, with adrenaline (epinephrine) to identify intravascular injection seems ideal, but pain-induced tachycardias produce false-positive results. Thus, no single test-dose injection is ideal, and every epidural dose should be treated as a test. Remember that if no analgesia follows the initial therapeutic dose, this may be due to intravascular placement as well as placement in 'gristle'. Intrathecal or subdural catheterisation is excluded, but a definitive intravascular test dose such as 1 mg kg^{-1} lidocaine (lignocaine) should be used before giving further therapeutic doses. If in doubt, an epidural resite should be performed.

There are many drug regimens used to establish initial analgesia. We recommend 20 ml 0.1% bupivacaine with 2 μg ml^{-1} fentanyl, which can also be used for continuous infusion at 10 ml h^{-1}, and top-ups of 10–20 ml. This solution has the advantage of being available commercially in bags and syringes of various volumes, thereby avoiding contamination and admixture errors. Too many alternatives exist to be discussed individually.

COMBINED SPINAL–EPIDURAL ANALGESIA

As discussed above, there seems little justification for the routine use of CSE for labour pains given the rare but well reported risk of meningitis. However, the following are suggested indications for a technique comprising an initial single-shot spinal, followed by conventional epidural catheterisation:

- The distressed and uncooperative patient
- Pushing against an incompletely dilated cervix
- Severe rectal or perineal pain
- As a resite for a failing epidural.

Needle-through-needle techniques have the disadvantage of being slower to perform, and occasionally dural puncture with the spinal needle will not be achieved if the epidural needle enters the epidural space laterally. However, it does spare the patient a second injection and is a useful option when rapidity of onset is not the main indication for using a CSE. An example of this is would be establishing epidural analgesia when epidural scarring is likely, such as in women with a history of spinal surgery.

The intrathecal dose chosen most commonly in the UK is 2.5 mg plain bupivacaine mixed with 25 μg fentanyl. This usually produces effective analgesia within one or two contractions. Using 3 ml of a premixed solution of 0.1% bupivacaine with 2 μg ml^{-1} fentanyl is less effective, especially in advanced labour, but once again this avoids admixture errors. Both cocktails provide analgesia for about 90 min, with motor block receding after about 45 min.

Subsequent analgesia can be provided in the usual way. There is undeniable logic in allowing the spinal component to wear off before using the epidural component, and then beginning this phase with an epidural test dose. However, an epidural infusion can be started immediately to produce a seamless transition between spinal and epidural analgesia. Taking this choice, the anaesthetist must remember that an intravascular catheter might present as analgesic failure after 90 min. An intrathecal catheter will become apparent slowly over 2 h, with increasingly dense motor blockade.

EPIDURAL TROUBLESHOOTING

BLOODY TAP
An obviously intravenous catheter should be withdrawn to its desired length and the aspiration test repeated. Obviously, if still aspirating blood, the catheter should be resited. If aspiration proves negative, the tip of a blind-ended multiorifice catheter may still be intravascular. Catheter migration can lead to subsequent epidural top-ups, ending up in the blood. This will present as analgesic failure if a low-dose regimen is used, rather than the classical signs of intravascular toxicity. It is therefore essential to consider the possibility of intravascular catheter migration in a patient who had a bloody tap managed by catheter withdrawal, who subsequently needs a high-dose epidural top-up for any reason.

INADVERTENT DURAL PUNCTURE
This topic was covered in the Overview section.

18

THE FAILING EPIDURAL

The incidence of the failing epidural can be minimised by adopting a good catheter siting and fixation technique, and the use of an adequate drug regimen for the circumstances. This also speeds up the remedy, given that every manoeuvre to improve analgesia takes 30 min to assess. For example, the 30 min required to treat unilateral analgesia by withdrawing the catheter and giving a top-up can be eliminated by not passing so much catheter in the first place! To simplify the topic, there are three typical patterns of breakthrough pain with epidural analgesia, each with likely causes and a suggested remedy. These are summarised in Table 18.4.

By the time a rescue top-up has failed, the patient will probably have been in pain for more than 1 h. In order to regain her confidence, a CSE will establish analgesia quickly – and perhaps more reliably – by bypassing epidural problems such as fibrous septa.

TABLE 18.4

The failing epidural

Pattern of pain	Possible causes	Remedy
Fundal or global pain	Inadequate top-up or infusion rate. Catheter dislodged	Inspect catheter. If OK, large-volume rescue dose. Increase subsequent top-ups or infusion rate
Unilateral pain or missed segment	Poor catheter position. Epidural fibrous septa	Withdraw catheter if more than 4 cm in space. Top-up with bad side down
Perineal pain or rectal pressure	Occipitoposterior position of fetus. Big baby. Oxytocin usage	Warn that all remedies may fail. Sit patient up. Use strong cocktail with opioid, and warn of side-effects

EXAMPLE RECIPES FOR EPIDURAL ANALGESIA TECHNIQUES

The examples shown in Table 18.5 are used by the author, producing excellent patient satisfaction scores, acceptable side-effects and minimal complications. 'Bup–fent mix' refers to 0.1% bupivacaine plus 2 μg ml^{-1} fentanyl.

PATIENT-CONTROLLED ANALGESIA

This technique is not routinely used in obstetrics, because opioid drugs are not well suited to treating severe episodic pain. Even if they were, the onset of action of most agents would be too slow and the duration too long to match the pattern of contraction pain. Alfentanil is worth trying with boluses of 250 μg, but accumulation can result in sedation, dizziness and nausea between contractions. Remifentanil has the most promising pharmacokinetic profile, with no concerns about accumulation. However, wide interpatient variations in response mean that a dose-finding study is required for each patient, starting with doses of 0.2 μg kg^{-1} and increasing in increments until an effective dose is found. Again, sedation is common, so this is not a technique for wide dissemination,

TABLE 18.5

Suggested epidural recipes

Technique	Loading dose	Maintenance	Top-up
Epidural	20 ml bup–fent mix	10 ml h^{-1} bup–fent mix	10–20 ml bup–fent mix
Higher mobility epidural	20 ml bup–fent mix	None	10–20 ml bup–fent mix
CSE	2.5 mg bupivacaine plus 25 μg fentanyl	10 ml h^{-1} bup–fent mix	10–20 ml bup–fent mix
Higher mobility CSE	2.5 mg bupivacaine plus 25 μg fentanyl	None	10–20 ml bup–fent mix
PCEA	20 ml bup–fent mix	None	10 ml bup–fent mix, 30 min lockout

CSE, combined spinal–epidural; PCEA, patient-controlled epidural anaesthesia.

although it is of value for distressed women with contraindications to epidural analgesia.

BIBLIOGRAPHY

Dresner M, Bamber J, Calow C, Freeman J, Charlton P. Comparison of low-dose epidural with combined spinal–epidural analgesia for labour. British Journal of Anaesthesia 1999; 83:756–760

Hart EM, Ahmed N, Buggy DJ. Impact study of the introduction of low-dose epidural (bubivacaine 0.1%/fentanyl 2 μg ml^{-1}) compared with bupivacaine 0.25% for labour analgesia. International Journal of Obstetric Anesthesia 2003; 12:4–6

Hawthorne L, Slaymaker A, Bamber J, Dresner M. Effect of fluid preload on maternal haemodynamics for low-dose epidural analgesia in labour. International Journal of Obstetric Anesthesia 2001; 10:312–315

Van der Vyver M, Halpern S, Joseph G. Patient-controlled epidural analgesia versus continuous infusion for labour analgesia: a meta-analysis. British Journal of Anaesthesia 2002; 89:459–465

Volmanen P, Akural EI, Raudaskoski T, Alahuhta S. Remifentanil in obstetric analgesia: a dose-finding study. Anesthesia and Analgesia 2002; 94:913–917

CROSS-REFERENCES

18

Anaesthesia for elective caesarean section

M. Dresner

There are five practical methods of providing anaesthesia for elective caesarean section, each with pros and cons. These are summarised in Table 18.6, and short notes are presented on each. The decision regarding which technique to use will depend on the preference and health of the patient, the experience of the anaesthetist, any anticipated surgical difficulties, and perhaps also the experience and speed of the surgeon.

GENERAL ANAESTHESIA

The speed and reliability of this technique are sometimes forgotten in the detailed considera-

TABLE 18.6

Anaesthetic techniques for caesarean section

Technique	Advantages	Disadvantages
General anaesthesia	Quick, reliable, of unlimited duration	Poor recovery and pain control. Failed intubation, aspiration, awareness
Epidural anaesthesia	Slow onset reduces hypotension. Unlimited duration	Slow onset. Relatively high failure and discomfort rate due to missed segments
Spinal anaesthesia	Quick, reliable, good perioperative analgesia	Of limited duration. Severe hypotension common
Combined spinal–epidural	Combines reliability of spinals with adjustability of epidurals	Slower than a spinal; risk of dural tap with Tuohy needle
Spinal catheter	As for CSE, but increments act quicker	Fiddly technique. Probably a higher headache rate than CSEs

TABLE 18.7

Problems of general anaesthesia

Problem	Prevention
1 in 250 chance of failed intubation	Preoxygenate meticulously – provides more time Optimise head position before induction Use your favourite laryngoscope If incomplete view of larynx, always use gum elastic bougie Use size 7 tubes or smaller
Aspiration of stomach contents	No solid food during labour Lansoprazole 30 mg before surgery, or equivalent 30 ml 0.3 M sodium citrate before induction Aspirate stomach before reversal if not fasted Recover in lateral position
Awareness	Give generous dose of induction agent Over-pressure volatile agent until high end-tidal concentration achieved Do not worry about neonatal effects – these are temporary and easy to treat
Sedation of the baby	Do not let this make you give an inadequate anaesthesia

tion of its disadvantages. Once sensible precautions are taken to avoid these problems, we are left with a safe and reliable form of anaesthesia. The problems and methods of minimising these are summarised in Table 18.7.

The negative history of maternal deaths due to the sequelae of failed intubation and aspiration cannot be ignored. The gratifying fall in the number of such deaths in the UK over the past three decades has been assumed by many to be due to the rising rate of regional anaesthetic usage, and as a result some almost demonise the use of general anaesthesia. However, although the UK general anaesthesia rate might now be low, the dramatic increase in caesarean deliveries over this period means that the total number of general anaesthetics is still significant. The fall in anaesthetic-related deaths must therefore mean that general anaesthesia has become safer. This point is raised to discourage prolonged attempts at achieving regional anaesthesia if the mother is becoming distressed, and will be raised again in the section on emergency caesarean section.

INTRODUCTION TO REGIONAL ANAESTHESIA

- *Consent issues* – always document warnings of sensations during surgery, the possibility of failure, and the potential need for conversion to general anaesthesia.
- *Block height assessment* – there are medicolegal experts who argue that block height assessment must be made with light touch. You are vulnerable if a complaint about intraoperative pain is associated with any other method of assessment. T4 is required without opioids; T6 is satisfactory if a lipid-soluble opioid is used.
- *Escape route* – if a block cannot be sited or fails, general anaesthesia is the usual escape route. Do not, therefore, persuade women to have regional anaesthesia because general anaesthetics are dangerous!

EPIDURAL ANAESTHESIA

Anyone experienced in using spinal anaesthesia, particularly incorporating lipid-soluble opioids, finds epidural anaesthesia slow and unreliable in comparison. Incremental regional anaesthesia can be achieved more reliably with a CSE technique. The author cannot suggest any indication for the use of epidural analgesia in elective caesarean section.

SPINAL ANAESTHESIA

Spinal anaesthesia is a quick and reliable form of anaesthesia that has become the most popular choice for elective caesarean section in the UK.

WHICH SPINAL NEEDLE?
Spinal headache is now rare, thanks to small gauge pencil-point needles. There is no jus-

tification for the use of cutting edge needles other than lack of availability, in which case the incidence of headache can be reduced by orienting the needle bevel in parallel with the dural fibres. Even with pencil-point needles, 24 gauge is the maximum size that should be used in obstetrics.

WHICH SPINAL INTERSPACE?
If possible, dural puncture should be performed at or below the L3–4 interspace to avoid the risk of conus damage. However, there is plenty of neural tissue in the cauda equina, so a gentle, careful technique is still important. Difficult anatomy does justify the careful use of higher interspaces, but the reason for such a decision should be documented.

WHICH PATIENT POSITION?
Zealous advocates of every conceivable position exist, each implying that other positions do not work as well. The truth is that every position can be used effectively, but adjustments in drug dosage may be necessary. The key is to standardise the position of spinal insertion, the speed of injection, and the timing of moving to the left tilted supine position. Each practitioner will then find, through experience and analysis, the range of drug dosages that work for him or her.

WHICH LOCAL ANAESTHETIC?
In the UK, hyperbaric 0.5% bupivacaine is the most popular local anaesthetic agent, but some advocate the isobaric alternative. Publications have produced contradicting results, which suggests neither is superior, but that familiarity and experience with one is the key.

WHAT DOSE?
Pregnant women get a higher block for a given dose than non-pregnant patients. The dose used depends on patient height, abdominal size, whether an opioid is used, patient position during spinal injection, and many other minor, unquantifiable influences. One overriding principle applies: an inadequate dose will lead to surgical pain, which provides the commonest reason for litigation against obstetric anaesthetists. Total spinal from a single-shot technique with hyperbaric bupivacaine is vanishingly rare, and the symptoms of a high spinal are eminently treatable. If in doubt, err on the side of generosity. A starting suggestion for a dose regimen is 2.6 ml 0.5% heavy bupivacaine plus 300 μg diamorphine, and move to the left lateral position as quickly as possible.

18

18

AN OPIOID – IF SO, WHICH?

The addition of a lipid-soluble opioid to the spinal cocktail reduces intraoperative discomfort and allows the dose of local anaesthetic to be reduced slightly. Fentanyl 15–25 μg performs this function well, but contributes little to postoperative analgesia because of its short duration of action. Morphine, being less lipophilic, gives no intraoperative benefit but gives around 12 h of postoperative analgesia. Some practitioners combine the two agents, but this is unnecessary if diamorphine is available because it is sufficiently lipophilic to provide excellent intraoperative comfort and its action is of sufficient duration to provide postoperative analgesia for 12–24 h. With 300 μg, a postoperative nausea and vomiting (PONV) rate of 30% can be expected, reduced to 15% if 50 mg cyclizine is given prophylactically. Severe pruritus occasionally occurs, is not responsive to antihistamines, but can be treated with 0.1 mg kg^{-1} subcutaneous nalbuphine without antagonising analgesia. The author is unaware of any reported cases of respiratory depression with the doses described and, apart from avoiding additional parenteral opioids, no extra postoperative monitoring is necessary.

PREVENTING AND TREATING HYPOTENSION

Symptomatic hypotension (dizziness, nausea, vomiting) is universal if no precautions are taken. Fluid preloads reduce the incidence and severity of hypotension, but are slow. Colloids may cause anaphylaxis; crystalloids do not. Ephedrine is equally effective, does not delay the start of anaesthesia, and avoids unwanted fluid loading in vulnerable patients such as pre-eclamptics. Tachycardia from ephedrine is undesirable in some patients with heart disease. New work with phenylephrine infusions is promising, producing less hypotension, vomiting and fetal acidosis than an ephedrine infusion, but more research is required before it can be recommended for routine use.

STILL NOT CONFIDENT?

Do a CSE.

COMBINED SPINAL–EPIDURAL ANAESTHESIA

There are two basic approaches. The first is to give a full anaesthetic spinal dose, with the epidural component in place to protect against inadequate block height or to prolong anaesthesia if complicated surgery is anticipated. Indications for this approach include:

- Extremes of maternal stature which make determining the spinal dose difficult
- Reduced abdominal size, as in prematurity or growth retardation, when a lower block height can be expected for a given spinal dose
- Difficult surgery or slow surgeon.

The other approach is deliberately to reduce the spinal dose and to top up the block with epidural increments. This approach is used to reduce the incidence and severity of spinal-induced hypotension. There are pros and cons of the 'separate space, separate needle' technique and the needle-through-needle approach. The choice boils down to personal preference.

SPINAL CATHETERS

These were covered in the overview to this chapter.

OXYTOCIC DRUGS

Oxytocin (Syntocinon) causes profound vasodilatation for about 2 min, which can produce devastating hypotension in hypovolaemic women or in those with cardiac conditions that limit cardiac output. The standard dose is 5 international units, given slowly. This can be omitted and replaced with uterine massage if even brief haemodynamic instability cannot be tolerated. An oxytocin infusion of 10 units per h is haemodynamically benign. Ergometrine produces more profound uterine contraction but causes nausea, vomiting and hypertension. It should not, therefore, be used routinely or in hypertensive women.

POSTOPERATIVE ANALGESIA

REGIONAL ANAESTHESIA

This is achieved with a long-acting intraspinal opioid plus:
- Diclofenac 100 mg per rectum at the end of the operation (obtain consent)
- Diclofenac 50 mg orally 8 hourly thereafter
- Paracetamol 1 g 6 hourly
- Dihydrocodeine 30 mg 4 hourly as required.

GENERAL ANAESTHESIA:
- Diclofenac 100 mg per rectum at the end of surgery (obtain consent)
- Morphine patient-controlled analgesia
- Begin oral regimen as above as soon as possible to help wean from PCA.

Prophylactic peroperative cyclizine 50 mg i.m., followed by doses as required, will reduce the nausea and vomiting associated with these regimens.

BIBLIOGRAPHY

Collis RE, Plaat FS, Morgan BM. Comparison of midwife top-ups, continuous infusion and patient-controlled epidural analgesia for maintaining mobility after a low-dose combined spinal–epidural. British Journal of Anaesthesia 1999; 82:233–236

Hawthorne L, Slaymaker A, Bamber J, Dresner M. Effect of fluid preload on maternal haemodynamics for low-dose epidural analgesia in labour. International Journal of Obstetric Anesthesia 2001; 10:312–315

McKinlay J, Lyons G. Obstetric neuraxial anaesthesia: which pressor agents should we be using? International Journal of Obstetric Anesthesia 2002; 11:117–121

Mowbray P, Cooper DW, Carpenter M, Ryall DM, Desira WR, Kokri MS. Phenylephrine, ephedrine and fetal acidosis at caesarean delivery under spinal anaesthesia. International Journal of Obstetric Anesthesia 2002; 11(Suppl):1 (abstract)

Pinder AJ, Dresner M, Calow C, O'Riordan J, Johnson R. Haemodynamic changes caused by oxytocin during caesarean section under spinal anaesthesia. International Journal of Obstetric Anesthesia 2002; 11:156–159

Reynolds F. Placental transfer of drugs. Current Anaesthesia and Critical Care 1991; 2:108–116

Russell I. Assessing the block for caesarean section. International Journal of Obstetric Anesthesia 2001; 10:83–85 (editorial)

18

CROSS-REFERENCES

Local anaesthetic toxicity
    Anaesthetic Factors 31: 761

Anaesthesia for emergency caesarean section

M. Dresner

In theory, the five methods of anaesthesia described in the section on elective caesarean section can all be used in the emergency situation, but in practice the choice is limited by the time available to induce anaesthesia. Good communication between obstetrician and anaesthetist is therefore vital if unnecessarily rushed general anaesthesia and inappropriately prolonged attempts at achieving regional blockade are to be avoided. To clarify decision-making and improve data collection, the Royal College of Obstetricians and Gynaecologists and the Royal College of Anaesthetists have endorsed the following categorisation of caesarean section urgency, with the incidence of each as found in a national audit shown in parentheses:

1. An immediate threat to the life of the mother or fetus (16%)
2. Maternal or fetal compromise that is not immediately life threatening (32%)
3. The mother needs early delivery but there is no maternal or fetal compromise (18%)
4. Delivery is timed to suit the mother and the staff (31%).

CATEGORY 1

Consider the following points:

- This situation requires your fastest anaesthetic for that individual patient.
- An experienced anaesthetist can induce spinal anaesthesia as fast as a general anaesthesia in an anatomically favourable patient. If you cannot, give general anaesthesia.
- If general anaesthesia is associated with increased risk (e.g. a predicted difficult airway), regional anaesthesia is justified even if it is the slower option.

If you intend using regional anaesthesia for category 1 sections, despite there being no contraindication to general anaesthesia:

- Practise performing spinal anaesthesia as quickly as you can with elective sections.

- To reduce the onset time of spinal anaesthesia, increase the dose of local anaesthetic and include a lipid-soluble opioid.
- There is no time for fluid preloading, so a vasoconstrictor technique must be used, such as 6-mg increments of ephedrine.
- Warn that there may be some discomfort during the first few minutes of surgery.
- Set yourself a time limit for achieving regional anaesthesia, after which you must convert to general anaesthesia.
- Preoxygenate during the regional attempt so that conversion to general anaesthesia is not delayed.
- Document the time you took performing anaesthesia. If the neonate has a poor outcome, the assumption may be made that regional anaesthesia delayed the delivery.

CATEGORIES 2 AND 3

These categories include the failure to progress patients, as well as cases of moderate fetal distress, poor fetal growth and subacute maternal illness such as pre-eclampsia. Excluding maternal conditions that influence the choice of anaesthesia, these categories allow ample time to perform any technique. There is only one issue to be considered: how best to manage anaesthesia for women already receiving epidural analgesia.

CONVERTING EPIDURAL ANALGESIA TO ANAESTHESIA

The reliability and quality of spinal and CSE anaesthesia, particularly when lipid-soluble opioids are used, reveal the relative inadequacies of epidural anaesthesia. The slow onset and potential for missed segments have led to its almost complete abandonment from use in elective caesarean sections. However, when an epidural is *in situ* for labour analgesia, it seems sensible to attempt to avoid the risks of a new procedure if possible. The two problems to be considered are:

- Poor-quality anaesthesia
- The risk of unexpectedly high blockade if spinal anaesthesia is superimposed on an epidural.

The author's own audits quantify these problems in the following way:

- Intravenous or inhaled agent supplementation required in 15% of epidurals, compared with 2% for spinal anaesthesia
- Conversion to spinal or general anaesthesia required in 5%
- Spinals used after epidural analgesia cause high spinal blocks requiring respiratory support in 1.5%.

A strategy is required to minimise these risks (Table 18.8).

Better quality and more rapid results can be achieved with 2-chloroprocaine, but this agent is not available in the UK. Some advocate a combination of 2% lidocaine (lignocaine) mixed with fresh adrenaline (epinephrine) and bicarbonate as a top-up that is almost as quick and reliable as spinal anaesthesia. The author is too concerned about admixture errors to advocate such an approach.

SPINAL ANAESTHESIA AFTER EPIDURAL ANALGESIA

An audit of 342 spinals used in these circumstances revealed five high blocks (1.5%) that required respiratory support. There were no obvious patterns or predictors for these cases. Attempts to reduce the risk by reducing spinal doses simply increased the incidence of inadequate spinal blocks. The following conclusions were drawn:

- After epidural analgesia, high spinal block is a sporadic and unpredictable complication.
- Anaesthetic preparation should include assessment of the airway.
- Spinals should be performed in an anaesthetic area with full intubation equipment available.
- An appropriate warning needs to be included at consent.

TABLE 18.8

Strategy for converting epidural analgesia to anaesthesia

	Observation or action needed
In situ epidural prerequisites	Baby, mother and obstetrician can wait 30 min before delivery Good epidural analgesia, no missed segments
Contraindications	Rapid delivery required *In situ* epidural not working well
Warning to patient	Strong sensations during surgery likely 5% need conversion to spinal or general anaesthesia
Initial top-up	10 ml 0.5% bupivacaine + lipid-soluble opioid (e.g. 100 μg fentanyl or 3 mg diamorphine) Look for deepening block at 10 min
First 10 ml working at 10 min?	Continue topping up in 5-ml increments to achieve touch block at T6
First 10 ml has not done much	Don't waste more time High spinal less likely after 10 ml than after 30 ml! Offer spinal or general anaesthesia

In all cases, no adverse outcomes ensued. Blocks had receded sufficiently to enable all the women to be extubated at the end of surgery.

NOTES ON EMERGENCY GENERAL ANAESTHESIA

- Unless specific risks apply, general anaesthesia is a low-risk, rapid, reliable technique.
- Gastric emptying ceases in labour, so aspiration prophylaxis is vital.
- Remember to empty the stomach with a large-bore orogastric tube before extubation.

18

BIBLIOGRAPHY

Cole P, Dresner M, Stockwell J, Freeman J.
Anaesthesia for emergency caesarean section in
women already receiving epidural analgesia.
International Journal of Obstetric Anesthesia 2001;
10:215 (abstract)

Confidential Enquiry into Stillbirths and Deaths in
Infancy. 7th Annual Report. London: Maternal and
Child Health Research Consortium; 1998. Available:
http://www.cemach.org.uk 25 April 2003

Lucas DN, Borra PJ, Yentis SM. Epidural top-up
solutions for emergency caesarean section: a
comparison of preparation times. British Journal of
Anaesthesia 2000; 84:494–496

Lucas DN, Ciccone GK, Yentis SM. Extending low-dose
epidural analgesia for emergency caesarean section.
A comparison of three solutions. Anaesthesia 1999;
54:1173–1177

Lucas DN, Yentis SM, Kinsella SM et al. Urgency of
caesarean section: a new classification. Journal of the
Royal Society of Medicine 2000; 93:346–350

18

Serious complications of pregnancy

M. Dresner

THROMBOEMBOLISM

The pregnant woman is already in a hypercoagulable state and the risk of thromboembolism is increased by:
- Age above 35 years
- Weight greater than 80 kg
- Parity of four or more
- Gross varicose veins
- Current infection
- Pre-eclampsia
- Immobility
- Extended operation (e.g. caesarean hysterectomy)
- Personal or family history of thromboembolic disease
- Patients with antiphospholipid antibodies (cardiolipin or lupus anticoagulant).

All women with one or more of these risk factors should wear thromboembolism deterrent (TED) stockings and receive enoxaparin (Clexane) 40 mg daily, or an equivalent prophylaxis. Neuraxial block and removal of epidural catheters should be timed according to the guidelines in the Overview section of this chapter.

PRE-ECLAMPSIA

This multisystem endothelial cell disorder of hereditary, immunological and environmental aetiology affects 5% of pregnancies.

FETAL COMPLICATIONS:
- Reduced fetal growth
- Premature labour
- Abruption.

MATERNAL COMPLICATIONS:
- Thromboembolism
- Pulmonary oedema
- Cerebral and hepatic haemorrhage
- Coagulopathy
- Eclampsia
- Haemolysis, raised liver enzyme and low platelet (HELLP syndrome) levels.

CRITERIA OF SEVERE PRE-ECLAMPSIA:
- Systolic pressure > 170 mmHg, diastolic > 110 mmHg with 1+ protein
- Systolic pressure > 140 mmHg, diastolic > 90 mmHg with 2+ or more protein
- Headache or cerebral disturbances (including eclampsia)
- Visual disturbances
- Epigastric pain
- Pulmonary oedema or cyanosis
- Haemolysis, raised liver enzyme and low platelet (HELLP syndrome) levels.

Women with one or more of these criteria should be managed according to the unit's protocol, preferably in an obstetric high-dependency area.

MANAGEMENT OF SEVERE PRE-ECLAMPSIA

The general principles of management of women with severe pre-eclampsia are:
- Treatment of hypertension
- Careful control of fluid balance
- Thromboprophylaxis
- Treatment of eclampsia with magnesium sulfate
- Consideration of eclampsia prophylaxis with magnesium
- Delivery on the best day in the best way.

In the absence of fetal distress, emergency delivery of a poorly controlled hypertensive woman is rarely indicated, even after a convulsion.

Management of eclampsia should include:
- Basic airway support, oxygen therapy and lateral position during the convulsion.
- Give 5 g magnesium sulfate intravenously over 25 min.
- Most fits stop spontaneously, but use midazolam 2–10 mg if necessary.
- Avoid sedation and intubation if possible; if unavoidable, cerebral haemorrhage must be excluded by scanning.

18

- Continue magnesium by infusion of 1 g h^{-1}.
- If tendon reflexes are present, magnesium levels are not in the toxic range.
- Blood monitoring is indicated in the presence of renal dysfunction.

Anaesthetic considerations in pre-eclampsia include:

- Avoidance of fluid preloads and excessive fluid therapy associated with neuraxial block and caesarean section
- Prevention of hypertensive responses associated with general anaesthesia
- Use of neuraxial block in the presence of thrombocytopaenia (clotting is usually normal with platelet count as low as 50×10^9/litre
- Timing of neuraxial block in relation to thromboprophylaxis
- Severe hypotension after spinal anaesthesia – rare, but may occur if multiple antihypertensive agents and magnesium are being used
- Low spinal blocks in association with prematurity or growth retardation – consider increasing doses or use CSE.

A final learning point concerns HELLP syndrome complicated by severe disseminated intravascular coagulation (DIC) and anaemia. When large volumes of blood products are required, volume overload and pulmonary oedema are likely to occur if oliguria is present. Early renal support with dialysis may be necessary to prevent this, so nephrologists should be consulted at an early stage.

HAEMORRHAGE

Abruption, antepartum haemorrhage, postpartum haemorrhage and surgical bleeding are, of course, major considerations in obstetrics. Team management of these potentially catastrophic problems warrants careful planning and rehearsal drills. The medical and anaesthetic management of haemorrhage is the same as in other clinical situations, and will not therefore be detailed here. However, there are some aspects of diagnosis and management that warrant emphasis. Occult haemorrhage, without vaginal bleeding, is particularly important; the following points should be considered:

- Any patient with tachycardia and hypotension is potentially bleeding.
- Abruption is characterised by abdominal pain, a tense uterus and fetal distress.
- Abruption severe enough to kill the fetus is frequently followed by significant anaemia

and coagulopathy. Anticipate this during caesarean section for abruption.
- Postpartum haemorrhage is more likely with increased uterine size, as with twins and polyhydramnios. Use oxytocin infusions after caesarean deliveries in these circumstances.
- Post-delivery tachycardia, but no vaginal loss – check the fundal height for blood-filled uterus.
- Remember intra-abdominal bleeding after caesarean section.
- If possible, central lines should be inserted with ultrasonographic guidance, especially in the presence of coagulopathy.
- Know how and where to get hold of group O negative blood.
- Know how and where to get hold of rapid transfusion equipment and its operator.

AMNIOTIC FLUID EMBOLISM

Sudden fetal distress in labour, complicated by haemodynamic collapse, dysrhythmias, hypoxia and subsequent DIC, can be caused by amniotic fluid embolism. This is a diagnosis of exclusion which does not alter the supportive management necessary for the features described. This condition should be borne in mind when obvious coagulopathy is occurring during emergency caesarean section for sudden maternal collapse or fetal distress. The insertion of central venous access, communication with a haematologist and arrangement of an intensive care bed should be expedited.

PUERPERAL CARDIOMYOPATHY

- Onset can be between 6 months of gestation and 6 months postpartum
- More common in multiple pregnancies, multiparous and older women
- Presents as dyspnoea, palpitations, pulmonary and/or peripheral oedema, all of which are features of normal pregnancy
- Diagnosed by cardiomegaly and reduced left ventricular function on echocardiography
- Treatment includes delivery, anticoagulation, conventional heart failure drugs and, occasionally, heart transplantation
- 50% spontaneous and full recovery rate, but sudden death may occur.

18

ACUTE FATTY LIVER OF PREGNANCY

- Rare, but potentially fatal
- Associated with male fetuses, obesity and multiple pregnancies
- Usually presents after 30 weeks' gestation with nausea, anorexia, abdominal pain and malaise
- Often coexists with features of mild pre-eclampsia
- Can be hard to distinguish from HELLP, but differentiated by hypoglycaemia and marked hyperuricaemia
- Early delivery usually reverses the disease process
- Early consultation with intensivists and hepatologists is essential
- Fulminant hepatic failure with encephalopathy may necessitate transfer to a liver unit for multisystem support and even hepatic transplant.

BIBLIOGRAPHY

Eclampsia Trial Collaborative Group. Which anticonvulsant for women with eclampsia? Evidence from the collaborative eclampsia trial. Lancet 1995; 345:1455–1463

MAGPIE Trial Collaborative Group. Do women with preeclampsia, and their babies, benefit from magnesium sulphate? The MAGPIE Trial: a randomised placebo controlled trial. Lancet 2002; 359:1877–1889

Nelson-Piercy C. Handbook of obstetric medicine. Oxford: Isis Medical Media; 1997

Walker JJ. Pre-eclampsia. Lancet 2000; 356:1260–1265

18

19

UROLOGY
L. Bromley

Overview

L. Bromley

Patients presenting for urological operations are of all ages and degrees of fitness. Paediatric reconstructive urology is a highly specialised area in which operations are performed on newborn babies and repeated operations will take place throughout childhood and adolescence. This takes place in specialist centres and is not covered here.

The majority of urology patients are elderly men. The increased incidence of benign hyperplasia of the prostate gland with age is largely responsible. There is an association between cigarette smoking over long periods and bladder cancer. The combination of maturity-onset diabetes and incomplete bladder emptying predisposes to urinary tract infections. These three factors act to skew the population presenting for urological investigation and operation.

As with anaesthesia for any group of elderly patients, intercurrent diseases are of the utmost importance to the anaesthetist. Where obstruction of the lower urinary tract has been long-standing, it is of great importance to ensure that kidney function is normal and that levels of urea and creatinine are not rising. Formal preoperative assessment is essential, with particular reference to smoking-related diseases. Many patients return on a regular basis for repeat examination. It is a mistake, however, to assume that recent (e.g. 3 months ago) uneventful anaesthesia will allow the anaesthetist to omit a preoperative visit. Other important medical events are more likely in this age group, and a history should always be taken.

A number of urologists have an interest in the problems of continence in women. These problems sometimes arise after traumatic childbirth, or may be related to gynaecological surgery. There seems to be no hard and fast rule on who should deal with these conditions, and local practice is the deciding factor. It may therefore be the case that operations such as colposuspension, or Stamey's operation, may appear in one hospital on a urology list and in another on a gynaecology list.

Urologists were among the first surgeons to realise the potential of minimally invasive surgery. Transurethral prostatectomy was one of the first minimally invasive procedures and, although it is not without its problems and there is some doubt as to whether the mortality rate is lower over a 5-year period, the technique is now universally accepted. In the last 3 years there has been a growing interest in performing other operations, particularly nephrectomy, laparoscopically, and staging of advanced prostate cancer by laparoscopic sampling of para-aortic lymph nodes. The introduction of the flexible cystoscope has allowed urologists to perform many diagnostic cystoscopies without general anaesthesia in the outpatient clinic. This has enabled them to select patients for cystoscopy under general anaesthesia who need biopsy of the bladder mucosa, or more extensive examination.

The management of renal stones has been revolutionised in the past 10 years. Renal stones were formerly a major source of renal damage, and the passage of stones with associated renal colic is one of the commonest urological emergencies. Stones are now treated with a combination of minimally invasive techniques, and open operations are becoming rare. Ultrasonic lithotripsy, percutaneous nephrolithotomy and ureteric lasering of stones have virtually abolished use of the Dormia basket and open removal.

Major urological surgery falls into two groups: operations performed for malignant conditions of the genitourinary tract, and operations for reconstruction of congenital malformations. A number of attempts have been made in both areas to provide the patient with as normal a function as possible after operation. Previously, urinary diversion into an ileal conduit was used as a replacement for bladder function, but increasingly surgery is designed to refashion and replace the bladder with a pouch constructed from a piece of bowel (caecoplasty, ileoplasty or gastroplasty). This pouch can be attached to the trigone, if suitable, allowing normal voiding of urine after surgery. If the bladder neck is to be removed, a continent stoma may be fashioned with the appendix, allowing catheterisation of the stoma at regular intervals (Mitroffanof procedure).

A urologist is part of the team of specialists managing patients with spinal injury, in whom procedures to restore continence with artificial urinary sphincters and to restore erectile function with penile implants may be required. This group of patients has its own set of anaesthetic problems. Loss of erectile function is also found amongst diabetic men, and operations are performed to overcome this problem. Ligation of penile veins, implantation of rods or inflatable devices are undertaken. These patients are frequently long-standing diabetics and, when considering their anaesthetic management, the other sequelae of diabetes must be investigated, and blood sugar control managed perioperatively.

The most commonly performed urological procedures are reviewed in detail in this chapter.

CROSS-REFERENCES

Spinal cord injury (acute)
    Patient Conditions 1: 30
Spinal cord injury (chronic)
    Patient Conditions 1: 33
Diabetes Mellitus type 2
    Patient Conditions 2: 59
The elderly patient
    Patient Conditions 27: 606

19

Cystoscopy

L. Bromley

19

PROCEDURE

- Examination of the urethral and bladder mucosa using a rigid fibreoptic cystoscope passed through the urethra is the usual technique.
- Diagnostic cystoscopy is intended for initial investigation of symptoms, particularly haematuria or recurrent urinary tract infections.
- Check cystoscopy is performed after treatment of bladder cancer to look for recurrence, often combined with diathermy or resection of recurrences. The patients often return every few months for several years.
- The operation is frequently performed as a day case.
- Fibreoptic cystoscopy using a flexible cystoscope is usually performed under local anaesthesia.

PATIENT CHARACTERISTICS

Patients for cystoscopy are frequently:
- Men aged over 50 years
- Have a high incidence of chronic disease
- American Society of Anesthesiologists (ASA) status II and III.

PREOPERATIVE ASSESSMENT AND INVESTIGATIONS

- Assessment of cardiovascular and respiratory systems
- Assessment of renal function
- If repeat cystoscopy, ask whether there has been any change in health status since last visit
- Check previous anaesthetic records
- Assess suitability for day-case anaesthesia.

PREMEDICATION

Patients having day-case cystoscopies are frequently not premedicated. If required, a benzodiazepine is appropriate.

PERIOPERATIVE MANAGEMENT

MONITORING:
- ECG
- Non-invasive blood pressure
- SaO_2
- $EtCO_2$.

ANAESTHETIC TECHNIQUE:
- *General anaesthesia* – a spontaneously breathing technique is usual. Propofol is a suitable induction agent; maintenance is with a volatile agent of choice or use a total intravenous anaesthetic (TIVA) technique with propofol. A laryngeal mask is suitable for airway management. Biopsy and resection of tumour will require analgesic supplementation.
- *Regional anaesthesia* – may be indicated in severe respiratory disease. Caudal block may be sufficient, but filling of the bladder may cause discomfort that is not blocked by a caudal. A low spinal block is more reliable.

These anaesthetics, despite their simplicity, can be the most challenging to give smoothly. Unpremedicated patients who are elderly and frequently have respiratory disease can be very difficult to settle to spontaneously breathing anaesthesia. The combination of propofol and the laryngeal mask has made the anaesthetist's task easier, but there is still a great deal of skill to performing this anaesthetic well.

POSTOPERATIVE MANAGEMENT

Diagnostic and check cystoscopies where no resection has taken place do not result in significant postoperative pain. In the case of a

POSTOPERATIVE MANAGEMENT

The management of postoperative pain is best achieved via an epidural infusion of low-dose local anaesthetic and opioids. The local practice as to nursing and the management of epidurals containing opioids varies. It may be necessary to manage the patient on a HDU, in which case the patient should be electively booked for the HDU before surgery. Provided the patient is haemodynamically stable and normothermic at the end of the procedure, there is no other indication for HDU admission.

Where there is significant chest disease, postoperative physiotherapy is indicated. The combination of large abdominal incision and the use of opioids after operation is an indication for prescribing additional oxygen for the first three postoperative days and nights.

OUTCOME

This is a major operation and the postoperative mortality rate is between 3% and 5%.

BIBLIOGRAPHY

Beydon L, Hassapopoulos J, Quera MA et al. Risk factors for oxygen desaturation during sleep after abdominal surgery. British Journal of Anaesthesia 1992; 69:137–142

Hobbs GJ, Roberts FL. Epidural infusion of bupivacaine and diamorphine for postoperative analgesia use on general surgical wards. Anaesthesia 1992; 47:58–62

Morris RH. Influence of ambient temperature on patient temperature during intra abdominal surgery. Archives of Surgery 1971; 173:230–233

CROSS-REFERENCES

The elderly patient
    Patient Conditions 27: 606
Blood transfusion
    Anaesthetic Factors 31: 729
Postoperative pain management
    Anaesthetic Factors 31: 728

19

Nephrectomy

L. Bromley

PROCEDURE

- Removal of kidney with or without part of the ureter
- Performed with the patient positioned on the side
- Access for surgeon is improved by 'breaking' the table
- There is potential for considerable blood loss.

PATIENT CHARACTERISTICS

- The procedure can be undertaken at any age.
- In cases of chronic infection, the patient may be debilitated.
- ASA grade I–IV.

COMMON ASSOCIATIONS WITH NEPHRECTOMY

Nephrectomy is performed for tumour, hydronephrosis, chronic infection and, rarely, for staghorn calculi that cannot be treated by other means. Patients with renal tumours may have pulmonary metastases. Patients who have had chronic infections may have been in poor health for some time, and may be poorly nourished, with low albumin levels.

PREOPERATIVE ASSESSMENT

- Exclude associated conditions
- Systematic review of other medical conditions
- Discuss postoperative analgesia and obtain consent for epidural block
- Ensure availability of blood.

PREMEDICATION

Analgesic premedication, with or without an antisialagogue, is indicated.

PERIOPERATIVE MANAGEMENT

THEATRE PREPARATION

Careful positioning of patient for this operation is important. The patient is placed on the table with the side of operation uppermost, and great care must be taken to support the patient and prevent them rolling off the table. Supports that fasten to the table may be used, or alternatively use a bean-bag type of support. This latter type of support helps to reduce heat loss. Fluids should be warmed. Care must be taken to ensure that the legs are supported by pillows and that the arms are not touching any part of the metal supports.

ANAESTHETIC TECHNIQUE

The positioning of the patient on the side results in a ventilation–perfusion mismatch between the lungs; intermittent positive-pressure ventilation (IPPV) is mandatory. In addition, there is a risk of surgical disruption of the pleura during the dissection.

Epidural analgesia via a low thoracic or high lumbar catheter is the most effective form of postoperative analgesia in these cases. Thus, the combination of light general anaesthesia with IPPV with an epidural is the preferred method of anaesthesia. If an epidural is not possible, intercostal nerve blocks from T9 to T12 are a useful supplement to general anaesthesia and will give some postoperative pain relief.

The potential for blood loss during this operation is an indication for invasive monitoring. A large-bore cannula, a CVP line and an intra-arterial line are recommended. Monitoring should also include the following:

- ECG
- Sao_2
- $Etco_2$
- Blood loss
- Temperature.

At the end of the procedure, if there is any suggestion of damage to the pleura, several large-volume breaths may be given to attempt to detect any pleural leak. If there is a pneumothorax, it must be drained.

POSTOPERATIVE MANAGEMENT

Nephrectomy is a painful operation and requires optimal postoperative pain relief. This is best provided by continuous epidural infusion of a mixture of opioids and low-dose local anaesthetics. If local policy requires patients with epidural infusions to be nursed in a HDU, a bed should be booked before the operation.

There is a risk of atelectasis in the dependent lung and good physiotherapy is essential, for which good pain relief is also important.

OUTCOME

Long-term outcome depends largely on the aetiology of the renal damage. The operative mortality rate is of the order of 1%.

CROSS-REFERENCES

Blood transfusion
    Anaesthetic Factors 31: 729
Complications of position
    Anaesthetic Factors 31: 736

19

Open prostatectomy

H. Owen Reece

PROCEDURE

Open prostatectomy is performed in one of two ways:
- *Retropubic prostatectomy* – when a benign hypertrophic prostate is too large for transurethral resection
- *Radical prostatectomy* – for clearance of a malignant prostatic tumour and lymph nodes (if they are involved on frozen section; see below).

PATIENT CHARACTERISTICS

- Over 50 years of age
- High incidence of chronic disease
- ASA grade II–IV.

PREOPERATIVE ASSESSMENT AND INVESTIGATIONS

- Identification and assessment of chronic disease.
- Deep vein thrombosis prophylaxis – elasticated stockings are recommended; patients are not routinely heparinised because it is considered that, on balance, the decreased haemostasis may do more harm than good.
- Blood transfusion availability – 3 units for retropubic prostatectomy, 6 units for radical prostatectomy.
- Antibiotic prophylaxis – cefuroxime and metronidazole is a popular combination.
- Assessment of the suitability for spinal or epidural analgesia. This is a particularly valuable technique to use in conjunction with general anaesthesia for radical prostatectomy because it provides excellent postoperative analgesia, reduces the perioperative blood loss and decreases the quantity of inhalational agent required.

PREMEDICATION

An opioid premedicant is suitable. It has the advantage of pre-empting the nociceptive stimulus, although if an epidural technique is contemplated these are not necessary.

A benzodiazepine is a suitable alternative and will provide anxiolysis and amnesia. All elderly patients are at risk of becoming confused if anticholinergics that cross the blood–brain barrier (e.g. hyoscine) are employed.

THEATRE PREPARATION

- Patient positioning requires care, because the operation is often lengthy.
- Monitoring nasopharyngeal temperature is an easy and effective means of measuring body temperature. Body temperature should be maintained with a warming mattress, warm air overblanket, warmed intravenous fluids and a ventilator circuit humidifier.

PERIOPERATIVE MANAGEMENT

MONITORING:
- Arterial blood pressure – via an arterial line for radical prostatectomy
- ECG
- SaO_2
- $EtCO_2$
- Core temperature
- Fluid balance and blood loss
- CVP – for radical prostatectomy.

ANAESTHETIC TECHNIQUE
The combination of epidural and general anaesthesia with a muscle relaxant and volatile agent is a suitable technique. Retropubic prostatectomy can be performed under epidural analgesia alone if required.

During radical prostatectomy there will be an interval (which may be substantial) during

19

which a frozen section of pelvic lymph node is examined histologically. If the nodes contain metastatic deposits, the planned radical operation will not usually proceed.

Retropubic prostatectomy leaves the prostatic capsule intact, and bleeding – although significant – is not as great (1–2 litres) as in radical prostatectomy, in which the capsule is removed. In the latter case the blood loss may be as much as 4 litres. It has been suggested that fibrinolysins, which exacerbate bleeding, are released by prostatic handling.

POSTOPERATIVE MANAGEMENT

If an epidural infusion is already *in situ*, a combination of local analgesia and an epidural opioid will provide excellent analgesia for both procedures.

Postoperative blood loss and urine output should be monitored.

OUTCOME

With good case selection, the 5-year survival rate is 95%. The operative mortality rate is very low.

BIBLIOGRAPHY

Madsen RE, Madsen PO. Influence of anaesthesia on blood loss in transurethral resection of the prostate. Anesthesia and Analgesia 1967; 46:330–332

Richmond CE, Bromley LM, Woolf CJ. Preoperative morphine pre-empts postoperative pain. Lancet 1993; 342:73–75

Smart RF. Endoscopic injection of the vasopressor ornithine-8-vasopressin on transurethral resection. British Journal of Urology 1984; 56:191–197

CROSS-REFERENCES

The elderly patient
    Patient Conditions 27: 606
Blood transfusion
    Anaesthetic Factors 31: 729
Thrombotic embolism
    Anaesthetic Factors 31: 789
Preoperative assessment of pulmonary risk
    Anaesthetic Factors 27: 638

19

Percutaneous nephrolithotomy

J. Frossard

PROCEDURE

Percutaneous nephrolithotomy (PCNL) is a procedure whereby stones in the renal pelvis are removed with a nephroscope via a dilated percutaneous puncture made under radiological control.

PATIENT CHARACTERISTICS

Patients for PCNL are generally:
- Any age
- ASA I–IV
- May have compromised renal function.

PREOPERATIVE INVESTIGATIONS

- Exclusion of commonly associated medical conditions
- Review of renal function
- Blood transfusion availability
- Antibiotic prophylaxis.

PREMEDICATION

At the anaesthetist's discretion.

PERIOPERATIVE MANAGEMENT

MONITORING:
- ECG
- Non-invasive blood pressure
- Sao_2
- $EtCO_2$
- Estimation of blood loss
- Core temperature.

ANAESTHETIC TECHNIQUE:
- Intravenous induction, opioid and inhalational maintenance is a suitable technique.

- Muscular paralysis is required because the patient will be placed prone and coughing must be avoided during renal puncture.
- Use an armoured (reinforced) tracheal tube.

POSITIONING:
The patient is placed first in the lithotomy position and a retrograde catheter is placed in the ureter to allow for opacification of the percutaneous puncture and to prevent fragments of stone from passing down the ureter.

The patient is then turned to the prone position:
- Ensure that there is enough help to turn the patient.
- Protect the eyes, shoulders, knees, elbows.
- Place arm with intravenous access above the head – beware of brachial plexus strain.
- The other arm with the blood pressure cuff may be placed by the side.
- Place a pillow(s) under the chest and pelvis to free the abdomen for ventilation.
- Place a pad under the flank to prevent a mobile kidney from rotating anteriorly in the prone position.
- Turn the head to the side to be punctured in order to prevent neck strain.
- Drape the patient in a foil blanket (with a hole cut in it for the puncture site) because the patient often becomes wet (this will help to conserve heat; do not use a foil blanket if diathermy is to be used).
- Warm irrigation fluid.

COMPLICATIONS

HAEMORRHAGE
Tears in the parenchyma may occur if the rigid scope is not handled with care.

Bleeding requiring transfusion following percutaneous renal manipulation is rare; most reports quote 3%. About 0.5% of patients may require balloon tamponade of the tract or arterial embolisation. Transfusion is very rare in patients that have small stones, and bleeding is not related to the size of the track.

EXTRAVASATION

Any tear in the pelvicaliceal system will result in some extravasation of the irrigant fluid. It is important, therefore, that normal saline is used as the endoscopic irrigant. Water and glycine may cause fluid intoxication, because they are absorbed from the peritoneum.

PLEURAL COMPLICATIONS

If an intercostal puncture is performed to reach an upper calyceal calculus, the pleura may be entered and either a minor pleural reaction seen or, following endoscopy, there could be a massive collection of irrigant fluid and air within the thoracic cavity.

INFECTION

The most serious complication that must be guarded against is infection. Stones containing infection may be disintegrated at percutaneous nephrolithotomy, releasing bacteria into the urine and, therefore, potentially into the blood-stream. Prophylactic antibiotics should be used routinely. Bacteraemia is unavoidable, but the duration of the endoscopy should be limited. If a large infected stone is being disintegrated and infection is clearly present, endoscopy should be limited to 1 h. Endoscopy for a non-infected stone should be limited to 1.5 h. If Gram-negative septicaemia is suspected, the patient should be treated aggressively immediately.

POSTOPERATIVE MANAGEMENT

Intravenous fluids should be given to increase urine output and flush out any gravel via the nephrostomy left *in situ*. Analgesia, as required, with opioids and/or non-steroidal anti-inflammatory drugs (NSAIDs) if renal function is normal.

BIBLIOGRAPHY

Marberger M, Stackl W, Hruby W. Percutaneous litholapaxy of renal calculi with ultrasound. European Urology 1982; 8:236–237

Pollack HM, Banner MP. Percutaneous extraction of renal and ureteric calculi; technical considerations. American Journal of Roentgenology 1984; 143:778–784

Schultz PE, Hanno PM, Wein AJ et al. Percutaneous ultrasonic lithotripsy: choice of irrigant. Journal of Urology 1983; 130:858–860

CROSS-REFERENCES

Blood transfusion
    Anaesthetic Factors 31: 729
Complications of position
    Anaesthetic Factors 31: 736
TUR syndrome
    Anaesthetic Factors 31: 801

19

Transurethral prostatectomy

L. Bromley

PROCEDURE

- Some 95% of prostatectomies are performed endoscopically.
- The patient is placed in the lithotomy position.
- Continuous irrigation of the bladder with a solution of 1.5% glycine occurs during the resection.
- The operation may be performed as a repeat procedure.

PATIENT CHARACTERISTICS

- Over 50 years of age; male
- High incidence of chronic disease
- ASA status I–IV.

COMMON ASSOCIATIONS WITH TRANSURETHRAL PROSTATECTOMY

The patient may present with haematuria or may have long-standing obstruction, increasing the risk of renal failure. Urinary tract infection can complicate large residual volumes of urine. These patients have a higher incidence of cardiopulmonary problems, hypertension, obesity and diabetes mellitus.

PREOPERATIVE ASSESSMENT AND INVESTIGATIONS

- Exclude associated conditions
- Systematic review of intercurrent illness
- Discuss anaesthetic technique and decide on suitability for regional anaesthesia.

PREMEDICATION

Anxiolysis with a benzodiazepine is suitable for patients having a regional technique. For general anaesthesia, analgesic premedication may be preferred.

PERIOPERATIVE MANAGEMENT

THEATRE PREPARATION

Warm irrigating fluid should be used in order to maintain core temperature.

ANAESTHETIC TECHNIQUE

This operation can be conducted using a regional technique – either spinal or epidural anaesthesia. This method is commonly used, although a number of patients prefer to be asleep during the operation. There are advantages to a regional technique:

- These patients often have intercurrent chest disease, and benefit after surgery from not having a general anaesthetic.
- The awake patient is a better monitor of the onset of the 'transurethral (TUR) syndrome', as any confusion can be detected rapidly.
- There is a reduction in the incidence of postoperative thromboembolic disease.

If a general anaesthetic is to be used, paralysis and ventilation is not specifically required for this operation which can be performed with the patient breathing spontaneously through a laryngeal mask.

MONITORING:

- ECG
- Non-invasive blood pressure
- Sao_2
- Temperature.

THE TRANSURETHRAL SYNDROME

This is caused by the absorption of the irrigating fluid during resection of the prostate. Symptoms include hypertension, visual disturbances, dyspnoea, mental changes and circulatory collapse.

POSTOPERATIVE MANAGEMENT

The transurethral syndrome can develop at any stage in the postoperative period, and the nursing staff should be aware of this. The initial postoperative period is not characterised as particularly painful, the most painful period being when the catheter is removed.

OUTCOME

The reported hospital mortality rate is 0.2–2.5%, and may be as low as 0.5–1% in specialist centres. There is evidence of increased intermediate and long-term mortality and morbidity with transurethral prostatectomy compared with open prostatectomy, and with other minimally invasive operations in this age group. These reports can all be attributed to cardiovascular morbidity and mortality factors. Studies also suggest that haemodynamic changes relating to a drop in core temperature may be responsible.

BIBLIOGRAPHY

Evans J, Singer M, Chapple C, Macartney N, Walker M, Milroy E. Haemodynamic evidence for cardiac stress during transurethral prostatectomy. British Medical Journal 1992; 304:666–670.

Hahn R. Prevention of TUR syndrome by detection of trace ethanol in the expired breath. Anaesthesia 1990; 45:577–581

Roos NE, Wennberg JE, Malenka DJ et al. Mortality and reoperation after open and transurethral resection of the prostate for benign prostatic hyperplasia. New England Journal of Medicine 1989; 320:1120–1123

19

20

VASCULAR SURGERY
A. J. Mortimer

Overview

A. J. Mortimer

Vascular surgery comprises the major operations of carotid endarterectomy, infrarenal aortic reconstruction and leg salvage by either arterial grafting or amputation of the distal limb when gangrene or infection is present.

The commonest underlying pathological condition is atherosclerotic disease of the main conducting arteries, often with associated aneurysm formation. The occlusive disease causes ischaemic symptoms when the oxygen delivery is insufficient to satisfy tissue oxygen consumption, whereas aneurysm formation causes pain due to stretching or acute rupture and the possibility of sudden death when the aorta is involved.

The commonest symptom of peripheral vascular disease is intermittent claudication, which occurs when blood flow is reduced by 75% or more (this corresponds to a 50% or more reduction in arterial diameter as seen on angiography). The presence of permanent rest pain in a leg indicates that blood flow is reduced by 90% or more, which corresponds to a 70% or greater reduction in arterial diameter as seen on an angiogram. A patient in this condition requires urgent treatment, usually amputation.

PATIENT CHARACTERISTICS

AGE

The majority of patients are between 60 and 80 years of age. Younger patients with severe arterial disease usually have a strong family history (genetic predisposition), diabetes mellitus or a history of heavy cigarette smoking.

SEX

Although the incidence of arterial disease is higher in males than females, the gap between the sexes is closing. This is attributed to the increased proportion of females who smoke.

SMOKING

Cigarette smoking is a major causative factor in the pathogenesis of atherosclerosis. More than 95% of patients are previous or present smokers.

MORTALITY

Both elective and emergency vascular operations have high morbidity and mortality rates (5–50%) because of the presence of co-existing cardiac, pulmonary or endocrine disease.

ASA PHYSICAL STATUS

Advanced age plus the presence of coexisting disease places patients into American Society of Anesthesiologists (ASA) group III (the majority), IV or V (ruptured aortic aneurysm).

COEXISTING DISEASE

Ischaemic heart disease (angina 15%, previous myocardial infarction 50%)

Approximately two-thirds of all patients have atherosclerotic disease of the coronary arteries. This manifests as angina or previous myocardial infarction (MI). Subendocardial infarction, as opposed to transmural infarction, is the most frequent problem and is more likely to occur in hypertensive patients. Perioperative MI occurs mostly in the first postoperative week. The incidence is highest on the third postoperative day and ranges from 3% to 8% in published series. Myocardial performance is the single most important determinant of outcome following a major vascular operation. Some 70% of all patients who experience a perioperative MI do not survive.

Hypertension (50%)

Hypertensive disease affects the conducting arteries supplying the heart, brain and kidneys, as well as the arteriolar resistance vessels throughout the circulation. In the heart this results in left ventricular hypertrophy, reduced ventricular compliance, and the need for filling pressures higher than normal to ensure adequate cardiac output. In the brain and kidneys, autoregulation of blood flow is shifted to the right, exposing these vital organs to reduced blood flow when the perfusion pressure is reduced. The widespread increase in arteriolar resistance means that patients manifest exaggerated

20

responses to excess induction agents (hypotension) and light anaesthesia (hypertension).

Heart failure (10%)
Failure of one or both ventricles occurs in up to 10% of patients. Left ventricular failure (pulmonary oedema) or right ventricular failure (dependent oedema) and associated symptoms must be treated prior to surgery. The pharmacological management of heart failure has improved markedly over recent years.

Pulmonary disease (25–50%)
Chronic obstructive pulmonary disease (COPD) is common because of the high incidence of smokers. Preoperative lung function tests are rarely of help as the symptoms are obvious. The most useful assessment of cardiorespiratory function is arterial blood gas estimation. Whilst hypoxia ($PaO_2 < 7$ kPa) is found occasionally, hypercarbia ($PaCO_2 > 7$ kPa) is uncommon. Regular use of nebulisers with or without physiotherapy should be considered.

Renal disease (5–10%)
Chronic renal failure caused by hypertensive disease, congestive cardiac failure, and renal artery stenosis and/or aneurysmal disease is detected by increased preoperative plasma concentrations of creatinine and urea. A baseline 24-h urinary creatinine clearance estimation is useful before aortic surgery is carried out.

Endocrine disease: diabetes mellitus (10%)
Diabetic patients comprise a large number of those undergoing peripheral arterial reconstruction. The microvascular circulation is affected predominantly and, as a consequence, revascularisation is sometimes inappropriate. Amputation of toes and limbs is commonly undertaken to control local infection, which may be affecting diabetic management adversely. Good control of blood glucose levels, adequate hydration and attention to blood loss are essential in the perioperative period. Insulin-dependent patients should be managed on an intravenous fluid and a sliding-scale insulin regimen. Patients taking oral antidiabetic agents should omit the dose on the morning of operation. These agents sometimes have a long duration of action (up to 24 h) and it is advisable to commence a glucose intravenous infusion with hourly blood glucose monitoring in order to avoid hypoglycaemia.

CONCURRENT MEDICATION

All patients are taking medication from one or more of the groups listed below:

- Antianginal agents
- Antihypertensive agents
- Antiarrhythmic drugs
- Antiplatelet drugs
- Anticoagulants
- Bronchodilators.

Usually, all medication should be continued during and after surgery, with the following exceptions:

- *Clopidogrel* – this antiplatelet drug appears to cause undue bleeding. It may be stopped up to 7 days before planned surgery.
- *Warfarin* – this anticoagulant needs to be stopped 3 days prior to planned surgery. Its therapeutic effect can be replaced with either intravenous heparin or subcutaneous unfractionated heparin.
- *Angiotensin-converting enzyme (ACE) inhibitors* – some authorities recommend that this type of drug be omitted on the day of operation to minimise hypotensive episodes.
- *Oral antidiabetic agents* – these must be omitted on the day of surgery. Monitoring of blood glucose concentration and good control (4–8 mmol l^{-1}) with intravenous insulin can be performed if necessary.

RECENT DEVELOPMENTS

CAROTID ANGIOPLASTY AND STENTING (CAS)
CAS has been compared to conventional carotid endarterectomy (CEA) and found to be more expensive and to have a higher stroke rate. CEA currently remains the treatment of choice for patients with symptomatic carotid artery disease.

AVOIDANCE OF PERIOPERATIVE HYPOTHERMIA
Mild perioperative hypothermia (34.0–36.5°C) is associated with significant adverse outcomes such as increased blood loss, wound infection and cardiac arrhythmias, plus prolonged duration of action of anaesthetic agents. All patients undergoing arterial surgery should be covered with a heated air warming blanket for the duration of the operation.

INTERNAL JUGULAR CANNULATION
Cannulation of the right internal jugular (RIJ) vein is routinely performed for operations where significant blood loss may occur. Because the RIJ is absent in 2.5% of the population, it is recommended that the vein be identified with a portable ultrasonographic device rather than relying on the landmark technique of RIJ location.

20

BIBLIOGRAPHY

Kaplan JA, ed. Vascular anaesthesia. New York: Churchill Livingstone; 1991

Mortimer AJ. Anaesthesia for vascular surgery. In: Healey TEJ, Cohen PJ, eds. A practice of anaesthesia. 6th edn. London: Edward Arnold; 1995:1119–1147

Smith G. Anaesthesia for vascular surgery. In: Bell PRF, Jamieson CCV, Ruckley CV, eds. Surgical management of vascular disease. London: WB Saunders; 1992:291–307

CROSS-REFERENCES

Diabetes Mellitus type 1
   Patient Conditions 2: 56
Diabetes Mellitus type 2
   Patient Conditions 2: 59
Preoperative assessment of cardiovascular risk in non-cardiac surgery 27: 634

20

Abdominal aortic reconstruction: open repair

J. M. Hopkinson and A. J. Mortimer

PROCEDURE

This is a major surgical procedure performed on a high-risk patient group, aimed at reducing the mortality rate from rupture (aneurysm) or the unpleasant symptoms of claudication (occlusive disease).

The procedure involves aortic cross-clamping with resultant haemodynamic and ischaemic complications. A tube graft (aneurysm) or a bifurcation graft (occlusive disease) is inserted below the origin of the renal arteries. The principal perioperative complication is myocardial infarction.

PREOPERATIVE ASSESSMENT AND INVESTIGATIONS

AIMS:
- Correct patient selection for surgery to improve outcome. Identify a low-risk subgroup – either no coronary artery disease or mild coronary artery disease with normal investigations.
- Optimise general condition by treating coexisting problems, particularly congestive cardiac failure, tachyarrhythmias and hypertension.
- Defer patients with a recent (less than 6 months) history of MI.
- On the basis of surgical and anaesthetic assessment, conservative management may be indicated.

GENERAL ASSESSMENT:
- Routine clinical assessment of cardiovascular and respiratory systems
- Full anaesthetic and drug history.

INVESTIGATIONS:
- Haemoglobin, platelets, white cell count
- Urea, creatinine, electrolytes, glucose
- Cross-match 6 units of blood
- Resting 12-lead ECG
- Chest radiography

- Respiratory function tests (peak expiratory flow rate (PEFR), forced expiratory volume in 1s/forced vital capacity (FEV_1/FVC) ratio) if history of chronic obstructive airway disease
- Echocardiography (left ventricular and valvular function, ejection fraction)
- Abdominal computed tomography to define diameter and the limits of the lesion.

Further investigations may be considered to quantify the degree of coronary artery disease and myocardial dysfunction.

FURTHER INVESTIGATIONS:
- Ambulatory 24-h ECG to detect conduction abnormalities and silent myocardial ischaemia
- Radionuclide dipyridamole–thallium scanning (MUGA scan) to detect abnormalities of coronary perfusion
- Angiography and coronary revascularisation prior to aortic surgery, if indicated, by the presence of severe coronary artery disease
- Carotid artery surgery prior to aneurysm repair if asymptomatic with > 90% stenosis or symptomatic with > 70% stenosis.

Arrange for HDU or ITU bed for postoperative cardiorespiratory monitoring and provision of optimal analgesia.

PREMEDICATION

- Explanation to the patient about the procedure, anaesthetic management and postoperative care
- Anxiolytic drugs (amnesic properties useful) – for example temazepam or lorazepam
- Continue usual cardiac medication, especially antianginal and antihypertensive drugs – consider omission of ACE inhibitors and stop clopidogrel
- Administer a beta-blocker for 2 days before surgery (e.g. atenolol 25–50 mg) – has been shown to reduce morbidity and mortality rates

20

- Aspirin (cyclo-oxygenase 1 and 2 inhibitor) may be continued through the perioperative period, but clopidogrel (phosphodiesterase inhibitor) should be stopped before operation to minimise blood loss.

PERIOPERATIVE MANAGEMENT

ANAESTHETIC ROOM:
- Reassure patient, maintain a calm environment
- Oxygen (2 l min^{-1}) via a Hudson mask
- Establish initial monitoring:
  —ECG
  —pulse oximetry
  —invasive arterial pressure line inserted under local analgesia (radial artery)
  —central venous pressure (CVP) catheter or pulmonary artery (PA) catheter in the right internal jugular vein (preferably ultrasonographically assisted). A PA catheter is generally reserved for patients with a very poor left ventricle to assist with optimising filling pressures (ejection fraction < 30%).

A useful technique is to insert a PA catheter sheath at the same time as a CVP multilumen line. A PA catheter can then be inserted without delay if required perioperatively.

Regional techniques for perioperative and postoperative use (epidural) should be performed well before heparin is administered (may be done awake or anaesthetised).

INDUCTION OF ANAESTHESIA:
- Preoxygenate the patient
- Maintain haemodynamic stability during induction and tracheal intubation
- Insert a nasogastric tube – postoperative ileus is common
- Insert a urinary catheter to monitor urine output.

MAINTENANCE OF ANAESTHESIA:
- A balanced anaesthetic technique with intermittent positive-pressure ventilation (IPPV) to normocapnia is required to promote cardiovascular stability.
- Total intravenous anaesthesia (TIVA) using propofol and remifentanil, or inhalational anaesthesia with a volatile agent (isoflurane or sevoflurane) and intravenous opioids, are suitable techniques.
- Remifentanil infusions have the benefit of assisting with rapid control of cardiovascular parameters.

- Sevoflurane may confer benefits over isoflurane – less likely to cause tachycardia and hypotension, both of which impair myocardial oxygen delivery. In prolonged procedures, however, metabolism of sevoflurane can lead to significant fluoride ion production (care regarding renal function), but this does not appear to be a practical problem.
- Regional anaesthesia and analgesia may be used in combination with either TIVA or volatile agent techniques.
- Vasopressors or vasodilators may be required (metaraminol or glyceryl trinitrate).
- Heat loss must be minimised by humidifying inspiratory gases, warming intravenous fluids, and using a warming mattress and heated air blanket.

INTRAOPERATIVE MONITORING:
- ECG – leads II and V5 with ST segment analysis for early detection of subendocardial ischaemia
- Sa_{O_2}
- Capnography
- Fi_{O_2}
- Volatile agent
- Core temperature
- Invasive arterial pressure
- CVP
- PA and pulmonary artery wedge pressure (PAWP) if severe left ventricular dysfunction identified before surgery (ejection fraction < 30%)
- Oesophageal Doppler imaging (non-invasive haemodynamic parameters) – in place of a PA catheter – monitors the response to cross-clamping and release, and guides fluid and vasoactive or inotropic drug administration
- Fluid balance – intravenous fluids and measured blood loss and urine output.

POSITIONING
Supine with arms out for access (care to avoid brachial plexus injury). Potential pressure areas padded. Table break may be required.

SPECIFIC POINTS:
- Antibiotic prophylaxis (cefuroxime 1.5 g intravenously or similar broad-spectrum drug).
- Heparinisation (5000 units) is generally requested prior to aortic cross-clamping.
- Have a vasodilator (e.g. glyceryl trinitrate) and a vasopressor (e.g. metaraminol) available.

20

- Aortic cross-clamping produces a marked increase in left ventricular afterload in patients with aneurysmal disease. It is not generally a problem in patients with occlusive aortoiliac disease who have a well developed lumbar collateral circulation. An increased left ventricular end-diastolic pressure may precipitate myocardial ischaemia due to reduced coronary blood flow. Techniques for management include:
  —Regional technique with subsequent sympathetic block reduces the response to cross-clamping.
  —Add or increase the inspired concentration of volatile agent (e.g. isoflurane). This will produce a dose-dependent reduction in myocardial contractility and help off-load the heart by dilatation of vascular beds proximal to the cross-clamp.
  —In TIVA, increase the infusion rate of propofol and/or remifentanil.
  —Use an infusion of a vasodilator (e.g. glyceryl trinitrate).
- Aortic cross-clamp release may cause profound hypotension and myocardial ischaemia. Techniques for management include:
  —Prior to cross-clamp release, volume-load the patient, guided by either CVP/PAWP (to approximately 5 mmHg above baseline value) or oesophageal Doppler measurements.
  —Request controlled cross-clamp release by the surgeon.
  —Rapid fluid infusion guided by cardiovascular monitoring.
  —Use a vasopressor if necessary (e.g. metaraminol).
- In elective surgery, blood loss is usually between 2 and 4 units. Although it is routine practice in many hospitals for 6 units of homologous blood to be cross-matched, the need for blood transfusion can be reduced by the following measures:
  —Normovolaemic haemodilution following induction of anaesthesia (up to 3 units)
  —Use of intraoperative red cell salvage
  —Acceptance of postoperative haemoglobin concentration as low as 80 g l^{-1}.
- In the few instances where blood loss is great, the need for fresh frozen plasma and platelets needs to be considered.

POSTOPERATIVE MANAGEMENT

- HDU or ITU care is required, depending on the operation and the patient's co-morbidity.
- A short period of ventilatory support may be required in high-risk patients to enable haemodynamic stability, normothermia and adequate analgesia to be attained.
- Supplementary face-mask oxygen should be administered for a minimum of 3 days after surgery, ideally.
- Chest physiotherapy should be commenced early in an attempt to minimise basal atelectasis and sputum retention.

ANALGESIA
There are various suitable techniques – these may be used alone or in combination:
- Regional analgesia – local, with or without opioid:
  —continuous epidural infusion analgesia (CEA) – a widely used technique
  —patient-controlled epidural analgesia (PCEA) – a widely used technique
  —bolus epidural administration
  —continuous spinal analgesia (spinal catheter).
- Systemic analgesia:
  —intravenous or intramuscular opioids
  —patient-controlled intravenous analgesia (PCA).
- Wound infiltration with local anaesthetic by the surgeon
- Regular paracetamol in addition to any of the above regimens (avoid non-steroidal anti-inflammatory drugs (NSAIDs) because of potential for renal impairment) to provide opiate-sparing effect.
- Bilateral intercostal nerve blocks – may be repeated (risk of pneumothorax).

POSTOPERATIVE COMPLICATIONS

SURGICAL:
- Ischaemic limb due to embolisation
- Haemorrhage from graft anastomosis
- Ischaemia of the gastrointestinal tract
- Graft or wound infection
- Return to theatre may be required with all the attendant risks.

MEDICAL:
- Subendocardial ischaemia and myocardial infarction
- Renal failure – depends on preoperative renal function, site of cross-clamping, and

20

postoperative respiratory and cardiac function
- Pulmonary complications – basal atelectasis, sputum retention, hypoxaemia, respiratory failure.

OUTCOME

- The mortality rate ranges from 5% to 15% (compare with the rate for adult elective cardiac surgery of 1–3%).
- Outcome depends on age, coexisting disease and the nature of the surgical procedure.
- Perioperative myocardial infarction is the principal cause of death.

BIBLIOGRAPHY

Cunningham AJ. Anaesthesia for abdominal aortic surgery – a review (Part 1). Canadian Journal of Anaesthesia 1989; 36:426–444

Cunningham AJ. Anaesthesia for abdominal aortic surgery – a review (Part 2). Canadian Journal of Anaesthesia 1989; 36:568–577

Hessell EA. Intraoperative management of abdominal aortic aneurysms: the anaesthesiologist's viewpoint. Surgical Clinics of North America 1989; 69:775–793

Mortimer AJ. Anaesthesia for vascular surgery. In: Healy TEJ, Cohen PJ, eds. A practice of anaesthesia. 6th edn. London: Edward Arnold; 1995:1119–1147

CROSS-REFERENCES

Preoperative assessment of cardiovascular risk in non-cardiac surgery
    Patient Conditions 4: 129
Coronary artery disease
    Anaesthetic Factors 27: 634

20

Abdominal aortic reconstruction: endovascular aneurysm repair (EVAR)

S. L. Wilmshurst and A. J. Mortimer

INTRODUCTION

Endovascular aneurysm surgery provides an alternative to conventional open abdominal repair. The technique was first described in 1969 and was first used clinically in 1990. Peripheral, thoracic and abdominal aneurysms, diffuse aortoiliac occlusive disease, arterial dissections and traumatic lesions have all been repaired using the endovascular technique. Although there are obvious initial advantages, long-term outcome is unclear and local vascular complication rates appear to be higher than with conventional open repair.

ADVANTAGES OVER OPEN REPAIR:
- Surgically less invasive (no abdominal wound)
- Consequent reduced anaesthetic and analgesic requirements
- Reduced aortic cross-clamp-associated cardiovascular instability
- Reduced blood loss
- Reduced visceral manipulation with minimal postoperative ileus
- Much earlier eating, ambulation and discharge (only 3–4 days compared with 7–8 days for open repair).

PATIENT SELECTION:
- Patients have the same high-risk profile as for open surgical repair.
- Each patient must meet the anatomical criteria for endovascular aneurysm repair (EVAR).
- Specific aneurysm characteristics:
  —a straight aneurysm neck more than 15 mm below the origin of the renal arteries
  —minimal artherosclerotic plaque inside the neck to enable a good seal to be made between the stent graft and the wall of the aorta
  —relatively disease-free ileofemoral vessels with good run-off

  —one of the femoral arteries should exceed 8 mm in diameter to enable the collapsed stent to be inserted (diameter up to 7.5 mm).
- Approximately one-third of infrarenal aneurysms meet these criteria.

SURGICAL TECHNIQUE

- The procedure may be performed in an X-ray department or operating room, depending on local provision of space and facilities.
- Fluoroscopic equipment is bulky and takes up floor space.
- The procedure is usually performed jointly by a surgeon and radiologist.
- Preparation must be made for open repair and dealing with complications.
- Surgical access is made via bilateral femoral arteriotomies.
- Proximal dissection to the iliac vessels may be necessary.
- A guidewire is inserted under fluoroscopic guidance, after which:
  —the stent–graft delivery system is inserted over the guidewire and advanced to the diseased segment, where it is deployed
  —rarely, access to the left axillary artery may be required to gain access above the aneurysm.

COMPLICATIONS:
- Arterial rupture
- Aortic injury from instruments, occlusion or embolisation
- Distal organ embolisation
- Renal injury from radiographic contrast or ischaemia
- Conversion to open repair (3% – high mortality rate)
- Endoluminal leaks from either proximal or distal anastomosis

20

- Postimplantation syndrome – fever, leukocytosis, raised C-reactive protein (CRP) level; rarely disseminated intravascular coagulation (DIC) and shock.

OUTCOME:
- 80% successful
- 4-year survival rate 77%
- High incidence of subsequent interventions due to leaks.

ANAESTHETIC CONSIDERATIONS

MAJOR GOALS:
- Anaesthesia required for surgical access of the femoral arteries
- Local and systemic analgesia
- Haemodynamic stability.

ASSESSMENT
As for open repair.

PREPARATION:
- Explanation of technique and anaesthetic to patient
- Consent for regional anaesthesia and documentation of risks
- Anxiolysis and premedication (temazepam), including usual cardiac medication except for ACE inhibitors and antiplatelet or anticoagulant drugs, which may be omitted on day of operation.

TECHNIQUES
Options include:
- Local infiltration anaesthesia with sedation
- Regional anaesthesia – spinal, epidural or combined spinal–epidural
- Light general anaesthesia plus regional anaesthesia
- General anaesthesia.

The procedure can be as short as 1.5 h, but may be up to 5 h if complicated or difficult and, although minimally invasive, a regional anaesthetic technique is usually required. Spinal anaesthesia alone or epidural anaesthesia may be considered, but a combined spinal–epidural (CSE) technique is most appropriate as the procedure may outlast the duration of single-shot spinal blockade. The offset of the spinal may be delayed by the addition of diamorphine or by giving a larger dose than usual of local anaesthetic drug.

General anaesthesia may be required to supplement regional block, for extensive groin dissection or upper-limb access sites, or for uncooperative patients.

MONITORING:
- Intra-arterial blood pressure via the right radial artery
- Urine output
- Core temperature
- Usual monitoring as for any anaesthetic – cardiorespiratory and anaesthetic delivery parameters.

POSTOPERATIVE:
- Nurse on HDU for first 24 h
- Analgesia requirement is usually minimal
- Early mobilisation (next day).

BIBLIOGRAPHY

Baxendale BR, Hutchinson A, Chuter TA, Wenham PW, Hopkinson BR. Haemodynamic and metabolic response to endovascular repair of infra-renal aortic aneurysms. British Journal of Anaesthesia 1996; 77:581–585

Khan RA, Moskowitz DM: Endovascular aortic repair. Journal of Cardiothoracic and Vascular Anesthesia 2002; 16:218–233

Linerberger CK, Robertson KM. Vascular stenting. Current Opinion in Anaesthesiology 2002; 15:37–44

CROSS-REFERENCES

Preoperative assessment of cardiovascular risk in non-cardiac surgery
    Anaesthetic Factors 27: 634
Coronary artery disease
    Patient Conditions 4: 129
Abdominal aortic recombination-open repair
    Surgical Procedures 30: 497

20

Abdominal aortic reconstruction: emergency repair

J. M. Hopkinson and A. J. Mortimer

PROCEDURE

A ruptured or leaking aortic aneurysm is fatal if untreated. Emergency repair is the patient's only chance of survival. Patients, by definition, are ASA grade IV or V (E) and urgent operation in a specialist unit is required. Rapid decisions by experienced surgeons and anaesthetists need to be made on the benefit of surgery because the mortality rate is high, even in specialist units – 50% or more.

PREOPERATIVE ASSESSMENT AND INVESTIGATIONS

- Identify patients for whom surgery is appropriate – criteria such as age, premorbid condition, response to initial resuscitation and urine output may be useful.
- Formal detailed assessment and investigations are rarely possible, but attempts should be made to establish the severity of any coexisting disease. Recent hospital admissions and their documented findings in hospital records may prove useful.
- Portable abdominal ultrasonography can be useful, if time permits.
- A 12-lead ECG may be helpful where a differential diagnosis of aneurysm leak or rupture and massive myocardial infarction is being considered.
- While assessing the patient, establish reliable intravenous access with two large-bore peripheral venous cannulae (14 G). If feasible, insert a percutaneous pulmonary artery catheter sheath in the right internal jugular vein (preferably ultrasonographically assisted).
- Send blood for haemoglobin, platelets, baseline coagulation tests, and urea and electrolytes. Baseline renal function measurement is useful for postoperative management.
- Request urgent cross-match of 12 units blood and 4 units fresh frozen plasma.
- Use crystalloid or colloid solutions to maintain a systolic arterial pressure greater than 80 mmHg and transfer to the theatre suite. There is little to be gained by increasing the blood pressure above 100 mmHg, as the incidence of haemorrhage may be increased.
- Insert an indwelling urinary catheter.

PERIOPERATIVE MANAGEMENT

- Notify ITU of the potential need for a bed.
- Ideally have two anaesthetists to manage the case in theatre, although the procedure may need to commence while awaiting arrival of the second anaesthetist.
- Transfer the patient into the operating theatre, with high-flow face-mask oxygen.
- Try to reassure a terrified patient and explain what is happening.
- No time should be wasted in attempting to set up invasive arterial monitoring or central venous lines at the beginning; it is important for the surgeon to cross-clamp the aorta as soon as possible.
- Colloid, blood, blood products and rapid infusers with warming coils should be prepared for use.
- Draw up induction drugs and have available a vasopressor (metaraminol) and an inotrope (adrenaline, epinephrine).
- The anaesthetist leads the theatre team and needs to ensure that the patient is on a warming mattress, on the operating table with both arms out, that the surgeons and assistants are scrubbed, and that all anaesthetic equipment is available prior to induction.
- When the patient has been prepared and draped for surgery and is preoxygenated with 100% oxygen, the anaesthetic can commence.

20

INDUCTION:

- Use a standard rapid sequence induction with minimum dose of induction agent, as in any hypovolaemic patient. An opioid-based induction with fentanyl or remifentanil may have fewer cardiodepressant effects.
- As soon as the airway is secure, instruct the surgeon to proceed.
- Anticipate sudden hypotension as the abdominal tamponade effect is lost at laparotomy.

MAINTENANCE:

- A balanced anaesthetic technique with IPPV and 100% oxygen (initially) is appropriate.
- Fentanyl and small increments of volatile agent can be used. There is probably little to choose between isoflurane and sevoflurane in these circumstances.
- Alternatively TIVA with propofol and remifentanil can be used.
- When the aorta has been cross-clamped, a degree of haemodynamic stability can usually be obtained, and this period is suitable for the insertion of invasive monitoring lines.
- Heat loss must be minimised by humidifying inspiratory gases, warming intravenous fluids, using a warming mattress and heated air blanket.
- A nasogastric tube is required because postoperative ileus is common.
- Recheck patient positioning with specific reference to brachial plexus (both arms out) and all pressure points.

INTRAOPERATIVE MONITORING:

- ECG – leads II and V5 with ST segment analysis – early detection of subendocardial ischaemia
- SaO_2 – limitations in hypovolaemic patients with poor peripheral perfusion
- Capnography – indication of changes in cardiac output; care required in interpreting values, which will not accurately reflect arterial carbon dioxide in these shocked patients
- FiO_2
- Volatile agent
- Core temperature
- Invasive arterial pressure
- CVP
- Rarely, a pulmonary artery (PA) and wedge pressure to guide therapy in patients with suspected left ventricular dysfunction – may be required after operation

- Oesophageal Doppler imaging (non-invasive haemodynamic parameters) – in place of a PA catheter; monitors the response to haemorrhage, cross-clamp release, fluid and vasoactive or inotropic drug administration
- Fluid balance – intravenous fluids and measured blood loss and urine output
- Arterial blood gases, haematocrit and haemoglobin, coagulation profile and serum potassium level.

SPECIFIC POINTS:

- Antibiotic prophylaxis – cefuroxime 1.5 g or similar.
- Haemorrhage, continuing during surgery, is common and large volumes of blood may need to be administered. A dilutional coagulopathy may occur and require correction with fresh frozen plasma and platelets. The use of the antifibrinolytic agent aprotinin may need to be considered.
- Cross-clamp release may cause severe hypotension despite best efforts to replace blood loss.
- Controlled cross-clamp release by the surgeon is the best option. Further fluid and vasopressor or inotropic support can be administered, guided by trends in invasive and/or oesophageal Doppler monitoring.

POSTOPERATIVE MANAGEMENT

- Transfer to ITU with continued ventilatory support.
- Attain haemodynamic stability, normothermia and correct coagulopathy if present.
- Formulate a plan for analgesia. Initially this is usually an intravenous opioid regimen. Regional analgesia may be considered after correction of coagulopathies and will depend on the risk : benefit assessment for the particular patient.
- Extubate when the patient's condition allows. Continuous humidified face-mask oxygen and frequent physiotherapy will be necessary, possibly for several days.
- Close monitoring of renal function is required as renal failure occurs commonly in this patient group.
- Recovery depends on the success of the surgical repair and the occurrence of complications such as myocardial infarction, respiratory failure and renal failure.

20

POSTOPERATIVE COMPLICATIONS

SURGICAL:
- Uncontrollable haemorrhage.
- Limb ischaemia due to embolisation.
- Gastrointestinal or spinal cord ischaemia.

MEDICAL:
- Myocardial infarction.
- Hypoxaemic lung failure which may progess to adult respiratory distress syndrome.
- Renal failure.

OUTCOME

- The mortality rate among patients who undergo emergency surgery is 60% or more.
- It is imperative that patients are not subjected to operation when there is no real hope of survival. Patient selection is difficult: only experienced surgeons and anaesthetists should be involved in the care of these patients.
- Effective analgesia and nursing care should be provided for patients in whom operation is not appropriate, so they may die peacefully and with dignity.

BIBLIOGRAPHY

Cunningham AJ. Anaesthesia for repair of abdominal aortic aneurysms. In: Atkinson RS, Adams AP, eds. Recent advances in anaesthesia and analgesia. London: Churchill Livingstone; 1992:49–69

Mortimer AJ. Anaesthesia for vascular surgery. In: Healey REJ, Cohen PJ, eds. A practice of anaesthesia. 6th edn. London: Edward Arnold; 1995:1119–1147

Rutherford RB, McCroskey BL. Ruptured abdominal aortic aneurysms: special considerations. Surgical Clinics of North America 1989; 69:859–868

CROSS-REFERENCES

Preoperative assessment of cardiovascular risk in non-cardiac surgery
    Anaesthetic Factors 27: 634
Blood transfusion
    Anaesthetic Factors 31: 729
Massive transfusion
    Patient Conditions 7: 214
Disseminated intravascular coagulation
    Patient Conditions 7: 205

20

Leg revascularisation and amputations

J. M. Hopkinson and A. J. Mortimer

PROCEDURES

Various surgical bypass techniques are used in an attempt to revascularise legs that are ischaemic as a result of occlusive vascular disease:

- Acute ischaemia due to an embolism is often dealt with by femoral embolectomy – local infiltration anaesthesia is generally used for this procedure.
- Chronic ischaemia due to atheromatous disease requires bypass procedures to improve blood flow to distal regions.
- Aortoiliac disease may require an aortic bifurcation graft (see section on Abdominal aortic reconstruction – open repair).
- The procedure commonly encountered is femoropopliteal bypass, although many variations are performed. Axillofemoral bypass is generally reserved for the high-risk patient with severe occlusive aortic disease.
- Usually prolonged procedures in a high-risk patient group, although the operation is relatively non-invasive.
- Patients may present for repeated procedures in an attempt to salvage ischaemic limbs, sometimes culminating in progressive proximal amputation in the following sequence: (1) toes, (2) forefoot, (3) below knee, (4) above knee.
- Diabetic patients are frequently encountered. Infected and necrotic tissue disturbs blood sugar control and amputation can be life-saving.
- A high proportion of patients with peripheral vascular disease are heavy smokers.

PREOPERATIVE INVESTIGATION AND ASSESSMENT

AIMS:

- Optimise general condition by treating coexisting problems, in particular congestive cardiac failure, tachyarrhythmias, hypertension and respiratory disease. Diabetics should have their blood glucose level tightly controlled, between 6 and 8 mmol l^{-1}.
- Formulate the anaesthetic management plan according to the findings and risk assessment.

GENERAL ASSESSMENT:

- Routine clinical assessment of cardiovascular and respiratory systems
- Full anaesthetic and drug history.
- Investigations:
  —haemoglobin, platelets and white cell count
  —blood group and save serum
  —urea, creatinine, electrolytes and glucose
  —coagulation studies if indicated by drug therapy
  —resting 12-lead ECG
  —recent chest radiography
  —respiratory function tests – peak expiratory flow rate, FEV_1/FVC if history of chronic obstructive airway disease or smoking
  —echocardiography if indicated (e.g. known aortic stenosis or suspected poor left ventricular function).

PREMEDICATION

- Discuss the procedure and anaesthetic management with the patient.
- Consider the use of an anxiolytic drug, for instance a benzodiazepine such as temazepam.
- Sedative drugs may be avoided in some already obtunded patients.
- Continue the usual cardiac and respiratory medication.
- Intravenous management of diabetes, where appropriate.
- A perioperative plan needs to be made for the management of anticoagulant medication.

PERIOPERATIVE MANAGEMENT

The choice of anaesthetic technique will depend on anaesthetic expertise, the individual patient and the particular procedure, including likely duration of surgery. The options are:

- General anaesthesia – spontaneous respiration or controlled ventilation (volatile agent or TIVA)
- Regional anaesthesia – single-shot spinal, continuous spinal or epidural anaesthesia (local anaesthetic with or without opioids)
- Combined general and regional anaesthesia
- Local anaesthesia with femoral and sciatic nerve blocks
- General anaesthesia combined with femoral and sciatic nerve blocks.

There is probably little to chose between the above techniques for the majority of patients. However, a regional technique (spinal or epidural) is better than general anaesthesia for amputations because of effective initial analgesia. Of paramount importance is the maintenance of haemodynamic stability and adequate oxygenation during anaesthesia and surgery.

Factors that need consideration are the severity of coexisting cardiovascular and respiratory disease. This may be particularly important; for example, in a patient with severe aortic stenosis and poor lung function an incremental regional block using a spinal catheter may be an appropriate technique.

ANAESTHETIC ROOM

- Patient reassurance and a calm environment
- Commence monitoring – ECG, pulse oximetry and non-invasive blood pressure are adequate in most cases. Invasive arterial pressure monitoring may be required in some high-risk cardiac patients, such as those with aortic stenosis
- Intravenous access
- Induction of general or regional anaesthesia maintaining oxygenation and cardiovascular stability.

OPERATING THEATRE

MAINTENANCE OF ANAESTHESIA:

- Balanced anaesthetic technique – if general anaesthesia, use a volatile agent (isoflurane or sevoflurane) and opioid or TIVA (propofol and remifentanil). Sevoflurane may confer benefit over isoflurane in having less tendency to cause tachycardia and hypotension.
- Maintain cardiovascular stability.
- Heat loss must be minimised during a prolonged procedure by humidifying inspiratory gases, warming intravenous fluids, and using a warming mattress and heated air blanket.
- Blood loss is usually minimal.
- Surgeon will request intravenous heparin (5000 units) for reconstructive procedures.
- Antibiotic prophylaxis – cefuroxime 0.75–1.5 g intravenously

MONITORING:

- ECG – leads II and V5 with ST segment analysis; early detection of subendocardial ischaemia
- Sao_2
- Capnography (and volatile agent)
- Fio_2
- Non-invasive blood pressure (invasive where indicated).

POSTOPERATIVE MANAGEMENT

- Observe in a recovery area until stable and adequate analgesia established
- Oxygen via face-mask – for 3 days in the high-risk patient
- Chest physiotherapy in appropriate cases.

ANALGESIA

There are various suitable techniques:

- Regional analgesia – local analgesia with or without opioid:
  —continuous epidural infusion
  —bolus epidural administration
  —patient-controlled epidural analgesia
  —spinal opioid – long-acting (e.g. diamorphine)
  —continuous spinal analgesia – spinal catheter.
- Systemic analgesia:
  —intravenous opioid infusion
  —patient-controlled intravenous analgesia.

Paracetamol and NSAIDs may be given concurrently (care with NSAID and renal function). Patients undergoing amputation, in particular, benefit from the excellent analgesia afforded by the regional techniques. Consider instituting regional anaesthesia before operation in patients with significant rest pain.

20

POSTOPERATIVE COMPLICATIONS

SURGICAL:
- Persistent ischaemia causing severe pain
- Progression to gangrene with localised or systemic infection
- Reoperation may be required, including amputation
- Poor wound healing predisposing to infection
- Reperfusion injury following revascularisation of the critically ischaemic limb.

MEDICAL:
- Myocardial ischaemia or infarction
- Problematic diabetic control
- Respiratory problems – atelectasis, retention of secretions and hypoxaemia.

OUTCOME

- Outcome depends on the successful bypassing of the obstructions and the severity of the distal arterial disease.
- Multiple procedures and anaesthetics are often required in this high-risk patient group.
- All too often the result is the requirement to amputate the limb of a patient with ASA grade 4 because of severe rest pain and/or gangrene.

- Risk increases with the number of procedures carried out.
- Analgesia should be given high priority to minimise patient suffering.
- The mortality rate from leg amputation is high (25%), as this is a near end of life operation.

BIBLIOGRAPHY

Christopherson R, Beattie C, Frank SM et al. Perioperative morbidity in patients randomised to epidural or general anaesthesia for lower extremity vascular surgery. Anesthesiology 1993; 79:422–434

Foex P, Reeder MK. Anaesthesia for vascular surgery. Baillieres Clinical Anaesthesiology 1993; 7:97–126

Ruckley CV. Amputations in peripheral vascular disease. Hospital Update 1992; 1:126–133

CROSS-REFERENCES

Diabetes Mellitus type 1
    Patient Conditions 2: 56
Preoperative assessment of cardiovascular risk in non-cardiac surgery
    Anaesthetic Factors 27: 634

20

Carotid endarterectomy

S. L. Wilmshurst and A. J. Mortimer

Carotid artery disease causes symptoms of cerebral ischaemia which may be reversible (transient ischaemic attacks; TIAs) or irreversible (stroke or cerebrovascular accident; CVA). It is caused by atheromatous plaques in the carotid vessels, thereby narrowing the arterial lumen and resulting in a reduction in blood flow or causing platelet or clot embolism into the distant cerebral vessels. Carotid endarterectomy is a prophylactic operation but carries high morbidity and mortality rates due to the patient population and operative complications. Consequently, risk–benefit analysis is important in patient selection.

Controversy exists in the fields of patient selection, anaesthetic technique (local or general) and cerebral monitoring during operation.

PRESENTATION

- Incidental, asymptomatic finding during the investigation of arterial disease
- TIAs – lasting less than 24 h
- Reversible ischaemic neurological deficit – lasting less than 3 weeks
- Permanent ischaemic neurological deficit (stroke, CVA)
- Stroke has a 30% 1-year mortality rate.

PATIENT SELECTION

ASYMPTOMATIC PATIENTS:

- Asymptomatic carotid artery surgery – showed benefit if stenosis greater than 60% in low-risk male patients only. This criterion is used mostly by surgeons in North America.

SYMPTOMATIC PATIENTS:

- North American Symptomatic Carotid Endarterectomy Trial (NASCET) – patients with more than 70% stenosis and TIAs show clear benefit from surgery
- European Carotid Surgery Trial (ECST) – no benefit if less than 30% stenosis even with symptoms; unclear benefit if stenosis

30–69%, but significantly reduced stroke incidence in patients with more than 70% stenosis.

SURGICAL PROCEDURE

- Reverse Trendelenburg position – head up with feet up to minimise venous pooling
- Head turned away from operating side
- Shoulders raised with support between shoulder blades
- Head ring
- Incision along anterior border of sternomastoid muscle between ear and sternal notch
- Carotid and internal jugular vessels are dissected
- Heparin 5000 i.u. after exposure of the common carotid and bifurcation
- Cross-clamps applied sequentially to the common, internal and external carotid arteries
- The need for a shunt (common to internal carotid artery bypass) to be inserted is determined either by surgical preference or from the estimated magnitude of cerebral perfusion as given by cerebral monitoring (awake patient, local anaesthesia; transcranial Doppler imaging, general anaesthesia)
- After the endarterectomy, the artery is either repaired directly or a patch angioplasty is performed
- Following arterial repair the arterial clamps are removed sequentially from the external, common and internal carotid arteries. This sequence is used to prevent any debris from entering the cerebral circulation.

POSTOPERATIVE PROBLEMS

- Neurological deficit (3%)
- Altered blood pressure regulation. The pressure may be higher or lower than before operation

20

- Wound haematoma
- Tracheal compression and deviation
- Cranial nerve damage.

ANAESTHESIA

GOALS:
- Maintenance of adequate cerebral blood flow
- Maintenance of normal blood pressure, PaO_2 and $PaCO_2$ throughout the procedure
- Avoidance of cardiac ischaemia and infarction.

PREOPERATIVE ASSESSMENT:
- Ischaemic heart disease – 60% have asymptomatic coronary artery disease. Perioperative MI occurs in up to 3% of patients, and the degree of carotid stenosis correlates with the incidence of perioperative myocardial ischaemia. Assessment of the patient is covered elsewhere (see section in Ch. 27 on Preoperative assessment of cardiovascular risk in non-cardiac surgery).
- Cerebrovascular disease – the severity of preoperative symptoms is a predictor of the risk of stroke.
- Age and sex – advancing age correlates with an increased incidence of cardiac and neurological complications, as does female sex.
- Hypertension – systolic blood pressure greater than 180 mmHg increases the risk of stroke and postoperative death.
- Diabetes and renal failure are relatively common.

ANAESTHETIC TECHNIQUE
The choice of anaesthetic technique is controversial with either general or local anaesthesia being the preferred technique in different centres. General anaesthesia reduces cerebral oxygen consumption the most. However, postoperative neurological deficits are usually due to emboli rather than ischaemic events. Cerebral autoregulation is impaired by volatile anaesthetic agents, but the stress response to surgery is suppressed, providing some protection from cardiac ischaemia.

Local anaesthesia allows the patient's cerebral function to be monitored constantly, providing 'gold standard' cerebral function monitoring. Blood pressure and therefore cerebral perfusion are largely unaltered, but the patient may exhibit a greater stress response, and cerebral and cardiac oxygen consumption may be increased, causing ischaemic complications.

PREMEDICATION
Avoid long-acting agents such as lorazepam. Short-acting benzodiazepines are preferable when premedication is required.

CAROTID ENDARTERECTOMY UNDER GENERAL ANAESTHESIA

Induction:
- Avoid hypotension by choice of induction agent (etomidate) and its slow administration
- Blunt hypertensive responses to laryngoscopy and intubation with fentanyl.

Maintenance:
- Isoflurane and sevoflurane are agents of choice.
- Nitrous oxide is safe but does not need to be used. An air–oxygen mixture is preferable.

Muscle relaxants:
- Avoids the need for high-dose volatile agents.

Opioids:
- Low incidence of postoperative pain – only a superficial surgical procedure
- Small doses of opioids required – no need for more than 200 μg fentanyl
- Remifentanil infusion is ideal.

Equipment:
- Normal or armoured tracheal tube, depending on local preferences
- Warming equipment for operating table, intravenous fluids and hot air blanket for patient
- Non-glucose-containing fluids (Hartmann's solution ideal)
- Vasoactive agents – mostly vasopressors such as ephedrine, metaraminol or adrenaline (epinephrine) for increasing the blood pressure during general anaesthesia.

Monitoring:
- Standard – ECG, FiO_2, SaO_2, $EtCO_2$ and volatile agent
- Intra-arterial blood pressure
- Cerebral function monitors:
  —awake patient – 'gold standard' monitor during local anaesthesia
  —stump pressure and waveform – not reliable and no longer widely used

—transcranial Doppler imaging
—cerebral oximetry
—EEG or processed EEG
—somatosensory evoked potentials
—jugular venous oxygen saturation.

With the exception of the awake patient, cerebral function monitoring requires dedicated equipment and accompanying technical staff. In the awake patient, no new neurological symptoms following a test clamp of 1 min indicates adequate collateral flow.

Special considerations:
• Cross-clamping requires a 10–20% increase in mean arterial pressure (MAP) to preserve cerebral perfusion pressure (CPP).
• Surgical stimulation of the carotid sinus may cause bradycardia plus hypotension and rarely asystole. This can be treated with anticholinergics drugs or prevented by injection of lidocaine (lignocaine) around the carotid sinus nerve, or by asking the surgeon to cease operating temporarily.

Postoperative care:
• HDU, ideally for 24 h, to observe cerebral and cardiovascular function
• Direct arterial monitoring continued for 4–6 h.

CAROTID ENDARTERECTOMY UNDER LOCAL ANAESTHESIA

Currently, there is no overwhelming evidence for better results with either general or local anaesthesia.

Advantages:
• Reliable cerebral monitor
• Better postoperative recovery
• Less blood pressure fluctuation
• Lower incidence of MI
• Fewer vasoactive drugs required because of blood pressure stability.

Disadvantages:
• Patient and surgeon cooperation required
• Discomfort or restlessness during operation necessitating intravenous sedation
• Higher perioperative blood pressure
• Loss of control if cerebral ischaemia occurs with difficulty controlling the airway.

Technique of local anaesthesia
C2–C4 blockade by:
• Deep cervical plexus block
• Superficial cervical plexus block
• Combination of the above
• Cervical epidural.

Deep cervical plexus block:
• Head turned away, neck extended
• Palpate C2 transverse process below mastoid and C6 at level of cricoid
• C3 and C4 are at 2-cm intervals along line joining the above
• 5–8 ml local anaesthetic at each of C2, C3 and C4
• Major complications include phrenic nerve block, vertebral artery injection and injection into the cerebrospinal fluid.

Superficial cervical plexus block
Infiltrate along posterior border of sternomastoid muscle. Usually this block alone is sufficient, with additional analgesia being provided by local injection by the surgeon.

COMBINATION OF GENERAL AND LOCAL ANAESTHESIA

An alternative technique is to use superficial a cervical plexus block in combination with a light general anaesthesia. This is the technique favoured in the authors' centre.

BIBLIOGRAPHY

Garrioch MA, Fitch W. Anaesthesia for carotid endarterectomy. British Journal of Anaesthesia 1993; 71:561–579

O'Hare DJ, Bodenham AR. Carotid endarterectomy under local anaesthesia. Hospital Medicine 1999; 60:271–276

Wilke HJ, Ellis JE, McKinsey JF. Carotid endarterectomy: perioperative and anaesthetic considerations. Journal of Cardiothoracic and Vascular Anesthesia 1996; 10:928–949

20

CROSS-REFERENCES

Preoperative assessment of cardiovascular risk in non-cardiac surgery
    Anaesthetic Factors 27: 634
Brain monitoring
    Patient Conditions 10: 321

21

TRANSPLANTATION
S. Cottam
M. J. Boscoe

Overview

S. Cottam

THE ROLE OF THE ANAESTHETIST

In relation to transplant surgery, the anaesthetist has several roles to play. Before the operation the recipient will require selection, assessment and preparation for surgery. The success of organ transplantation and a relative decrease in the numbers of organs from heart-beating donors has led to the introduction of techniques that maximise the use of the precious resource of donated organs. The anaesthetist is increasingly called on to assess and support patients and donors for living related kidney, liver or lung transplants. The relative shortage of cadaveric organs has also led to the use of so called 'marginal' donors where satisfactory early postoperative graft function cannot be guaranteed. Organ shortages may also increase the interval between initial patient assessment and transplantation; during this wait the patient's underlying condition may deteriorate significantly. Intraoperative management will demand close cooperation with the surgical team, an understanding of the physiological stresses imposed by the procedure, and a detailed knowledge of surgical technique.

Intensivists have an important contribution to make in the early identification and management of potential donors, either before and after confirmation of brainstem death or, increasingly, in the identification and management of non-heart-beating donors, both of which will involve sympathetic support of the patient's family.

Management of the donor before and during the retrieval operation will influence the function of the transplanted organs and the course and outcome for the recipient.

PATIENT SELECTION

Each transplant team has its own organ-specific criteria for listing patients for transplantation,

which will depend upon the pathological diagnosis, severity of illness, technical anaesthetic and surgical factors, and an assessment of prognosis in relation to availability of organs.

PATIENT ASSESSMENT

Patient assessment depends on the severity of organ failure, the availability and effectiveness of medical support, and the impact of the primary organ failure on other systems. The anaesthetist needs to have an understanding of the surgical procedure, and the stresses imposed by it, in assessing the chances of survival. In individual patients, as opposed to statistical groups, this remains a very inexact science.

PATIENT PREPARATION

Preparation of the patient for surgery includes:
• Medical supportive therapy for the primary organ failure
• Prompt treatment for complications as they arise
• Psychological and emotional support for the patient and their family while on the waiting list
• Anaesthetic reassessment
• Short-term measures immediately before operation.

The constraints of organ ischaemia time do not allow much scope for immediate preoperative interventions, but dialysis, haemofiltration or plasma exchange to correct metabolic, biochemical or coagulation derangements are possible. Some patients with acute organ failure will be receiving intensive care and multiple forms of support prior to surgery.

ANAESTHETIC MANAGEMENT

General principles of anaesthetic management apply:

- Appropriate premedication
- Reduction of aspiration risk
- Induction titrated to individual requirements
- Early control of the airway
- Multiple venous access of sufficient calibre to cope with anticipated transfusion requirements
- Monitoring of patient and equipment
- Maintenance with minimal depression of vital functions
- Appropriate level of postoperative care
- Postoperative analgesia and, if needed, sedation.

Organ-specific requirements:
- Monitoring effects of explantation
- Support during the explantation phase of surgery
- Management of the reperfusion phase
- Antibiotic and immunosuppressive therapy.

POSTOPERATIVE CARE

All transplant patients need careful post-operative monitoring and intensive or high-dependency care, with varying degrees of support of respiratory, circulatory or renal function.

Monitoring includes:
- Cardiovascular system for hypovolaemia
- Clinical examination and microbiological surveillance for sepsis
- Graft function, for signs of rejection, impaired perfusion sometimes requiring biopsy, Doppler scanning or angiography
- Secondary organ function for signs of multiple organ failure syndrome
- Drug toxicity – assays of immunosuppressive drugs and antibiotics in plasma.

Renal failure is perhaps the most common complication in all transplant patients, and may be related to poor perfusion and/or drug toxicity.

SEDATION AND ANALGESIA

Sedation and analgesia should be titrated to individual needs using methods appropriate to the case that will not compromise respiration. As in other forms of major surgery, intravenous infusion, under staff or patient control, and regional techniques are the commonest methods of analgesia. Intravenous infusion of propofol or a benzodiazepine is suitable if continued sedation is required.

The length of ITU/HDU stay and complication rates varies widely, but urgent exploration for bleeding or retransplantation may be necessary, often in a very sick patient.

Later complications or unrelated surgical pathology may also necessitate anaesthesia for the transplanted patient.

DONOR MANAGEMENT

The interval between recognition, confirmation and retrieval may extend over 48 h or more. The management of the donor during this period and during the retrieval operation has a significant effect on the subsequent function of the donated organs. The most important considerations are:
- Maintenance of adequate perfusion pressures and normovolaemia
- Optimisation of electrolyte and glucose levels, and acid–base status
- Maintenance of normothermia.

The retrieval operation itself may be protracted, especially if multiple organs are involved, and it is important to maintain levels of monitoring and support in the preliminary phases of the operation right up to the application of clamps and cold perfusion of the organs.

21

Heart transplantation

M. J. Boscoe

PROCEDURE

- Median sternotomy with cardiopulmonary bypass.
- Orthotopic transplant – anastomoses of left atrium, right atrium, donor and recipient aorta and pulmonary artery. Alternative technique uses bicaval anastomosis with possible advantages in function. Virtually all heart transplants are now orthotopic.
- Heterotopic heart transplant: also known as 'piggyback'. The native heart is not removed and the heterotopic heart becomes a left heart assist device. Particularly a possible use for a small donor heart in presence of pulmonary hypertension.

Box 21.1 lists the selection criteria for heart transplant donors.

BOX 21.1

Selection criteria for heart transplant donors

Relative contraindications:

- Age > 55 years
- Diabetes
- Smoking history
- Hypertension
- Prolonged hypotension – blood pressure < 60 mmHg for > 3 h

Absolute contraindications:

- Prolonged high-dose inotropic support
- Prolonged cardiac arrest
- Severe left ventricular hypertrophy on ECG
- Protracted cardiac arrhythmias
- Poor function on echocardiography
- Negative findings by surgeon at retrieval stage

Matching of possible donor to possible recipient is critical

PATIENT CHARACTERISTICS

- New York Heart Association (NYHA) functional class III or IV with end-stage heart failure.
- Increasing number of recipients are over 65 years age, reflecting better medical and surgical management early in disease process.
- About half have ischaemic cardiomyopathy and are not amenable to revascularisation. Most of the rest have dilated cardiomyopathy on maximal medical therapy, sometimes necessitating intra-aortic balloon pump, artificial internal cardiac defibrillators, paracorporeal ventricular assist devices and ventilation. Many have had cardiac surgery such as revascularisation, and an increasing number will have implanted left ventricular assist devices.

PREOPERATIVE ASSESSMENT AND INVESTIGATIONS

Assessment to determine relative and absolute contraindications:

- Relative contraindications – vascular and other complications of diabetes, peripheral vascular disease, cerebrovascular disease, some inflammatory bowel disease, lack of support, age over 60 years
- Absolute contraindications – malignancy, persistent hepatitis B, active tuberculosis, serious psychosis, cachexia
- Functional status is more important than ejection fraction
- Cardiopulmonary exercise testing: myocardial oxygen consumption (MV_{O_2}) must be < 14 (usually < 10) ml kg^{-1} min^{-1}
- Right heart catheter to determine pulmonary vascular resistance is < 4 Wood units. Transpulmonary gradient (mean Pulmonary artery pressure – Pulmonary

21

artery wedge pressure) should be < 15 mmHg, and patients with raised values should be subjected to pharmacological tests of reversibility

- Renal – creatinine clearance should be > 50 ml min^{-1} or 30 ml min^{-1} m^{-2}. Mild renal dysfunction may be reversible but postoperative renal failure increases the mortality rate by 10%.

PREMEDICATION

- Patients are anxious but looking forward to the operation. If cardiac output is reasonable, the patient will usually tolerate an oral benzodiazepine, if time permits.
- H$_2$ antagonist
- Oxygen by face-mask following premedication if in heart failure.

THEATRE PREPARATION

- Coordination with retrieval team is essential. Do not anaesthetise recipient until donor heart has been assessed as acceptable by the retrieval team.
- Strict aseptic technique for vascular access; otherwise clean anaesthetic preparation.
- History of anticoagulants, previous mediastinal surgery, complex procedures, all tend to complicate surgery leading to delay in preparation for implantation and possible lengthening of ischaemic time. Consider use of high-dose aprotinin or tranexamic acid. Platelets should be made available for repeat operations and fresh frozen plasma in presence of coumarin anticoagulants.
- Facilities to maintain body temperature are critical as wound closure may be prolonged, Consider sterile forced warm air blankets on operating table, blood warmer, silver hats.

PERIOPERATIVE MANAGEMENT

MONITORING:

- Intra-arterial radial artery cannula and 14-gauge peripheral venous line under local anaesthesia
- SpO_2, ECG, $EtCO_2$, urinary catheter
- Left-sided neck lines if possible, as cardiologists may need to perform endocardial biopsy in postoperative period via right internal jugular vein. Pulmonary artery catheter sheath with side arm in left internal jugular or left subclavian vein

allows access for rapid filling and also passage of pulmonary artery catheter, for later measurement of cardiac output and pulmonary blood saturation. Left atrial line should be inserted by surgeon. Transoesophageal echocardiography (TOE) should be used in all cases. May be useful before bypass to detect clot in left ventricle, and after implantation it is essential to examine and monitor the new heart.

ANAESTHETIC TECHNIQUE
Induction

- Cardiac resuscitation drugs drawn up; preparation for emergency cardiopulmonary bypass.
- Etomidate or propofol, fentanyl, sevoflurane or isoflurane. Modified rapid sequence induction is occasionally necessary if not starved, but not as a routine.
- Sudden removal of endogenous catecholamine drive may cause hypotension. Many are relatively dehydrated due to loop diuretics and vasodilators. Usually volume suffices with small doses of metaraminol or phenylephrine, adequate to maintain systemic pressure.

Maintenance:
Aim to preserve perfusion of vital organs until smoothly on cardiopulmonary bypass.

- *Drug interactions* – although various drug interactions between immunosuppressants and anaesthetic drugs have been reported, these are rarely of importance in practice.
- *Immunosuppression* – see Table 21.1. Anaesthetist administers methylprednisolone during operation. Other drugs are given orally before surgery or after operation via a nasogastric tube or intravenously.
- *Coagulation* – can be a problem if the patient was taking aspirin or coumarins in reoperations. Use of aprotinin is routine but beware the risk of anaphylaxis due to previous exposure for cardiac surgery. Oozing occurs if the patient is allowed to cool below 34°C. Thromboelastography can be useful in detecting fibrinolysis and platelet dysfunction.

POSTOPERATIVE MANAGEMENT

WEANING FROM BYPASS
Most hearts are in sinus rhythm. Atrial and ventricular pacing wires (two each) are placed

21

TABLE 21.1

Drugs used for immunosuppression in heart and lung transplantation

Time	Type	Example	Complications
Induction	Anti-T cell agent, biological	Antithymocyte globulin	Opportunistic infections, lymphoproliferative disease
	Murine monoclonal	OKT3	As above
	Biologically engineered	Daclizumab, basiliximab	Few side-effects
Maintenance	Calcineurin inhibitor	Ciclosporin, tacrolimus	Renal failure
	Inhibitor of DNA synthesis	Azathioprine	Bone marrow suppression (both) Liver dysfunction. (azathioprine) Nausea (both)
	Inhibitor of DNA synthesis	Mycophenolate	Diarrhoea; more specific Better for heart transplant
	Corticosteroids	Methylprednisolone, prednisolone, prednisone	All the many complications of steroids, especially hyperglycaemia, hypokalaemia, fluid retention, osteoporosis

because donor heart may enter nodal rhythm or A-V block. A-V sequential pacing may be required to optimise output with stiff left ventricle. There has been a serious reduction in donors over the past decade, necessitating the use of marginal hearts. Immediate cardiac support is graded from low-dose dopamine through to noradrenaline (norepinephrine) and adrenaline (epinephrine). Newly transplanted hearts are very sensitive to volume and are difficult to recover if overloaded. TOE is useful at this stage, particularly in demonstrating a failing right ventricle associated with an empty left ventricle, or even the reverse situation with a failing left ventricle. Milrinone administration (combined with noradrenaline) may be helpful, particularly in the former situation, but also with left ventricular diastolic dysfunction. Intra-aortic counterpulsation will aid left ventricular function, and the common event of a failing right ventricle is best managed with inhaled nitric oxide, sometimes together with isoprenaline, glyceryl trinitrate and a phosphodiesterase inhibitor. Prostaglandin E_1 is used much less often. Acute right heart dysfunction is associated with pre-existing pulmonary hypertension, a long ischaemic time (> 4 h) and donor–recipient size mismatch.

Many transplant programmes now have co-existing facilities to insert left and right ventricular assist devices. For left ventricular failure, an intra-aortic balloon pump may be followed by a paracorporeal device. A right-sided device may be required, either alone or in combination with a left-sided device (e.g. Thoratec, Abiomed).

OUTCOME:

Some 90% of transplant patients are extubated within 24 h and can be managed similarly to routine open-heart surgery patients.

Actuarial survival figures are:
- 85% at 1 year
- 75% at 5 years
- 55% at 10 years.

Some 86% of survivors are NYHA class I at 1 year. Major causes of long-term mortality are chronic rejection causing coronary artery disease, malignancy and infection.

BIBLIOGRAPHY

Banner NR, Boscoe MJ, Khaghani A. Postoperative care of the adult heart transplant patient. In: O'Donnell J, Nacul F, eds. Surgical intensive care. Kluwer Academic; 2001

Baumgartner WA, Reiz B, Kasper E, Theodore J. Heart and lung transplantation. 2nd edn. Philadelphia: WB Saunders; 2002

Dash A. Anesthesia for patients with a previous heart transplant. International Anesthesiology Clinics 1995; 33(2):1–9

Hertz MI, Taylor DO, Trulock EP et al. The Registry of the International Society for Heart and Lung Transplantation. Nineteenth official report – 2002. Journal of Heart and Lung Transplantation 2002; 9:950–970

Kirklin JK, Young JB, McGiffin DC. Heart transplantation. Churchill Livingstone; 2002

21

Kidney transplantation

J. Broadfield

PROCEDURE

Kidney transplantation may be from either a live or a cadaver donor. A live donor must be fit and well (American Society of Anesthesiologist (ASA) grade I), and is subjecting him or herself to a major operation for no personal gain. If there is any query about the donor's relationship to the recipient, the problem should be referred to the Unrelated Live Transplant Regulating Authority (ULTRA).

Donor tissues must be immunologically compatible. The details of the tests and their significance are changing regularly as more information emerges. The donor should also be free of tumour and infection (including human immunodeficiency virus; HIV).

The graft is usually transplanted extraperitoneally to an iliac fossa because of the proximity of the bladder and suitable blood vessels (iliac artery and vein). There is also poor viability of the distal end of the donated ureter as its blood supply is from the donor's bladder.

PATIENT CHARACTERISTICS

- Any age group – transplantation is unusual in small babies
- The patient will suffer from the dual pathophysiology of:
  —chronic renal failure
  —the underlying disease process (e.g. diabetes, systemic lupus, hypertension).

PREOPERATIVE ASSESSMENT AND INVESTIGATIONS

There are important aspects of the pathophysiology to note:
- Cardiovascular system:
  —Anaemia – there are many contributing factors; reversed by erythropoietin
  —Circulating volume – usually increased (look for congestive cardiac failure); may be decreased with polyuria or recent enthusiastic dialysis
  —Hypertension – could be either the result or the cause of the renal failure
  —Ischaemic heart disease.
- Uraemia – pericardial effusion and tamponade (improves with good dialysis). Confirm with echocardiography if suspicious. Aspirate before surgery if compromising the cardiac output.
- Water and electrolyte imbalance.
- Neuropathy – including autonomic.

Assessment of all of the above points and treatment, where appropriate, is very important.

These patients may be on large doses of a diverse selection of drugs.

Vascular access is often difficult because:
- Veins that may be needed for shunts or fistulae should not be used, especially the antecubital fossa and radial aspect of the forearm
- Years of therapy and venesection may have taken its toll of veins.

PREMEDICATION

As appropriate, but remember there will be problems of excreting drugs and active metabolites until the grafted kidney works. These patients are often frail.

THEATRE PREPARATION

- Ensure that drugs specific to kidney transplantation are available, e.g. renal perfusion solution for live related transplantation, and immunosuppressive agents.
- A sterile trolley is required for central venous pressure (CVP) catheter insertion.
- Maintenance of body temperature is important – warming blanket, warm fluids, humidification.

PERIOPERATIVE MANAGEMENT

MONITORING:

- ECG
- Non-invasive blood pressure – avoid arms with fistulae
- SaO_2
- $EtCO_2$
- CVP – triple lumen is helpful for drug administration
- Fluid balance and blood loss
- Body temperature.

ANAESTHETIC TECHNIQUE

Regional techniques may be used, but there are problems:

- Duration of procedure – and hence comfort of patient
- Occasional bleeding problems
- Patient apprehension.

These often make general anaesthesia the method of choice.

GENERAL ANAESTHESIA

The modern armamentarium of anaesthetic drugs and monitoring have greatly reduced the problems of general anaesthesia in these patients.

- Hypnotics:
  - —Propofol gives good postoperative recovery
  - —Etomidate gives good cardiovascular stability.
- Muscle relaxants:
  - —Atracurium avoids any problems of renal excretion of neuromuscular blocking drugs
  - —Suxamethonium has been cited as causing problems with high serum potassium levels.
- Analgesia – renal excretion of opioids and metabolites needs consideration. Buprenorphine, in theory, offers the best metabolic profile.
- Volatile agents – in theory, enflurane provides the highest free fluoride levels. Isoflurane is better.

VASCULARISATION OF THE GRAFT

Maintain optimal circulating volume (CVP and peripheral temperature) with a good cardiac output at the time of revascularisation. This is important:

- For perfusion and early function of the graft
- Because this can also be a time of sudden blood loss.

Beware of excess potassium (e.g. in stored blood).

Beware of fluid overload.

NB: The last two factors may necessitate early dialysis.

POSTOPERATIVE MANAGEMENT

- Fluids to keep graft well perfused
- Avoid haemodialysis if possible, because of the problem of heparinisation immediately after operation
- Dopamine (2–3 µg kg^{-1} min^{-1}) may help renal function, but this has been questioned.

OUTCOME

Successful transplantation improves quality of life radically.

GRAFT SURVIVAL:

- Live related – 90% at 1 and 5 years
- Cadaver – 80–85% at 1 year and 70% at 5 years.

OTHER PROBLEMS:

- Rejection
- Malignant disease, especially lymphoma
- Steroid-induced cataracts.

21

CROSS-REFERENCES

Blood transfusion
    Anaesthetic Factors 31: 729
Fluid and electrolyte balance
    Anaesthetic Factors 27: 624
Postoperative oliguria
    Anaesthetic Factors 31: 774

Liver transplantation

S. Mallett

PROCEDURE

- Laparotomy by bilateral subcostal incision, occasionally with extension to xiphisternum (Mercedes' incision).
- Surgery is divided into three phases:
  —Dissection phase, with skeletonisation of native liver
  —Anhepatic phase, with removal of liver and implantation of donor organ by anastomosis of vena cava (suprahepatic and infrahepatic) and portal vein, or by anastomosis of hepatic vein of donor organ to cuff of native hepatic vein (piggyback procedure)
  —Reperfusion phase with graft reperfusion, haemostasis, completion of hepatic arterial anastomosis and biliary drainage.
- Venovenous bypass may be used in the anhepatic phase to maintain venous return, cardiac output and renal perfusion when the inferior vena cava (IVC) and portal vein are clamped. With the increasingly used piggyback technique the liver is dissected off the IVC, which remains *in situ*, this technique allows a segment of liver rather than a whole organ to be implanted. It allows living related liver transplantation.
- Orthotopic liver transplantation (OLT) , with a whole or 'split' liver, is the most common procedure (90%), although auxiliary grafting (either orthotopic or heterotopic) may be performed for patients with acute liver failure or children with isolated enzyme defects.

PATIENT CHARACTERISTICS

Patients are aged from 1 week to 70 years and fall into two distinct patient groups.

ACUTE LIVER FAILURE (ALF)

Jaundice and encephalopathy developing in a patient with no history of chronic liver disease.

- Hyperacute liver failure – encephalopathy within 7 days of onset of jaundice
- Acute liver failure – encephalopathy 8–28 days from onset of jaundice
- Subacute liver failure – encephalopathy 5–12 weeks from onset of jaundice.

In the UK emergency transplantation is reserved for patients with a poor prognosis without OLT, as defined by O'Grady et al (1993) (Box 21.2).

CHRONIC LIVER DISEASE (CLD)

A wide variety of congenital and acquired disease in both adults and children may lead to end-stage liver disease. Transplantation is frequently required, as medical treatment fails to control life-threatening complications such as gastrointestinal bleeding.

BOX 21.2

Emergency transplant criteria

Paracetamol induced

- pH < 7.3 after volume repletion (irrespective of grade of encephalopathy)

or

- Prothrombin time > 100 s
- Creatinine > 300 µmol l^{-1}
- Grade 3 or 4 encephalopathy

Non-paracetamol induced

Any three of the following (irrespective of grade of encephalopathy):

- Age < 10 or > 40 years
- Non-A, non-B hepatitis
- Halothane hepatitis
- Idiosyncratic drug reaction
- Jaundice to encephalopathy time > 7 days
- Prothrombin time > 50 s
- Bilirubin level > 300 mmol l^{-1}

COMMONLY ASSOCIATED PATHOLOGY

CENTRAL NERVOUS SYSTEM:
- Encephalopathy (CLD)
- Cerebral oedema (ALF).

RESPIRATORY:
- Restrictive defect due to massive ascites (50% of CLD)
- Hypoxia due to ventilation perfusion defect (15% of CLD)
- Pulmonary hypertension (1–2% of CLD) – relative contraindication to transplantation
- Acute lung injury may progress to adult respiratory distress syndrome (ALF).

CARDIOVASCULAR:
- High cardiac output with low systemic vascular resistance (75%, CLD and ALF)
- Pericardial effusion
- Cardiomyopathy, especially in alcoholic liver disease or myocardial involvement in disease process (e.g. amyloid). Cirrhotic cardiomyopathy may be difficult to detect before operation as the signs may be masked by the concurrent afterload reduction.

RENAL:
- Pre-renal or renal failure
- Hepatorenal syndrome both ALF and CLD.

GASTROINTESTINAL:
- Portal hypertension and ascites (CLD).

HAEMATOLOGY:
- Anaemia
- Coagulopathy
- Abnormal fibrinolysis.

PREOPERATIVE ASSESSMENT

A multidisciplinary approach is essential to assess risk, aimed at precisely defining the multisystem involvement described above. Occult cardiovascular disease is a major cause of perioperative death; rigorous cardiac investigation, including angiography, is indicated.

PREMEDICATION

A short-acting benzodiazepine (preferably not dependent on phase I elimination) is tolerated in the absence of hepatic encephalopathy.

PREOPERATIVE PREPARATION

- Detailed patient and relative counselling.
- When an organ becomes available, liaison with donor team is essential.
- Success is dependent on support services such as blood bank and laboratory services, anaesthetic technical back-up and clinical perfusionists for rapid infusion devices, cell saver and bypass equipment.
- Theatre temperature is important; patient warming devices, infusion equipment and monitoring must all be available and ready.

PERIOPERATIVE MANAGEMENT

MONITORING:
- ECG
- Invasive arterial pressure
- CVP
- Pulmonary artery catheter or alternative measurement of cardiac output such as with PiCCO is useful
- Intracranial pressure (ALF)
- Core temperature
- Sp_{O_2}
- Et_{CO_2}
- Urine output and blood loss.

BLOOD SAMPLES:
- Arterial and mixed venous gases
- Full blood count
- Clotting screen
- Sodium, potassium, calcium and blood glucose levels
- Thromboelastography.

INTRAVENOUS ACCESS
- Wide-bore venous access is mandatory for rapid infusion.
- Internal jugular access is safer than subclavian in the presence of severe coagulopathy.

ANAESTHETIC TECHNIQUE

- Rapid sequence induction is advisable if patient is not fully fasted, or in the presence of massive ascites.
- Induction with narcotic (fentanyl) and sleep dose of thiopental.
- Insert a wide-bore nasogastric tube and a fine-bore enteral feeding tube for early postoperative enteral nutrition.
- Maintenance with oxygen–air–desflurane or isoflurane, narcotic and relaxant infusion.

21

Total intravenous anaesthesia (TIVA) techniques are well described. Remifentanil has achieved popularity in some centres to facilitate early extubation.

- Intermittent positive-pressure ventilation (IPPV) with ventilator capable of minute volumes of up to 20 l min^{-1}.
- Aim to maintain renal perfusion. Inotropes, mannitol and the use of venovenous bypass in the anhepatic phase are all advocated. We no longer use 'low-dose dopamine'.
- Maintenance of cardiac output and oxygen transport, especially in the anhepatic phase. During operation, cardiac output increases, especially on reperfusion with profound systemic vasodilatation. Adequate volume loading is essential. Pressor inotropes are required occasionally, as guided by cardiac output and systemic vascular resistance. Beware of the deleterious effects of vasoconstrictors on already limited oxygen extraction.
- Intraoperative monitoring of coagulation by thromboelastography and laboratory parameters of coagulation and appropriate blood product replacement. Ionised calcium concentrations will fall due to administered citrate and will require supplementation.
- Prophylactic antibiotic administration and intraoperative doses of immunosuppressive agents.

POSTOPERATIVE MANAGEMENT

- Continue invasive monitoring.
- 90% of patients with CLD are extubated within 24 h.
- In ALF, ITU stay may be prolonged.
- Early complications include bleeding (now < 5%) and hepatic artery or portal vein thrombosis, which will require early re-exploration.
- Early liver function is monitored by resolution of metabolic and lactic acidosis and resolution of coagulopathy (falling international normalised ratio; INR).
- Poor initial graft function may be treated with prostaglandins or with N-acetylcysteine.
- Primary non-function of the liver is rare in UK centres (1–2%), but will entail emergency retransplantation. Initial poor function is relatively common with the increasing use of 'marginal' donors.

- Acute rejection is common – suggested by changes in aspartate aminotransferase (AST) concentration and INR and confirmed by biopsy if coagulation permits. Additional steroids and/or modification of immunosuppressive regimen may be required.
- Ciclosporin or tacrolimus may be introduced early if renal function is satisfactory.

OUTCOME

- Patients with acute liver failure are selected for OLT if their chances of survival with medical treatment are less than 10%. The 1-year survival rate following emergency OLT is currently 74%.
- Patients with chronic liver disease currently have a 1-year survival rate of 85–90% following OLT.
- Quality of life is improved; the majority of patients are severely incapacitated prior to transplantation.
- The majority of deaths are in the early postoperative period due to infection and multiple organ failure. Later deaths are due to complications of immunosuppression, chronic rejection or recurrence of the primary liver disease.
- Retransplantation will be required in 5–10% of patients.

BIBLIOGRAPHY

Eason J, Potter D. Anaesthesia for liver transplantation (2). In: Kaufmann L, ed. Anaesthesia review, vol 7. Edinburgh: Churchill Livingstone; 1990: ch 10

Elias E. Liver transplantation. Journal of the Royal College of Physicians of London 1993; 3:224–232

Ginsburg R, Peachey T. Anaesthesia for liver transplantation (1). In: Kaufmann L, ed. Anaesthesia review, vol 7. Edinburgh: Churchill Livingstone; 1990: ch 9

O'Grady J, Schalm SW, Williams R. Acute liver failure: redefining the syndromes. Lancet 1993; ii:273–275

Plevak D, Southorn PA, Narr BJ, Peters SG. Intensive care unit experience in the Mayo liver transplantation program: the first 100 cases. Mayo Clinic Proceedings 1989; 64:433–445

21

Lung and heart–lung transplantation

M. J. Boscoe

PROCEDURE

Heart–lung transplant (HLT) is performed through a median sternotomy or clam-shell (transverse sterno-bithoracic incision) under cardiopulmonary bypass (CPB). This operation is becoming less common internationally, the preference being to preserve the native heart if possible. Single-lung transplant (SLT) via a posterolateral thoracotomy may be used in the absence of a suitable heart–lung block.

Bilateral sequential single-lung transplant (BSSLT) is usually performed via a clam-shell incision with bronchial anastomoses with or without cardiopulmonary bypass. Less commonly, surgery is via a median sternotomy.

Living lobe transplant (LLT) uses a lower lobe from each of two donors to replace an entire lung in a child or small adult. The operation is performed through a clam-shell incision and is usually done using CPB.

Box 21.3 shows the selection criteria for lung transplant donors.

BOX 21.3

Selection criteria for lung transplant donors

- Hepatitis B, HIV negative
- Normal chest radiograph, except minor lung contusion sometimes allowable
- Smoking history variable acceptance, but should be < 20 a day
- $Pa_{O_2} > 300$ mmHg on 5-cm positive end-expiratory pressure (PEEP) with an Fi_{O_2} of 1.0 for 5 min
- Blood gases should be repeated frequently up to the point of retrieval
- Normal lung compliance with tidal volume of 10 ml per kg bodyweight
- Mild lung contusion injury may be considered
- Age criteria vary from centre to centre, but usually < 55 years
- Absence of pus in airways following bronchoscopy
- Absence of history of aspiration
- Retrieval surgeon's final examination is critical

21

PATIENT CHARACTERISTICS

This is the only treatment for end-stage parenchymal lung disease and pulmonary vascular disease. Half of lung transplants are bilateral and half unilateral. HLT is the operation of choice for patients with congenital heart disease with Eisenmenger's complex. It is also used for primary pulmonary hypertension (PPH) and some parenchymal lung disease. PPH is less often an indication than previously owing to new medical approaches, and parenchymal disease is usually managed with BSSLT or SLT. If the recipient heart is healthy, it may be used as a 'domino' heart for another recipient with end-stage heart disease. SLT is undertaken for non-infective parenchymal lung disease, i.e. emphysema (chronic obstructive airway disease and α_1-antitrypsin disease) and pulmonary fibrosis.

BSSLT is the technique of choice for septic lung disease including cystic fibrosis and bronchiectasis, and also for pulmonary vascular disease or Eisenmenger's complex (with cardiac repair).

LLT replaces both lungs, typically of small patients with cystic fibrosis, but also has been used for pulmonary fibrosis as a substitute for SLT. It has been used in paediatric lung transplantation. Rigorous protocols for the screening of donors and recipients must take account of the ethical issues.

PREOPERATIVE ASSESSMENT AND INVESTIGATIONS

Investigations include chest radiography, pulmonary function tests, computed tomography

(CT), V/Q scanning and estimation of blood gases while breathing air.

RESPIRATORY

Lung function tests are severely abnormal in parenchymal lung disease. A typical forced expiratory volume in 1 s (FEV_1) < 30% is predicted in obstructive lung disease. Chest radiography shows emphysematous bullae, and CT shows the worst side to transplant. A high-resolution CT scan to exclude malignancy is needed in older age groups. A quantitative ventilation perfusion scan helps to guide the choice of target lung in SLT.

Baseline arterial blood gases confirm hypoxic respiratory drive in many patients with parenchymatous lung disease.

CARDIOVASCULAR

Many patients are at risk of cardiovascular system disease, including ischaemic heart disease, for example with smoking. ECG, echocardiography and coronary angiography are indicated in patients > 50 years of age. Right heart catheter studies to measure pulmonary vascular resistance and pulmonary artery pressure should be performed. Severe pulmonary hypertension will make the need for CPB in SLT more likely. A multiple gated acquisition (MUGA) scan is useful to assess left heart function.

OTHER:

- Renal assessment is essential as some immunosuppressives are nephrotoxic. Patients should have a creatinine clearance > 50 ml min^{-1}. Hyperbilirubinaemia > 2.5 mg dl^{-1} is a predictor of poor outcome when associated with right heart failure.
- Patient satisfies the criteria for donor lung selection. Donor and recipient sputum analysis may be guide to antibiotic therapy, especially in cystic fibrosis.
- Previous intrathoracic procedures such as lung biopsy, drainage of pneumothorax or lobectomy increase risk of intraoperative bleeding. Prolonged preparation for implantation may lead to an undesirably long ischaemic time.
- Complex congenital heart disease, particularly pulmonary atresia, is associated with the presence of extensive collateral vessels. Bleeding during dissection and after surgery is a serious cause of morbidity and mortality.
- Preoperative drugs may include antiplatelet and anticoagulant drugs, steroids, nifedipine and prostaglandin infusions to reduce pulmonary hypertension.

PREMEDICATION

- Usually none as patients already have borderline respiratory function. Premedication prevents stress-related crises in the presence of pulmonary hypertension.
- Close co-operation with the donor retrieval team is important. Ischaemic time for lungs is optimally < 5 h.

THEATRE PREPARATION

- Clean anaesthetic equipment. Prepare to aspirate thick secretions.
- Attention to sterility with line insertion. All resuscitation drugs as for heart transplantation, but also aminophylline for bronchospasm and 1 : 100 000 adrenaline (epinephrine) for pulmonary hypertensive crisis.
- Preparations for emergency chest drainage and CPB.
- Fibreoptic bronchoscope available for every patient.
- Additional padding to protect peripheral nerves in patients with poor nutrition (e.g. cystic fibrosis).

PERIOPERATIVE MANAGEMENT

MONITORING
Before induction:
- ECG
- SpO_2
- Intra-arterial line
- Baseline blood gases.

After induction:
- Quadruple-lumen internal jugular line
- Pulmonary artery sheath with side arm
- $EtCO_2$
- Urinary catheter
- Consider second arterial line in femoral artery, particularly in clam-shell incision, as arms may be placed together over head and line may be precarious
- Transeosophageal echo probe.

ANAESTHETIC TECHNIQUE
Induction:
- Surgeon's presence in theatre is essential. Wait until retrieval team confirms that

donor lung meets criteria before inducing recipient.

- A balanced technique using etomidate or propofol, fentanyl and pancuronium is usually well tolerated. In patients with emphysema, volume preloading lessens chance of hypotension once positive-pressure ventilation is commenced.
- Hypotension in patients with emphysema requires immediate differential diagnosis of a tamponade of the heart by overexpanded lungs (treat with volume and constrictor, for instance metaraminol or phenylephrine) or a tension pneumothorax. Ventilation may be difficult in either; stethoscope, chest movement, $EtCO_2$ all help.
- Choice of airway management. Single-lumen tube for HLT and BSSLT if on CPB. Left-sided double-lumen tube for either left or right SLT (as surgeon leaves long left main bronchus stump). Always check position with fibreoptic bronchoscope.
- Have pre-rehearsed plan for emergency sternotomy (to relieve tamponade), chest drainage (for pneumothorax) or CPB.
- Acute pulmonary hypertensive crisis may occur in patients with previous pulmonary hypertension despite smooth induction with 100% oxygen. Adrenaline (epinephrine) is usually effective in improving right heart contractility.
- Use of high-dose aprotinin is routine to minimise postoperative bleeding.

Maintenance

- Most patients will tolerate moderate doses of a volatile agent. Avoid nitrous oxide. Keep narcotic dose low if early extubation is planned. Propofol and remifentanil infusions are used, to minimise possibility of awareness.
- A high I : E ratio (e.g. 1 : 5) may be required in obstructive airway disease, but this is not predictable and some variation may be tried. Manual ventilation allowing 'permissive hypercapnia' is often necessary during dissection with pH as low as 7.15.
- The need for CPB during operation is indicated by: (1) difficulty in mechanical ventilation, (2) unacceptable blood gases, (3) haemodynamic instability to right heart dysfunction in pulmonary hypertensive crisis Check fibreoptic bronchoscopy and TOE are useful diagnostic aids but must not be used to delay rapid progress to CPB when necessary.

Post-implantation and weaning from bypass

- Keep crystalloid fluid infusions to a minimum as new lungs are devoid of lymphatics and are also prone to fluid-induced injury.
- Maintain $FiO_2 < 0.5$ to avoid theoretical toxic lung damage associated with free radicals (not always possible).
- Methylprednisolone 1 g at anaesthetic induction or on reperfusing the lung.
- Avoid overinflation and barotrauma.
- Evaluate heart with TOE for signs of right heart failure or raised pulmonary artery pressure; may need milrinone (to improve diastolic function), adrenaline (epinephrine) or noradrenaline (norepinephrine).
- Insert pulmonary artery catheter in most cases.
- Inhaled nitric oxide for early postoperative period in most cases, but outcome data still awaited.
- Evaluate lungs for signs of primary graft failure and reperfusion injury: Tracheal tube for pulmonary oedema, serial blood gas assessment, decreased lung compliance.
- Surgeon will want to examine bronchial anastomoses with a large fibreoptic bronchoscope at the end of the operation. This will require exchange of double-lumen for single-lumen tube.
- Consider insertion of thoracic epidural at end of operation to enable early extubation in SLT for emphysema as spontaneous ventilation minimises complications of mediastinal shift and compromise of native lung.

POSTOPERATIVE MANAGEMENT

- A high $PaCO_2$ should be expected after surgery (may be due to carbon dioxide retention before operation). Extubation policy should regard pH as more important. Long ischaemic time or poor-quality organ may result in early graft dysfunction. Failure of gas exchange due pulmonary oedema, infection or rejection.
- Early mediastinal shift in ventilated SLT recipients for emphysema is caused by hyperinflated remaining native lung compressing new lung. Independent lung ventilation using a double-lumen tube and two ventilators may be necessary to replace mediastinum centrally.

21

- Perioperative problems include primary graft failure, bleeding, pneumothorax, blood clot in airway.
- Temporary right heart failure may occur following primary graft failure of the lungs leading to increased pulmonary vascular resistance.
- Diagnosis of cause of graft failure may require transbronchial biopsy.
- Immunosuppressive regimen – see Table 21.1. Long-term problems affecting airway include healing and infection, and necessitate multiple anaesthetics for diagnostic bronchoscopy, bronchial dilatation, cryotherapy and, occasionally, stent insertion. Bronchial anastomosis complications are rare with new surgical techniques.
- Obliterative bronchiolitis, an obstructive lung disease caused by chronic rejection, occurs in up to 40% at 4 years with no effective cure except retransplantation – no longer an option due to scarcity of donors.

There are some special considerations in regard to HLT:

- There is a loss of carinal reflex below anastomosis in HLT. Patients fail to cough on endobronchial suction. Physiotherapy is important.
- Global myocardial dysfunction following HLT may be due to poor preservation or long ischaemic time (see section on Heart transplantation).

OUTCOME

About 60–70% of both ventilation and perfusion go to the new lung following SLT. The 1-year survival rate for SLT and BSSLT is in the range of 65–70%. There is a better outcome for BSSLT than SLT in patients with emphysema at 5 years, when the survival rate is around 45–50%. Patients with cystic fibrosis do best at 1 and 5 years. The 1-year survival rate for HLT is about 60% (reflects serious pathology). The major cause of mid-term mortality is acute rejection and obliterative bronchiolitis, and late mortality is usually due obliterative bronchiolitis, caused by chronic rejection. Malignancy occurs in 4% of survivors at 1 year and in 13% at 5 years.

BIBLIOGRAPHY

Baumgartner WA, Reiz B, Kasper E, Theodore J. Heart and lung transplantation. 2nd edn. Philadelphia: WB Saunders; 2002

Boscoe MJ. Anesthesia for patients with transplanted lungs and heart and lungs. International Anesthesiology Clinics 1995; 33(2):21–44

Boscoe MJ, George SJ. Anaesthesia and perioperative care. In: Banner NR, Polak J, Yacoub MH, eds. Lung transplantation. Cambridge: Cambridge University Press; 2003 (in press)

Farrimond JG, Boscoe MJ. Anaesthesia for living donor lobe of lung transplantation. Current Anaesthesia and Intensive Care 2000; 11(4):217–222

Hertz MI, Taylor DO, Trulock EP et al. The registry of the International Society for Heart and Lung Transplantation. 19th official report – 2002. Journal of Heart and Lung Transplantation 2002; 9:950–970

Smiley R, Navedo A. postoperative independent lung ventilation in a single lung patient. Anesthesiology 1991; 74:1144–1148

21

Management of the organ donor

B. J. Pollard

Demand for donor organs continues to exceed supply and there is no likely change in this situation. Patients still die on the waiting list for transplantation. Early recognition of a potential donor and organ-oriented support after all prospect of patient survival has been lost is one important factor in attempting to redress this imbalance.

DONOR SELECTION

In general, a donor must be brainstem dead from a known cause. Following identification of a potential organ donor, cardiovascular and respiratory support should be maintained while the viability of the brainstem is being assessed. The criteria for assessment of brainstem function differ between countries and are described on page 6.

General donor assessment:
- Full history, including social aspects
- Complete physical examination
- Laboratory investigations (see below).

The following are contraindications to organ donation:
- Age > 75 years – variable, depending on individual unit policies
- Patients with untreated sepsis
- Those testing positive for HIV
- Those testing positive for viral hepatitis B or C
- Patients with active tuberculosis, malaria or rabies
- Patients with malignant disease (excluding primary brain tumours)
- A risk of rare viral disease such as Creutzfeldt–Jakob disease (CJD)
- Patients who have received human pituitary growth hormone.
- Patients who have been, or are, intravenous drug abusers or who are sex workers
- Those who have had sex in the previous 2 years with anyone from Africa (except for Morocco, Algeria, Libya or Egypt) or (men) with another man
- Those who have suffered from a neurological disease of unknown cause.

In certain situations, donors from high-risk groups such as sex workers or intravenous drug abusers, who are HIV antibody negative may be considered on an individual basis together with the status and needs of the potential recipient.

Cardiac arrest and prolonged hypotension do not necessarily contraindicate organ donation; the suitability of individual organs depends on post-resuscitation function. These patients should be considered on an individual basis.

Certain organs, for example heart valves, bone, skin and cornea, may be removed from a donor up to 24 h after death. Formal brainstem testing may therefore not always be necessary in these patients.

Every hospital should have a transplant coordinator, either on-site or available at another hospital nearby, who will advise on the suitability and management of a potential donor as necessary. The transplant coordinator should be involved at an early stage when brainstem tests are being performed.

HEART DONOR SELECTION

EXCLUSIONS:
- History of hypertension, ischaemic heart disease, cardiomyopathy or valvular disease.
- Excessive inotrope requirement. Exogenous and endogenous catecholamines have a deleterious effect on myocardial energy stores and post-transplant function.

INCLUSIONS:
- Age < 50 years
- Normal chest radiograph
- Normal 12-lead ECG

21

PULMONARY DONOR SELECTION

EXCLUSIONS:
- Chronic lung disease, heavy smoking, pulmonary aspiration and parenchymal trauma.
- High alveolar–arterial oxygen gradient – $PaO_2 < 300$ mmHg (40 kPa) breathing 100% oxygen with PEEP $< +5$ cmH$_2$O
- Respiratory sepsis – tracheal colonisation with fungus or bacteria adversely affect the outcome by increasing the morbidity and mortality rates.

INCLUSIONS:
- Age < 50 years. However, physiological age is more important than absolute age and elderly fit donors >60 yrs are frequently considered suitable.
- Normal chest radiograph – minor chest radiographic abnormalities are noted in 27% of donors and do not contraindicate the possibility of lung donation
- Normal bronchoscopic findings.

LIVER DONOR SELECTION

EXCLUSIONS:
- Age > 60 years. However, physiological age is more important than absolute age and elderly fit donors > 60 yrs are frequently considered suitable.
- History of chronic liver disease and/or viral hepatitis. Alcohol abuse with potential liver disease is more difficult to assess from history and liver function tests, unless the latter are widely deranged. Marked increases in serum transaminase levels can occur in donors subjected to short periods of hypotension or asystole. If the level of transaminase decreases in the subsequent 48 h, the liver can be used.

KIDNEY DONOR SELECTION

EXCLUSIONS:
- History of chronic renal insufficiency or recurrent urinary tract infection
- Serum creatinine level > 170 μmol l^{-1} is associated with decreased graft survival.

MEDICAL MANAGEMENT OF THE POTENTIAL ORGAN DONOR

The principal goals include early recognition and treatment of haemodynamic instability, mainte-nance of a systemic perfusion pressure to max-imise post-transplantation allograft function, and the prevention and treatment of complications related to brainstem death and supportive care.

ROUTINE ICU CARE:
- Pulmonary artery catheterisation or TOE may be necessary to help to optimise cardiac function and minimise inotrope requirement.
- Warming blankets to maintain a temperature above 35°C – hypothermia impairs cardiac, renal and hepatic function.

LABORATORY INVESTIGATIONS:
- Haematology:
  —ABO and Rhesus blood group
  —full blood count
  —coagulation profile.
- Biochemistry:
  —electrolytes
  —glucose
  —urea
  —creatinine
  —liver function tests
  —arterial blood gases.
- Microbiology:
  —blood cultures
  —urine cultures
  —sputum cultures.
- Serology:
  —hepatitis B serum antigen
  —hepatitis C screen
  —cytomegalovirus screen
  —HIV screen
  —HLA tissue typing.

OTHER INVESTIGATIONS:
- Chest radiography
- Electrocardiography
- Echocardiography may be requested for potential heart donors.

CARDIOVASCULAR SUPPORT
The predominant haemodynamic abnormality seen in brainstem dead patients is hypotension due to the destruction of pontine and medul-lary vasomotor centres. A systolic pressure of less than 80 mmHg is inadequate for optimal liver function. Maintaining a minimum systolic pressure of 90–100 mmHg is necessary to ensure adequate perfusion to all vital organs.

Hypovolaemia should be corrected and inotropic support added judiciously, using a pulmonary artery catheter if necessary. Dopa-mine is often used as the vasopressor because of its potential for maintaining renal and mesenteric blood flow. Although dopamine at a

21

dose higher than 10 μg kg^{-1} min^{-1} does not seem to affect early cardiac allograft survival, doses above this range can increase the risk of acute tubular necrosis and reduce renal allograft survival. If additional inotropic support is required, dobutamine is preferred to minimise any increase in myocardial oxygen demand. Exogenous and endogenous catecholamines have a deleterious effect on myocardial energy stores and post-transplant function, and inotropic dosage should be kept to the minimum compatible with adequate perfusion pressures by optimising volume status.

RESPIRATORY SUPPORT

Adequate oxygenation should be maintained by controlled ventilation, with PEEP < 5 cmH$_2$O and FiO$_2$ < 0.5. Excessive PEEP impairs liver perfusion and increases the risk of pulmonary barotrauma. Acid–base status should be optimised as far as possible.

RENAL AND METABOLIC SYSTEMS

A urine output of at least 100 ml h^{-1}, especially in the hour preceding retrieval, has been shown to be one of the most important factors determining renal allograft function in the recipient. If urine output is inadequate after volume expansion at a systolic pressure of 90–120 mmHg, mannitol or furosemide (frusemide) may be administered to establish a diuresis. Dopamine at 1–2 μg kg^{-1} min^{-1} may be helpful to maintain urine output.

Hypernatraemia should be avoided and adequate stores of intrahepatic glycogen maintained by using hypotonic saline with dextrose as maintenance fluid. Destruction of the hypothalamic–pituitary axis results in central diabetes insipidus. Desmopressin is the preferred vasopressin analogue because of its long duration of action and low pressor activity. The high pressor activity of other vasopressin preparations can result in reduced blood flow to the liver and cause post-transplant acute tubular necrosis and impaired renal function.

INTRAOPERATIVE MANAGEMENT FOR ORGAN DONATION

- Anaesthetic agents are not required.
- Full cardiovascular and respiratory support should be maintained up to the time of clamping vessels.
- Administer a neuromuscular blocking agent.
- Full systemic heparinisation will be requested.
- Maintain body temperature.

SURGICAL PROCEDURE DURING ORGAN DONATION

The surgical procedure varies depending on the number of organs to be retrieved. It also requires the cooperation of a number of different hospital departments. The donor operation usually takes place in an operating theatre at the hospital where the donor is a patient. Surgeons from a different hospital (the retrieval team) may attend to remove the donated organs. Remember to carry out the routine procedures with respect to death of a patient including referral to the coroner (or equivalent official) if necessary.

The salient features of multiple organ retrieval, in which at least two teams are usually involved, are:
- Chest and abdomen are opened through a midline incision
- Organs are examined for suitability
- The liver is mobilised first, and the anatomy of the hilar structures determined
- Distal abdominal aorta and superior mesenteric vein are prepared for cannulation
- Descending thoracic aorta is prepared for cross-clamping
- Cardiac team prepares the superior and inferior vena cavae
- Ascending aorta is cannulated for infusion of cardioplegia
- Heparin (300 units per kg bodyweight) is given
- Antibiotics and steroids may be requested
- Abdominal aorta and superior mesenteric vein are cannulated
- Inferior vena cava is incised within the pericardium
- Heart and liver are allowed to empty
- Thoracic aorta is cross-clamped at the arch and above the diaphragm
- Cold perfusion of abdominal and thoracic organs is started simultaneously
- Pericardium and peritoneum are irrigated with chilled saline
- Organs are removed in the following order: heart (with lungs *en bloc* if required), liver, pancreas, kidneys
- Spleen and lymph nodes are removed for tissue typing, and iliac artery and vein for possible use in vascular reconstruction.

This sequence may be modified in an unstable donor or according to individual team protocols. When heart and lungs are being retrieved, full cardiopulmonary bypass and whole-body cooling may be used.

21

BIBLIOGRAPHY

Booij LHDJ. Brain death and care of the brain death patient. Current Anaesthesia and Critical Care 1999; 10:312–318

Darby JM, Stein K, Grenvik A, Stuart S. Approach to the management of the heart beating 'brain-dead' organ donor. Journal of the American Medical Association 1989; 261:2222–2228

Harjula A, Starnes VA, Oyer PE, Jamieson SW, Shumway NE. Proper donor selection for heart–lung transplantation. Journal of Thoracic and Cardiovascular Surgery 1987; 94:874–880

Intensive Care Society. Donation of organs for transplantation – the management of the potential organ donor. A manual for the establishment of local guidelines. London: Intensive Care Society; 1999

Jordan CA, Snyder J. Intensive care and intra-operative management of the brain-dead organ donor. Transplantation Proceedings 1987; 19:21–25

Pruim J, Klompmaker IJ, Haagsma EB, Bijleveld CMA, Sloof MJH. Selection criteria for liver donation: a review. Transplant International 1993; 6:226–235

21

22

ORTHOPAEDICS
A. Loach

Overview

A. Loach

Orthopaedic surgery is a successful and expanding specialty concerned with elective surgery of bones and connective tissue. Great success has been achieved with the replacement of diseased or worn joints in elderly patients with synthetic prostheses leading to restoration of almost normal mobility. Advances over the past 5 years have been incremental rather than dramatic, with a steady increase in the scope of orthopaedic surgery.

JOINT REPLACEMENT

One-fifth of the population in the UK is aged 65 years or over, and this proportion is increasing alarmingly. In 2001, more than 50 000 joint replacements were performed and there remains a backlog of cases for surgery. Hip and knee replacements make up the bulk of operations, but increasing numbers of shoulder, elbow and interphalangeal joints are also being replaced, particularly in patients with rheumatoid arthritis. Increasing numbers of patients are also presenting for revision surgery due to loosening of the original prosthesis, infection of the prosthesis or, more rarely, fracture. Revision operations may be very complex and lengthy, involving bone grafting and custom-made prostheses. Recent improvements in primary replacement have focused on using resurfacing procedures, which conserve bone stock for future revision, rather than elaborate hinge prostheses.

ARTHROSCOPY

Arthroscopy of all major joints is undertaken including shoulder, elbow, ankle and wrist. Machine tools are available to permit many procedures without open operation. Trimming of meniscal tears or osteophytic deposits can be performed as day cases – an area where orthopaedic surgery has, in the past, trailed behind other fields of surgery.

SPINAL SURGERY

Surgery to the spine may involve decompressive laminectomy or discectomy (although percutaneous injection of the disc under radiological control, with a proteolytic enzyme, chymopapain, is gaining popularity), while more extensive surgery is undertaken to improve scoliosis and correct congenital deformity. Monitoring of cord function by detection of evoked responses during these procedures is necessary to avoid ischaemic injury or traction injury to the cord.

INTERNAL FIXATION

Internal fixation of fractures of long bones soon after trauma has been shown to improve recovery and reduce the requirement for ITU care. Such cases, therefore, increasingly appear on daily elective accident service lists. Patients are commonly young and fit, and pose few problems for anaesthesia during internal fixation by either plating or intramedullary nailing procedures. However, manipulation of long-bone fractures is known to liberate fat from marrow cavities into the circulation, and reaming of the medullary cavity for nailing may be followed by fat embolism syndrome of varying severity. The use of non-steroidal anti-inflammatory drugs (NSAIDs) for analgesia may be contraindicated after surgical treatment of malunion because of a suggestion that these drugs inhibit osteoblast activity.

OTHER OPERATIONS

These procedures may include: resection of tumours of bone or connective tissue (sometimes involving huge fore- or hind-quarter amputation); debridement and removal of sequestra for the treatment of osteomyelitis; reconstructive repair of trauma with nerve repair, tendon transplantation; limb straightening, lengthening or shortening with a variety of external fixators.

22

PROBLEMS IN ORTHOPAEDIC ANAESTHESIA

BLEEDING

The commonest error in orthopaedic anaesthesia is to underestimate blood loss. Cut bone surfaces ooze steadily and control is difficult, so that bleeding persists throughout an operation and may reach major proportions if surgery is lengthy. It is essential to keep a running total of loss from the weighing of swabs and sucker contents (then add one-third). Extensive bleeding can be expected during resection of tumours, which may be very vascular, and during operations on patients with Paget's disease. Procedures such as excision arthroplasty (Girdlestone's procedure) that leave an unfilled space may be followed by huge occult bleeding into the space.

INFECTION

Infection of bone is difficult to eradicate even over many years, so surgeons take every possible precaution to avoid it. Arthroplasties may be carried out in a sterile (Charnley) enclosure, which tends to isolate the anaesthetist and makes monitoring of surgical progress and blood loss more difficult. Comprehensive patient monitoring is vital. Prophylactic antibiotics are employed when metal is implanted and must be given before a limb tourniquet is applied. If deep-seated infection is suspected, antibiotics are generally withheld until samples have been collected for bacteriological examination.

VENOUS THROMBOEMBOLISM

Orthopaedic patients are particularly at risk of venous thromboembolism because of their age, their immobility and sluggish circulation in the legs during surgery, especially if the legs are placed in an awkward position, as in hip replacement, which might kink vessels. Needless mortality continues to be incurred by ignoring this hazard (Campling et al 1993). Prophylaxis should be used: correctly fitted graduated compression stockings, postoperative anticoagulation, adequate hydration and early mobilisation. Central neural blockade improves leg blood flow.

AGE

Many patients are elderly: two-thirds of joint replacements are in patients over 65 years of age. These are elective operations to improve the quality of life, and preoperative selection is vital to avoid death or damaging morbidity due principally to cardiovascular events, stroke and renal failure. Some patients have already undergone heart valve replacement, coronary artery surgery or renal transplantation, and require careful assessment.

SPLINTS

The effect of splints and fixators must be anticipated. When applied to the legs, they make turning a patient difficult and may contribute to deep vein thrombosis (DVT). Poorly applied hip spicas may cause a restrictive ventilatory defect by impeding abdominal movement, particularly during anaesthesia; halotraction from chest to head may make tracheal intubation difficult.

COOLING

Loss of 1°C body temperature per hour of surgery is common and caused by:

- Laminar down-draught in a Charnley enclosure
- Exposure of large areas of the patient
- Evaporation from large wounds
- Ventilation with non-humidified gases
- Endothermic effect of curing plasters
- Use of regional blocks and resulting vasodilatation.

Elderly patients and very young patients compensate poorly for heat loss and all available means of warming should be employed with monitoring of patient temperature. Even hot air blowers may be only marginally effective when large surfaces are exposed.

BIBLIOGRAPHY

Campling EA, Devlin HB, Hoile RW, Lunn JN. The report of the National Confidential Enquiry into Perioperative Deaths 1991/1992. London: NCEPOD; 1993

Loach A. Orthopaedic anaesthesia. London: Edward Arnold; 1993

22

Arthroscopy

A. Loach

PROCEDURE

Arthroscopy is the percutaneous internal examination of a joint using a fine-bore telescope similar to a laparoscope. The internal anatomy of the joint may be viewed through a video camera attached to the arthroscope with the magnified image displayed on a television screen.

Miniature power tools can be introduced through separate ports and therapeutic procedures performed under visual control without opening the joint.

This type of operation is easily possible as day surgery, and can often be performed under regional anaesthesia.

All of the larger joints may be examined.

PATIENT CHARACTERISTICS

Most patients are either fit young sportspersons for assessment of joint injury, or older patients undergoing arthroscopy for assessment of distribution and severity of joint damage prior to total joint arthroplasty.

PREOPERATIVE ASSESSMENT AND INVESTIGATIONS

Fit sportspersons present few problems. Anabolic steroid intake may be by injection with the remote risk of transmitted diseases.

In older patients, undertake a systematic review for likely chronic diseases.

Day surgery preparation when booked as a day case.

PREMEDICATION

Seldom required and may delay recovery of day cases.

THEATRE PREPARATION

Arthroscopy of hip, knee, ankle and wrist is performed with the patient supine. Elbow arthroscopy is usually performed with the patient in the lateral position and the arm draped over a support. Shoulder arthroscopy is performed in the 'deckchair' position.

PERIOPERATIVE MANAGEMENT

MONITORING:
- ECG
- SaO_2
- Non-invasive blood pressure
- Inspired and expired gas analysis for general anaesthesia.

REGIONAL ANAESTHESIA
Regional anaesthesia is suitable for knee, elbow, shoulder and wrist. It is particularly good for day cases. Postoperative analgesia is good and postoperative vomiting rare. Regional anaesthesia permits demonstration to a patient of any pathology (or its absence) on the television monitor.

Intra-articular regional anaesthesia is ineffective in the presence of active synovitis.

GENERAL ANAESTHESIA
Standard techniques suitable for day surgery are adequate.

22

TECHNIQUES OF REGIONAL ANAESTHESIA FOR ARTHROSCOPY

Knee
- Marcaine (0.5%) with adrenaline (epinephrine) (20 ml) into joint
- Infiltrate portals of entry of instruments with lidocaine (lignocaine) and adrenaline
- Surgeon must be prepared to work without a tourniquet (not necessary if adrenaline-containing solution is used) and accept poor relaxation of the joint.

Shoulder
- Interscalene brachial plexus block and superficial blockade of supraclavicular nerves.

Elbow and wrist
Interscalene or axillary brachial plexus block
Sedation is seldom required.

POSTOPERATIVE MANAGEMENT

If bupivacaine is left in the joint at the end of the operation, rectal diclofenac and simple analgesics are adequate for analgesia, and the patient may go home that day.

OUTCOME

Arthroscopic surgery will increase as financial pressures militate against inpatient treatment, and also as hardware improves with technical development.

BIBLIOGRAPHY

Allum RL, Ribbans WJ. Day case arthroscopy and arthroscopic surgery of the knee. Annals of the Royal College of Surgeons of England 1987; 69:225

CROSS-REFERENCES

22

Manipulation under anaesthesia

A. Loach

PROCEDURE

Manipulation under anaesthesia (MUA) is performed:
- To correct deformity due to a fracture before plastering
- To overcome stiffness in a total joint replacement caused by postoperative adhesions
- To improve movement after patellectomy
- To improve position after an osteotomy, before replastering.

PATIENT CHARACTERISTICS

Fractures occur in patients of any age, especially after the first frosts of winter. Manipulation after joint replacement is most commonly required after knee replacement.

MUA for fracture is semi-urgent to reduce pain; it is urgent if there is any vascular impairment. These patients may therefore be unprepared.

MUA is required after joint replacement and patellectomy in the elderly.

PREOPERATIVE ASSESSMENT AND INVESTIGATIONS

For elective procedures after joint replacement, patients are fasted. Other considerations are as for total hip arthroplasty.

For fractures, ascertain:
- Time since last meal and relation to accident
- Brief medical history (even sportspersons may be asthmatic or diabetic)
- Drug intake and allergy.

For large-bone fracture, establish an intravenous infusion.

PREMEDICATION

Not required.

THEATRE PREPARATION

MUA is often performed in the anaesthetic room.

PERIOPERATIVE MANAGEMENT

MONITORING:
- SaO_2
- ECG
- Non-invasive blood pressure.

ANAESTHETIC TECHNIQUE

Regional or general anaesthesia is suitable.

For the arm, regional anaesthesia is often preferred because it is simple and saves an outpatient from having a general anaesthetic. Axillary brachial plexus block or intravenous regional anaesthesia (IVRA) are both acceptable (Box 22.1).

For the leg a general or regional anaesthetic is suitable. General anaesthesia is carried out as for day cases. Use an epidural and a catheter or a brachial plexus catheter if the patient is

---

BOX 22.1

Intravenous regional anaesthesia (IVRA) technique

- Establish intravenous line in both hands or forearms
- Check cuff connections and place cuff around upper arm
- Exsanguinate limb as thoroughly as possible
- Inflate cuff to systolic blood pressure plus 100 mmHg
- Slowly inject 40 ml local anaesthetic through a cannula as far distally as possible
- Do not release cuff until 30 min has elapsed from injection
- Monitor pulse continuously following release of cuff
- A dedicated individual is needed to monitor cuff pressure throughout

to receive continuous passive motion after operation.

POSTOPERATIVE MANAGEMENT

MUA after joint replacement or after patellectomy gives rise to great pain. Therefore, consider:
- A suitable regional block
- Patient-controlled analgesia.

MUA for fracture usually relieves pain, and simple analgesics only are required.

BIBLIOGRAPHY

Davis AH, Hall ID, Wilkey AD, Smith JE, Walford AJ, Kale VR. Intravenous regional anaesthesia. The dangers of the congested arm and the value of occlusion pressure. Anaesthesia 1984; 39:416

Grice SC, Norell RC, Balestrieri FJ, Stump DA, Howard G. Intravenous regional anaesthesia, evaluation and prevention of leakage under the tourniquet. Anesthesiology 1986; 65:316

22

Repair of fractured neck of femur

P. McKenzie

PROCEDURE

Repair of fractured neck of femur is performed via the supine, lateral or intermediate position. A number of different operations may be performed, for example:

- Screws to femoral head
- Screw and femoral plate
- Other 'pin-and-plate' methods
- Cemented or uncemented primary femoral prosthesis
- Total hip replacement (rarely).

PATIENT CHARACTERISTICS

- 65–95+ years old
- Female : male ratio 2 : 1
- Very high incidence of chronic disease
- Dementia and confusional states common
- Multiple medication common
- Dehydration common – extent often difficult to assess accurately
- Fracture may be pathological.

PREOPERATIVE ASSESSMENT

- Assess the state of hydration; rehydrate intravenously if required
- Full history, examination and routine investigations
- Blood cross-match
- Antibiotic prophylaxis and allergy history.

PREMEDICATION

Analgesia and acid aspiration prophylaxis, if necessary. Sedative and anticholinergic drugs should be avoided.

PERIOPERATIVE MANAGEMENT

MONITORING:
- ECG
- Non-invasive blood pressure
- SpO_2
- $EtCO_2$
- Fluid balance.

ANAESTHETIC TECHNIQUE

Operative blood loss moderate (200–300 ml); unaffected by choice of regional or general anaesthesia.

Regional anaesthesia is most commonly by the subarachnoid route. Spinal anaesthesia can be technically difficult in the elderly. Analgesia for positioning the block can be provided by a small dose of intravenous ketamine (20–30 mg). Profound falls in arterial pressure may occur because patients are often more hypovolaemic than they appear; this is best treated with a vasopressor such as methoxamine in 2-mg increments. This can cause bradycardia, and pretreatment with glycopyrrolate is wise.

Supplemental oxygen should be given to all patients, despite the fact that there is no change in blood gases except when a prosthesis is inserted.

Advantages of regional anaesthesia are:
- Reduction in DVT rate
- Useful in the presence of severe respiratory disease
- Avoids postoperative deterioration of SpO_2 if patients breathe air.

For general anaesthesia, any careful technique is suitable, and there is no difference in outcome between controlled and spontaneous ventilation. Avoidance of hypoxia and hypocarbia and use of short-acting muscle relaxant drugs (e.g. atracurium), if required, are important.

PROBLEMS ASSOCIATED WITH PROSTHESIS INSERTION

The insertion of a prosthesis may be associated with a fall in blood pressure and oxygen saturation, which may be severe. Treatment with vasopressors and high FiO_2 are most appropriate. Causes are embolism of one or more of: fat, air, thromboplastins and acrylic monomer.

DEEP VENOUS THROMBOSIS

The incidence measured by objective methods is extremely high (approximately 75%). If spinal anaesthesia is used, this is reduced to around 40%.

General anaesthesia increases the risk of DVT by:

- Reducing venous return
- Increasing blood viscosity by reduction in red cell deformability (flexibility).
  Spinal anaesthesia reduces the risk of DVT by:
- Increasing venous flow
- Reducing blood viscosity by decreased haematocrit and increased deformability.

POSTOPERATIVE MANAGEMENT

Severe hypoxaemia can occur after general anaesthesia if the patient does not receive added oxygen. This is most severe in the period between 5 and 10 min after the end of anaesthesia. The aetiology is unclear.

Postoperative confusional states have now been shown not to relate to the type of anaesthesia but to episodes of hypoxaemia. It is thus essential that all patients breathe added oxygen continuously for at least 6 h and preferably for 24 h after surgery. Patients are usually in less pain after operation than before. Judicious use of opioids or appropriate nerve blocks are satisfactory in the control of pain. The use of NSAIDs is potentially hazardous in this type of patient.

OUTCOME

There is no significant difference in long-term outcome whether spinal or general anaesthesia is used.

The mortality rate at 1 month is variously reported, from 32% in older studies to 5.2% in recent studies. At 6 months, the mortality rate is around 15%. After 6 months, the death rate has returned to that predicted by actuarial data.

BIBLIOGRAPHY

Coleman SA, Boyce WJ, Cosh PH, McKenzie PJ. Outcome after general anaesthesia for repair of fractured neck of femur: a randomised trial of spontaneous versus controlled ventilation. British Journal of Anaesthesia 1988; 60:43–47

McKenzie PJ. Anaesthesia and the prophylaxis of thromboembolic diseases. Current Anaesthesia and Critical Care 1993; 4:26–30

McKenzie PJ. Anaesthesia for orthopaedic surgery. In: Smith G, Nimmo WS, Robotham DJ, eds. Anaesthesia. 2nd edn. Oxford: Blackwell; 1993

McKenzie PJ. Anaesthesia and the accident service. In: Loach A, ed. Anaesthesia for orthopaedic patients. Edinburgh: Longman; 1993

McKenzie PJ, Wishart HY, Smith G. Long-term outcome after repair of fractured neck of femur. Comprising of subarachnoid and general anaesthesia. British Journal of Anaesthesia 1984; 56:581–585

22

Total hip arthroplasty

A. Loach

PROCEDURE

Total hip arthroplasty (THA):
• Requires the lateral, semilateral (most commonly) or supine position
• Uses a posterior or anterolateral incision (L4–S3)
• Uses a cemented or screw-in acetabular prosthesis followed by a cemented, or in younger patients an uncemented, modular femoral prosthesis
• Is increasingly performed as a revision procedure following loosening, infection or fracture of an earlier prosthesis.

PATIENT CHARACTERISTICS

• Age group 50–90+ years
• May have unsuspected accompanying disease (Table 22.1)
• American Society of Anesthesiologists (ASA) status I–IV
• Many are extremely active old people; farmers have a particularly high incidence of hip disease.

COMMON ASSOCIATIONS WITH THA
• Primary osteoarthritis or secondary to fractured neck of femur

TABLE 22.1	
Incidence of chronic disease in the elderly	
Medical condition	Incidence (%)
Systemic hypertension	45
Previous myocardial infarction	21
Rhythm other than sinus	18
Angina	13
Chronic obstructive airway disease	20
Renal disease	5

• Rheumatoid arthritis and ankylosing spondylitis (to give upright posture)
• Avascular necrosis after fractured neck of femur or steroid therapy, for example for immunosuppression after transplantation, or NSAIDs.

PREOPERATIVE ASSESSMENT AND INVESTIGATIONS

• Exclude commonly associated medical conditions (e.g. anaemia from analgesic gastropathy)
• Systematic review of likely chronic diseases, especially those of the myocardium, which are the major cause of postoperative death (angina is often masked by inactivity), hypertension, renal failure from analgesics, possible incidental carcinoma (e.g. bronchus)
• Blood transfusion availability
• Plan DVT prophylaxis – compression stockings, regional block, anticoagulant
• Antibiotic prophylaxis.

PREMEDICATION

Seldom necessary in the elderly, and likely to cause confusion. If essential, give a minimal dose of a benzodiazepine.

THEATRE PREPARATION

Take care with positioning; elderly patients are particularly fragile. Ample padding; evacuated bean-bag ensures good support. Do not forget items (e.g. diathermy plate). If using a Charnley enclosure, patients are subsequently inaccessible.

Maintain body temperature with warm fluids and a hot-air blower; humidification if intubated.

Blood loss measured during THA ranges from 300 to 1500 ml, and is doubled in the first 24 h after operation. Blood loss during THA is strongly related to anaesthetic technique and is reduced by regional anaesthesia and induced hypotension. This reduction may subsequently be cancelled by increased postoperative loss.

PERIOPERATIVE MANAGEMENT

MONITORING:
- Sao_2
- Direct blood pressure if history of cardiovascular disease, otherwise non-invasive blood pressure monitoring is adequate
- Blood loss and fluid balance
- ECG
- Core temperature
- $Etco_2$.

ANAESTHETIC TECHNIQUE
Regional anaesthesia is the method of choice (Box 22.2), because the risk of venous thromboembolism is reduced as a result of increased leg blood flow and better venous drainage. There is excellent postoperative analgesia, decreased blood loss and attenuation of the stress response. Cementing may be improved because of reduced bleeding from bone.

Spinal and epidural techniques may be difficult in the elderly (look at hip radiographs for the lower spine); positioning may be impeded by pain.

Sedation during surgery may be needed. Use a light general anaesthetic or an infusion of propofol in low dosage ($1-2$ mg kg^{-1} h^{-1}). Added oxygen should be provided throughout.

General anaesthesia may be necessary if the patient rejects regional anaesthesia or block is impossible (ankylosing spondylitis, previous spinal fusion, gross scoliosis). Venous and arterial bleeding may be reduced with the modest hypotension from a volatile anaesthetic agent. Intravenous antibiotics may produce severe hypotension if given in bolus.

CEMENT-INDUCED HYPOTENSION
Hypotension, occasionally severe, may occur during cement and prosthesis insertion, particularly into the femoral shaft. This is probably due to air embolism during impaction of the prosthesis. It does not occur if the surgeon uses a cement gun to layer the cement from the bottom of the cavity. Absorption of liquid polymer cellular debris and fat also occurs, marked by lasting hypoxaemia and a rise in pulmonary vascular resistance. Hypotension is amplified by hypovolaemia and undertransfusion. Fat embolism syndrome has been reported when press-fit prostheses have been cemented. Intravenous fluid therapy must be adequate at this stage and the Fio_2 increased to 0.5 at least.

THROMBOEMBOLISM
This is common after THA, principally due to femoral vein thrombosis (80%), possibly caused by the kinking of vessels as a result of extreme flexion and adduction during surgery, or by the heat of cement curing. Apart from cardiac causes, venous thromboembolism is the commonest cause of death following THA; prophylaxis is mandatory. Spinal and epidural anaesthesia reduce the incidence of DVT significantly.

POSTOPERATIVE MANAGEMENT

Pain relief may be provided by continuous epidural analgesia with epidural opioids or slow infusion of local anaesthetics. Blood pressure should be monitored carefully during epidural infusions. Urinary retention is common and up to 30% of patients need catheterisation. Patient-controlled analgesia is also effective; usually only small doses are required.

Rewarming may cause a fall in blood pressure, but beware severe bleeding into the operation site.

Urinary output should be monitored and added fluids given, if necessary, to maintain urinary output.

BOX 22.2

Regional anaesthesia used for total hip arthroscopy

Spinal or epidural

- Sole agent or with sedation
- One-shot gives limited postoperative analgesia
- Catheter technique continuous.

Combined spinal and epidural

- Usually used with a catheter
- Sedation may be needed
- Continuous postoperative analgesia.

Lumbar plexus block

- Used with general anaesthesia
- Less autonomic block.

Paravascular inguinal block

- Used with general anaesthesia
- Poor postoperative analgesia.

22

OUTCOME

The overall mortality rate from THA is 1–2%, rising with age to 5% at 90 years. Few studies include death at home. No reduction in the mortality rate at 6 months has been demonstrated with regional anaesthesia, and studies to date have been unable to show any difference in postoperative confusion.

BIBLIOGRAPHY

Evans RD, Palazzo MGA, Ackers JWL. Air embolism during total hip replacement: comparison of two surgical techniques. British Journal of Anaesthesia 1989; 62:243

Michel R. Air embolism in hip surgery. Anaesthesia 1980; 35: 858

Seagroatt V, Tan HS, Goldacre M, Bulstrode C, Nugent I, Gill L. Elective total hip replacement: incidence, fatality and short-term readmission rates in a defined population. British Medical Journal 1991; 303:1431

Watson JT, Stulberg BN. Fat embolism associated with cementing of femoral stems designed for press-fit application. Journal of Arthroplasty 1989; 4:133

22

23

ENDOCRINE SURGERY
A. Batchelor

General considerations

A. Batchelor

- Some endocrine disorders are amenable to surgical correction. Such patients are exposed to hazards in addition to those associated with the surgical procedure.
- The presence of an endocrine disorder may, in itself, make anaesthesia and surgery especially hazardous. For example, patients with uncorrected hyperthyroidism are likely to develop dangerous tachydysrhythmias regardless of the type of surgical intervention.
- The surgical procedure may provoke the release of hormones and their precursors into the general circulation. This is a particular problem in the case of phaeochromocytoma, where massive quantities of catecholamines may be released causing life-threatening hypertension, tachycardia and heart failure.
- When a hormone-excreting tumour has been removed, the patient may be faced with the consequences of acute withdrawal. Thus removal of a phaeochromocytoma may lead to severe hypotension and hypoglycaemia.

- Removal of functioning endocrine tissue may leave the patient with a secretory mass which is smaller than that required to maintain normal health. Thus total adrenalectomy, thyroidectomy or parathyroidectomy will lead to the development of typical hyposecretory syndromes that threaten survival unless corrected by immediate replacement therapy.
- Minimally invasive surgery is altering the anaesthetic techniques needed, for adrenalectomy, parathyroidectomy and, no doubt, other procedures in the near future.

CROSS-REFERENCES

Iatrogenic adrenocortical insufficiency
   Patient Conditions 2: 71
Multiple endocrine neoplasia
   Patient Conditions 2: 77
Hypertension
   Patient Conditions 4: 151

23

Parathyroid surgery

A. Batchelor

Parathyroidectomy is usually undertaken for removal of a parathyroid adenoma.

DIAGNOSIS

The clinical picture is due to hypercalcaemia. The commonest presentation results from deposition of insoluble calcium salts in the kidney, leading to stone formation.

Patients often are hypertensive and develop progressive renal impairment with increased serum urea and creatinine concentrations. In more advanced cases, patients suffer severe skeletal pain and even pathological fractures as a result of calcium mobilisation.

Parathyroid tumours may be visualised using computed tomography (CT), ultrasonography or scintigraphy, but the distinction between normal and abnormal glands often rests finally on surgical exposure and frozen-section microscopy.

ASSOCIATED CONDITIONS:
- Peptic ulceration
- Anaemia
- Myopathy.

In multiple endocrine neoplasia type I, parathyroid adenoma is associated with pancreatic islet cell tumour and adenoma or hyperplasia of the anterior pituitary.

LABORATORY FINDINGS

- Raised serum urea
- Raised serum creatinine
- Raised serum calcium
- Raised serum parathyroid hormone
- Reduced serum phosphate
- Raised urinary calcium
- Reduced urinary phosphate.

PREOPERATIVE PREPARATION

Some patients present with severe hypercalcaemia which should be corrected before surgery is considered. Such patients often suffer from fluid and electrolyte depletion as a consequence of intractable vomiting. In patients with adequate renal function these disturbances may be corrected using intravenous fluid therapy with a loop diuretic to promote calcium clearance. Hypocalcaemic drugs such as sodium pamidronate and calcitonin may be used.

Steroids have been used, but are of very limited value. Rarely, life-saving surgery may be required when these measures fail to abate severe hyperparathyroidism. The elderly may be very debilitated by hypercalcaemia and surgery should be expedited.

SURGICAL PROCEDURE

Exploration of all four parathyroid glands is essential, as both adenomas and simple hyperplasias may be solitary or multiple. Rarely, parathyroid adenomas appear at ectopic sites and can be localised only by scintigraphy.

PREMEDICATION AND ANAESTHESIA

The surgeon requires a quiet, bloodless field in order to identify the tiny glands. This does not necessitate hypotensive anaesthesia, but does place a high premium on good technique. Avoidance of coughing and straining during the induction sequence are high priorities.

The procedure may be prolonged, and so effective heat conservation and fluid replacement should be maintained from the outset. In patients with major preoperative electrolyte disturbances, serum potassium levels should be monitored throughout surgery. Blood loss usually is minimal.

Patients should be positioned with great care in order to avoid pathological fractures.

MONITORING:

- ECG
- SaO_2
- $EtCO_2$
- Non-invasive blood pressure
- Core temperature
- Peripheral nerve stimulation.

POSTOPERATIVE COMPLICATIONS

- Accidental division of the recurrent laryngeal nerve
- Acute hypocalcaemia may follow total parathyroidectomy.

BIBLIOGRAPHY

Mihai R, Farndon JR. Parathyroid disease and calcium metabolism. British Journal of Anaesthesia 2000; 85:29–43

Chen H, Parkerson S, Udelsman R. Parathyroidectomy in the elderly: do the benefits outweigh the risks? World Journal of Surgery 1998; 22:531–536

CROSS-REFERENCES

Hyperparathyroidism
    Patient Conditions 2: 61
Multiple endocrine neoplasia
    Patient Conditions 2: 77
Prolonged anaesthesia
    Anaesthetic Factors 30: 713

23

Phaeochromocytoma

A. Batchelor

Phaeochromocytomas are catecholamine-secreting tumours of chromaffin tissue. They may be benign (usually) or malignant, solitary or multiple, and occur most commonly within the adrenal gland, but can be found in a wide variety of paraganglionic sites ranging from the base of the bladder to the base of skull. Some 13% are associated with genetic problems such as multiple endocrine neoplasia (MEN) type 2, either type 2A associated with thyroid carcinoma and parathyroid hyperplasia or, more rarely, type 2B associated with Marfan-like features and mucosal neuroma. There are also associations with neurofibromatosis and von Hippel–Lindau syndrome. Some 10% are extra-adrenal, multiple, bilateral, or malignant.

Occasionally, phaeochromocytoma develops in childhood, more commonly in boys than in girls. The prevalence of extra-adrenal sites is greater than in adults.

DIAGNOSIS

Patients commonly present with the following:
- Hypertension – this may be paroxysmal (50%) or continuous
- Headache
- Sweating
- Cardiovascular problems ranging from arrhythmias to catecholamine cardiomyopathy
- Headache, palpitations, sweating and hypertension are 90% predictive of phaeochromocytoma
- Hyperglycaemia and glycosuria – some patients may even require insulin therapy.

Ectopic tumours in the neck may be provoked by head movement, and those at the base of the bladder by micturition.

The presentation depends on the relative proportion of adrenaline and noradrenaline secreted into the bloodstream. Patients with predominantly noradrenaline-secreting tumours present with hypertension, headache and pallor, whereas those with adrenaline-secreting tumours tend to present with tachycardia and arrhythmias. Some patients develop a hypermetabolic state similar to that seen in severe hyperthyroidism.

INVESTIGATIONS

Confirmation of diagnosis is achieved by estimation of:
- 24-h or overnight urine collection for met-adrenaline and nor-met-adrenaline
- Plasma catecholamines are less reliable.

Tumour localisation depends on CT, magnetic resonance imaging (MRI) and [131I]m-iodobenzylguanidine (MIBG) scintigraphy. Radiological contrast media may precipitate a crisis in unblocked patients.

Genetic analysis can determine abnormalities of the *RET* oncogene.

SURGICAL PROCEDURE

Some 90% of tumours occur in the adrenal medulla, so the surgical approach of choice is laparoscopic resection of the adrenal gland.

As extra-adrenal tumours may be found anywhere from the base of skull to the pelvis, usually along the paraganglionic line, their removal may require a variety of surgical approaches.

PREOPERATIVE MANAGEMENT

Multisystem preoperative assessment is necessary, with special emphasis on the cardiovascular system. All patients should have echocardiography, as cardiomyopathy is often symptomless and unsuspected.

PREOPERATIVE BLOCKADE

Published recommendations range from nothing to many weeks of alpha blockade with

23

or without β-adrenergic blockade. Other agents used include calcium channel blockers, magnesium and metyrosine. No adequate trials of preoperative preparation exist in the literature, but a reduction in the mortality rate from 50% to 0–3% was coincident with the introduction of preoperative alpha and beta blockade. Both selective and non-selective alpha-blockers have been used.

Adrenergic blockade does not prevent the release of catecholamines, but does obtund the physiological response, producing unimpaired myocardial performance and tissue oxygen delivery.

RECOMMENDATIONS FOR PREOPERATIVE BLOCKADE

Alpha blockade using phenoxybenzamine (10 mg orally, twice daily) increased as tolerated.

- *Aim*: stabilisation of blood pressure. Increase dosage until symptoms abate and the blood pressure and heart rate are adequately controlled as assessed on 24-h recording; maximum blood pressure 140/90 mmHg and heart rate 100 b.p.m. The object is to allow restoration of normal circulating volume, and in patients with cardiomyopathy a period of cardiac rest which may allow some recovery.
- *Side-effects*:
  —stuffy nose
  —dizziness on standing (initial treatment should be as an inpatient)
  —drowsiness and blurred vision (the patient should not drive)
  —tachycardia, which can be controlled with a beta-blocker (propranolol or atenolol) introduced after alpha blockade is established.

At least 7–10 days of established blockade is required, but many patients benefit from a longer period of treatment, particularly those with cardiomyopathy or ST–T-wave changes. Plasma volume may increase during blockade, thus preventing severe hypotension after tumour removal.

PREMEDICATION

- An anxiolytic such as temazepam. Avoid atropine because of tachycardia.
- Deep venous thrombosis prophylaxis.
- Discontinue blockade on the evening before surgery.

PERIOPERATIVE CARE

DRUGS AND INFUSIONS PREPARED:

- Sodium nitroprusside infusion for control of hypertensive surges during surgery
- Noradrenaline (norepinephrine) for postresection hypotension
- Adrenaline (epinephrine) in case of decreased cardiac output associated with an abrupt fall in circulating catecholamines levels
- Bolus doses of propranolol for control of tachycardia.

MAINTENANCE OF TEMPERATURE IN A VASODILATED PATIENT:

- Warm all intravenous fluids.
- Use a warming blanket on the operating table.
- Use a forced-air warmer over exposed parts of the patient if possible.
- Warm and humidify inspired gases.

ANAESTHESIA

Aim to avoid provocation of catecholamine release by anaesthetic drugs or manoeuvres, to suppress the adrenergic response to surgical stimulation, and to minimise haemodynamic responses to tumour handling and devascularisation.

MONITORING:

- ECG – CM5 lead preferred
- Arterial line for continuous blood pressure measurement
- Central venous pressure – triple-lumen catheter
- A pulmonary artery flotation catheter is optional
- Sp_{O_2}
- Et_{CO_2}
- Core temperature.

ANAESTHETIC TECHNIQUE

For laparotomy, use a high lumbar epidural block plus general anaesthesia. Combined opioid and regional blockade provides postoperative analgesia. As these patients already have peripheral vasodilatation, it is most unusual for the epidural to cause hypotension.

For laparoscopic surgery, general anaesthesia alone is sufficient.

Avoid histamine-releasing drugs such as morphine and atracurium. Most anaesthetic drugs have been reported as being used successfully, but the combination used by the author is alfentanil, etomidate, vecuronium and isoflurane.

CONTROL OF ARTERIAL PRESSURE AND HEART RATE DURING SURGERY

Despite preoperative preparation, marked swings in blood pressure and heart rate may be seen during manipulation of the tumour. These should be controlled with short-acting agents such as nitroprusside and propranolol.

Alpha blockade leads to increased plasma volume, but even then it is usually necessary to administer additional intravenous fluids during the dissection phase if hypotension following tumour devascularisation is to be prevented.

After ligation of all venous drainage from the tumour, arterial pressure commonly declines. This may be associated with a high cardiac output and very low systemic vascular resistance, requiring noradrenaline (norepinephrine) treatment, low cardiac output requiring inotropic support, or both. A pulmonary artery flotation catheter simplifies decision-making during this phase. An adequate period of preoperative blockade, combined with generous intraoperative fluid loading, may obviate the need for postresection catecholamines.

POSTOPERATIVE CARE

The patient should be managed in a critical care area by nursing staff familiar with the special problems posed by these patients for the first few postoperative hours.

BLOOD PRESSURE

Despite persisting alpha and beta blockade, arterial pressure usually stabilises remarkably quickly, and vasoactive medication can be withdrawn rapidly. In some cases, hypertension persists for several days before settling down, but in a small minority hypertension may persist, raising the possibilities of residual tumour or underlying essential hypertension.

BLOOD GLUCOSE

High catecholamine levels increase blood glucose concentration and block the secretion of insulin. Tumour removal and loss of catecholamines may result in hypoglycaemia, either via a rebound increase in insulin secretion and/or via a decrease in lipolysis and glycogenolysis. Persisting beta blockade will mask the signs of hypoglycaemia. Failure to detect severe hypoglycaemia has led to disastrous outcomes. Blood glucose levels should be monitored every half hour for the first 6 h, and corrected promptly if subnormal.

STEROIDS

If bilateral adrenalectomy has been carried out, steroid replacement will be required.

ANALGESIA

Abrupt withdrawal of catecholamines and residual concentrations of blocking drugs may cause marked somnolence. Such patients are very sensitive to the sedative actions of opioids, such that conventional doses may result in dangerously deep sedation. Patient-controlled analgesia, either epidural or intravenous, avoids this problem.

UNEXPECTEDLY ENCOUNTERED PHAEOCHROMOCYTOMA

Very occasionally, a patient will exhibit severe hypertension with a tachycardia and possibly arrhythmias and pulmonary oedema during surgery for an unrelated condition. Once the possibility of an undiagnosed phaeochromocytoma has been raised, alpha blockade with phentolamine should be instituted immediately. Surgery should be completed as rapidly as possible and no attempt made to resect the tumour unless this is essential to the patient's immediate survival. Then, diagnosis, localisation and preparation may be undertaken as usual.

Acute non-operative presentation may include hypotension as heart failure supervenes; in these circumstances diagnosis may be difficult.

Presentation in pregnancy is associated with increased risks to both mother and fetus; both early intervention and conservative management until delivery have been reported.

OUTCOME

In adequately prepared patients, the mortality rate is 0–3% in reported series. The mortality rate is high (of the order of 50%) in patients diagnosed during operation. In a series of 40 000 post-mortem examinations, phaeochromocytoma was found in 0.13%. Of patients whose tumours were identified at autopsy, 27% died in the perioperative period from a cardiovascular collapse of unknown cause.

23

BIBLIOGRAPHY

Hull CJ. Phaeochromocytoma. British Journal of Anaesthesia 1986; 58:1453–1468

Joris JL, Hamoir EE, Hartstein GM et al. Hemodynamic changes and catecholamine release during laparoscopic adrenalectomy for pheochromocytoma. Anesthesia and Analgesia 1999; 88:16–21

Prys-Roberts C. Phaeochromocytoma – recent progress in its management. British Journal of Anaesthesia 2000; 85:44–57

Roizen MF, Hung TK, Beaupre PN et al. The effect of alpha-adrenergic blockade on cardiac performance and tissue oxygen delivery during excision of phaeochromocytoma. Surgery 1983; 946:941–945

Sutton MG, Sheps SG, Lie JT. Prevalence of clinically unsuspected phaeochromocytoma: review of a 50 year autopsy series. Mayo Clinic Proceedings 1981; 56:354–360

CROSS-REFERENCES

Iatrogenic adrenocortical insufficiency
    Patient Conditions 2: 71
Multiple endocrine neoplasia
    Patient Conditions 2: 77
Hypertension
    Patient Conditions 4: 151
Prolonged anaesthesia
    Anaesthetic Factors 30: 713
Intraoperative hypertension
    Anaesthetic Factors 31: 755

23

24

PAEDIATRICS
G. H. Meakin

Overview

G. H. Meakin

The fundamental differences between paediatric patients and adults with regard to anaesthesia have been discussed previously. This section deals with the practical aspects of anaesthetic management.

PREOPERATIVE PREPARATION

Children should be admitted to a dedicated children's ward that is suitably decorated and equipped with a selection of books and toys. The child's nickname, if one is used, should be entered in the nursing notes and used by the carers. At the preoperative visit, the anaesthetist should explain the proposed procedure in simple terms, avoiding words that may cause alarm. For example, if intravenous induction of anaesthesia is planned, it is more tactful to describe this as a 'scratch on the hand' rather than a 'prick from a needle'. A parent should be invited to accompany the child at induction of anaesthesia.

ANAESTHETIC ASSESSMENT

The case notes should be reviewed with particular attention to:

- Age and weight (is the weight appropriate?)
- History of prematurity
- Previous illnesses and medications
- Allergy and any unusual syndrome
- Previous anaesthetics
- History of upper respiratory tract infection.

Children with a history of upper respiratory tract infection within 4 weeks of operation are at increased risk of respiratory complications during or after anaesthesia. Ideally, elective surgery should be postponed for 4–6 weeks, but this is not always practical as symptoms tend to recur. Moreover, many children with recurrent symptoms will be suffering from allergy. If a decision is made to proceed, it may be prudent to intubate and ventilate the patient during anaesthesia to minimise the risk of coughing or laryngospasm. Careful monitoring and supplemental oxygen will be required during recovery.

Physical examination should be carried out with particular attention to:

- Loose deciduous teeth
- Signs of difficult intubation (limited mouth opening, micrognathia, large tongue, noisy breathing)
- Signs of lower respiratory tract infection (pyrexia, cough, malaise and abnormal breath sounds).
- Possible venepuncture sites.

When signs of lower respiratory tract infection are present, elective surgery must be postponed for 4–6 weeks to allow hyperactive airways to return to normal.

Investigations are not required routinely in healthy children undergoing relatively minor surgery. Estimation of haemoglobin concentration is required in patients at increased risk of anaemia, although the significance of anaemia should be judged by its clinical effects. Because of compensatory mechanisms, symptoms rarely appear until the haemoglobin level falls below 6 g dl^{-1}.

A formal assessment of the risk of anaesthesia should be made using the American Society of Anesthesiologists (ASA) classification and entered into the patient's notes.

FASTING AND PREMEDICATION

Patients are fasted before operation to minimise the volume of gastric contents at induction of anaesthesia. The recommended fasting times for liquids and solids are summarised in Table 24.1.

The routine use of atropine as prophylaxis for bradycardia in infants has declined following the introduction of sevoflurane for gaseous induction. Some older children may benefit from sedative premedication with oral midazolam: 0.5 mg kg^{-1}, maximum 20 mg, 30–45 min before surgery. A topical local anaesthetic preparation, such as EMLA cream or Ametop gel, should be applied over possible venepuncture sites.

TABLE 24.1

Preoperative fasting times for different types of liquids and solids in infants and children

Age	Minimum fasting period (h)			
	Clear fluids[a]	Breast milk	Formula or cow's milk	Solids
> 3 months	2	4	6	6
< 3 months	2	4	4	6

[a]A clear fluid is one you can read newsprint through.

TABLE 24.2

Laryngeal mask sizes for children aged over 1 year

Size	Weight (kg)	Maximum inflation volume (ml)
2	10–20	10
2.5	20–30	15
3.0	30–50	20
4.0	> 50	30

MANAGEMENT OF ANAESTHESIA

INDUCTION

Both intravenous and inhalation methods have advantages in children and a flexible approach is required. Much will depend on the age and preferences of the child.

Inhalation induction is often more convenient for infants and toddlers, who frequently have poor venous access and difficulty cooperating with an intravenous induction. Inhalation induction is also rapid in these very young patients owing to a relatively large minute volume ventilation in relation to the functional residual capacity, and a relatively high cardiac output. Sevoflurane is used most commonly because of its relative lack of pungency, rapid uptake and elimination, and reduced incidence of cardiovascular effects. For older children with visible veins, intravenous induction of anaesthesia with thiopental or propofol is quicker and creates less operating room pollution.

AIRWAY MANAGEMENT

The laryngeal mask (LM) is fast becoming the most common method of managing the airway in children aged over 1 year undergoing relatively short procedures under anaesthesia with spontaneous ventilation. The appropriate sizes for children together with their maximum recommended inflation volumes are given in Table 24.2. Overinflation of the cuff must be avoided because it may cause trauma to the pharynx and larynx or herniation of the cuff. The LM is usually inserted during moderately deep anaesthesia without the aid of a muscle relaxant. It can be left *in situ* at the end of the operation and removed by the recovery nurse when the child is fully awake.

Despite the increasing popularity of the LM, tracheal intubation remains the 'gold standard' for paediatric airway management. Infants and children are intubated with the head in a neutral position because raising the head on a pillow does not improve the view of the larynx. The most effective manoeuvre is the application of external pressure at the level of the cricoid cartilage to push the larynx into view.

In infants, a flat-blade laryngoscope such as the infant Magill, which passes posterior to the epiglottis, may be more suitable than a curved one, as it flattens out the U-shaped curvature of the epiglottis and can be used to lift it forwards to expose the larynx. In children aged over 1 year, laryngoscopy can usually be accomplished with a medium-sized Macintosh blade with the tip placed in the vallecula.

As the narrowest part of the larynx before puberty is the cricoid ring, cuffed tracheal tubes are not usually required in infants and children. The correctly sized tube is one that passes easily through the cricoid ring and leaks minimally or not at all in the working range of 0–20 cmH$_2$O. The following formula may be used as a guide in children aged 2 years and over:

Tube size (internal diameter in mm) = (Age in years/4) + 4.5

Tube sizes in infants and children aged less than 2 years have to be memorised. A normal neonate weighing 3 kg requires a 3-mm tracheal tube; premature and low-weight babies may require a 2.5-mm tube. Other tube sizes can be interpolated.

Tracheal tubes should be cut to a length that allows the tip of the tube to be placed in the mid-trachea while 2–3 cm protrudes from the mouth for fixation. The following formula may be used to estimate orotracheal tube length in children aged over 2 years:

24

Orotracheal tube length (cm) =
(Age in years/2) + 13

Orotracheal tube lengths for patients aged less than 2 years have to be memorised. The length for neonate is 10 cm, and that for a 1-year-old is 12 cm; other tube lengths can be interpolated. The position of the tracheal tube should be checked by auscultation of the lung fields.

MAINTENANCE OF ANAESTHESIA

In general, infants are poor candidates for anaesthesia with spontaneous ventilation because of poor pulmonary mechanics. In these patients, the combination of tracheal intubation and balanced anaesthesia with full doses of muscle relaxants, controlled ventilation, minimum concentrations of volatile anaesthetics and reduced doses of opioids is recommended. This regimen provides ideal surgical conditions with minimal cardiovascular depression and rapid return of laryngeal reflexes at the conclusion of anaesthesia.

Children aged over 1 year undergoing long operations will also benefit from balanced anaesthesia. However, for many children undergoing operations lasting less than 30–40 min, simple inhalation anaesthesia with 66% nitrous oxide in oxygen and sevoflurane (2–3%) may be adequate. This may be combined with an opioid analgesic, local infiltration or a regional block to provide analgesia in the postoperative period.

ANAESTHETIC BREATHING SYSTEMS

Anaesthetic breathing systems may be classified broadly into those that do not contain a chemical means of absorbing carbon dioxide and those that are equipped with such units. In the past, concerns about resistance to breathing and apparatus deadspace with the use of absorber systems led paediatric anaesthetists to use mainly non-absorber breathing systems. However, recent concerns for economy and environmental pollution have led to a renewed interest in the use of circle absorber systems in paediatric anaesthesia.

The Jackson Rees T-piece is a popular breathing system for paediatric anaesthesia because of its compact size, low resistance to breathing and low apparatus deadspace. The low compressible volume of the T-piece gives a good 'feel' for the lung compliance in an infant, and facilitates hand ventilation even in the face of a decrease in lung compliance or partial respiratory obstruction. Notable disadvantages of the system include its high fresh gas requirements (3–8 l min^{-1}) and the inability to scav-

enge waste gases. The practical advantages of the T-piece outweigh its disadvantages when the system is used for induction of anaesthesia and anaesthesia of short duration.

The main advantages of circle absorber systems are economy in the use of anaesthetic agents and gases, conservation of heat and moisture in the respiratory tract, and reduced operating room pollution. These advantages are most evident when the circle system is used for maintenance of anaesthesia of intermediate to long duration. Fears that these systems invariably impose unacceptable resistance to breathing and apparatus deadspace for paediatric use appear to have been unfounded. Moreover, the ready availability of anaesthetic gas monitors and oxygen saturation monitors has greatly improved the safety of low-flow anaesthesia techniques. The main disadvantage of circle systems in paediatric anaesthesia is their high compression volume, which gives a poor 'feel' for the lung compliance in infants and may make it difficult to hand-ventilate these patients in the event of an unexpected decrease in lung compliance. Accordingly, a low compression volume system such as the T-piece should always be readily available when using a circle system in children.

MONITORING

Routine monitoring should include:
- ECG
- Non-invasive blood pressure
- Pulse oximetry
- Respiratory gases.

A range of paediatric cuffs must be available for measurement of blood pressure; the correctly sized cuff is one that covers two-thirds of the upper arm. Temperature measurement is mandatory in infants and young children, who are at especially high risk of developing hypothermia. Heating devices such as water mattresses and warm air blowers should be available to counter heat loss in these patients.

INTRAOPERATIVE FLUID THERAPY

An intravenous infusion should be established for all but minor procedures. A 22-gauge cannula can generally be sited in a peripheral vein in an infant, whereas a 20-gauge cannula is suitable for children. Maintenance fluid and electrolyte requirements can be calculated from the equation given on p. 611. A balanced salt solution, such as Ringer lactate, should be given to replace third-space losses.

Blood loss should be determined by swab weighing or colorimetry. In general, losses less than 10% of the blood volume (estimated at 80 ml kg^{-1}) either require no replacement or can be replaced by crystalloid solution. Losses of 10–20% can be replaced by colloids or blood, but losses of more than 20% must be replaced by blood.

POSTOPERATIVE MANAGEMENT

At the conclusion of anaesthesia, the child should be turned into the lateral position and transported, breathing oxygen, to a fully equipped recovery room. Details of the operative procedure and any special instructions should be given to the recovery nurse assuming care of the child. Recovery room protocol should include airway maintenance, provision of oxygen therapy, monitoring of oxygen saturation, pulse, respiration and blood pressure, and the completion of a postanaesthetic recovery chart. The anaesthetist should ensure that the child is fully awake and that postoperative fluids and analgesics have been ordered before the child is returned to the surgical ward.

BIBLIOGRAPHY

Meakin G. Low flow anaesthesia in infants and children. British Journal of Anaesthesia 1999; 83:50–57

Meakin GH, Welbourn LG. Anaesthesia for infants and children. In: Healy TEJ, Cohen PJ, eds. Wylie and Churchill Davidson's a practice of anaesthesia. 7th edn. London: Edward Arnold; 2003 (in press)

Steward DJ. Screening tests before surgery in children. Canadian Journal of Anaesthesia 1991; 38: 693–695

Westhorpe RN. The position of the larynx in children and its relationship to the ease of intubation. Anaesthesia and Intensive Care 1987; 15:384–388

CROSS-REFERENCES

Infants and children
    Patient Conditions 22: 610

24

Circumcision

D. Patel

PROCEDURE

Circumcision is excision of the foreskin from around the penis. It is usually performed on an elective day-case basis.

PATIENT CHARACTERISTICS

Approximately 12200 boys each year in England are circumcised in the hospital setting. Pathological phimosis is the only absolute indication for circumcision. This affects 0.6% of boys, with a peak incidence at 11 years of age, and is rarely encountered before the age of 5 years. In addition, many procedures are performed by non-medical practitioners for religious and cultural reasons.

PREOPERATIVE ASSESSMENT

- Exclude active respiratory tract infection with productive cough or pyrexia.
- Exclude those with a recent exposure to childhood infections.
- Ensure no history of bleeding diathesis or anaesthetic problems.

PREOPERATIVE INVESTIGATIONS

None necessary unless clinically indicated.

PREOPERATIVE PREPARATION

- Fasting of solids (including milk) for 6 h and clear fluids for 2 h
- Obtain informed consent and explain to parents when a local anaesthetic procedure and/or rectal analgesics are to be used during surgery
- A parent should be invited to accompany the child at induction of anaesthesia.

PREMEDICATION

- Topical local anaesthetic preparation (e.g. EMLA or Ametop cream) over possible venepuncture sites
- Oral paracetamol 20 mg kg^{-1} and/or ibuprofen 5 mg kg^{-1}, 30–45 min before operation to enhance intraoperative and postoperative analgesia
- If anxiolytic required, oral midazolam (0.5 mg kg^{-1}) may be given 30–45 min before surgery.

PERIOPERATIVE MANAGEMENT

Routine non-invasive monitoring.

GENERAL ANAESTHESIA:
- Intravenous or inhalation induction
- Spontaneous ventilation via laryngeal mask for children aged over 1 year
- Intermittent positive-pressure ventilation (IPPV) via tracheal tube for children under 1 year.

LOCAL ANAESTHESIA:
- The local anaesthetic block should be performed after induction to provide intraoperative and postoperative analgesia.
- Penile nerve block using plain 0.25% levobupivacaine (1–3 ml) for babies aged less than 1 year and plain 0.5% levobupivacaine (3–5 ml) for those older than 1 year (Box 24.1). Do not use solutions containing adrenaline (epinephrine) or other vasoconstrictors.
- Alternatively, a single-shot caudal extradural block, using 0.25% levobupivacaine (0.5 ml kg^{-1}) is suitable (Box 24.2).
- Clonidine (1–2 µg kg^{-1}) or preservative-free ketamine (0.5 mg kg^{-1}) additives may be used to prolong the caudal block.

24

BOX 24.1

Penile nerve block

- The nerves lie deep and superficial to Buck's fascia and may be separated by a midline septum
- Supine position
- Aseptic technique
- 21-SWG regional block needle
- Palpate the lower border of the symphysis pubis with the index finger and retract the penis
- Insert the needle between finger and arch of pubis until there is a slight 'give' or bone is struck; if bone is struck, 'walk' the needle inferiorly until it is free
- Local anaesthetic solution should be injected either side of the midline by directing the needle from a single puncture
- Aspirate before injecting deep and superficial to Buck's fascia
- Minimal swelling should be seen
- Analgesia should last about 4–6 h

BOX 24.2

Caudal extradural block of the sacral nerves

- The sacral hiatus is located by placing the child on his side with legs flexed at the hips and palpating the cornua and sacral notch at the lower end of the vertebral column.
- A 22-SWG cannula or regional block needle is used.
- The cannula or needle is advanced through the sacrococcygeal membrane at the apex of the hiatus until a 'give' is felt. The cannula or needle should be advanced only a few millimetres to avoid dural puncture.
- A single-shot caudal block does not cause hypotension in children.
- Analgesia should last about 4–6 h, and up to 12 h with caudal additives.

POSTOPERATIVE MANAGEMENT

- Good postoperative analgesia is essential for smooth recovery; be prepared to supplement with oral or intravenous opiates.
- Provide an information leaflet, contact details and oral analgesia on discharge.

OUTCOME

Discharge may be delayed by:
- Failure to micturate (more likely with inadequate analgesia; penile block has a higher failure rate than caudal)
- Bleeding
- Unsteady when walking (occasionally with caudal epidural, but should not delay discharge in young children)
- Nausea and vomiting.

BIBLIOGRAPHY

Brown TCK, Fisk GC. Regional and local anaesthesia. In: Brown TCK, Fisk GC, eds. Anaesthesia for children. 2nd edn. Oxford: Blackwell Scientific; 1992:301–323

Rickwood AMK, Walker J. Is phimosis over diagnosed in boys and are too many circumcisions performed in consequence? Annals of the Royal College of Surgeons of England 1989; 71:275–277

Shankar KR, Rickwood AMK. The incidence of phimosis in boys. British Journal of Urology 1999; 84:101–102

24

Congenital diaphragmatic hernia

A. J. Charlton

PRESENTATION

Incidence 1 in 2–4000 live births. Probably a primary defect of lung growth. Right-sided hernia (10%) associated with higher mortality rate.

The child presents with respiratory failure at birth but the condition is frequently detected by antenatal ultrasonography. Patients have bilateral pulmonary hypoplasia and tend to revert to fetal circulation with severe right–left shunting.

Death occurs due to:
- Pneumothorax
- Inadequate gas exchange surface
- Fixed high pulmonary vascular resistance (decreased vascular cross-sectional area, normal cardiac output)
- Reversible pulmonary hypertension (abnormal muscularity of vessels)
- Additional anomalies (5%).

RESUSCITATION

Mask inflation distends herniated viscera, worsening mediastinal shift and risks pneumothorax. Use immediate tracheal intubation, with muscle relaxants to facilitate IPPV. Pass nasogastric tube to deflate gut and keep on free drainage.

PREOPERATIVE PREPARATION

Surgery often worsens lung mechanics. Time (days) should be taken to stabilise gas exchange by meticulous medical management aiming to avoid trigger factors for pulmonary vasoconstriction (hypoxia, hypercarbia, acidosis) and allowing the physiological fall in pulmonary vascular resistance to occur. Precise indicators of optimal surgical timing have not been established.

MONITORING

Peripheral arterial cannulation allows pressure and blood gas monitoring with minimal disturbance. Published predictive indices require postductal oxygen values. Transcutaneous oxygen and carbon dioxide transducers aid continuous monitoring. Pulse oximeters placed pre- and post-ductally may demonstrate the variability of shunting.

VENTILATION:
- Risk of pneumothorax from high inflation pressures and asynchrony
- Muscle relaxants (such as atracurium or cisatracurium) by infusion give optimal control and decrease oxygen consumption
- No evidence that high-frequency IPPV improves outcome
- Surfactant therapy may be indicated.

ACID–BASE STATUS

Metabolic acidosis should be corrected with buffers. Moderate alkalosis by systemic alkalinisation (to pH 7.5–7.6) or hyperventilation (Pa_{CO_2} 30–35 mmHg) may enhance pulmonary circulation.

PULMONARY CIRCULATION

Refractory hypoxaemia may respond to pulmonary vasodilators. Nitric oxide has superseded other agents.

FLUID BALANCE

Preoperative restriction (6 ml kg^{-1} per 24 h) avoids fluid retention. Circulating volume should be maintained with plasma or blood (maintain haemoglobin level above 14 g dl^{-1}).

SEDATION

Lability in response to handling (unusual) may be helped by a narcotic (e.g. morphine infusion).

24

SURGERY

Usually undertaken via an upper abdominal incision, which permits correction of the gut malrotation. In about 5% of cases, closure can be achieved only with a prosthetic patch or latissimus dorsi muscle flap.

ANAESTHESIA

- Surgery causes little disturbance if delayed to permit inspired oxygen requirement to stabilise below 50%.
- The exact pattern of preoperative ventilation should be continued.
- Volatile agents should be avoided – cardiovascular depression.
- Fentanyl in large doses (up to 25 μg kg^{-1}) obtunds response to surgery (even with 100% oxygen) and has negligible cardiovascular effect.
- Monitoring should include ECG, direct or indirect arterial pressure, pulse oximetry, capnography and body temperature.

POSTOPERATIVE CARE

General intensive care with attention to fluid and nutritional requirements (enteral or parenteral) must continue. Weaning from IPPV in severe cases may take months. After tracheal extubation a period on continuous positive airway pressure (CPAP) is usual. The most severely affected survivors have little respiratory reserve, require long-term oxygen therapy and may die in infancy from respiratory infection.

EXTRACORPOREAL MEMBRANE OXYGENATION (ECMO)

ECMO has little impact on survival statistics. Consider in severely ill patients (oxygenation index (OI) > 0.4; OI = $F_{I}CO_2$ x Mean airway pressure/$P_{a}O_2$) who have shown potential for survival on conventional treatment (best post-ductal P_{O_2} > 100 mmHg). Transport to an ECMO centre is hazardous.

OUTCOME

Current management has evolved without controlled trials. The mortality rate in large series ranges from 29% to 55%. Survivors may exhibit chronic lung disease and developmental impairment.

BIBLIOGRAPHY

Charlton AJ. The management of congenital diaphragmatic hernia without ECMO. Paediatric Anaesthesia 1993; 3:201–204

Charlton AJ, Bruce J, Davenport M. Timing of surgery in congenital diaphragmatic hernia. Anaesthesia 1991; 46:820–823

Moyer V, Moya F, Tibboel R, Losty P, Nagaya M, Lally KP. Late versus early surgical correction for congenital diaphragmatic hernia in newborn infants (Cochrane Review). In: The Cochrane Library, Issue 3. Oxford: Update Software; 2003

Rice LJ, Baker SB. Congenital diaphragmatic hernia. Does extracorporeal membrane oxygenation (ECMO) improve survival? Paediatric Anaesthesia 1993; 3:205–208

Sakai H, Tamura M, Hosokawa Y, Bryan AC, Barker GA, Bohn DJ. Effect of surgical repair on respiratory mechanics in congenital diaphragmatic hernia. Journal of Pediatrics 1987; 111:432–438

Wilson JM, Lund DP, Lillehei CW, O'Rourke PP, Vacanti JP. Delayed repair and preoperative ECMO does not improve survival in high-risk congenital diaphragmatic hernia. Journal of Pediatric Surgery 1992; 27:368–375

24

CROSS-REFERENCES

Infants and children
    Patient Conditions 27: 610

Congenital hypertrophic pyloric stenosis

R. Walker

PROCEDURE

Repair of congenital hypertrophic pyloric stenosis (Ramstedt procedure) is performed:
- Via either a transverse incision in the right upper quadrant or a hemicircumferential supraumbilical incision (both in a skin crease)
- By a longitudinal serosal and muscular incision down to the mucosa of the pylorus
- Patency is checked by passage of air through the pylorus injected via a nasogastric tube at operation.

PATIENT CHARACTERISTICS

- Typically first-born male children (more males affected than females)
- Age 3–8 weeks
- Incidence 1 in 300 live births, but considerable regional variation
- Symptoms and signs are shown in Box 24.3.

COMMON ASSOCIATIONS:
- Renal anomalies
- Increased unconjugated bilirubinaemia (17%).

BOX 24.3

Clinical features

- Bile-free vomiting after every feed, becoming projectile
- Hungry
- Dehydrated – may vary from mild to severe hypovolaemia
- Visible peristalsis in left upper quadrant from left to right
- Palpable tumour

Diagnosis confirmed by palpation of tumour (with or without test feed); if in doubt, confirm by abdominal ultrasonography

PREOPERATIVE ASSESSMENT, INVESTIGATIONS AND RESUSCITATION

The operation is never urgent and full resuscitation is imperative. This may take several days. Preoperative management involves the cessation of oral feeding, passage of a nasogastric tube, and correction of the fluid and electrolyte status.

There are two main problems:
- Dehydration – assessment of volume status (NB: 1 litre water is approximately equal to 1 kg bodyweight) (Table 24.3).
- Biochemical defect – hypochloraemic metabolic alkalosis, hypokalaemia.

Loss of hydrochloric acid in the vomitus results in metabolic alkalosis. Correction of this defect depends on retention of hydrogen ion by the kidney. As hydrogen and potassium ions are exchanged for sodium in the distal renal tubule, retention of hydrogen ions results in increased potassium excretion and hypokalaemia. If dehydration becomes severe, increased reabsorption of sodium ions increases excretion of both hydrogen and potassium, exacerbating hypokalaemic alkalosis.

TABLE 24.3

Assessment of hydration in the infant

	Mild	Moderate	Severe
Loss of bodyweight (%)	5	10	15
Clinical signs	Dry skin and mucous membranes	Mottled cold periphery Loss of skin turgor Sunken fontanelle Oliguria, low blood pressure	Shocked Moribund
Replacement (ml kg^{-1})	50	100	150

Treatment requires replacement of the calculated fluid deficit using 0.9% saline with potassium (40 mmol l^{-1}).

In severe dehydration, up to half of the calculated fluid deficit may be required in the first hour, and 20 ml kg^{-1} may be given as salt-poor albumin. Once the circulation is restored and urine output of at least 1 ml kg^{-1} h^{-1} is established, the remaining deficit can be replaced over 24–48 h. Maintenance fluid requirements should also be given as 0.18% saline in 5% dextrose.

The serum electrolytes and acid–base status must be normal before surgery takes place.

PREMEDICATION

Usually nil. The custom of giving intramuscular atropine (20 μg kg^{-1}) as prophylaxis for bradycardia has declined following the introduction of sevoflurane for gaseous induction.

THEATRE PREPARATION

Increase ambient temperature in theatre to 24–26°C. Warming blanket, warm gamgee padding, fluid warmer and warm-air blower should be available.

PERIOPERATIVE MANAGEMENT

MONITORING:

- ECG
- Non-invasive blood pressure
- Spo$_2$
- E$t$co$_2$
- Core temperature
- Peripheral nerve stimulator
- Fluid balance and blood loss.

ANAESTHETIC TECHNIQUE

General anaesthesia should be induced in the operating theatre with all efforts made to maintain the infant's body temperature. All precautions protecting against a full stomach should be employed. The nasogastric tube should be aspirated prior to induction. Two techniques are commonly used:

- A rapid sequence induction with preoxygenation, cricoid pressure, thiopental (5–7 mg kg^{-1}), suxamethonium (1.5–2 mg kg^{-1})
- An inhalational induction with oxygen and sevoflurane followed by tracheal intubation.

Both techniques of induction should be followed by muscle paralysis (e.g. atracurium 0.5 mg kg^{-1}) and IPPV.

Following the relatively short procedure, the infant should be extubated awake and vigorous in the left lateral position.

POSTOPERATIVE MANAGEMENT

Postoperative pain relief can be provided by wound infiltration with local anaesthetics (e.g. 0.25% levobupivacaine 1 ml kg^{-1}) and oral or rectal paracetamol. Only rarely are more potent analgesics required.

The infant can be fed 8 h after surgery; 70% of infants tolerate this. Graduated feeding regimens are of no proven benefit.

OUTCOME

Recurrence of the disease reflects inadequate surgery. Morbidity in other areas is associated with related disease pathology.

BIBLIOGRAPHY

Atwell JD, Levick P. Congenital hypertrophic pyloric stenosis and associated anomalies in the genitourinary tract. Journal of Pediatric Surgery 1981; 16:1029–1035

Daley AM, Conn AW. Anaesthesia for pyloromyotomy: a review. Canadian Anaesthetists Society Journal 1969; 16:316–320

Dawson KD, Graham D. The assessment of dehydration in congenital pyloric stenosis. New Zealand Medical Journal 1991; 104:162–163

Steven IM, Allen TH, Sweeney DB. Congenital hypertrophic pyloric stenosis: the anaesthetist's view. Anaesthesia and Intensive Care 1973; 1:544–546

Vivori E, Bush GH. Modern aspects of the management of the newborn undergoing operation. British Journal of Anaesthesia 1977; 49:51–57

Winters RW. Metabolic alkalosis of pyloric stenosis. In: Winters RW, ed. The body fluids in paediatrics. Boston: Little Brown; 1973:402

Wooley MM, Felsher BF, Asch MJ, Carpio N, Isaacs H. Jaundice, hypertrophic pyloric stenosis and glucuronyl transferase. Journal of Pediatric Surgery 1974; 9:359–363

24

CROSS-REFERENCES

Infants and children
    Patient Conditions 27: 610

Tracheo-oesophageal fistula and oesophageal atresia

S. G. Greenhough

PROCEDURE

Tracheo-oesophageal fistula (TOF) and oeso-phageal atresia repair is performed as follows:
- Left lateral position (right side up)
- Axillary skin crease or axillary longitudinal incision
- Extrapleural approach, if possible
- Requires compression collapse of right lung
- In the presence of oesophageal atresia, closure of TOF and either primary oesophageal anastomosis or oesophagostomy and gastrostomy is required.

PATIENT CHARACTERISTICS

- Generally less than 1 week old
- Incidence of 1 in 3500 live births
- 30% of babies are premature.

There are several different combinations of fistula and atresia. The three most common are oesophageal atresia and lower pouch fistula (80%), oesophageal atresia with no fistula (10%), and tracheo-oesophageal fistula with no oesophageal atresia (2%) (Fig. 24.1).

COMMON ASSOCIATIONS WITH TOF

- 20–25% have associated major cardiac anomalies
- Polyhydramnios in the mother is common
- Increasing antenatal diagnosis.

PREOPERATIVE ASSESSMENT AND INVESTIGATIONS

ROUTINE:
- Haemoglobin
- Urea and electrolytes
- Cranial ultrasonography
- Single radiograph of chest and abdomen
- Cross-match blood.

SPECIFIC:
- Rectal examination
- Renal ultrasonography
- Echocardiography
- Blood gases if indicated, especially if premature.

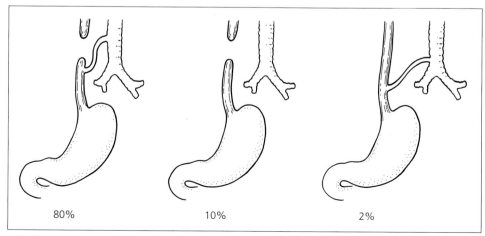

80%   10%   2%

Fig. 24.1 Common presentations of oesophageal atresia.

PREOPERATIVE MANAGEMENT

- Replogle tube to prevent aspiration of saliva
- A small number of premature babies may require positive-pressure ventilation. If lung compliance is low and the fistula large, immediate surgery may be the only method of achieving adequate ventilation.

THEATRE PREPARATION

- High theatre temperature
- Warming blanket
- Humidification of inspired gases.

PERIOPERATIVE MANAGEMENT

INDUCTION:
- In the operating theatre
- Awake intubation or thiopental and atracurium.

TRACHEOSCOPY:
- Requires a ventilating bronchoscope to identify the fistula position
- A small proportion of patients will have upper and lower pouch fistulas.

MONITORING:
- ECG
- SaO_2
- Non-invasive blood pressure
- $EtCO_2$
- Core temperature.

Care should be taken with siting the monitors. The axillary artery in the uppermost arm may be compressed by surgical traction.

MAINTENANCE
Oxygen and nitrous oxide with 0.2–0.5% halothane. Inspired oxygen may occasionally need to be increased during lung collapse.

SPECIAL CONSIDERATIONS

Many authors stress the importance of tracheal tube placement relative to the fistula in order to prevent excessive quantities of gas being forced into the stomach. In the author's unit, this risk is believed to be overstated, and normal-length tracheal tubes are sited irrespective of fistula position. Gastric distension is much more commonly the result of overvigorous ventilation with high airway pressures. Gentle hand ventilation is the best way of avoiding this. Lung collapse is produced by surgical retraction, which has the advantage of compressing both alveoli and blood supply together, making ventilation–perfusion mismatch uncommon. This method of collapsing the lung does, however, commonly result in intermittent tracheal obstruction caused by overenthusiastic retraction by the assistant. Hand ventilation using a Jackson Rees modified T-piece allows obstruction to be detected instantly, and also allows reinflation of the compressed lung periodically during periods of surgical inactivity.

IMMEDIATE POSTOPERATIVE PERIOD

Although TOF repairs can be managed without elective postoperative ventilation, it may be difficult to predict which patients will require ventilation and which will not. In order to decrease the risk of collapse requiring emergency ventilation, often during the hours of darkness, patients with a TOF repair are now electively ventilated overnight in the author's unit. A small number of patients, particularly preterm babies, may require longer periods of ventilation. It is common surgical practice to request ventilation for patients with a difficult TOF repair for between 5 and 10 days after surgery. If the baby is ventilated, care should be taken with both tracheal suction and physiotherapy to avoid the risk of disruption of the repair.

OUTCOME

- Good in TOF with no other abnormalities
- Overall survival rate is about 90%
- If there are associated anomalies, the mortality rate is much higher
- A small number have tracheal weakening at the site of the fistula and may require aortopexy, trachelopexy or, in severe cases, tracheoplasty before extubation is possible.

24

BIBLIOGRAPHY

Goh DW, Brereton RJ. Success and failure with neonatal tracheo-oesophageal anomalies. British Journal of Surgery 1991; 78:834–837

Waterston DJ et al. Oesophageal atresia: tracheo-oesophageal fistula. A study of survival in 218 infants. Lancet 1962; i:819–822

CROSS-REFERENCES

Infants and children
    Patient Conditions 27: 610

25

CARDIAC SURGERY
A. Vohra

Cardiopulmonary bypass: principles, physiology and biochemistry

A. Vohra

The objective of cardiopulmonary bypass (CPB) is to allow surgery on the heart and great vessels while the rest of the body is perfused with oxygenated blood and the products of metabolism are removed. Bypass necessitates anticoagulation with heparin (usually 3–4 mg kg^{-1}) and haemodilution. Abnormal surface interactions between blood, air and plastics damage cells and denature proteins. Air and particulate microemboli may enter the bypass circuit via suction, so blood filters are essential.

THE CPB CIRCUIT

This is shown diagrammatically in Fig. 25.1 Venous cannulae are inserted into either the right atrium, the venae cavae, or (more rarely) the femoral vein or pulmonary artery. The large-bore venous return line drains blood, under gravity, from the patient on the table to the reservoir of the bypass machine on the floor.

The reservoir is either a rigid casing or a bag (soft cell). Blood is then pumped through the oxygenator, where it is oxygenated and carbon dioxide is removed. In addition, a heat exchanger allows heating and cooling of the blood. The pumps driving the flow may be compression roller devices or use centrifugal force (centrifugal pumps). The blood is returned to the body via an aortic or (more rarely) a femoral cannula after passing through a filter.

There are additional auxiliary roller pumps that feed blood into the circuit. One – sometimes called the 'coronary sucker' or 'cardiotomy sucker' – acts as a sucker to return blood in the operative field to the bypass circuit. The other, sometimes called the 'vent', aspirates gently from the left ventricle, or pulmonary artery to prevent ventricular distension, and from the aortic root when retrograde cardioplegia is used. During bypass, when the heart is arrested and there is no effective ejection, blood draining from the bronchial and thebesian veins and retro-

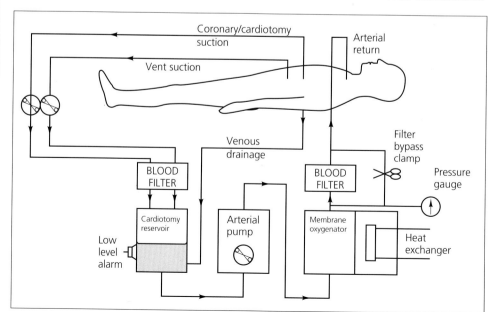

Fig. 25.1 The CPB circuit.

gradely across the aortic valve collects in the left ventricle. Ventricular distension causes mechanical damage, impairs subendocardial perfusion and can result in subendocardial infarction.

Poor venous return is occasionally a problem and can result from kinks, air locks, drainage tube malposition, decreased circulating blood volume, sequestration of blood into body cavities and tissues, or vasodilator therapy. When the heart is rotated by the surgeons operating on the circumflex arteries, not only can venous return be impaired, but also venous drainage from the brain may be sufficiently obstructed to cause jugular venous hypertension with an acute rise in central venous pressure (CVP). This obviously needs immediate correction. Complications of aortic cannulation are embolisation (from air and wall debris), haemorrhage, dissection and malposition (abutting the aortic wall), and can be detected by high arterial supply line pressures in the presence of normal flow rates. Venous return is usually amenable to repositioning. Complications of venous cannulae are haemorrhage, reduction of venous return, arrhythmias, and atrial or caval damage.

MANAGEMENT OF ANTICOAGULATION

The activated clotting time (ACT) should be kept three times greater than the baseline, or over 450 s, by the use of heparin. The patient must be anticoagulated adequately before the arterial return cannula is inserted, or a clot will form on its tip and within its lumen. At the end of bypass the action of the heparin is reversed with protamine. Protamine is a potent vasodilator and decreases in blood pressure should be anticipated and treated. No blood should be returned to the pump via suction after this. If it is, clot formation can occur in the pump making an emergency return to bypass impossible and preventing the blood being used later for autotransfusion.

Aprotinin is frequently used for patients with a high risk of bleeding. Regimens range from 500 000 to 2 000 000 KIU to the patient and 2 000 000 KIU in the pump, and occasionally 500 000 KIU h^{-1} infusion. Some units use tranexamic acid as an alternative. Problems of graft occlusion associated with these two drugs are as yet inconclusive.

THROMBOELASTOGRAPHY (TEG)

TEG is a method of evaluating the formation and breakdown of a clot. A small amount of blood is placed into the machine to obtain values for the following parameters:

- R time – the period of time to initial fibrin formation
- K time – a measure of the speed with which a particular level of clot strength is reached
- α – measures the rapidity of fibrin build-up and cross-linking (clot strengthening)
- Maximum amplitude (MA) – the ultimate strength of the fibrin clot
- LY30 – the rate of amplitude reduction 30 min after MA.

TEG may be used to evaluate platelet function, plasma factors, and activators or inhibitors of coagulation. Thus, it may be of use as a guide to appropriate therapy for postoperative bleeding.

TEMPERATURE, FLOW AND PRESSURE ON CPB

There are many controversies surrounding the management of CPB. For instance, some centres routinely use normothermic bypass whenever possible, whereas others invariably use hypothermic bypass. The advantages claimed for normothermic bypass are reduced bypass time (no cooling or warming needed), and reduced postoperative cooling and shivering with its increased metabolic demand and tissue hypoxia. For normothermic bypass, flow rates greater than 2.2 l min^{-1} m^{-2} are usually used. Hypothermic bypass reduces metabolism, and oxygen consumption falls by a factor of 2.5 (known as the Q10), for every 10°C fall in temperature. Moderate hypothermia (25–30°C) is commonly used for adult coronary and valve work, with an associated reduction in flow rate. For some operations (e.g. on the aortic arch), circulatory arrest is needed. The brain will tolerate approximately 1 h of arrest during deep hypothermia at 15–18°C. Even moderate hypothermia permits a brief (approximately 12 min) period of circulatory arrest, which may be life-saving if there is a catastrophic mechanical failure or circuit disruption.

Management protocols vary considerably in relation to the perfusion pressure to be maintained on bypass. When the aorta is clamped and the heart protected by cardioplegia, as far as the heart is concerned myocardial perfusion pressure is irrelevant. If the aorta is not cross-clamped, the heart is less likely to suffer ischaemic damage if it is kept empty, beating and well perfused. During intermittent

25

cross-clamping techniques, the fibrillating ventricle consumes more oxygen than the beating but unloaded heart. At normothermia, with autoregulation, cerebral blood flow is maintained at a mean perfusion pressure of 50 mmHg. Under hypothermia, with reduced metabolic demand, lower perfusion pressures can be tolerated; many regard 40 mmHg as satisfactory. A number of retrospective studies have indicated no relationship between hypotension during bypass and postoperative neurological dysfunction. Typical UK practice is to fix the flow rate and then keep the mean perfusion pressure above 50 mmHg and below 80 mmHg. Pharmacological management of blood pressure centres around the use of α agonists – metaraminol, phenylephrine, noradrenaline (norepinephrine) – and smooth muscle relaxants, such as sodium nitroprusside, glyceryl trinitrate and phentolamine.

The use of pulsatile flow is controversial and outcome data on its benefits are lacking. Physiological models suggest that such flow improves perfusion and oxygen uptake; achieving it requires intermittent roller pump action or external reservoir compression, both of which add complexity to the circuit. Pulsatile flow is not commonly used.

BIOCHEMICAL AND HAEMATOLOGICAL CONTROL OF CPB

For adult patients the CPB is primed with 1.5–2 litres of balanced asanguinous salt solution (e.g. 1000 ml Gelofusin plus 800 ml Hartmann's solution and 200 ml mannitol 10%), to which heparin is added. This causes significant haemodilution with a reduction in the total oxygen-carrying capacity per millilitre.

On the other hand, by reducing viscosity, haemodilution improves blood rheology and prevents microcirculatory sludging during hypothermia. Most anaesthetists consider a haematocrit of more than 15% to be satisfactory for bypass.

Oxygen flow into the oxygenator should be sufficient to maintain an arterial Pao_2 of over 14 kPa. If this produces unacceptable hypocapnia, carbon dioxide will need to be added to the oxygenator gas flow to reduce carbon dioxide washout. Some centres now use in-line electrodes to monitor both arterial and venous blood gas status, the oxygen saturation in the venous line being used to confirm acceptable blood flow rates, with the A–V difference across the pump confirming satisfactory oxygenator function. Guidelines for minimal monitoring during bypass have been published recently.

There is controversy over the optimum method of blood gas management during hypothermic CPB. The alpha stat method aims to achieve a pH of 7.4 and a $Paco_2$ of 40 mmHg when blood drawn from the hypothermic patient is measured at 37°C: the pH stat method aims to achieve a pH of 7.4 and a $Paco_2$ of 40 mmHg when blood drawn from the hypothermic patient is measured at the in vivo temperature. A comparison between the two methods is shown in Table 25.1. Alpha stat management is thought to preserve autoregulation and coupling of flow and metabolism in the brain better than pH stat, and therefore is currently gaining favour.

The most important electrolyte to monitor on CPB is potassium, because correct levels optimise contractility and suppress dysrhythmias. High levels can be reduced by haemofiltration, diuresis, and insulin and dextrose, and countered by calcium. Low levels can be

TABLE 25.1

Alpha stat versus pH stat blood gas management (Hindman et al, 1993)

| In vivo temperature (°C) | Measured and reported at 37°C | | | | Corrected to in vivo temperature | | | |
| | pH$_a$ | | $Paco_2$ (mmHg) | | pH$_a$ | | $Paco_2$ (mmHg) | |
	Alpha stat	pH stat	Alpha stat	pH stat	Alpha stat	pH stat	Alpha stat	pH stat
37	7.40	7.40	40	40	7.40	7.40	40	40
33	7.40	7.34	40	47	7.44	7.40	35	40
30	7.40	7.30	40	54	7.50	7.40	29	40
27	7.40	7.26	40	62	7.55	7.40	26	40
23	7.40	7.21	40	74	7.60	7.40	22	40
20	7.40	7.18	40	84	7.65	7.40	19	40

corrected by giving incremental doses of 10–20 mmol potassium chloride. These need to be corrected near the end of the bypass phase, just before coming off bypass.

TEMPERATURE MEASUREMENTS ON BYPASS

It is vital to measure the body temperature on bypass. The temperature of the nasopharynx is generally used to approximate to that of the brain. Thorough rewarming is essential. Normal central blood temperatures at the end of bypass after the patient has been rewarmed do not, however, represent the temperature in peripheral, poorly perfused, tissues. After the discontinuation of CPB an 'afterdrop' is usually seen, which is caused by the opening up of cold, vasoconstricted tissue beds, particularly muscle. This can lead to postbypass shivering with its high metabolic load.

BIBLIOGRAPHY

Association of Cardiothoracic Anaesthetists. Recommendations for standards of monitoring and alarms during cardiopulmonary bypass. Available: http://www.acta.org.uk/publications_cpb.asp 29 May 2003

Hindman BJ, Lillehaug SL, Tinker JH. Cardiopulmonary bypass and the anesthesiologist. In: Kaplan JA, ed. Cardiac anesthesia. 3rd edn. Philadelphia: Saunders; 1993:919–950

25

The sequelae of cardiopulmonary bypass

A. Vohra

During CPB, normal physiology and biochemistry are significantly altered by changes in blood pressure and flow, temperature and haemodilution. The blood is in contact with abnormal surfaces in the oxygenator, heat exchanger, reservoir, tubing, cannulae and filters. These factors can lead to systemic and cerebral complications. Fortunately, the incidence of serious morbidity from them is sufficiently low (0.5–1%) for CPB to be regarded as a safe procedure in the majority of patients. There is, however, a much higher incidence of more minor and subtle effects, which are usually temporary and which the patient may not notice.

Blood flow, pressure and temperature are abnormal during CPB. At the onset of CPB using a crystalloid prime there can be a sharp drop in the blood pressure. This is caused by the lower systemic flow and the sudden fall in blood viscosity as the crystalloid is pumped into the circulation. Subsequently during bypass the systemic vascular resistance (SVR) usually gradually increases towards the normal range. A further reduction may be seen when the cross-clamp is removed, particularly in patients receiving blood cardioplegia.

Although the endocrine response cannot be separated from that due to anaesthesia and surgery, during CPB there is a generalised increase in serum catecholamine levels in excess of those seen in operations not utilising CPB. There is no pulmonary metabolism of noradrenaline; renin secretion is increased, and with this follows angiotensin activation and aldosterone secretion. Vasopressin levels increase considerably during CPB and remain raised for up to 48 h after surgery. These increased levels of catecholamines, angiotensin and vasopressin, together with local tissue vasoconstrictor agents, lead to arteriolar constriction. A mild hyperglycaemia may be seen following CPB, due to increased gluconeogenesis, peripheral insulin resistance, a decrease in serum insulin concentration, and raised ACTH and cortisol levels.

Total body water is increased at the end of CPB, the extra water being contained in the extracellular and extravascular spaces. Haemodilution and the increased capillary permeability resulting from activation of inflammatory mediators are the major factors causing this fluid shift.

DAMAGING EFFECTS OF THE CPB CIRCUIT

The exposure of blood to abnormal surfaces during CPB causes platelet activation and aggregation, the net effect being a reduction in platelet numbers and impairment in function of those that remain. Platelet damage is probably the most important factor in the bleeding diathesis associated with CPB. Proteins are denatured by contact with foreign surfaces, and this can lead to activation of various clotting and fibrinolytic cascades with consumption of clotting factors, microcoagulation, fibrin generation and complement activation. The complement cascade results in the production of powerful anaphylotoxins which increase capillary leakage, mediate leukocyte chemotaxis and facilitate leukocyte aggregation and enzyme release. There is mechanical damage to leukocytes and erythrocytes from the shear stresses caused by turbulence from the pumps, suckers, abrupt changes in velocity of blood flow and cavitation around the cannula tip. Damage to blood produces fibrin microemboli, aggregates of denatured protein and lipoproteins, and platelet and leukocyte aggregates. Particulate emboli in spilt blood are aspirated by suckers and returned to the bypass circuit. There can be significant air emboli during aortic cannulation, during filling of the beating heart after removal of the aortic cross-clamp and during discontinuation of CPB despite meticulous de-airing techniques. In about 1 in 1000 procedures a critical incident will occur from malfunction of the extracorporeal circuit.

SPECIFIC ORGAN DAMAGE ASSOCIATED WITH CPB

HEART
CPB *per se* has only a minor effect on cardiac dysfunction unless there has been inadequate myocardial protection or perfusion. Post-bypass cardiac function is more closely related to the preoperative condition of the heart and the success of the operation.

LUNGS
Abnormalities of lung function following CPB are frequent, with clinical manifestations of atelectasis and pulmonary oedema. Acute lung injury leading to adult respiratory distress syndrome (ARDS) occurs in 1–2% of patients. A reduction in functional residual capacity (FRC) with an increased A–a difference may persist for up to 10 days. Sputum retention and ineffective coughing, which contribute to pulmonary morbidity, are consequences of the operation and postoperative care, rather than the CPB.

KIDNEYS
Renal dysfunction occurs to some degree in 1–4% of patients following CPB. It is usually due to acute tubular necrosis and, although potentially reversible, is associated with a high mortality rate. Factors associated with an increased risk of renal failure are pre-existing renal impairment, long bypass times and low cardiac output. Drugs such as aminoglycoside antibiotics and non-steroidal anti-inflammatory drugs (NSAIDs) may be contributory.

GASTROINTESTINAL TRACT
Gastrointestinal tract complications develop in less than 2% of patients following CPB, but the associated mortality rate is high. The commonest problem is upper gastrointestinal bleeding and is maximal on the tenth postoperative day. Hyperbilirubinaemia has been reported in up to 20% of patients. Rare complications are ischaemic bowel and ischaemic pancreatitis.

NEUROLOGICAL
These can be divided into global, focal or neuropsychological complications. Global damage often presents as a prolonged depression of conscious level unrelated to sedation and is seen in up to 3% of patients. In serious cases, signs of widespread neurological dysfunction are frequently present. Patients in coma for over 24 h have a high mortality rate; poor prognostic signs include extensor posturing, the absence of motor responses, and seizures. Choreoathetosis is a rare but serious complication occurring almost exclusively in paediatric patients who have had total circulatory arrest. Sensorineural hearing loss is often missed clinically, but up to 13% of patients have been reported to have a hearing loss of greater than 10 dB following CPB.

Focal events or strokes, defined as a focal CNS deficit of relatively sudden origin that lasts for more than 24 h, are the major cause of persisting neurological disability following cardiac surgery. They are usually seen as an acute hemiparesis or visual field defect and have been reported as occurring in 1–6% of patients after coronary artery bypass grafting (CABG). Approximately 70% of cardiac-related strokes occur during surgery, and 30% in the early postoperative period. Acute focal deficits due to air emboli usually resolve steadily over the first 24 h. Membrane oxygenators have been shown to produce fewer microemboli than bubble oxygenators, and there are fewer microvascular occlusions seen in the retinal microcirculation when using a membrane oxygenator compared with a bubble oxygenator.

The most important risk factors for cerebral damage during CPB are increasing age, a previous cerebrovascular event, pre-existing carotid or cerebrovascular disease, aortic atherosclerosis, valve surgery, left ventricular thrombus, poor preoperative cardiac function, the occurrence of microemboli and long bypass times. Current evidence suggests that the best way to reduce the sequelae of CPB is to perform the operation meticulously and expeditiously, with minimal suction of shed blood, using a membrane oxygenator and a 40-μm main arterial filter.

25

CROSS-REFERENCES

Cardiopulmonary bypass: principles, physiology and biochemistry
  Surgical Procedures 25: 568

Coronary artery bypass grafting

A. Vohra

PHYSIOLOGICAL CONSIDERATIONS

Coronary artery disease (CAD) is the leading cause of death in Western societies and CABG comprises 50–60% of most cardiac surgical programmes. The heart extracts oxygen to a greater extent than any other organ, with only minimal increases in oxygen extraction possible; therefore, any increase in oxygen demand must be met by increasing flow. In health this is done by autoregulation, and in the absence of CAD maximal flow is four to five times as great as at rest. The coronary arteries arborise on the surface of the heart to form a mass of smaller epicardial arteries from which 'B' branches perforate directly through the myocardium to reach the endocardium (Fig. 25.2). These vessels are subject to torsion and pressure during muscular contraction, which in the left ventricle results in the majority of useful myocardial perfusion occurring during diastole. The only collateral circulation exists at subendocardial level and becomes of importance if there is a blockage in an epicardial vessel. Patients with classical CAD are asymptomatic at rest. As the severity of the stenosis increases, coronary flow reserve declines, resting coronary blood flow (CBF) is preserved by progressive vasodilatation of the microcirculation, and the onset of angina of effort occurs with in-creased demand. CABG aims to bypass epicardial blockages using either the internal mammary artery or vein grafts taken from the leg, and so increase myocardial blood flow and oxygen delivery.

GENERAL ANAESTHETIC CONSIDERATIONS

PREOPERATIVE ASSESSMENT

This comprises history, examination and investigations. The history should concentrate on the symptoms of ischaemic heart disease (i.e. degree of angina pectoris – Canadian Heart Association classification) and, when it occurs, previous infarction, exercise tolerance, shortness of breath and orthopnoea leading to functional debility (American Heart Association classification). Diabetes mellitus, renal disease, hypertension, vascular disease and pulmonary disease are common associated problems. These are all added risk factors for patients having CABG. Knowledge of perioperative medication is essential, with antianginal agents and anticoagulant or platelet-inhibiting drugs being of particular importance. While the patient should continue with the usual antihypertensive and/or antidysrhythmic medication, platelet-inhibiting drugs, such as aspirin and clopidogrel, should be stopped 1 week before

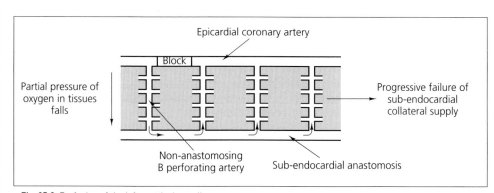

Fig. 25.2 Perfusion of the left ventricular wall.

operation to avoid antiplatelet effects at surgery. Angiotensin-converting enzyme (ACE) inhibitors have been associated with low SVR in the perioperative period and should, therefore, be omitted on the day of surgery.

On examination, physical findings are often few in this group of patients, but look for signs of right and left ventricular failure and check the arterial pulses. If there is a marked difference in right- and left-sided pulses, the strongest should be used for monitoring, as this will be the better reflection of aortic root pressure. If carotid bruits or stenoses are present, make a note to avoid jugular lines on that side.

Investigations involve routine preoperative tests, which include urea and electrolytes, haemoglobin, chest radiography and ECG, as well as more invasive procedures, such as cardiac catheterisation. The latter can give information on left ventricular function and ejection fraction. A low ejection fraction, the presence of ventricular dys-synergy, high left ventricular end-diastolic pressure (LVEDP) and pulmonary hypertension suggest a strong possibility of post-CABG myocardial dysfunction. All patients must have a baseline 12-lead ECG for postoperative comparison.

PREMEDICATION

The purpose of premedication is pharmacologically to reduce apprehension, fear and the stress of painful events, such as insertion of an intra-arterial catheter prior to induction. Commonly used drugs include benzodiazepines (e.g. oral diazepam or temazepam) and intramuscular opiates (e.g. morphine or papaveretum). Metoclopramide and ranitidine may be used to reduce the volume and acidity of the gastric contents. Heavy premedication should be supplemented with face-mask oxygen in a safe clinical environment.

INTRAOPERATIVE MANAGEMENT
Remember antibiotic prophylaxis.

MONITORING

Commence by establishing good peripheral venous access, an arterial line and a multilead ECG (leads II and V5). Following induction, additional monitoring will involve insertion of a central venous catheter, using the internal jugular or subclavian routes, temperature probes and urinary catheter. The use of a pulmonary artery catheter (PAC) varies from centre to centre, but one would be indicated in patients with abnormal left ventricular function, recent myocardial infarction or postinfarc-

tion sequelae (e.g. ventricular septal defect, left ventricular aneurysm, mitral regurgitation). In some patients, who may or may not need a PAC, it is sensible to insert a PAC sheath to facilitate easy insertion of a PAC after surgery if required. Use of transoesophageal echocardiography is increasing, particularly for mitral valve repair surgery.

ANAESTHESIA

The fundamental principle of any anaesthetic technique is to minimise myocardial ischaemia and prevent awareness. Experience in the use of the available drugs is probably of greater importance than the particular agent itself. Prior to induction of anaesthesia the patient should be preoxygenated. Induction of anaesthesia needs to be smooth with cardiovascular stability, but simultaneously adequate to prevent the sympathetic response to laryngoscopy and intubation. Agents that have been used successfully for induction with or without opioid supplementation include propofol, etomidate, thiopental and ketamine. Some centres use high-dose opioid techniques (fentanyl 50 μg kg^{-1}) for the whole procedure, with very modest benzodiazepine supplementation.

Probably the most commonly used induction technique in UK practice is a slow bolus of opioid (fentanyl 10–15 μg kg^{-1}) followed by a small dose of induction agent. Maintenance is usually provided by an opioid infusion (e.g. remifentanil 1–3 μg kg^{-1} min^{-1} or alfentanil 50 μg kg^{-1} h^{-1}), combined with a low dose of either a volatile or an intravenous agent. Propofol by infusion can be used for maintenance at a rate of 5–6 mg kg^{-1} h^{-1} to achieve adequate serum levels during CPB. Of the volatile agents, isoflurane has received much attention because its known vasodilator properties have been implicated in causing myocardial ischaemia through the coronary steal mechanism. However, this has been shown not to be of relevance at concentrations less than 1.5%. Both enflurane and halothane have been and are still used for maintenance in CABG anaesthesia. If there is poor urine flow in the presence of an adequate circulating fluid volume and blood pressure, commence a furosemide (frusemide) infusion. All the currently available muscle relaxants have been used to produce adequate intubating and maintenance conditions during anaesthesia for CABG. The cardiovascular side-effects of pancuronium are sometimes used therapeutically to counter the bradycardias caused by the fentanyl group of drugs.

25

During dissection of the internal mammary artery, blood pressure should be observed during insertion of the Chevalier retractor. There may be a genuine fall due to right ventricular compression or, if the arterial cannula is in the ipsilateral arm, an artefactual fall due to stretching of the subclavian artery.

The management and sequelae of bypass are described in other sections. Adjust serum potassium concentration to between 4.5 and 5.5 mmol l^{-1} before cessation of bypass.

In addition to the goals of providing anaesthesia and muscle relaxation, in the pre- and post-bypass periods myocardial ischaemia must be minimised by the anaesthetist; this requires constant observation of the ECG. If ischaemic changes do occur (which can be manifested by dysrhythmias and low cardiac output as well as by ST-segment changes), always make sure immediately that the patient is ventilating well with a satisfactory FiO_2 and SpO_2. The mainstays of good cardiovascular management are meticulous attention to fluid balance – using information from direct visual inspection of the heart, CVP, PAC (if present), left atrial catheter (if present) and surgical palpation of the pulmonary artery – and tight control of the cardiac output and blood pressure. The latter can best be achieved by the appropriate combination of vasodilators (e.g. glyceryl trinitrate, sodium nitroprusside or phentolamine), inotropes (e.g. enoximone, dobutamine, adrenaline (epinephrine)), vasopressors (noradrenaline (norepinephrine), metaraminol) and a volatile anaesthetic agent. In the absence of severe hypotension or tachycardia causing poor coronary perfusion, glyceryl trinitrate infusion can be used to treat ischaemic changes. Rapid increases in diastolic coronary perfusion pressure are easy to achieve with short-acting α agonists (e.g. metaraminol), but these do of course also increase systolic work and may constrict vital microvasculature. The key to post-bypass care is to optimise the intravascular volume by transfusion from the pump and then, if cardiac output and blood pressure are still poor, to introduce an inotropic agent.

Following cessation of CPB and the heart taking over the circulation, the true cardiac performance is usually not seen for several minutes because energy stores have often accumulated within the myocardium while it was perfused and beating but with no load on full bypass. A heart that had good initial ventricular performance and was satisfactorily grafted can be expected to continue to beat well. The heart can, however, be disadvantaged by poor myocardial protection during CPB and/or by reperfusion injury. This can result in the 'stunned myocardium', which functions badly and needs a period of hours to days to recover fully. Perioperative infarcts may also occur. In both of these situations inotropes are usually necessary. If drug therapy shows no alleviation of the ischaemic picture (from continued ST-segment change, reduced cardiac output, increased pulmonary artery wedge pressure (PAWP), increasing acidosis), this is usually an indication for a balloon pump. This is the only treatment modality that simultaneously increases myocardial oxygen supply whilst decreasing demand. In the immediate post-bypass period, calcium antagonists and beta-blockers are relatively contraindicated and must be used with extreme caution because their negative inotropic effects are both magnified and unpredictable.

OFF-PUMP CORONARY ARTERY BYPASS SURGERY

This involves the use of stabilising devices such as the Octopus 3 (Medtronic, Minneapolis, Minnesota, USA). The grafts to the coronary arteries are performed on the beating heart with that area stabilised by the use of the Octopus, so named because it has eight suction pads that attach to the heart and fix that small area. The assistant blows carbon dioxide (4 l min^{-1}) on the site of coronary suturing, to ensure a relatively bloodless field. Patients may be turned to various head-down and lateral positions to optimise the view for the surgeon. Slow heart rates (50–60 beats per min) would be ideal in these patients. This technique avoids the complications associated with bypass.

25

Postoperative care of adult patients after cardiopulmonary bypass

A. Vohra

The increase in demand for cardiac surgery, caused mainly by coronary artery disease, has led to a marked rise in the number of patients presenting to postoperative ITUs. The trend has been towards the development of specialised postcardiac surgery units, with protocol-based care becoming the norm. The protocols used and the duration of postoperative ventilation, etc., vary considerably from one unit to another. However, the basic principles of postoperative care are common to all patients and are summarised below. For convenience the postoperative period has been divided into transfer, early and late phases.

TRANSFER PERIOD

After the completion of surgery, patients are usually transferred to their intensive care bed within theatre and transported on it to the ITU. The distances involved vary enormously from one hospital to another. This is a period of great potential instability and, unless the transfer distance is very short indeed, at the very least ECG and intra-arterial pressure monitoring should be continued. The development of modern transport monitors has made this a much easier task.

EARLY POSTOPERATIVE PERIOD (0–6 H)

The essentials of the early postoperative care of these patients are summarised in Box 25.1.

ANALGESIA AND SEDATION

Adequate opioid analgesia is essential, but there is wide variability in the drugs and routes of administration used; fentanyl, alfentanil, pethidine and morphine are all popular. The use of high doses of fentanyl (40–60 μg kg^{-1}) during operation provides analgesia well into the postoperative period; alfentanil is a potent short-acting agent and is given by continuous

> **BOX 25.1**
>
> Care in the early postoperative period
>
> - Analgesia and sedation
> - Assisted ventilation ± PEEP
> - Measurement of arterial blood gases, potassium, haemoglobin, etc.
> - Adjustment of inspired oxygen concentration
> - Maintenance of cardiac rhythm; treatment of arrhythmias
> - Control of postoperative hypertension
> - Haemodynamic monitoring
> - Manipulation of cardiac filling pressures
> - Maintenance of adequate cardiac output
> - Maintenance of adequate renal perfusion and urine output
> - fluid management; colloid replacement, crystalloids
> - Monitoring and treatment of clotting and platelet abnormalities
> - Reduction of heat loss; assisted rewarming

infusion. Remifentanil appears to be associated with an acute withdrawal syndrome, sometimes requiring higher initial doses of opioid at the cessation of infusion. Morphine is widely available, cheap and has useful additional sedative properties, but care should be taken in patients with poor renal function owing to the accumulation of active metabolites. Epidurals are used at some centres. The NSAIDs are now widely used after general surgery, but they all inhibit the renal protective actions of prostaglandins during hypotension and should be used with great caution in the early postoperative period. In some patients, despite adequate analgesia, additional sedation may be required; propofol, midazolam and isoflurane (0.4–0.6%) are popular and combine a short duration of action with acceptable haemodynamic stability. Shivering is an important complication in the early postoperative period as it markedly increases oxygen consumption and must be suppressed

25

by adequate analgesia and sedation (e.g. pethidine 10–20 mg).

ASSISTED VENTILATION

The duration of mechanical ventilation after cardiac surgery is very variable even in routine patients, varying from none (extubation on the operating table) to several hours. Improvements in surgical and anaesthetic techniques with a reduction in cardiopulmonary bypass times, less hypothermia, epidurals, etc., have led to a trend towards earlier extubation in many centres. Safety is an important consideration and it seems prudent to continue mechanical ventilation until adequate rewarming (at the least to central normothermia), adequate analgesia, haemostasis and haemodynamic stability have been achieved.

A degree of atelectasis is common after cardiac surgery, especially if the pleura has been breached during internal mammary dissection. Low levels of positive end-expiratory pressure (PEEP) (2.5–5 cmH$_2$O) are widely used after cardiac surgery; they improve oxygenation in the presence of pulmonary oedema and may play a role in reversing atelectasis. The adverse haemodynamic effects of PEEP are exacerbated by hypovolaemia.

Most modern intensive care ventilators incorporate the facilities for weaning in the form of synchronised intermittent mandatory ventilation (SIMV) with inspiratory assist. Mandatory breaths are gradually reduced to zero and, if adequate ventilation is maintained, the patient is then extubated. Many factors may precipitate more prolonged periods of mechanical ventilation. These include previous lung pathology, haemodynamic instability, persistent pulmonary oedema, delayed neurological recovery and pulmonary infection.

MONITORING

Box 25.2 lists the basic monitoring required in the postoperative period.

HAEMODYNAMIC MANIPULATION

Skilled haemodynamic monitoring and manipulation are essential after cardiopulmonary bypass. In UK practice, most routine patients do not have pulmonary artery catheters inserted and the adequacy of cardiac output has to be estimated from a combination of arterial blood pressure, urine output, peripheral rewarming and the absence of a metabolic acidosis. Early hypotension is most commonly due to hypovolaemia exacerbated by the vasodilatation that occurs during the rewarming phase. CVP should be maintained by the infusion of col-

---

BOX 25.2

Basic monitoring after cardiopulmonary bypass

- ECG (rate, rhythm, ST changes)
- Intra-arterial blood pressure
- Central venous pressure
- F_{IO_2}, respiratory rate, airway pressures, tidal and minute volumes
- Arterial blood gases
- Pulse oximetry
- Serum potassium level
- Blood loss
- Haemoglobin level, clotting screen, platelet count
- Blood sugar level
- Core and peripheral temperatures
- Chest radiography
- Urine output

---

loids, including blood, if indicated. The pressure required is variable, but in the absence of significant ventricular dysfunction, pulmonary hypertension, etc. a level of 5–8 mmHg is a reasonable starting point. Hypertension after cardiopulmonary bypass is also common and should be treated to avoid excessive left ventricular workloads, suture-line disruption and bleeding. Having ensured adequate analgesia and sedation, nitrodilators (glyceryl trinitrate, sodium nitroprusside) form the mainstay of treatment.

Arrhythmias are common after cardiac surgery and require aggressive treatment because of their effects on cardiac output and blood pressure. When they occur, always quickly ensure that the patient has not become acutely hypoxic from a simple cause such as ventilator disconnection. Hypokalaemia is a common contributing factor and serum potassium concentration should be maintained at 4.5–5.0 mmol l^{-1}. After cardiopulmonary bypass, ventricular function is often impaired and many patients have relatively fixed stroke volumes. Persistent bradycardias should be avoided by making use of pacing, isoprenaline or dobutamine infusions, for example to maintain the heart rate; a rate of 60–100 beats min^{-1} is usually considered optimal.

The absolute indications for the instigation of more complex haemodynamic monitoring in the form of PAWP measurements and thermodilution cardiac output measurements are difficult to define. Failure to rewarm, oliguria, worsening metabolic acidosis and persistent hypotension despite apparently adequate filling pressures are all good indications. Pericardial tamponade should be high on the list of suspected causes if these conditions develop in the postoperative period.

Inotropic agents such as enoximone, dobutamine and adrenaline (epinephrine) are indicated if the cardiac index is low despite adequate filling. A low SVR occurring after prolonged bypass may require the use of norepinephrine.

RENAL FUNCTION

Acute renal failure requiring dialysis is rare after uncomplicated cardiac surgery, but a degree of oliguria is common. Although there is little scientific evidence, dopamine at 'renal' doses (e.g. 3 μg kg^{-1} h^{-1}) is still used both during and after operation. Dopexamine may be a suitable alternative. It is important to maintain a diuresis in the postoperative period in order to reverse the anaemia from haemodilution caused by the bypass prime and the cardioplegia. If oliguria persists despite an adequate cardiac output and blood pressure, small doses of a loop diuretic are indicated.

FLUID MANAGEMENT

Cardiac filling pressures should be maintained by the infusion of colloid solutions, including the modified gelatins, albumin solutions and blood. Free water is required for the formation of urine, and in the absence of pulmonary oedema the authors' routine practice is to give all patients 1 ml kg^{-1} h^{-1} of crystalloid (dextrose saline, saline or Hartmann's solution). Although circulating hypovolaemia is common, tissue dehydration is rare in the immediate postoperative period, the usual problem being an increase in total body water.

LATE POSTOPERATIVE PERIOD (AFTER 6 H)

In a routine case, following extubation, the activities described above are continued, but the emphasis shifts towards preparing the patient for return to the HDU or ward. Most patients require oxygen to be administered by face-mask to maintain arterial saturations above 95%. Oral or rectally administered analgesics may be prescribed and the patient undergoes regular chest physiotherapy. Where postoperative complications develop, or if the patient's progress is slow, the intensive care administered during the first few hours is continued. In these circumstances every effort must be made to look for correctable causes of the failure to progress. Observing the deterioration closely but without intervention achieves nothing.

CROSS-REFERENCES

Cardiopulmonary bypass
    Surgical Procedures 25: 568
Postoperative oliguria
    Anaesthetic Factors 31: 774
Postoperative pain management
    Anaesthetic Factors 31: 778

25

Aortic valve surgery

A. Vohra

AORTIC STENOSIS

PHYSIOLOGICAL CONSIDERATIONS

Aortic stenosis can be either congenital (in which case the valve is abnormal and bicuspid in more than 50% of cases) or acquired (usually from rheumatic involvement of a previously normal valve). In the absence of other valvular disease, aortic stenosis is almost always congenital in origin. If it is of rheumatic aetiology there is usually involvement of the mitral valve as well. The normal aortic valve area (AVA) is 2.5–3.5 cm². 'Severe' aortic stenosis has an AVA of less than 0.7 cm² and 'moderate' aortic stenosis has an AVA of 0.7–1.2 cm².

As aortic stenosis develops there is a progressive increase in outflow obstruction to the left ventricle. Systolic pressures within the left ventricle rise and a pressure gradient develops between the left ventricle and the aorta. Increased systolic chamber pressure stimulates parallel replication of sarcomeres with consequent wall thickening and concentric ventricular hypertrophy. The consequences of this are twofold. First, the ventricle relaxes poorly during diastole, so that left ventricular end-diastolic pressure (LVEDP) rises and higher filling pressures are needed to maintain cardiac output. The ventricle becomes increasingly dependent on atrial contraction to ensure diastolic filling, and the atrium (in sinus rhythm) contributes up to 40% of LVEDV in aortic stenosis, compared with 10–15% in normals. The sudden onset of atrial fibrillation (which suggests a rheumatic aetiology) can precipitate a major fall in cardiac output. Second, the balance between myocardial oxygen supply and demand becomes precarious. This is because increased myocardial bulk and high cavity pressures increase myocardial oxygen demand, while increased wall thickness and raised LVEDP predispose to subendocardial ischaemia. The relationship between diastolic time (determined by heart rate), LVEDP and the systemic diastolic pressure available for coronary perfusion (determined by cardiac output and SVR) is therefore critical. Coincident coronary artery disease is a serious added risk factor for these patients.

With aortic stenosis there is usually a long (can be up to 50 years or more) asymptomatic period and sudden death may be the first presenting feature. The most common symptoms are angina, syncope, dyspnoea and dysrhythmias. When symptoms finally occur, the stenosis is severe. Their significance, particularly signs of left ventricular failure (LVF), are ominous; if the stenosis is not surgically corrected death occurs within a few years.

The ECG will show left ventricular hypertrophy if aortic stenosis is significant, often with ST-segment changes of left ventricular strain. Unless there is LVF, chest radiography will show a normal transverse diameter of the heart. If LVF has supervened there will be cardiomegaly and lung field changes. Specialist investigation is by coronary angiography and ultrasonography.

GENERAL ANAESTHETIC PRINCIPLES

Anaesthetic technique is similar to that described for CABG. The physiological objective is to maintain the basic haemodynamic state by carefully managing heart rate, filling pressure and systemic blood pressure. Give antibiotic prophylaxis.

Hypotension

Very dangerous. Caused by low cardiac output, hypovolaemia or vasodilatation. It implies that a ventricle generating high intracavity pressures is being perfused by a low-pressure arterial system. Needs immediate correction with an α agonist, while the underlying cause is remedied.

Tachycardia

Dangerous. Produces myocardial ischaemia (sometimes acute LVF), and reduces cardiac output by increasing dynamic impedance of stenosis. Treat cause (light anaesthesia, hypovolaemia, etc.). Do not give beta-blockers. Persistent dysrhythmias affecting cardiac output may need d.c. countershock.

Bradycardia
Moderate degrees tolerated. Reduces dynamic impedance of stenosis. If severe with very low diastolic pressures, use tiny doses of glycopyrrolate and avoid overcorrection at all costs.

Preload on left ventricle
Must be maintained to ensure filling of hypertrophied ventricle.

Afterload on left ventricle
Changes have little effect on valve pressure gradient and hence left ventricular load, but the effect on systemic blood pressure in the aortic root significantly changes coronary perfusion.

MONITORING
Invasive arterial monitoring is mandatory prior to induction. ECG monitoring must be able to detect left ventricular ischaemia and diagnose dysrhythmias; use V_5 and standard lead 2 leads. In practice, it may be difficult to interpret 'ischaemic' changes due to pre-existing ST abnormalities caused by left ventricular hypertrophy (strain pattern).

CVP is a poor indicator of left ventricular filling when left ventricular compliance is reduced. A flotation catheter, however, may cause severe and persistent dysrhythmias as it passes through the right ventricle.

Persistent ischaemia in the face of appropriate corrective measures necessitates early institution of cardiopulmonary bypass. In the event of cardiac arrest, defibrillate immediately. Only internal massage is effective because of valve stenosis, and emergency bypass may be required. Do not commence anaesthesia unless a theatre and bypass facilities are immediately available.

Intraoperative care, management of bypass and postoperative care are as described elsewhere for CABG and ITU care.

AORTIC REGURGITATION

PHYSIOLOGICAL CONSIDERATIONS
Aortic regurgitation may be acute or chronic. Chronic causes are rheumatic valve disease, connective tissue disorders or a congenital bicuspid valve. Acute aortic regurgitation is most commonly caused by infective endocarditis or trauma. The basic problem is volume overload of the left ventricle caused by blood leaking through the incompetent aortic valve during diastole. The degree of regurgitation is determined by the size of the regurgitant orifice and the diastolic time interval. Systemic vasodilatation, increased inotropy and tachycardia all contribute to increased forward flow in patients with aortic regurgitation and may explain the phenomenon of mild exercise tolerance with symptoms at rest. Over a period of time, eccentric left ventricular hypertrophy, gross cardiomegaly and impaired oxygen supply result.

Mild to moderate degrees of chronic regurgitation are well tolerated and there is a long asymptomatic period. Symptoms, when they arise, are usually those of LVF or angina. The life expectancy of patients with significant aortic regurgitation is about 9 years. Sudden death is rare. In acute aortic regurgitation there is a sudden volume overload of the left ventricle with a dramatic rise in the LVEDP. Ventricular dilatation enlarges the mitral valve annulus resulting in functional mitral regurgitation. Pulmonary oedema is marked and refractory. Very severe aortic regurgitation with gross distortion of the valve ring can result in dissection, which may involve the coronary arteries.

GENERAL ANAESTHETIC PRINCIPLES
Anaesthetic technique is as for CABG. Only severe aortic regurgitation is a major anaesthetic risk. If there is an associated dissection, refer to the appropriate section. Remember antibiotic prophylaxis.

Bradycardia
Allows time for back flow into the ventricle and increases regurgitant fraction. Treat carefully with glycopyrrolate or very small dose of adrenaline (epinephrine) or isoprenaline.

Tachycardia
If mild, tachycardia is well tolerated, because it increases dynamic impedance of reverse flow through valve.

Preload
This needs to be maintained to keep the dilated ventricle full.

Afterload
This needs to be kept low to enhance forward flow. A balance has to be found between good cardiac output and an aortic perfusion pressure adequate to perfuse the coronary arteries of the dilated ventricle.

25

MONITORING

As for aortic stenosis. In severe cases, use of a pulmonary artery flotation catheter allows cardiac output to be maximised by afterload reduction, whilst maintaining preload by titrating fluid replacement to pulmonary artery capillary wedge pressure (PCWP).

Principles of intraoperative and postoperative management are as for CABG and ITU care.

CROSS-REFERENCES

Aortic valve disease
    Patient Conditions 4: 115
Elective surgery
    Anaesthetic Factors 27: 614
Premedication
    Anaesthetic Factors 27: 621

25

Mitral valve surgery

A. Vohra

MITRAL STENOSIS

PHYSIOLOGICAL CONSIDERATIONS

Patients with mitral stenosis continue to present regularly to specialist units, despite the success of antibiotic therapy against acute rheumatic fever. The history of the condition is a gradual deterioration over many years. By the time surgical intervention is required these patients are classically dyspnoeic and exhibit a relatively fixed, low cardiac output, often in association with atrial fibrillation. The area of the normal adult mitral orifice is 4–6 cm^2 and the severity of mitral stenosis is graded by reduction in this area into mild (1.5–2.5 cm^2), moderate (1.1–1.5 cm^2) and severe (0.6–1.0 cm^2). The narrowed mitral valve restricts flow between the left atrium and ventricle, and the degree of stenosis thus limits both early diastolic ventricular filling and the contribution of atrial contraction to late diastolic ventricular filling. Increased left atrial work inevitably causes dilatation of the thin-walled left atrium. In the normal heart the two phases of diastole are clearly distinguishable using echocardiography, but in mitral stenosis the echocardiographic pattern shows a plateau and loss of late diastolic filling because the dilated left atrium generates less force than normal. In the presence of atrial fibrillation the uncoordinated movements of the left atrium no longer contribute to this second diastolic phase, reducing end-diastolic ventricular volume by up to 30%. Duration of diastole is therefore of great importance in mitral stenosis, and excessive tachycardia compromises cardiac output, especially in the presence of atrial fibrillation. Many of these patients will be on long-standing digitalis therapy and this should be continued into the perioperative period, along with appropriate potassium supplementation. The primary purpose of this therapy is to control ventricular rate, rather than to enhance myocardial contractility. Mean left atrial pressure (LAP) is usually greater than 15 mmHg, and factors causing increased filling of the left atrium are liable to precipitate pulmonary oedema. The natural history of the condition is progression to pulmonary hypertension and, eventually, to cor pulmonale as a response to left- and then right-sided heart failure.

GENERAL ANAESTHETIC PRINCIPLES

The main areas of anaesthetic consideration for this group are heart rate, rhythm and preload. Anaesthetic technique is similar to that described for CABG and must include antibiotic prophylaxis.

Bradycardia:
- Causes a decrease in cardiac output due to a fixed stroke volume.

Tachycardia:
- Decreases ventricular filling time and thus cardiac output
- Increases LAP and may result in pulmonary oedema.

Atrial fibrillation:
- Will further decrease ventricular filling by up to 30%
- Is often long standing and, if so, will be highly resistant to cardioversion
- May be induced by anaesthesia
- Digitalis toxicity may be induced by intraoperative hypokalaemia.

Preload:
- Hypovolaemia may result in reduced LAP, and thus a further reduction in left ventricular filling.
- Excessive fluid load may result in pulmonary oedema.

Afterload:
- A large decrease in SVR may cause severe hypotension due to a relatively fixed cardiac output.

25

MONITORING CONSIDERATIONS

The pressure gradient across the mitral valve means that PAWP overestimates the LVEDP. However, in the absence of significant changes in heart rate, PAWP trend measurements reliably track left-sided filling pressure. A reflex tachycardia following excessive blood loss will make this technique inaccurate, and in some cases it may be more appropriate to place a LAP catheter at operation for postoperative monitoring.

SUMMARY

Cardiac anaesthesia for mitral stenosis is guided by the principles of any good anaesthetic, but requires greater care in preventing extremes of heart rate and changes in circulating volume. It is often complicated by the presence of, or a tendency to develop, atrial fibrillation. This may precipitate sudden, rapid drops in cardiac output. This dysrhythmia is often extremely resistant to both external and internal cardioversion, and inotropic support may be required to support systemic blood pressure. Inotropes may in turn cause tachycardia, thus worsening the situation, and should be administered with caution. These patients also have a relatively fixed cardiac output, and severe reductions in SVR may be associated with a severe reduction in systemic blood pressure. Potent vasodilators including the nitrovasodilators should be used with extreme caution in this group.

MITRAL INCOMPETENCE

PHYSIOLOGICAL CONSIDERATIONS

Mitral incompetence results in dilatation of both the left atrium and the left ventricle. During systole the regurgitant flow causes high pressure to be transmitted to the left atrium and increases left ventricular work. In contrast to mitral stenosis, there is no obstruction to forward flow through the valve, with the exception of a combined stenotic and regurgitative lesion. Any increase in SVR will limit left ventricular forward ejection and thus encourage retrograde flow into the more compliant atrium. An increased afterload causes decreased forward flow and increased regurgitant flow, and in this respect these patients are sensitive to peripheral vasoconstrictors. The magnitude of regurgitant flow is determined by the size of the regurgitant orifice and the pressure gradient across it; the orifice size tends to parallel ventricular size. Increased preload produces left atrial dilatation and further stretching of the mitral valve orifice, which may result in a decrease in ventricular forward flow due to an increased regurgitant flow into the atrium. In common with mitral stenosis, these patients may progress to pulmonary hypertension and cor pulmonale. It is important to realise that acute mitral incompetence may be due to posterior left ventricular papillary muscle damage induced by myocardial infarction. In this case the left atrium may be small, making replacement of the valve technically difficult. This group are especially sensitive to increases in SVR. Patients with mitral regurgitation caused by coronary artery disease, including those with recent myocardial infarction, require extremely careful anaesthesia.

GENERAL ANAESTHETIC PRINCIPLES

Anaesthetic technique is similar to that described for CABG and must include antibiotic prophylaxis. The anaesthetic aims for these patients are centred around the maintenance of forward flow through the left ventricle.

Systemic vascular resistance:
- An increased SVR increases the tendency for regurgitative flow, and vasoconstrictors should be avoided.

Preload:
- A large increase in preload causes atrial distension and the relatively rapid onset of pulmonary oedema.

Heart rate:
- Bradycardia reduces ventricular filling and increases the degree of regurgitation; however, a moderate tachycardia increases forward flow, and is thus preferable.

MONITORING CONSIDERATIONS

It has been suggested that faster, fuller and vasodilated are the principles on which forward flow in mitral regurgitation may be maintained. In these circumstances (especially when using potent vasodilators and with the dangers of vascular overfilling) a pulmonary artery catheter allows assessment of intravascular filling, measurement of cardiac output and evaluation of therapeutic intervention. In patients with high pulmonary artery pressures, evidence of tricuspid regurgitation should be looked for in the CVP trace. Passive tricuspid regurgitation results from right ventricle dilatation in the face of increased afterload from pulmonary hypertension. There are few attractive therapies for this combination of pulmonary hypertension and right ventricular failure, and attention should be paid to basic principles, including the avoidance of hypoxia, hypercarbia and acidosis. One promising therapeutic strategy for the treatment of pulmonary hypertension is the use of prostaglandin E_1 (prostacyclin), a potent dilator of pulmonary arterial smooth muscle. It has been noted that prostacyclin is also a systemic vasodilator. However, it has the theoretical advantage of having pulmonary endothelial first-pass metabolism, and may be considered as a 'pulmonary specific' vasodilator when given via the right atrium. Enoximone and milrinone may be used as they reduce systemic and pulmonary vascular resistance as well as improving inotropy.

SUMMARY

Anaesthesia for replacement of an incompetent mitral valve is dominated by the need for a relatively low SVR allowing the left ventricle to eject the majority of its output into the systemic circulation and reducing regurgitant flow into the left atrium. A high end-systolic LAP increases the incidence of pulmonary oedema and inhibits diastolic left atrial filling. Valve repair is becoming increasingly more common. Transoesophageal echocardiography may be helpful in assessing the repair.

BIBLIOGRAPHY

Braunwald E. Valvular heart disease. In: Braunwald E, ed. Heart disease. Philadelphia: WB Saunders; 1992

Chaffin JS, Dagget WM. Mitral valve replacement: a nine year follow up of risks and survivals. Annals of Thoracic Surgery 1979; 27:3–12

CROSS-REFERENCES

Mitral valve disease
    Patient Conditions 4: 133
Cardiopulmonary bypass: principles, physiology and biochemistry
    Surgical Procedures 26: 568
Premedication
    Anaesthetic Factors 27: 621

25

Thoracic aorta surgery

A. Vohra

PHYSIOLOGICAL AND PATHOLOGICAL CONSIDERATIONS

AORTIC DISSECTION

Aortic dissections are characterised by an intimal tear followed by a longitudinal separation within the media of the wall that extends parallel with the lumen. The condition usually presents acutely with severe anterior or posterior chest pain. Depending on position and progression, dissections can cause aortic valve incompetence, interruption of the coronary, cerebral, spinal, subclavian, mesenteric, renal or femoral arteries. Clinical presentation may be related to these secondary effects. Young patients may have an associated connective tissue disorder such as Marfan's syndrome. The major classification is into types A (involving the ascending aorta) and B (distal to the origin of the left subclavian), as shown in Fig. 25.3. The characteristics of type A and B dissections are shown in Table 25.2.

ANEURYSMAL DILATATIONS

These are usually asymptomatic until they leak or produce symptoms due to compression on surrounding structures such as the superior vena cava, left main bronchus or lung. Intimal deterioration can occlude smaller arteries; paraplegia, for example, may be the presenting symptom. There is often a history of hyperten-

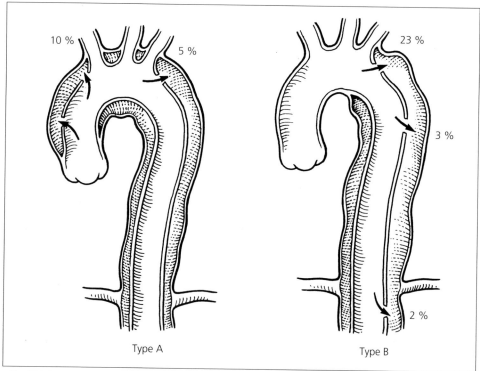

Fig. 25.3 Type A and type B aortic dissections. (From Ergin et al 1985).

TABLE 25.2

Characteristics of type A and type B aortic dissections

	Type A	Type B
Frequency (%)	65–70	30–35
Male : female ratio	2 : 1	3 : 1
Average age (years)	50–55	60–70
Associated hypertension (%)	50	80
Hypertension on admission	±	++
Associated atherosclerosis	±	++
Aortic regurgitation (%)	50	10
Intimal tear	Always present	Absent in 5–10%
Acute mortality (%)	90–95	40

From Ergin et al (1985), with permission.

sion and diabetes together with aneurysmal dilatation of the abdominal vessels.

Although clinical presentation and plain chest radiography may suggest a diagnosis, accurate diagnosis depends upon special investigations such as aortography, computed tomography, magnetic resonance imaging and echocardiography.

ANAESTHETIC CONSIDERATIONS

PREOPERATIVE

Perform a full neurological assessment and record any deficits. Reduce hypertension with the use of vasodilators (e.g. sodium nitroprusside, nitrates and beta-blockers). Catheterise and check renal function.

Insert two large-bore cannulae and an arterial line in the arm least affected by the lesion. Order at least 10 units of blood. Accompany patient to scan room, etc., and be prepared to resuscitate. Continued or suddenly increasing pain may indicate further dissection and the need for immediate surgery.

PERIOPERATIVE

Antibiotic prophylaxis is essential. Provide renal protection with furosemide (frusemide) and mannitol. The anaesthetic technique is as for CABG.

Type A with involvement of ascending aorta only:
- Full cardiopulmonary bypass (CPB) is necessary with cardioplegia for myocardial protection.

- Replacement of the aortic valve and reimplantation of the coronary arteries may be required in addition to grafting of the ascending aorta.

Type A with involvement of aortic arch:
- As above, but in addition the operation on the cerebral vessels requires total circulatory arrest at <18°C.

Type B with involvement of the descending aorta:
- Does not require CPB and is approached via a left thoracotomy. A double-lumen tube is preferred, to allow deflation of the left lung.

All of these operations necessitate cross-clamping of the aorta. When the clamp goes on there may be proximal hypertension, requiring the use of vasodilators. Unclamping produces a sudden fall in left ventricular afterload and systemic blood pressure. Fluid loading and/or vasoconstrictor agents will be required.

Some of the type B dissections may be corrected with the use of endoluminal stents. This involves an approach through the femoral or iliac arteries and therefore avoids the aforementioned problems leading to a reduction in perioperative morbidity. It involves an approach through the femoral artery with radiology for ensuring correct placement, and can be performed under local anaesthesia and sedation. Arterial monitoring is helpful.

POSTOPERATIVE

Ensure stable haemodynamics. Monitor and preserve renal function wherever possible. The incidence of renal failure is 5% and is related to preoperative renal function and the cross-clamp ischaemia time. Central and peripheral neurological function need careful observation, although there is little that can be done to affect the course of intraoperative damage from ischaemia or embolisation. The incidence of paraplegia is 5–10%. Postoperative hypotension should be avoided because it may contribute to the incidence of late-onset paraplegia.

ENDOLUMINAL STENTING OF AORTA

This involves the use of stents specifically designed for each patient on the basis of spiral computed tomography. Not all patients are suitable for this form of surgery. A stent is passed through the femoral route and placed in the aorta under radiographic control. This

25

avoids the need for bypass or one-lung anaesthesia. There is minimal effect on the cardiovascular system because cross-clamping of the aorta is avoided. This procedure is usually performed in theatre under general anaesthesia, although some centres are performing it under sedation in the X-ray department. These patients require direct arterial monitoring, but central venous monitoring may not always be necessary. Occasionally the left subclavian artery is occluded. This may, on rare occasions, necessitate carotid to axillary artery bypass surgery. Patients can be sent to the HDU.

BIBLIOGRAPHY

Ergin MA, Galla JD, Lansman S, Griepp RB. Acute dissections of the aorta. Current surgical treatment. Surgical Clinics of North America 1985; 63:721–741

CROSS-REFERENCES

Diabetes mellitus
    Patient Conditions 2: 56
Hypertension
    Patient Conditions 4: 151
One-lung anaesthesia
    Anaesthetic Factors 30: 710
Blood transfusion
    Anaesthetic Factors 31: 729

25

Regional anaesthesia and cardiac surgery

A. Vohra

The clinical use of spinal opioids originated in the late 1970s when, following the description of opioid receptors in the spinal cord, various opioid drugs were administered both intrathecally and epidurally. The application of these techniques to cardiac surgery followed soon afterwards and, although the majority of the clinical experience to date in cardiac anaesthesia has been with intrathecal morphine, epidural opioids have also been used. Typically, 0.03 mg kg^{-1} morphine diluted with 10 ml normal saline is administered to the lumbar CSF using a 25-gauge bevelled or 24-gauge Sprotte needle.

The advantages claimed for intrathecal morphine in cardiac surgery are:

- Excellent analgesia, which can persist well into the postoperative period following ITU discharge
- Reduced vasodilator use in the ITU
- Less respiratory depression when compared to intravenous opioid use
- Reduced hormonal stress response to surgery
- Reduction in cardiac ischaemia and arrhythmias.

Epidural analgesia may be a better option when compared to single-shot spinal anaesthesia because it may be continued for a number of days after surgery. This varies between 2 to 5 days. The needles are inserted at the T1–T4 levels (usually (T2–T3) in order to provide sympathetic blockade of the cardiac sympathetic fibres. The timing of the insertion is debatable. Some institutes insert them the day before the operation in order to reduce the worries of bloody tap. Logistically this is problematic because of the need for appropriate sterile area and staffing during insertion. It is more logical to insert the needles on the day of surgery in the anaesthetic room in an adequately premedicated patient with full invasive monitoring. This also allows the procedure to be used in unstable patients, allowing more time to stop any preoperative anticoagulants.

As heparin is not a fibrinolytic agent, there should be no problem in administering it an hour after the epidural has been inserted. There have been no problems in the author's department over the past 5 years in nearly 700 patients (unpublished data). A 16-gauge Tuohy needle and catheter are inserted at the T2/3 level with the patient in the supine position. We have used a combination of local anaesthetic (bupivacaine or ropivacaine) and opioid (diamorphine or fentanyl) to initiate and maintain the anaesthesia. With such high epidurals it is mandatory to monitor ascending blockade towards the phrenic nerve (C3–C5). This may be performed with the Epidural Scoring Scale for Arm Movement (ESSAM). This utilises the handgrip, wrist flexion and elbow flexion (C5–T1) to assess ascending motor blockade.

It should be noted that, although intrathecal morphine results in a reduction in the patient's demand for analgesia, there have been few controlled studies comparing this technique with other methods of analgesia and no studies have conclusively proven that intrathecal morphine provides better analgesia. Furthermore, although intrathecal morphine is associated with a modest improvement in respiratory parameters, such as peak expiratory flow rate and postoperative arterial carbon dioxide tension, it has not been shown to reduce time to extubation or length of ITU stay.

Many anaesthetists will not utilise regional anaesthesia because it is deemed to add a new potential for complications, ranging from the undesirable to the life threatening. Spinal and epidural anaesthesia are procedures that require a significant amount of skill, and should be associated with a low failure rate, particularly in the elderly, as well as the rare complications of infection and neurological sequelae. Postspinal headache does not appear to be a problem in the cardiac surgical patient; urinary retention is not an issue owing to the necessity for catheterisation; and backache attributable

25

to dual puncture has not been reported. In common with intravenous opioids, up to 20% of patients will suffer from nausea and/or vomiting, and a much smaller number experience pruritus, which is often confined to the facial dermatomes and which may be severe.

The two most important problems associated with the use of spinal opioids in cardiac surgery are respiratory depression and the potential for spinal haematoma formation. Respiratory depression is characteristically delayed following the use of hydrophilic drugs such as morphine. It is believed to be due to slow rostral spread of the drug by bulk flow in the cerebrospinal fluid, which acts on the respiratory centre in the floor of the fourth ventricle many hours after administration. Several papers have attested to the fact that the phenomenon does not occur after the first 24 h, during which time close respiratory monitoring is clearly required. This prerequisite is easily provided in the postcardiac surgical patient, as it is usual practice to nurse these patients in an ITU, HDU or step-down unit during this time. The respiratory depression associated with intrathecal morphine may be precipitated by the concomitant use of opioids by other routes (including premedication drugs), which should be given with caution, if at all. It is easily reversed with a carefully titrated dose of intravenous naloxone, which is insufficient to antagonise analgesia. The use of diamorphine, which is very lipophilic, until it breaks down to monoacetylmorphine within the spinal cord, may be a better alternative. There are no reports of it causing delayed respiratory depression.

The controversy surrounding the use of spinal and epidural blocks in patients with abnormalities of coagulation reaches its zenith in cardiac surgery, as the patient is required to be fully anticoagulated. Spontaneous epidural haematomata in the presence of a coagulopathy, and haematomata following axial blocks, although rare, have been reported in the literature, and may lead to irreversible neurological damage. However, several large series from the 1980s have demonstrated the safety of axial blockade in patients who have subsequently been heparinised for vascular surgery. Indeed, there have been no reports of epidural haematoma following intrathecal morphine for cardiac surgery. Current practice in the author's department is to insert epidurals on the day of the operation. There have been no major problems in 5 years of practice.

Notwithstanding the above argument, it is generally accepted that the pre-existence of an iatrogenic or other coagulopathy is an absolute contraindication to regional anaesthesia, although if there were very strong indications some anaesthetists might proceed in a patient receiving low-dose heparin or antiplatelet drugs. The other contraindications to spinal puncture – local infection, spinal deformity, neurological disease, raised intracranial pressure and patient refusal – also apply.

BIBLIOGRAPHY

Aun C, Thomas D, St John-Jones L et al Intrathecal morphine in cardiac surgery. European Journal of Anaesthesiology 1985; 2:426–429

El-Baz N, Goldin M. Continuous epidural infusion of morphine for pain relief after cardiac operations. Journal of Thoracic and Cardiovascular Surgery 1987; 93:878–883

Mathews ET, Abrams LD. Intrathecal morphine in open heart surgery. Lancet 1980; ii:543

Odoom JA, Sih IL. Epidural analgesia and anticoagulant therapy: experience with one thousand cases of continuous epidurals. Anaesthesia 1983; 38:254–259

Razek E, Scott N, Vohra A. An Epidural Scoring Scale for Arm movements (ESSAM) in patients receiving high thoracic epidural analgesia for coronary artery bypass grafting. Anaesthesia 1999; 54:1104–1109

CROSS-REFERENCES

Epidural and spinal anaesthesia
    Anaesthetic Factors 30: 696
Postoperative pain management
    Anaesthetic Factors 21: 778

25

Congenital heart disease: general principles and preoperative assessment

A. Vohra

CONGENITAL HEART DISEASE (CHD)

- Incidence 6–8 per 1000 live births
- Two to three times more common in premature infants
- Often associated with other abnormalities – diaphragmatic hernia, gastroschisis, tracheo-oesophageal fistula, imperforate anus
- Often accompanies specific genetic disorders or known teratogens – Down's syndrome (40%), maternal alcohol (25%), rubella (35%), diabetes (3–5%).

SIMPLE PATHOPHYSIOLOGICAL CLASSIFICATION OF CHD

- Is there obstruction to blood flow (e.g. coarctation of the aorta, valvular stenoses)? Increased work needed to overcome obstruction; flow decreased distal to obstruction
- Is there shunting between pulmonary and systemic circulations and, if so, in which direction?
  —Shunting left to right (L–R) with increased pulmonary blood flow. Acyanotic (e.g. atrial septal defect (ASD), ventricular septal defect (VSD), patent ductus arteriosus (PDA). Risk of volume or pressure overload to pulmonary circulation.
  —Shunting right to left (R–L) with decreased pulmonary blood flow. Cyanosis occurs because of anatomical reduction in flow (e.g. tetralogy of Fallot) or physiological mixing of saturated and desaturated blood (e.g. single ventricle).

PRESENTATION

Depending on the defect, may present in neonatal period, infancy or childhood. Some defects have little effect on function and are picked up on routine medical checks.
- Cardiac failure presents as breathlessness on feeding and exertion, failure to thrive, pallor, sweating and hepatomegaly.
- Cyanosis may be intermittent (crying, exercise) or continuous (at rest).

AIMS OF SURGERY

- Total correction
- Palliation
- Preparation for future palliative or definitive repair.

PREOPERATIVE ASSESSMENT

Anatomy and function are very variable and individual assessment is essential.

HISTORY AND EXAMINATION:
- Level of activity (cardiac reserve) and symptoms
- Murmurs, peripheral pulses and skin temperature.

INVESTIGATIONS:
- Chest radiography – heart position, size and shape; increased or decreased pulmonary vascular markings
- ECG – R-axis deviation normal in infancy
- Echocardiography – anatomy, function, cardiac output
- Catheterisation – site and magnitude of shunts, pressures, saturations
- Haematocrit – increased in lesions with decreased pulmonary flow; significant risk of thrombosis if greater than 60%.

MEDICATIONS:
- Diuretics, digoxin, captopril
- Warfarin, aspirin
- Antibiotics (see Endocarditis prophylaxis).

25

PREVIOUS SURGERY

Review records. Note airway problems, dental hygiene.

INDUCTION

The aim is for a smooth induction, with impeccable airway control and balanced systemic and pulmonary vascular resistances. Consider sedative and antisialagogue premedication, EMLA cream. Intravenous induction is generally preferred, although children with mild functional impairment (e.g. ASD, small VSD) will tolerate inhalational induction.

L–R SHUNTS:

- An increase in SVR increases L–R shunting. An increase in PVR reduces L–R shunting.
- Intravenous induction may be prolonged because of recirculation in the lung.
- Inhalational uptake is minimally influenced by L–R shunt unless there is poor cardiac output. An agent with low blood gas solubility coefficient will then show increased speed of uptake. Pulmonary congestion increases incidence of atelectasis.

R–L SHUNTS:

- Avoid prolonged starvation times. Polycythaemia and increased blood viscosity increase risk of thrombosis.
- Pay scrupulous attention to avoiding air and particulate embolisation.
- The aim is to avoid worsening the shunt – hypoxia, hypotension.
- Raised intrathoracic pressure decreases pulmonary blood flow.
- Cyanotic patients have a blunted ventilatory response to hypoxia which may persist after lesion is corrected.
- Intravenous induction is rapid, but reduce dose to avoid precipitous drop in SVR.
- Volatile anaesthetic uptake is slow.

OBSTRUCTIVE LESIONS:

- Avoid dehydration, as reduced heart volume may worsen functional stenosis.
- Similarly, avoid tachycardia.

MONITORING

- ECG
- Pulse oximetry – consider pre- and post-ductal sites (see Coarctation of aorta)
- Temperature – multiple sites for cardiopulmonary bypass: heart (oesophageal), brain (nasopharyngeal or tympanic) and peripheral skin. Monitors cooling and rewarming of specific organs and helps to assess perfusion
- Invasive pressures, arterial and venous – in small children pulmonary artery and left atrial pressure lines can be brought out directly through the surgical field
- Capnography – note increased arterial to $EtCO_2$ gradient with R–L shunting and reduced pulmonary blood flow
- Urine output
- Arterial blood gases, electrolytes, glucose and ionised calcium (especially for neonates)
- Activated clotting times
- Ventilation (FiO_2, airway pressure, PEEP, tidal volume).

25

Management of specific congenital cardiac conditions

A. Vohra

PATENT DUCTUS ARTERIOSUS

Failure of the duct to close can cause a significant left–right (L–R) shunt. Symptoms include recurrent chest infections. Medical management involves treating heart failure (diuretics) and pharmacological closure of the duct (prostaglandin inhibitor such as indomethacin). Interventional management includes surgical ligation or 'umbrella' device closure, via cardiac catheterisation.

ANAESTHETIC CONSIDERATIONS:
- Relatively quick operation via left thoracotomy
- Postoperative ventilation may be necessary, especially if heart failure is present
- Avoid hypothermia – many infants small and premature
- Cross-match blood – vessels may be damaged during ligation.

AFTER CORRECTION
May be assumed to have normal cardiovascular systems and do not require routine endocarditis prophylaxis for subsequent surgery.

COARCTATION OF THE AORTA

The presentation depends on the age of the child and on the degree and site of stenosis. There are often other cardiac anomalies. Neonates may present acutely with heart failure and absent femoral pulses. In this group the lesion is proximal to the ductus, so blood flow to the lower body is dependent on flow through the ductus arteriosus. Prostaglandin E infusion is required before operation to keep the duct open. Repair involves left thoracotomy, resection of the stenosed segment and end-to-end anastomosis, or a subclavian 'flap' to increase the aortic size. More complicated lesions (e.g. interrupted aortic arch) are repaired on bypass.

ANAESTHETIC CONSIDERATIONS:
- Arterial line and SpO_2 probe sited preductally (right arm). Additional postductal (lower limb) blood pressure cuff or arterial line and SpO_2 probe useful for comparison.
- Aorta is cross-clamped. In infants and older children, vasodilators (e.g. sodium nitroprusside) may be required to control upper body hypertension.
- Hypotension may occur on release of the clamps, requiring volume or inotrope (e.g. calcium) administration.
- Document cross-clamp times – risk of spinal cord ischaemia.

ATRIAL SEPTAL DEFECT

Generally well tolerated in children, most having mild or no symptoms. Atrial pressures are low, hence degree of L–R shunting is small. However, if the defect is large or remains unrepaired, increased pulmonary blood flow causes vascular damage, increased pulmonary vascular resistance (PVR), and risk of shunt reversal. The most common defect is the secundum atrial septal defect (ASD), lying at the fossa ovalis. An ostium primum ASD occurs lower down in the atrial septum and may be associated with abnormal atrioventricular valve function, particularly mitral regurgitation.

ANAESTHETIC CONSIDERATIONS:
- Surgery is generally straightforward, with a short bypass time; hence early awakening and extubation is appropriate
- Rhythm problems occur if atrioventricular node compromised
- Risk of paradoxical embolus.

AFTER CORRECTION:
- Most children will have normal function.
- Atrioventricular valve malfunction can persist.

25

- Simple secundum defects (repaired without use of prosthetic material) do not require endocarditis prophylaxis for subsequent surgery. Prophylaxis is required following repair of ostium primum defects.

VENTRICULAR SEPTAL DEFECT

The effect of a VSD on cardiovascular function depends on its size. Small lesions (many of which close spontaneously during the first year) may cause few symptoms, with only moderate amounts of L–R shunting. More severe shunting occurs with larger defects, depending on the ratio of systemic to pulmonary vascular resistance. If left uncorrected, increased pulmonary blood flow eventually leads to obstructive vascular disease, R–L shunting (Eisenmenger's syndrome) and systemic desaturation.

ANAESTHETIC CONSIDERATIONS:

- The aim is to minimise shunting by balancing SVR and PVR.
- Good airway control during induction is very important. Hypoxia increases PVR and may cause reversal of shunt – systemic desaturation.
- Risk of air and particulate embolisation.
- Impaired left ventricular function may persist.
- Endocarditis prophylaxis is required.

TETRALOGY OF FALLOT (TOF)

Tetralogy of Fallot (TOF) is the association of a VSD with an obstruction to the right ventricular outflow tract (usually infundibular stenosis), together with right ventricular hypertrophy and a mal-aligned aorta 'over-riding' the VSD. Pulmonary blood flow is reduced by a variable amount: some children have few symptoms unless stressed, whereas others present in early infancy with cyanosis, particularly if the pulmonary arteries are also small. Cyanotic 'spells' are due to infundibular spasm and cause an increased shunt across the VSD to the systemic circulation. Such cyanotic spells are precipitated by catecholamines (fear, anxiety, exercise) and handling of the heart at operation. Preoperative treatment includes beta-blockade. In infants with small pulmonary arteries, a systemic to pulmonary shunt (e.g. Blalock–Taussig, subclavian to pulmonary artery) is inserted via a thoracotomy in the neonatal period, to ensure pulmonary blood flow while the vasculature develops. Definitive correction is usually per-

formed towards the end of the first year of life. Correction consists of patch repair of the VSD and relief of the obstruction to the right ventricular outflow tract.

ANAESTHETIC CONSIDERATIONS:

- Preoperative hydration (see R–L shunts, above)
- Sedative premedication (helps reduce cyanotic spells)
- As in VSD repair, avoid hypotension and hypoxia on induction, which tend to increase R–L shunting
- NB: Intraoperative desaturation and reduced $EtCO_2$ values also occur in other acute situations such as hypovolaemia and air embolus
- Treatment of infundibular spasm:
  —increased FiO_2
  —analgesia
  —beta-blockade – propranolol 0.1 mg kg^{-1} i.v.
  —volume ± α-agonist (noradrenaline; norepinephrine) to increase SVR
- Risk of embolisation.

AFTER CORRECTION:

- Usually totally corrected, but risk of residual VSD and outflow tract obstruction; rhythm disturbance
- Impaired left and right ventricular function may persist
- Endocarditis prophylaxis.

TRANSPOSITION OF THE GREAT ARTERIES

In transposition of the great arteries (TGA), the aorta arises from the right ventricle and the pulmonary trunk from the left ventricle. To be compatible with life, mixing must occur through a septal defect or patent ductus. If the neonate has an intact septum, an atrial communication (Rashkind balloon septostomy) is performed. Physiological correction involves septating the atria such that systemic venous return flows preferentially into the left ventricle, then into the pulmonary trunk (Senning or Mustard operation). Anatomical correction involves switching the aorta and pulmonary trunk (with reimplantation of the coronary arteries). In the longer term, the right ventricle is unable to power the systemic circulation indefinitely and right ventricular failure may occur. Cardiovascular function is usually good following anatomical correction, although the long-term outcome is yet to be determined.

25

CROSS-REFERENCES

25

Postoperative care of paediatric patients after cardiopulmonary bypass

A. Vohra

GENERAL PRACTICE POINTS

- Analgesia – an opioid infusion is recommended
- Sedation.

CARDIOVASCULAR

- Contractility is reduced with a long bypass time or ventriculotomy. Consider early use of inotropes (dobutamine, dopamine) ± vasodilator (nitroprusside) to reduce afterload. Use right and left atrial pressures and heart rate as a guide to volume loading.
- Dysrhythmias may be the result of surgical damage. Exclude a metabolic cause (pyrexia, potassium) or irritation by invasive monitoring. Treat by cardioversion (d.c. shock, adenosine), antidysrhythmics or pacing.
- Cardiac tamponade is usually secondary to blocked chest drains. Look for pulsus paradoxus, rising right atrial pressure and systemic hypotension. Treatment is urgent surgical evacuation.
- Adequacy of cardiac output assessed by peripheral perfusion, core–skin temperature gradient, urine output, acid–base balance.

RESPIRATORY

- Mechanical ventilation until fully rewarmed and haemodynamically stable.
- Ensure tracheal tube is correctly positioned (chest radiography) and secure (nasotracheal route in small children).
- Use PEEP and regular physiotherapy to prevent atelectasis.
- Ventilatory requirements may alter because of pulmonary oedema (capillary leakage if bypass time long) or altered pulmonary flow (V/Q mismatch).
- Limit peak inspiratory times and PEEP to minimise risk of barotrauma.

RENAL

- Postoperative fluid and electrolyte disturbances are more likely if the child was previously hypoxic, hypertensive or receiving diuretic therapy.
- Hypovolaemia is unmasked by vasodilatation on rewarming.
- Hormonal responses cause sodium and water retention.
- Potassium and calcium losses increase, so monitor carefully.
- Maintenance fluids are initially restricted (50–60 ml kg^{-1} daily), increasing to normal (120 ml kg^{-1} daily) by day 3.
- If oliguric (< 0.5 ml kg h^{-1}), check patency of catheter and review volume replacement and systemic pressures. Consider furosemide (frusemide) and dopamine. A few children may require peritoneal (cross-flow) dialysis.

NEUROLOGICAL

- Complications are infrequent but may be secondary to periods of hypoxia, electrolyte disturbance, hypoglycaemia and embolisation.
- Phrenic nerve damage – surgical trauma, or from ice used for topical cooling.

GASTROINTESTINAL

- Opioids, nitrates and hypokalaemia all reduce smooth muscle tone and increase risk of abdominal distension.
- Hepatic failure is uncommon, but may occur secondary to congestion or hypoxia. Monitor liver function.
- Start enteral nutrition on first postoperative day and parenteral nutrition within 3 days if absorption is poor.

25

BIBLIOGRAPHY

Cote CJ, Todres ID, Goudsouzian NG, Ryan JF, eds. A practice of anaesthesia for infants and children. 2nd edn. Philadelphia: WB Saunders; 1993

Katz RL, Steward DJ, eds. Anaesthesia and uncommon pediatric diseases. 2nd edn. Philadelphia: WB Saunders; 1993

Lake C. Pediatric cardiac anesthesia. New York: Appleton & Lange; 1988

25

26

NON-THEATRE PROCEDURES
B. J. Pollard

Electroconvulsive therapy

O. Abdelatti

HISTORY

Seizure therapy, first introduced for the treatment of schizophrenia in 1934, employed drugs such as metrazol. Electrically induced seizure was introduced in 1938. The early ECTs were unmodified, that is they used no sedation, anaesthesia, relaxation, ventilation or supplemental oxygen. In 1963 the treatment was modified by the use of intravenous anaesthetic agents, neuromuscular blockade and ventilation with oxygen.

Despite almost 70 years of use of ECT, the mechanism of action is still uncertain. What is not in doubt is the efficacy and dramatic improvement in the treatment of endogenous depression and acute schizophrenic states.

PROCEDURE

Modern ECT devices deliver brief electrical stimuli, have two electrodes, and are equipped with controls to adjust the duration and frequency of the stimulus. The electrodes can be attached either on both sides of the head for bilateral ECT or on the dominant hemisphere for unilateral ECT. A typical setting would be a pulse of 60 Hz and duration of 0.75 ms, with a total stimulus duration of 1.25 s.

PHYSIOLOGICAL EFFECTS OF ECT

One of the major effects of ECT is on the autonomic nervous system. First there is stimulation of the parasympathetic system followed by intense stimulation of the sympathetic system. This can give rise to bradycardia followed by tachycardia, hypertension and increased myocardial oxygen demands, and, in susceptible patients, myocardial ischaemia. These changes are, however, transient and rarely require treatment. ECT also raises intracranial pressure, intraocular pressure and intragastric pressure.

PREANAESTHETIC ASSESSMENT

Patients for ECT are all adult and, with the growth of psychogeriatrics, many are in the older age group. History taking can be difficult and is often unreliable. In the elderly many cases of depression are brought on by the patient's poor general health. Patients can therefore be suffering from many chronic conditions and are often on many different medications for respiratory, cardiac and musculoskeletal disorders. In addition, they will almost certainly be on drugs for their psychiatric condition.

Drug interactions are not normally a problem. Monoamine oxidase inhibitors can be withheld and/or substituted with the reversible and short-acting drug moclobemide, which can be withheld on the day of the procedure. Lithium is likely to cause problems and should therefore be discontinued before treatment. The use of propofol in patients on long-acting benzodiazepines (e.g. diazepam) may result in delayed recovery; consequently, long-acting benzodiazepines should be withheld prior to ECT.

Contraindications to treatment by ECT include recent stroke, intracranial mass lesion and recent intracranial surgery. Other contraindications are recent (less than 3 months) myocardial infarction and aortic aneurysm.

ANAESTHETIC MANAGEMENT

ECT should be undertaken only where full anaesthetic and resuscitation facilities are available, and preferably in a specially designated room with a fully monitored recovery area.

Patients should be prepared, starved and investigated, as for any other anaesthetic procedure.

PREMEDICATION

Sedative premedication is not usually required. Anticholinergics are not now given prior to

ECT, but should be readily available in case of an exaggerated vagal response.

MONITORING:

- ECG
- Non-invasive blood pressure
- SaO_2
- Duration of seizure.

INDUCTION

Methohexitone was the induction agent of choice but it is currently unavailable commercially in the UK. Currently, there is increased reliance on propofol. Propofol has a direct shortening effect on seizure duration, but this has minimal effect on the therapeutic effectiveness of ECT in clinical practice. Etomidate is another alternative but the increased muscle tone and pain on injection have limited its use for ECT.

Muscle relaxation is used to reduce the incidence of fractures related to ECT. Succinylcholine (0.5 mg kg^{-1}) is the drug of choice. Following modified ECT, only 2% of patients suffer muscle pain.

Intubation is not normally necessary and the airway can be maintained by correct head position and an oral airway. Assisted ventilation with 100% oxygen is mandatory until spontaneous respiration returns. Because of the seizure and clamping of jaws that occurs with ECT, it is advisable to insert a mouth gag to prevent damage to the teeth and injury to lips and the tongue.

After administration of ECT, bradycardia and even asystole may occur, and atropine or glycopyrrolate may be required. These drugs may accentuate the sympathetic response that invariably follows, putting undue stress on the myocardium. The use of a short-acting beta-blocker such as esmolol has been advocated to attenuate the sympathetic response to ECT, and should be available to treat arrhythmias and hypertension that persist into the recovery period. Prolonged seizure following ECT is uncommon and can easily be aborted with diazepam.

POST-ECT MANAGEMENT

Patients who have had ECT should be monitored closely until fully recovered.

OUTCOME

The mortality rate following ECT is 0.02–0.04%. Arrhythmias, myocardial infarction, congestive cardiac failure and sudden cardiac arrest are the commonest causes of death, nearly always occurring during the recovery period.

Morbidity following ECT include memory loss, confusion, drowsiness, muscular aches, weakness, anorexia and amenorrhoea.

BIBLIOGRAPHY

Carney S, Geddes J. Electroconvulsive Therapy. BMJ 2003; 326:1343–1344

Gaines GY, Rees DI. Anaesthetic consideration for electroconvulsive therapy. Southern Medical Journal 1992; 85(5):469–482

Matters RM, Beckett WG, Kirkby KC, King TE. Recovery after electroconvulsive therapy: Comparison of propofol with methohexitone. British Journal of Anaesthesia 1995; 75(3):297–300

Mayur PM, Shree RS, Gangadhar BN et al. Atropine premedication and the cardiovascular response to electroconvulsive therapy. British Journal of Anaesthesia, 1998; 81(3):466–470

O'Flaherty D, Giesecke AH. Electroconvulsive therapy and anaesthesia. Current Opinion in Anaesthesiology 1991; 4:436–440

O'Flaherty D, Husain MM, Moore M et al. Circulatory responses during electroconvulsive therapy. The comparative effect of placebo, esmolol and nitroglycerine. Anaesthesia 1992; 47:563–567

Simpson KH, Lynch L. Anaesthesia and electroconvulsive therapy. Anaesthesia 1998; 53(7):615–617 (editorial)

26

PART 3

ANAESTHETIC FACTORS

27

PREOPERATIVE ASSESSMENT
B. J. Pollard

The elderly patient

A. M. Severn

DEMOGRAPHY AND DEFINITIONS

Various definitions of the 'elderly' serve only to confuse, and offer nothing to the anaesthetist to identify particular needs or characteristics. From a social perspective, the term can refer to someone aged 65 years who is in receipt of an 'old age' pension, but this is not a useful definition in medical practice. The fact that the decline in physiological fitness varies between individuals is used as an argument by some against the idea of there being a relevant definable population of interest. In the UK, the adoption of the term 'older person' in lieu of the term 'elderly' reflects this difficulty in definition. What is quite clear, however the definition is made, is that the population of the Western world is growing older. The term 'oldest old' is used for the population over 85 years of age. The term 'ageism' refers to the practice of making an arbitrary – and possibly discriminatory – decision on matters of health care based on the age of a patient without considering other factors.

ANAESTHETIC CONSIDERATIONS IN THE ELDERLY

While elderly patients do become recruited into medical research and feature in case reports and other published literature, the paucity of data is out of proportion to the number of cases in the population. There is a recruitment bias against elderly patients in clinical trials, not only in anaesthesia, but also in other medical specialties. This is sometimes for apparently legitimate and humane reasons, such as the desire to spare a very elderly patient a number of trips to hospital to visit a researcher, but may be because the patient is perceived as being unrewarding for the researcher. Ethics committees are currently advised to ensure that unnecessary and arbitrary age limits are not written into research trial protocols. It is also recognised that a simple investigation of, for example, a new anaesthetic drug is undertaken most easily in a homogeneous, fit young population, rather than an older population with multiple and diverse pathology and variation of physiological status.

A consequence of the paucity of research data is the use of drugs or techniques that have been assessed in a younger population without due consideration of the altered physiological state or advanced pathology of the older patient. Such inappropriate extrapolation of a technique of anaesthesia to the older population is commented upon in studies of mortality.

The influence of cultural factors should not be underestimated. The older patient who has suffered the privations of one (or possibly two) world war(s) and a disadvantaged upbringing with dignity may suffer in silence in a modern health service unless particular care is taken to establish the presence of pain. Deafness may make communication difficult. Preoperative rituals, such as removal of underwear, wedding rings or dentures, may cause great distress to those who may have never been seen without them. There is a case for local policies and sympathetic management of patients who may be distressed in this way.

It is appropriate to consider the challenge of the older patient by looking at two separate issues: first, the presence of age-related pathology, and second but no less important, the physiological effect of ageing in the apparently well person.

AGE-RELATED PATHOLOGY RELEVANT TO ANAESTHETISTS:

- Conditions that present in adulthood and progress with age – examples are the progression of atherosclerosis and rheumatoid arthritis. The anaesthetic management of such conditions is well described (see other chapters) and needs no special consideration here.
- Conditions that are diseases of ageing of a particular system – examples are isolated systolic hypertension and neurodegenerative

disease such as Parkinson's disease and Alzheimer's dementia.

- Conditions in which surgery is required in old age for complications of disease acquired earlier in life. An example is fractured neck of femur as a consequence of osteoporosis.

PHYSIOLOGICAL DISTURBANCES OF AGEING

These should be considered to be occurring universally with age but to varying degrees. The concept that the oldest old are exempt from such physiological deterioration (i.e. that they are indestructible) is a dangerous myth. The consequence of age-related physiological deterioration is that a patient has less physiological reserve. The apparently fit 90-year-old who plays a round of golf is still a 90-year-old who will have suffered in part some of the changes detailed below. Relevant changes in homeostasis that occur with ageing are described below.

Cardiovascular system

There is fibrotic myocardial infiltration and loss of large artery elasticity. The autonomic control of the circulation is underdamped. The response to adrenergic stimulation is altered: changes in cardiac output are obtained through an increased inotropic, rather than chronotropic, action and indirectly acting catecholamines such as ephedrine may be ineffective.

Respiratory system

Closing capacity increases with age. Forced expiratory volume in 1 s (FEV_1) reduces by up to 10% per decade, and there is a linear relationship between the decline of arterial oxygen tension and age. Pulmonary elasticity reduces with age.

Metabolism

Liver mass reduces with age and there is a reduction of glomerular filtration rate of approximately 8% per decade of life. This may result in delayed drug elimination. In health, the reduced filtration rate is compensated for by a lower rate of protein breakdown. Thermoregulation is impaired.

Nervous system

Neuronal death and dysfunction is progressive and manifest by reduced conduction velocity and deafferentation. Transmitter deficiencies may result in specific neurological syndromes (e.g. dopamine deficiency, Parkinson's disease; acetylcholine deficiency, dementia). Transmitter deficiency syndromes may be symptomless until an advanced degree of neurological deterioration has occurred. They may be unmasked by inappropriate drug usage (e.g. antidopaminergics and anticholinergics) in the perioperative period.

ISOLATED SYSTOLIC HYPERTENSION

The pathology of this condition of ageing of the arterial system is distinct from that of atheroma and hypertension (primary and secondary), although the coexistence of either of these may hasten the development of arteriosclerosis. In arteriosclerosis, the arterial system is characterised by degeneration of the elastic laminae. This loss of elasticity results in a reduction of the 'damping' action on the systolic pulse wave, with a corresponding increase in its velocity. The end result is observed as an increased systolic blood pressure, pulse pressure and rate of change of pressure during the cardiac cycle. Factors that raise the stroke volume, such as apprehension or surgical stimulation, will raise the systolic blood pressure, and factors that reduce it or cause vasodilatation (e.g. general or regional anaesthesia) may precipitate sudden falls in blood pressure.

PARKINSON'S DISEASE

See Chapter 1, section on Movement disorders.

COGNITIVE IMPAIRMENT

Dementia

Alzheimer's disease is the commonest dementia. Its importance lies in the observation that its pathology is primarily a degeneration of the 'processing' functions of the brain, rather than the 'somatosensory' functions. From a practical point of view this means that pain threshold and pain 'signalling' are unimpaired, but the ability to rationalise about a painful stimulus may be affected. The patient with Alzheimer's may therefore suffer acutely with every painful movement (such as with coughing after abdominal surgery or rib fractures) and be unable either to take any measures to lessen the pain or understand what is happening. It has been claimed that this could lead to a state of continuous arousal of the central nervous system pain pathways. Dementia as a diagnosis must be distinguished from other causes of apparent cognitive dysfunction in the elderly patient. The presence of corroborating evidence from, for example, a nursing home is important. The differential diagnosis of dementia includes acute confusional states (due to pain, infection, hospitalisation, withdrawal of alcohol or caffeine), depression and deafness. The distinction is important because acute confusional states may improve with

27

27

successful management of the underlying condition. Dementia presents to varying degrees, and the patient who is mildly demented may live safely in the community. However, the added stress of hospitalisation, together with the risk of perioperative cerebrovascular complications or unsuitable drug use (e.g. anticholinergics), may make it difficult for full rehabilitation to be achieved.

Postoperative cognitive deficit

A degree of cognitive deficit is common after surgery in the elderly, and age is an independent risk factor for its appearance. Some 14% of those aged over 60 years without pre-existing neurological disease having major surgery involving more than 4 days in hospital have been shown by a battery of neuropsychological tests to have a degree of cognitive deficit up to 3 months after discharge. The use of regional anaesthesia compared with general anaesthesia does not alter the incidence of cognitive deficit at 3 months, although the situation at 7 days may support the use of regional anaesthesia. In the immediate postoperative period, cognitive impairment may be a consequence of unrelieved pain, or the effect of certain drugs associated with anaesthesia. Long-acting benzodiazepines and pethidine have been suspected as being responsible. The use of anticholinergic medication, often used in anaesthetic practice, is also suspected and indeed is a well known contributory factor to confusion in elderly patients admitted to medical wards. A distinction should be made between the acute confusional state or delirium occurring in the immediate postoperative period, and the more insidious, longer term and poorly understood phenomenon of postoperative cognitive deficit for which there is, on current evidence, no clear risk factor.

ANAESTHESIA FOR HIP FRACTURE SURGERY

Hip fracture surgery demonstrates many of the problems with anaesthesia for the elderly. This group of patients presents with a variety of medical problems. Some patients have tripped while undertaking normal independent activities out of the home; others may have suffered stroke or cardiac arrhythmia leading to a fall. It is important to ascertain the circumstances behind the injury. A degree of delirium is not unexpected as a consequence of pain or hospitalisation: in one series up to 44% of such patients were so described. Dementia is regularly recorded in case notes, sometimes without justification. These patients have traditionally been operated on late at night by junior medical staff, after an excessively long preoperative fast. The 30-day mortality rate is reported in large series as 13%. Some of these deaths are a natural progression of a disease process that has led to the fall, but not all the deaths can be so justified. In selected series, very low hospital mortality rates have been reported by implementing a policy of active management of the cardiac output or HDU admission with continuous regional anaesthesia. The practice of 'inappropriate extrapolation of technique' in respect of spinal anaesthesia for hip fractures is discussed in the 1999 Confidential Enquiry into Perioperative Deaths: failures of technique due to fluid overload and hypotension are reported. Systematic review of trials comparing regional with general anaesthesia has demonstrated that regional anaesthetic techniques are associated with improved short-term survival and reduced thromboembolic complication rates.

The surgical service for fractured neck of femur has been subject to review processes of which the anaesthetist needs to be aware. The National Service Framework for Older People set a 'target' of a maximum of 24 h wait for surgery for fractured neck of femur. The Audit Commission, working with the Royal College of Physicians, has stipulated the requirement for 'experienced' anaesthetists to be involved in the management of fractured neck of femur. Useful though these guidelines are in raising the profile of the service, they do not necessarily help the management of the individual patient, who may require specific investigation or treatment of medical conditions. Nor do they consider that in many hospitals the surgical service cannot provide a 24-h recovery or HDU service, and that without these facilities there are dangers in operating late at night just to fit in with a 24-h 'target'.

BIBLIOGRAPHY

Audit Commission. United they stand: coordinating care for elderly patients with hip fracture. London: Audit Commission; 1995

National Confidential Enquiry into Perioperative Deaths. Extremes of age. The 1999 Confidential Enquiry into Perioperative Deaths. London: NCEPOD; 2000

Prys-Roberts C. Isolated systolic hypertension: pressure on the anaesthetist. Anaesthesia 2001; 56:505–511

Rasmussen LS, Johnson T, Kuipers HM et al. Does anaesthesia cause postoperative cognitive dysfunction? Acta Anaesthesiologica Scandinavica 2003; 47:260–266

Sharrock NE. Fractured femur in the elderly: intensive perioperative care is needed. British Journal of Anaesthesia 2000; 84:139–140

Urwin SC, Parker MJ, Griffiths R. General versus regional anaesthesia for hip fracture surgery: a metaanalysis of randomized controlled trials. British Journal of Anaesthesia 2000; 84:450–455

CROSS-REFERENCES

27

Infants and children

G. H. Meakin

Infants and children differ from adults in size, bodily proportions and maturity. Small size presents practical problems for the anaesthetist, while differences in proportion and the maturation of organ systems have complex effects on the responses to anaesthetic drugs.

SIZE

Size is usually measured by weighing patients. The following formula gives average values for children aged less than 13 years:

$$\text{Weight (kg)} = [(\text{Age} + 3) \times 5]/2$$

Many physiological processes are related to body surface area. As the surface area : weight ratio of the infant is approximately twice that of the adult (Fig. 27.1), there is a proportionate increase in metabolic rate, water, electrolyte and ventilation requirements, and some drug dosages. These differences decrease gradually throughout childhood.

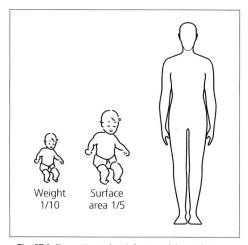

Weight   Surface
1/10   area 1/5

Fig. 27.1 Proportions of an infant aged 6 months relative to an adult, with respect to weight and surface area.

RESPIRATORY SYSTEM

Oxygen consumption is 7 ml kg^{-1} min^{-1} in the neonate compared with 3.5 ml kg^{-1} min^{-1} in the adult; similarly, ventilation is increased to 200 ml kg^{-1} min^{-1} compared with 100 ml kg^{-1} min^{-1} in the adult. As tidal volume remains constant at around 7 ml kg^{-1}, the increased ventilation in younger patients is brought about by an increase in respiratory rate; this is approximately 30 breaths min^{-1} at birth, 24 breaths min^{-1} at 1 year and 12 breaths min^{-1} in the adult.

Lung compliance is reduced in infants, and small airways tend to close at end-expiration. This tendency is increased during anaesthesia, thus increasing the risk of absorption atelectasis and hypoxaemia. To prevent these effects, it is customary to control ventilation in infants by using large tidal volumes (12 ml kg^{-1}) and applying up to 5 cm H_2O end-expiratory pressure.

Premature infants, especially those with a postconceptual age of less than 60 weeks and a postnatal age of less than 4 months, are at increased risk of apnoea following anaesthesia. These patients require careful monitoring for 24 h after operation, and should not be accepted as day cases.

CARDIOVASCULAR SYSTEM

Changes in the cardiovascular system mirror those in pulmonary ventilation (Fig. 27.2). The increased cardiac output in younger patients is brought about by an increase in heart rate; stroke volume remains constant at 1 ml kg^{-1} throughout life.

Parasympathetic control is well developed at birth, but sympathetic control is incomplete. This may explain the normally reduced blood pressure in infants and their increased susceptibility to reflex bradycardia and hypotension. Bradycardia during anaesthesia can be pre-

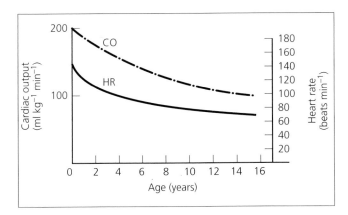

Fig. 27.2 Variation in cardiac output (CO) and heart rate (HR) with age.

vented or treated with intravenous atropine (20 μg kg^{-1}).

WATER AND ELECTROLYTES

Approximately 1 ml of fluid is required per kilocalorie of energy expended. Thus, maintenance fluid rate and metabolic rate may be calculated using the same formula (Table 27.1).

Maintenance requirements of electrolytes are 30 mmol sodium, 20 mmol chloride and 20 mmol of potassium per 1000 kcal. These will be supplied by 0.18% saline with 20 mmol potassium chloride per litre.

TEMPERATURE MAINTENANCE

This is a problem in infants because of their small size, large surface area : bodyweight ratio and lack of subcutaneous fat. During light to moderate anaesthesia, hypothermia increases oxygen demand, which may result in hypoxia, lactic acidosis, bradycardia, hypotension and cardiac arrest. Hypothermia can be prevented by increasing the temperature of the operating room and using heating devices such as warming mattresses and warm-air blowers.

TABLE 27.1	
Maintenance fluid (and energy) requirements	
Bodyweight (kg)	**Amount and rate**
0–10	4 ml kg^{-1} h^{-1}
10–20	40 ml + 2 ml kg^{-1} h^{-1} for each kilogram over 10 kg
> 20	60 ml + 1 ml kg^{-1} h^{-1} for each kilogram over 20 kg

PSYCHOLOGICAL FACTORS

Childhood is a period of great emotional lability and impressionability. Stressful experiences in hospital make a more lasting impression on children, and behavioural disturbances frequently occur after they return home. The following may reduce the stress of hospitalisation:
- Preadmission visit to the hospital
- Video presentation showing hospital procedures
- Preoperative visit of the anaesthetist
- Parental presence at induction of anaesthesia
- EMLA cream to venepuncture sites 1 h before surgery
- Oral sedative premedication, such as midazolam 0.5 mg kg^{-1}, maximum 20 mg, 30–45 min before operation.

DRUG DOSAGE

Paediatric drug dosage is determined by pharmacokinetic and pharmacodynamic variables that change independently of one another during development. Consequently, there is no general rule of converting adult doses to paediatric ones. The dosages of the following anaesthetic drugs were determined by clinical studies.

THIOPENTAL
Neonates require 4–5 mg kg^{-1}, infants 7–8 mg kg^{-1} and children 5–6 mg kg^{-1} of thiopental for induction of anaesthesia. The reduced requirements in neonates can be explained by decreased plasma protein binding. The increased requirements in infants and children compared with adults (usual dose 4 mg kg^{-1}) may be due to their increased cardiac output, as this would be expected to

27

reduce the first-pass concentration of thiopental arriving at the brain. Doses may be reduced by up to 50% by sedative premedication.

PROPOFOL

The use of propofol for induction and maintenance of anaesthesia is associated with rapid recovery and antiemesis. Average induction doses are 4 mg kg^{-1} for infants and 3–4 mg kg^{-1} for children. Pain on injection of propofol can be reduced by adding 20 mg lidocaine (lignocaine) to every 20 ml of 1% propofol.

MORPHINE

Infants aged less than 6 months appear to be sensitive to the respiratory depressant effects of morphine due to increased permeability of the blood–brain barrier. Balanced anaesthesia in neonates may be supplemented with 25 μg kg^{-1} of morphine followed by maintenance doses of 5–10 μg kg^{-1} h^{-1}. Infants aged more than 6 months and older children may be given a loading dose of 100 μg kg^{-1}, with maintenance doses of 25 μg kg^{-1} h^{-1}. Neonates and infants aged less than 6 months receiving morphine should be nursed in a high-dependency area with facilities for continuous monitoring of oxygen saturation and respiratory rate.

ATRACURIUM

The neuromuscular junction of the neonate is three times more sensitive to the effects of non-depolarising relaxants than that of the adult. However, because of the increased volume of extracellular fluid in younger patients, which approximates to the volume of distribution of muscle relaxants, the dosage does not vary significantly with age.

Atracurium 0.5 mg kg^{-1} produces about 30 min of neuromuscular blockade in children and adults. Recovery is slightly faster in neonates and infants owing to an increase in plasma clearance, which probably relates to the fact that 50% of the drug is eliminated by non-organ routes (e.g. Hofmann hydrolysis). Prompt recovery in patients of all ages makes atracurium an attractive drug for use in paediatric anaesthesia.

SUCCINYLCHOLINE

In view of reports of succinylcholine-induced cardiac arrests in children with undiagnosed muscular dystrophy, it is recommended that the use of succinylcholine in children should be reserved for emergency intubation or instances where immediate securing of the airway is necessary. Doses of 3 mg kg^{-1} in infants and 2 mg kg^{-1} in children produce reliable intubating conditions within 60 s, and the block resolves in 6–8 min. Succinylcholine is also effective when given intramuscularly in a dose of 4–5 mg kg^{-1}. This may be particularly helpful in the event of laryngospasm occurring during inhalation induction of anaesthesia, before intravenous access has been established. Control of the airway is usually gained within 60 s and the block resolves in about 20 min.

NEOSTIGMINE

Neostigmine antagonises non-depolarising neuromuscular blockade more rapidly in paediatric patients than in adults. The usual dose is 50 μg kg^{-1}. Increasing the dose does not increase the rate of reversal, which is unlikely to be satisfactory in the absence of a response to train-of-four stimulation.

SEVOFLURANE

Sevoflurane has replaced halothane for induction and maintenance of anaesthesia in many paediatric centres owing to its relative lack of pungency and low blood solubility leading to rapid induction and recovery. In neonates and young infants, the minimum alveolar concentration (MAC) of sevoflurane is 3.3%, declining gradually throughout childhood to about 2.0% in the adult. Although about 2% of sevoflurane is metabolised, peak plasma fluoride levels are generally well below the purported nephrotoxic threshold of 50 p.p.m. Similarly, while sevoflurane reacts with soda lime to produce the potentially nephrotoxic substance compound A, there have been no reports of sevoflurane-induced nephrotoxicity in humans during low-flow anaesthesia. Rapid emergence from sevoflurane anaesthesia may be associated with increased agitation in children who have not received adequate analgesia.

BIBLIOGRAPHY

Harris JS. Special pediatric problems in fluid and electrolyte therapy in surgery. Annals of the New York Academy of Sciences 1957; 66:966–975

Holliday MA, Segar WE. The maintenance need for water in parenteral fluid therapy. Pediatrics 1957; 19:823–832

Meakin G. Anaesthesia for infants and children. In: Healy TEJ, Knight P, eds. A practice of anaesthesia. 7th edn. London: Edward Arnold; 2003 (in press)

27

Day-case surgery

B. J. Pollard

A day-case (ambulatory) patient is one who is an inpatient for several hours for purposes of investigation or minor surgery and does not stay overnight in hospital. There are a number of advantages for the patient:

- Less disruption to family life
- More pleasant for patient and family
- Usually able to return to work or school earlier
- Waiting time is reduced
- Less risk of hospital-acquired infections in susceptible individuals
- Incidence of postoperative respiratory complications is decreased.

The principal advantages to the hospital are that waiting lists are reduced for many minor operations and day-case activity is generally cheaper per patient.

PATIENT SELECTION

This is very important. Inappropriate selection of patients will hamper the smooth working of

---

BOX 27.1

Guidelines for patient selection for general anaesthesia

- Age greater than 6 months
- Age less than 70 years
- ASA status I or II
- ASA III may be acceptable – should be discussed on an individual basis between surgeon and anaesthetist
- Patient should live or stay within a 1-h drive of the unit
- There must be a responsible adult to escort the patient home
- Avoid procedures that are likely to last for longer than about 60 min
- Avoid procedures where severe postoperative pain is likely
- Avoid procedures where significant postoperative bleeding is likely

---

the unit and lead to operations being cancelled or deferred. It is useful for the day-case unit to draw up a series of guidelines of patients and operations that are suitable (Box 27.1). The potential suitability for a local or regional block must also be remembered.

SUITABLE PROCEDURES

These are too numerous to list, but include most minor gynaecological, urological, general, dental, plastic and ENT procedures. The list is constantly growing as surgical techniques become more refined.

PATIENT ASSESSMENT

An anaesthetic assessment clinic approach is used in most centres. Patients should not be seen more than about 3–4 weeks before admission, or the patient's condition might have changed. Patients are usually seen and assessed by a nurse using a questionnaire-type instrument with further referral on to a consultant anaesthetist for advice on specific patients. Any blood tests or other investigations can be ordered at the clinic visit. If any doubt remains, the surgeon and anaesthetist should discuss the case individually. Patients should be advised to telephone to defer the operation if they develop an acute upper respiratory tract infection.

It is possible to conduct assessment using a self-assessment questionnaire, which is sent to the patient in advance of the admission date. Patients are requested to complete the questionnaire and return it to the day-case unit. This works well, provided the questions are relevant and well worded. The range of topics that can be covered is wide (Box 27.2); each day-case unit may have its own individual version of this sort of questionnaire.

Interactive assessment by computer may be the method of the future. This could take place in the general practitioner's surgery, for example, and save on travel to the day-case centre. It may be particularly valuable for

27

BOX 27.2

Example questionnaire topics

- Have you ever had previous inpatient treatment, general anaesthesia, surgery?
- Do you take any medicines on a regular basis (including the contraceptive pill)?
- Any allergies?
- Any bleeding problems?
- Breathlessness or chest pain?
- Previous or present serious illnesses, such as diabetes, epilepsy, asthma, hypertension, heart disease?
- Risk of pregnancy?
- Family problems with anaesthesia?
- Smoking habits, drinking habits?

patients who live some distance from the day-case unit.

AGE

Most day-case units accept patients between the ages of 6 months and 70 years. Some will go down to 1 month, provided the infant was not a preterm delivery. Patients aged over 70 years may be suitable on an individual basis depending on other co-morbidity factors.

PERSONAL CIRCUMSTANCES

There must be a responsible adult to accompany the patient home. Patients who live a long distance from the facility should stay overnight within about a 60-min journey from the facility.

PREOPERATIVE STARVATION

The normal rules apply. It is important to emphasise the importance of preoperative starvation to the patient because it is less easy to be certain that the patient has not had a meal than when the patient is already in hospital.

INVESTIGATIONS

The surgeon should have organised these at the original booking clinic; any additional tests can be organised at the day-case assessment clinic. With regard to anaesthesia, there are no routine investigations that are always indicated. There should be a valid reason for each test that is ordered. It may be necessary to repeat certain investigations (e.g. blood sugar, coagulation) on the morning of the operation; the day-case unit should have this facility available.

PATIENT INFORMATION

It is sensible practice for each patient to receive an information pack at the booking

clinic giving information about the procedure and the day-case unit. This is also an opportune time to list important points that the patient needs to know about the postoperative period (Box 27.3). The patient should also receive another information sheet on discharge, re-emphasising the essential points.

CONDUCT OF THE ANAESTHESIA

PREMEDICATION

Often unnecessary. If required, use an agent with a relatively short duration of action.

INDUCTION

Propofol is presently the intravenous induction agent of choice. Desflurane and sevoflurane are suitable if an inhalational technique is desired.

MAINTENANCE

There appears to be little to choose between the various volatile agents, although desflurane and sevoflurane may be associated with a better recovery profile than the older agents. A total intravenous technique using propofol is also suitable and may be associated with less postoperative nausea and vomiting in some patients.

ANALGESIA

Alfentanil or fentanyl are popular because of their potency and short duration of action. Remifentanil may also have a place. The newer non-steroidal agents are being used increasingly for day-case patients.

BOX 27.3

Example patient information sheet

- Date, time, place of admission
- Nature of procedure and anaesthetic
- Preoperative starvation rules and surgical preparation requirements
- What to do about taking any preoperative medication
- Must arrange for a responsible adult
- No driving, alcohol, operating machinery, etc. for 24 h
- Postoperative analgesic advice
- Day-case unit phone numbers – routine and emergency
- What to do if the patient develops a cold, thinks she might be pregnant, or has any acute change in health
- Advice on time off work, follow-up appointments, etc.

MUSCLE RELAXANTS

A non-depolarising agent of short or intermediate duration is recommended if relaxation is required. Mivacurium, atracurium, vecuronium and rocuronium are all suitable. The incidence of muscle pain following suxamethonium is very high in ambulatory patients, and this drug should be avoided if possible. Mivacurium does not always need to be reversed with an anticholinesterase agent, which avoids the potential adverse effects of this family of drugs.

DISCHARGE FROM THE DAY-CASE UNIT

Whereas early recovery is important, return to 'street fitness' is the most important factor. Batteries of complex psychomotor and cognitive performance tests have been undertaken in a number of centres. These are not possible in the routine day-case unit. Each day-case unit should have a list of guidelines for safe discharge of patients (Box 27.4). In general, most patients are fit enough to go home after about 3–4 h.

COMMON POSTOPERATIVE PROBLEMS IN DAY CASES

The facility should always exist for admission of a patient from a day-case unit for overnight stay in a hospital bed if necessary. Such reasons might include:

- Extended surgery or surgical complications (e.g. bleeding)
- Perioperative complications (e.g. arrhythmias)
- Problems with control of a pre-existing disease (e.g. diabetes)
- Persistent nausea and vomiting
- Difficulty with pain control
- Prolonged drowsiness
- Lack of suitable escort.

BOX 27.4

Discharge guidelines

- Vital signs stable for at least 1 h
- No respiratory depression or undue drowsiness
- Able to eat and drink and to pass urine
- Able to walk unaided
- No significant pain, bleeding, nausea or vomiting
- Written instructions have been given to the patient and read by either patient or escort, or both
- Responsible adult present

27

Elective surgery

B. J. Pollard

Every patient should be assessed by an anaesthetist before anaesthesia. This should ideally be the same anaesthetist who is going to administer the anaesthetic. Undertaking a full history and examination on every patient is time consuming and difficult in the context of a busy operating list. Time may be saved by confining attention to those systems of direct relevance to anaesthesia and by gaining additional information from the notes of the surgical house officer.

PREVIOUS HISTORY

ANAESTHETIC:
- Problems with previous anaesthetics must be identified.
- Difficulty with intubation or sensitivity to drugs are the commonest problems encountered.
- Knowledge of the approximate dates of previous anaesthetics will allow certain agents to be avoided if necessary (e.g. halothane).

SURGICAL:
- The existence of previous pathology that has an effect on anaesthesia (e.g. lung resection) should be sought.
- If this is a repeat operation for a recurrent problem, a more prolonged procedure may be expected.

MEDICAL
Seek information on all old or ongoing disease processes, in particular determining the severity, treatment and complications.

CARDIOVASCULAR SYSTEM

The following conditions are especially relevant:
- Hypertension
- Ischaemic heart disease
- Valvular heart disease
- Recent or previous myocardial infarction
- Cardiac failure
- Arrhythmias
- Exercise tolerance
- Dyspnoea and orthopnoea
- Presence of a pacemaker.

RESPIRATORY SYSTEM AND AIRWAY

Particular attention should be paid to:
- Chronic obstructive airway disease
- Productive cough
- Exercise tolerance
- Dyspnoea (grade it)
- Any tendency to develop bronchospasm
- Acute upper respiratory tract infection
- Mouth opening, jaw mobility, Mallampati, thyromental distance, etc.
- Presence of any dental crowns, dentures or loose teeth
- Any previous surgery or trauma to the airway.

DRUG AND ALLERGY HISTORY

What drugs the patient is taking (prescribed or self-medication) and their doses. This may give a clue to the presence of other accidentally forgotten or concealed medical problems. The severity of a known disease process may be related to the strength and number of drugs being taken. Potential drug interactions may be avoided or allowed for, and potential allergic reactions prevented.

SOCIAL AND FAMILY HISTORY

- Smoking habits
- Consumption of alcohol – units per week or day
- Use of addictive drugs – which ones, route of administration, how often?
- Any family history of anaesthetic problems (e.g. malignant hyperpyrexia)

27

- Might the patient be pregnant? Elective surgery should be postponed until after delivery if possible
- Assess nutritional status – the obese patient and the thin cachectic patient pose a number of particular problems
- Might the patient have any ongoing infections? Elective procedures may need to be postponed while these are treated. Remember the potential hazard to theatre staff of certain infections (e.g. hepatitis).

NEUROLOGICAL, MUSCULAR AND PSYCHIATRIC DISEASES

- Level of consciousness – chart it if necessary.
- Patients with neuromuscular disorders (e.g. myasthenia) are likely to respond in an unusual way to muscle relaxants.
- Patients with myopathies and dystrophies may have an associated cardiomyopathy.
- Psychiatric disorders themselves do not usually pose any particular problem. The drugs used to treat them are usually of more importance.
- Some patients are incapable of giving consent to surgery. This may introduce a potentially problematic legal situation because consent for an adult cannot normally be taken from another adult, whatever their relationship to the patient. With respect to a child, the legal guardian (usually the parent) can give consent. If in doubt, the advice of the hospital legal department should be obtained.

GASTROINTESTINAL DISORDERS

These do not usually have an important effect on anaesthesia. In patients with a hiatus hernia, or who are otherwise at risk from gastric reflux, appropriate precautions should be taken to prevent pulmonary aspiration of gastric contents. When there has been a period of diarrhoea or vomiting, or continuous drainage from a fistula or nasogastric tube, fluid and electrolyte imbalances are common. Patients who have had a 'bowel prep' with a powerful laxative may be significantly dehydrated and should receive an intravenous fluid infusion before induction to replace estimated fluid loss. Care should be taken with the use of nitrous oxide in the presence of gas-filled loops of bowel.

LIVER DISEASE

Many drugs used in anaesthesia are at least partly metabolised in the liver. Pre-existing liver disease is therefore of profound importance in anaesthesia. A reduction in serum albumin concentration will alter the protein binding of many drugs. Coagulopathies are common in liver disease. There is likely to be a reduced plasma cholinesterase level and so the action of suxamethonium and mivacurium is likely to be prolonged. Look for jaundice and take appropriate precautions if present. Consider the possibility of one of the infectious forms of hepatitis.

RENAL DISEASE

Many of the drugs used in anaesthesia are excreted via the kidney and their action will therefore potentially be prolonged. Avoid any drugs that are exclusively renally excreted. The dosage of certain drugs (e.g. gentamicin) needs to be reduced.

The patient may be hypertensive, chronically anaemic, and on regular dialysis. Levels of plasma electrolytes should be measured before operation.

ENDOCRINE AND METABOLIC DISORDERS

Diabetic patients should be managed according to the hospital guidelines. Patients with adrenocorticoid dysfunction may require steroid cover if they have been receiving a high dose for a prolonged period of time. Patients who have received only a recent short course of steroids should not need steroid cover. Look for a goitre in patients with thyroid disease and remember the possibility of a difficult intubation.

INVESTIGATIONS

Blood tests, ECG, radiography, pulmonary function tests, etc. should not be performed routinely without good reason. For example, the clinically anaemic patient should have a preoperative haemoglobin estimation and patients taking a diuretic should have the plasma electrolytes measured. Patients whose ethnic origin places them at risk of sickle cell disease should have a Sickledex and possibly haemoglobin electrophoresis performed. Remember to check

27

that blood has been cross-matched if need is anticipated.

A concentration of 10 g dl^{-1} is generally accepted as the lower limit for haemoglobin, below which elective surgery should be postponed. In certain cases, for example chronic anaemia of renal failure, lower levels are accepted.

PREOPERATIVE STARVATION

The normally accepted period of starvation has been 6 h for food and 4 h for drinks for many years. Evidence suggests that clear fluids (water and juices, not tea, coffee and milky drinks) are cleared more rapidly from the stomach. Most anaesthetists will accept clear fluids in moderation up to 2 h before anaesthesia. A prolonged period of starvation is unpleasant and may even be hazardous in infants and babies, and should be avoided.

PREOPERATIVE PREPARATION

- The correct patient should arrive in theatre with the correct notes and radiographs.
- Dentures, contact lenses, prosthetic limbs, etc. should have been left on the ward.
- Patients who are deaf or with impaired vision may benefit from retaining their hearing aid or glasses until the moment of induction of anaesthesia.
- All lipstick, nail varnish and cosmetics should have been removed.
- All jewellery should have been removed, or should be taped securely to the patient.

- Never remove the patient's identity badge unless absolutely essential, whereupon it must be reattached immediately to a different part of the patient.
- If there could be any confusion regarding the site or side of the operation, the patient should have been marked with an indelible ink marker by the surgeon before leaving the ward. It is good practice to ask the patient to identify the site and side of operation before inducing anaesthesia and to verify this with the operating list.

CROSS-REFERENCES

Diabetes mellitus
    Patient Conditions 2: 56
Malignant hyperthermia
    Patient Conditions 2: 75
Smoking and anaesthesia
    Patient Conditions 3: 106
Chronic liver disease
    Patient Conditions 5: 159
Obesity
    Patient Conditions 5: 173
Acute renal failure
    Patient Conditions 6: 184
Sickle cell syndrome
    Patient Conditions 7: 226
Pregnancy
    Surgical Procedures 18: 473
Difficult airway
    Anaesthetic Factors 28: 660
Preoperative assessment of cardiovascular risk in non-cardiac surgery
    Anaesthetic Factors 27: 634
Preoperative assessment of pulmonary risk
    Anaesthetic Factors 27: 638

27

Emergency surgery

B. J. Pollard

An emergency anaesthetic is one that is required as soon as possible. The implication is that there is not enough time available for the patient to be fully prepared for surgery. It is likely, therefore, that the patient's condition has not been fully optimised; there may be existing homeostatic disturbances and not all of the laboratory or other tests may be available before beginning the operation.

ASSESSMENT

In the initial assessment of the patient, the first decision that must be taken relates to the urgency of the procedure. If the nature of the operation is compelling and immediate, no time should be wasted. If it is possible to introduce some delay, however short, this should be done in order to allow the patient to be assessed more fully and for the patient's condition to be optimised.

Assessment should be the same as for elective procedures, if time permits. Assess as fully as possible within the constraints of the degree of urgency. If the patient cannot give any history, look for warning cards and 'Medic-Alert' tags, or bracelets. Look at any previous hospital notes and emergency department records. Ask friends or relatives, if present. Perform appropriate investigations, depending on available time. Obtain the results for those already instituted. Look for the presence of alcohol or drug intoxication, particularly in cases of trauma. Remember that in urgent procedures there is an increased chance of cardiac-related death in the presence of pre-existing cardiovascular disease. If the patient is of an ethnic origin where sickle disease is prevalent, treat as positive until proven to the contrary.

STARVATION

Assume that the patient has a full stomach. Even if the last food intake was over 6 h previ-ously, the stomach may not be empty. In cases of trauma in particular, the stomach ceases to empty at the time of injury and may still contain partly digested food after 12 h or more. Attempts at emptying the stomach with a nasogastric tube are not usually completely successful and should not be relied on.

PREPARATION

Trained assistance must be available in the operating theatre. Make sure everything is prepared and ready before starting, including drawing up any drugs that you might want. If possible, check that blood has been crossmatched and is immediately available in theatre. Consider anaesthetising the patient in the operating theatre and not in the anaesthetic room to minimise delays between induction and incision. Test all equipment before starting.

Insert at least one intravenous line (minimum size 16 gauge, preferably 14 gauge). If major blood loss is expected, or if the patient is markedly hypovolaemic, a second large peripheral line should be inserted and strong consideration given to inserting a central venous (CVP) line.

MONITORING

Attach all monitors before starting and obtain baseline readings. Standard minimum monitoring should consist of pulse oximetry, electrocardiography, non-invasive blood pressure and end-tidal carbon dioxide. Other monitors (e.g. nerve stimulator) should be added as necessary. Core temperature monitoring is advisable in all but the most minor emergencies. An arterial line should be considered for invasive arterial pressure monitoring. In general, time should not be wasted in securing additional monitoring lines (e.g. central line, pulmonary artery flotation catheter) unless this is deemed essential before

27

starting. It is usually acceptable to establish these when the patient is anaesthetised and while preparation for surgery is progressing. A urinary catheter should be inserted in major cases.

INDUCTION

Secure the airway as rapidly as possible. Use a rapid sequence induction technique with pre-oxygenation and cricoid pressure. Take a further blood sample, if necessary, for more tests, blood gases, cross-match, etc. Give drugs slowly, particularly in the hypotensive patient. Etomidate is a good choice in the high-risk patient. It should not, however, be used as an alternative to adequate preoperative fluid replacement if there is time for the latter.

MAINTENANCE

Almost any technique is suitable, depending on the fitness of the patient. Remember that volatile agents tend to produce vasodilatation and/or a fall in cardiac output. This may further reduce an already low blood pressure.

Do not waste time waiting for cross-matched blood to arrive, but give any available fluid if required, particularly colloids. All intravenous fluids should be warmed. Remember to order fresh frozen plasma, platelets, etc., if giving more than about 4 units of blood or if coagulation problems are suspected. The condition of most patients who require emergency surgery is dynamic, and close observation is essential because rapid changes may occur. Auto-transfusion using a cell saver should be considered if blood loss is likely to be considerable or if there is any reason to avoid blood transfusion. There is rarely a need to use uncross-matched type-specific or O-negative blood.

It must be remembered that the patient may have one or more disease processes that have not been discovered before surgery. Keep an open mind at all times whatever happens – the patient could have almost anything wrong with them. If the patient has suffered from trauma, remember that there may be additional unknown fractures or injuries, such as neck injuries, thoracic trauma. Continuing hypotension may mean continuing bleeding somewhere other than the operating site. Additional precautions apply if the patient has suffered a head injury.

RECOVERY

Antagonise any residual block and discontinue anaesthesia in a routine manner. The patient should be extubated in the lateral position if possible. Administer face-mask oxygen for at least the early recovery period and consider its use for the first 24–48 h in high-risk patients.

If the operation has been extensive, the patient has received a large transfusion, perioperative complications have occurred or there are other concerns, it is wise to transfer the patient to a high-dependency or intensive care unit for the early postoperative period. Overnight controlled ventilation may be advisable in certain cases.

CROSS-REFERENCES

Sickle cell syndrome
   Patient Conditions 7: 226
Elective surgery
   Anaesthetic Factors 27: 616
Difficult airway, aspiration risk
   Anaesthetic Factors 28: 668
Blood transfusion
   Anaesthetic Factors 31: 729
Failure to breathe or wake up after operation
   Anaesthetic Factors 31: 740
Intraoperative hypotension
   Anaesthetic Factors 31: 758
Thrombotic embolism
   Anaesthetic Factors 31: 789
Trauma
   Anaesthetic Factors 31: 797
Preoperative assessment of cardiovascular risk in non-cardiac surgery
   Anaesthetic Factors 27: 634

27

Premedication

B. J. Pollard

Premedication is short for 'preoperative medication' or 'preliminary medication'. A drug, or a combination of drugs (the premed), is administered to the patient before anaesthesia and surgery.

A number of reasons exist for administering a premed, the commonest of which is patient anxiety. Reasons may also vary from patient to patient and within the same patient at different times. If a patient did not require a premed last time, this does not mean that they do not need one on this occasion. Circumstances also alter. The patient who did not require a premed on one occasion for a minor cosmetic procedure may be extremely anxious when facing a laparotomy for suspected malignancy. It must also be remembered that not every patient needs pharmacological premedication: a visit from the anaesthetist and an explanation of the procedure may be all that is required.

Sedative premedication is usually inadvisable in the old or frail patient. Profound sedation, confusion or disorientation may result.

The administration of a sedative premed will lead to a reduction in the requirements for anaesthetic agents, reduce the potential for awareness during tracheal intubation and surgery, assist in maintaining anaesthesia and reduce certain unwanted side-effects of anaesthesia.

Children require a premed more often than adults. Remember to scale the dose down. Some drugs are prepared in a flavoured liquid formulation for children; others may have to be mixed with a small quantity of juice. Bigger children may be better taking a tablet as a large volume of sweet syrup may be quite nauseating! Infants and neonates are special cases.

The factors that it may be necessary to consider in premedication are listed in Box 27.5 and the common premedicant drugs in Table 27.2.

ANXIOLYSIS

Many patients are apprehensive of forthcoming surgery and anxiolysis is welcome in such cases. Anxiety is a subjective sensation and it may be difficult to determine whether a patient is

27

BOX 27.5

Potential factors that may be combined to construct an ideal premed for a particular patient

- Anxiolysis
- Amnesia
- Antiemesis
- Analgesia
- Antibiosis
- Antithrombosis
- Antisialogogue
- Antacid
- Antihistamine
- Antivagal

TABLE 27.2

Common premedicant drugs and combinations

	Dosage
Adults	
Diazepam	5–15 mg orally
Temazepam	10–30 mg orally
Lorazepam	1–3 mg orally
Children	
Diazepam	0.2 mg kg^{-1} orally
Midazolam	0.2 mg kg^{-1} orally

This list is not exhaustive and many anaesthetists have personal combinations of drugs for individual circumstances. Premeds are normally given about 1 h before operation.

Metoclopramide may occasionally be added as an antiemetic. Antacids and/or antibiotics may need to be added.

anxious or not. The patient who has had several previous anaesthetics may be more, not less, anxious. The severity and site of the operation are poor indicators of potential for anxiety. An anxiolytic premed will lessen the normal stress response to surgery and anaesthesia. Benzodiazepines and opioids are the agents most commonly used to secure anxiolysis in the preoperative period.

AMNESIA

Amnesia may be appropriate for a particularly traumatic occasion, especially if further procedures are planned. It is disliked by many patients, however, who are disturbed by the removal of part of a day of their life. Amnesic drugs will assist in reducing the incidence of awareness under general anaesthesia, but will not erase the memory of a period of awareness that has occurred. Amnesia may not be advantageous if it has been necessary to go to lengths to gain the patient's confidence for a procedure: the patient may also forget all the positive points that were emphasised on this occasion. The benzodiazepines are commonly used amnesics. Hyoscine is also a potent amnesic, although it may cause confusion in the elderly.

ANTIEMESIS

This is useful for the patient who complains of previous sickness following surgery and is advisable if an opioid is used for premedication. The effect of an antiemetic given with the premed may be waning by the end of the procedure, however, requiring an additional dose to be administered. Prochlorperazine, metoclopramide, cyclizine and hyoscine are those most commonly used. The 5-HT$_3$ antagonists are usually reserved for situations when the simpler drugs do not work.

ANALGESIA

Analgesia is desirable if the patient has pain before surgery. It also reduces the intraoperative requirements for anaesthetic agents and analgesics, and improves comfort in the early postoperative period. The opioids remain the most commonly used analgesics, although there is an increasing trend towards giving a dose of a non-steroidal anti-inflammatory drug (NSAID) as part of the premed. NSAIDs lack the mild

sedative and euphoric effect of the opioids which are useful as a part of the premed.

ANTIBIOTICS

These are used principally for prophylaxis against subacute bacterial endocarditis in susceptible individuals. The accepted regimens are given in the *British National Formulary*; the commonest are listed in Table 27.3. Antibiotics may also be given as a part of local surgical practice for prophylaxis against postoperative infection, particularly where foreign material is to be implanted.

ANTITHROMBOTIC AGENTS

These should always be considered in patients at risk of deep venous thrombosis. The newer low molecular weight heparins are regarded as more effective than unfractionated heparin. They are also more convenient as they only need to be given in a once-daily dosage and the standard prophylactic regimen does not normally require monitoring.

ANTISIALAGOGUES

These are essential for premedication in infants. They are useful when intraoral surgery

TABLE 27.3

Common antibiotic regimens for prevention of subacute bacterial endocarditis in susceptible individuals who are at no special risk (adult doses)

Antibiotic	Regimen
Amoxicillin	3 g orally 4 h before surgery, then a further 3 g orally immediately after operation
Amoxicillin	1 g i.v. at induction, then 500 mg orally 6 h after operation
Vancomycin	1 g i.v. by infusion over 100 min, then gentamicin 120 mg at induction

Doses should be reduced proportionately in children. Choice of antibiotic depends on patient tolerance (e.g. allergies), site and type of operation, whether or not the patient has an artificial heart valve, and expected bacterial contaminants.
For further details and current guidelines see the *British National Formulary*.

is to be undertaken and also when fibreoptic intubation is planned. The principal disadvantage is the unpleasant dry mouth experienced by the patient. Atropine, hyoscine and glycopyrrolate are all potent drying agents.

ANTACIDS

An antacid should be used if there is an increased risk of regurgitation of gastric contents. Particular risk factors include pregnancy, hiatus hernia with reflux and obesity. Sodium citrate is recommended because it is non-particulate. Ranitidine and cimetidine need to be given 1–2 h before surgery.

ANTIHISTAMINES

Administration of antihistamines is a relatively unimportant consideration, but may be useful for atopic individuals. It may offer partial protection against endogenously released histamine. Promethazine is a suitable agent.

ANTIVAGAL ACTION

An antivagal action is important in ophthalmic surgery, although many anaesthetists administer the antivagal agent at the induction of anaesthesia rather than with the premed. It is indicated if repeated doses of suxamethonium are to be administered. It is not necessary in all cases; however, if not used, the potential for a profound bradycardia during surgery must always be remembered and atropine should be ready to hand at all times. Atropine and glycopyrrolate are the most effective antivagal agents for general use.

CROSS-REFERENCES

Paediatric anaesthesia
    Surgical Procedures 24: 554
Thrombotic embolism
    Anaesthetic Factors 31: 789
Awake or blind nasal intubation
    Anaesthetic Factors 30: 694
Awareness
    Management Problems 31: 727

27

Water and electrolyte disturbances

I. T. Campbell

27

The body is roughly 60% water, which is contained almost exclusively in lean tissue. Adipose tissue is virtually anhydrous. The ratio of intracellular : interstitial : intravascular water is 10 : 3 : 1 or, as a percentage of bodyweight, 40 : 14 : 5.

Normal body water turnover is in the region of 2–3 litres per day. There is about 1200 ml from fluid intake, 1000 ml from solid food and about 400 ml daily is derived from oxidation of foodstuffs. Urine output amounts to 1500 ml, with 600–1000 ml insensible losses via the skin and respiratory tract, and 50 ml via the gut.

The principal extracellular ions are sodium and chloride, with a plasma osmolality of about 300 mOsm. Sodium and chloride ions permeate through the whole of the extracellular fluid.

The intracellular–extracellular fluid and electrolyte relationships are maintained via the relative permeabilities of sodium and potassium ions and the high protein content of the intracellular fluid with its negative charge. They are also maintained by activity of the Na^+ and K^+ pump.

Movement of fluid between the capillaries and the interstitial fluid is determined by the colloid oncotic and hydrostatic forces across the capillary wall.

REGULATION OF SODIUM AND WATER BALANCE

Total body sodium ion and water are controlled by a variety of mechanisms involving antidiuretic hormone (ADH) and atrial natriuretic peptide (ANP) – a 'hormone' released by the muscle cells of the heart (plasma levels correlate with right atrial pressures). ANP is thought to affect salt and water secretion via an effect on glomerular filtration and sodium absorption in the proximal tubule.

ADH is secreted in response to changes detected by osmoreceptors in the hypothalamus. An increase in osmolality stimulates ADH secretion and resorption of fluid in the collecting ducts due to an increase in their permeability; less water is excreted and the urine is more concentrated.

The atrial receptors also have an effect on ADH secretion. Stretching, as in hypervolaemia, inhibits ADH secretion; loss of volume, such as following haemorrhage, stimulates it.

RENIN–ANGIOTENSIN SYSTEM

Sodium and water balance are also controlled by the renin–angiotensin system. The juxtaglomerular cells are sensitive to:
• Plasma sodium concentration
• Blood pressure in afferent arterioles
• Input from sympathetic nerves.
That is, they are sensitive to indicators of plasma sodium concentration and plasma volume.

Renin secretion is stimulated by the three factors listed above. Renin cleaves angiotensin I from angiotensinogen in plasma, which is then converted to angiotensin II by converting enzyme and then to angiotensin III in the adrenal cortex, where it stimulates aldosterone secretion.

Aldosterone controls reabsorption of sodium from the distal tubule but the system responds slowly and is the 'fine tuning' of the sodium and water balance, controlling only the final 3% of the filtered load; its effect may take several days to become evident.

Disorders of the renin–angiotensin system may result in hypertension; failure of the aldosterone system results in sodium loss and hypotension.

ANP acts as a control both on the renin–angiotensin system and by inhibiting the reabsorption of sodium in the distal tubule; it is a vasodilator and thus also affects blood pressure directly.

WATER HOMEOSTASIS

The kidney, via the ADH response, has a huge reserve capacity to clear excess water, so excess intake normally results in only a transient decrease in osmolality. The sensation of thirst and the ADH, ANP and the renal–angiotensin system are all interlinked. Angiotensin II is a powerful thirst-causing substance, and ADH neurones and the thirst centre in the hypothalamus are closely associated.

EXTRACELLULAR FLUID HOMEOSTASIS

This involves gain or loss of isotonic sodium chloride (NaCl), pure water, or pure NaCl:

- Cell membranes are effectively impermeable to sodium ions, so addition or loss of isotonic saline results in changes to only the extracellular fluid compartment (75% interstitial, 25% plasma).
- Loss of extracellular water results in an increase in extracellular osmolality, which causes water to move from the cells. With a gain in pure water the reverse is true.
- Changes in the extracellular fluid NaCl content alone are compensated for by movement of fluid into or from the intracellular fluid compartment.

Thus a change in pure water or NaCl concentration alone affects both intracellular and extracellular fluid, whereas isotonic changes affect only extracellular fluid.

POTASSIUM HOMEOSTASIS

The potential across cell membranes is largely controlled by the differential potassium ion concentrations. Changes in extracellular potassium have a disproportionately marked effect on the size of this potential. Potassium is lost from the cells in catabolic states, and in critical illness. This leads to disturbances in cell membrane function. Sodium leaks in and potassium leaches out, with a decrease in membrane potential. This can be restored with glucose, insulin and supplementary potassium. Recent work in has shown that when insulin was used aggressively to control blood glucose levels there was a significant improvement in mortality rate. This was ascribed to the tight control of blood glucose concentrations, but it could equally have been due to a restoration of cell membrane function by the glucose and insulin.

Some 90% of potassium is reabsorbed from the kidney in the proximal tubule and the proximal part of the loop of Henle. The remaining 10% arrives in the distal tubule; it is via this 10% that all potassium regulation occurs. Reabsorption of potassium from the distal tubule is via an active pump in the tubular cells; in the presence of hyperkalaemia, aldosterone secretion increases in response to the direct effect of potassium on the adrenal cortex (a mechanism not involving the renin–angiotensin pathway). Sodium reabsorbed from this distal tubule is associated with secretion of potassium and hydrogen ions, the two cations being in competition with each other.

CALCIUM AND PHOSPHATE HOMEOSTASIS

The normal plasma concentration of calcium ions is 2.5 mmol l^{-1}, but the physiologically important part is ionic calcium, which constitutes just under 50%; 46% of plasma calcium is protein bound and 6% is bound to phosphate.

Calcium ions are important in membrane excitability and are sensitive to pH changes,

27

TABLE 27.4

Hormonal control of calcium metabolism

Hormone	Source	Trigger to stimulation	Effect
Calcitonin	Parafollicular cells of thyroid		Stimulates bone deposition Decreases plasma Ca^{2+}
Parathormone	Parathyroid glands	Low plasma Ca^{2+}	Release of Ca^{2+} from bone Reabsorption from renal tubule Decreases renal reabsorption of phosphate
1,25-Dihydroxy-cholecalciferol	Derivative of vitamins D_2 and D_3 via metabolic pathways in liver and kidney		Ca^{2+} and phosphate absorption from gut

with alkalinity decreasing calcium ion concentration and acidosis increasing it.

Increased [Ca²⁺]	Decreased [Ca²⁺]
Lethargy	Muscle cramps
Fatigue	Convulsions
Sensory loss	Increased neuromuscular excitability

Metabolism and control of calcium ion concentration are inextricably bound up with phosphate metabolism; most calcium ions are contained in bone, which acts as a massive reserve in the control of calcium ion concentration. Intestinal uptake of calcium ions is in the range of 20–70%, varying in response to changes in plasma concentration. Calcium and phosphate are excreted by the kidney – filtered out then absorbed under hormonal control (Table 27.4).

TABLE 27.5

Disturbances of water, sodium and potassium balance

Disorder	Causes	Clinical signs	Biochemical signs	Treatment
Water deficiency	Diabetes insipidus Hyperosmolar non-ketotic diabetic coma Nephrogenic diabetes insipidus Some types of chronic pyelonephritis	Loss of skin turgor Loss of eyeball tension Dry mucous membrane Low blood pressure Delirium Coma	Plasma Na⁺ and Cl⁻ increased Plasma hypertonic, Na⁺ conserved K⁺ and H⁺ excreted to produce hypokalaemic acidosis Haematocrit and plasma protein concentration increased Urine and plasma osmolality increased	Oral rehydration, if possible, or dextrose (5% i.v.)
Water excess	Heart failure Acute renal failure Iatrogenic (administration of 5% dextrose)	Abdominal and skeletal muscular twitching and cramps Stupor Convulsions In severe cases peripheral and pulmonary oedema	Low plasma Na⁺ and Cl⁻ Increased blood and plasma volume Low osmolality Low plasma proteins and haematocrit	
Sodium chloride deficiency	Decreased intake unusual, but may occur in diarrhoea, malabsorption, severe vomiting Increased Na⁺ loss in diabetic acidosis Chronic renal disease Excessive sweating Adrenal insufficiency	Symptoms develop as [Na⁺] drops below 115 mmol l⁻¹ Clouding of consciousness Convulsions Coma	Plasma Na⁺ and Cl⁻ drop after 4–5 days Decrease in blood volume K⁺ moves out of cells (to maintain tonicity) Na⁺ conservation via renin–angiotensin– aldosterone system Metabolic alkalosis Haematocrit and plasma proteins increased (decreased in dilutional hyponatraemia)	
Sodium chloride excess	Iatrogenic (particularly intravenous nutrition) Primary aldosteronism	Oedema Congestive heart failure Fluid retained so osmolality and [Na⁺] may be normal		

TABLE 27.5 - contd.

Disturbances of water, sodium and potassium balance

Disorder	Causes	Clinical signs	Biochemical signs	Treatment
Potassium deficiency	Gastrointestinal losses Renal disease Diuretics Hormonal (aldosteronism) Cushing's disease Steroids Diabetic acidosis Trauma Burns Intravenous feeding with no added K^+	Drowsy Muscular weakness Paralytic ileus Bradycardia Heart block ST depression Inverted T waves Prolonged QT and PR intervals U waves		
Potassium excess	Renal failure Iatrogenic (administration of K^+) Na^+-conserving diuretics Adrenal insufficiency Acidosis Hypoxia	Anxiety Agitation Stupor Weakness Hyporeflexia Paralysis of extremities Peaked T waves Widened QRS and prolonged PR interval Arrhythmias Cardiac arrest		Acute treatment with Ca^{2+} salts Glucose/insulin Ion exchange resins

DISTURBANCES IN FLUID AND ELECTROLYTES

Probably the commonest abnormality in clinical practice is hypovolaemia, i.e. loss of both fluid and electrolytes (Table 27.5), due either to blood loss or fluid loss such as in diarrhoea or vomiting, or to loss into the gastrointestinal tract in obstruction or burn injury. This is loss of both fluid and electrolytes, and is best replaced by balanced salt solution, Ringer's lactate (Hartmann's solution) or 0.9% saline, although the latter provides a large chloride load and tends to produce metabolic acidosis, and lactate is metabolised in the liver to carbon dioxide and water and tends to produce alkalosis. If the hypovolaemia is severe enough to produce problems with cardiac output and peripheral perfusion, intravascular volume is more effectively repleted with colloidal solutions such as albumin, or one of the synthetic colloids – or even blood.

The colloid versus crystalloid debate continues. The objection to the latter is that is takes, on average, three times as much crystalloid to produce a persistent increase in blood volume as it does colloid, because of rapid transfer of the former to the extracellular space. Colloid also eventually leaks into the extravascular space, but more slowly. The objection to colloid is that this type of problem is usually associated with an acute-phase response and an increase in capillary permeability, both generally and at the site of injury. Fluid that leaks from the intravascular space is sequestered in this 'third' or 'oedema space', which may include the lung. When the patient recovers, this fluid is remobilised and excreted. With colloid this remobilisation may be more protracted.

FLUID BALANCE DURING SURGERY AND ANAESTHESIA

Patients arriving for surgery may have been starved for up to 12 h and would be about 1 litre in deficit. This deficit is of both fluids and electrolytes, and so can be replaced with balanced salt solution. Fluid requirements during surgery depend on the extent of the operation. It is conventional practice in the normal individual to transfuse blood when about 20% of the circulating blood volume has been lost. With blood loss, fluid requirements (in addition to blood replacement) are in the

27

range 5–15 ml kg^{-1} h^{-1}, depending on the amount of blood loss and the extent of the operation. Hypotonic (glucose) solutions should not be given for volume replacement, as in the short term they produce significant hyperglycaemia (> 20 mol l^{-1}) and in the longer term persistent hyponatraemia.

Too aggressive a use of fluids can cause problems in the postoperative period. Fluid retention of about 3 litres after abdominal surgery is not uncommon, but it has been demonstrated that if sodium and water is restricted after operation (2 litres over 24 h and 70–80 mmol Na$^+$ rather than the traditional 3 litres and 150 mmol Na$^+$) recovery is quicker and the incidence of postoperative complications lower.

BIBLIOGRAPHY

Lobo DN, Bostock KA, Neal KR et al. Effect of salt and water balance on recovery of gastrointestinal function after elective colonic resection: a randomised controlled trial. Lancet 2002; 359:1812–1818

Martinez-Riquelme AE, Allison SP. Insulin revisited. Clinical Nutrition 2003; 22:7–15

27

Psychiatric disorders

B. J. Pollard

The incidence of psychiatric disorders within the general population is high. In general, the major relevance to anaesthesia is from the treatment and other patient co-morbidities rather than from the psychiatric illness itself.

ANXIETY DISORDERS

Almost every patient suffers, or has suffered, from mild anxiety disorders at some time. It is only when the anxiety is particularly severe or does not resolve spontaneously that treatment is required. The mainstay of treatment is a drug from the benzodiazepine family, although small doses of β-adrenergic blocking agents may be beneficial. There may be fear of anaesthesia and/or surgery present, and thoughtful preoperative counselling is valuable. The administration of a benzodiazepine premed is useful.

DEPRESSION

Depression is usually divided into two types, endogenous and reactive, although the distinction may not be clear. Reactive depression is usually triggered by external events such as bereavement. Symptoms include fatigue, mood disturbances, insomnia, loss of appetite, decreased ability to concentrate and a general feeling of loss of worth. Suicidal thoughts may also prevail. It is more common in women than men and familial tendencies exist. The exact pathophysiology is not known, but disturbances in central amine levels seem to be present. It may be difficult to distinguish from dementia in the elderly. Treatment of depression is with drugs and/or ECT.

TRICYCLIC ANTIDEPRESSANTS
This was the original treatment for depression, and has been largely superseded by other drugs. Tricyclic drugs include amitriptyline and imipramine. Side-effects include mild sedation, dry mouth, blurred vision, urinary retention (anticholinergic effects) and ECG changes (increased PR and QT intervals). An overdose may cause potentially fatal cardiac arrhythmias. Treatment with tricyclics need not be interrupted during the operative period. An increased requirement for anaesthetic agents has been reported. Ephedrine should be given with care because there may be an exaggerated vasopressor response. A directly acting agent such as metaraminol may be preferable. Ketamine and pancuronium should be avoided or used with care. The injection of local anaesthetic containing adrenaline (epinephrine) may result in increased blood pressure and cardiac rhythm disturbances.

SELECTIVE SEROTONIN-REUPTAKE INHIBITORS (SSRIs)
Members of this family (e.g. fluoxetine, paroxetine) are currently the most commonly prescribed drugs for depression. They are devoid of anticholinergic and cardiac side-effects. Fluoxetine in a potent inhibitor of the cytochrome P450 enzyme in the liver. This may affect the plasma levels and bioavailability of other co-administered drugs that rely on this pathway for metabolism. SSRIs should not affect anaesthesia and may be safely continued throughout the perioperative period.

MONOAMINE OXIDASE INHIBITORS (MAOIs)
These drugs tend not to be used as first-line treatment for depression. They do not have an anticholinergic effect or a significant cardiac effect themselves. It is no longer recommended that MAOIs should be stopped 21 days before a general anaesthetic. The consideration with these drugs is the effect of inhibiting monoamine oxidase on the responses of other drugs and chemicals. Foods containing tyramine (e.g. cheese) should not be eaten. Care should be exercised in the choice of all drugs. Indirectly acting vasopressors (e.g. ephedrine) and pethidine should be avoided. Care should be exercised with other opioids as a hypertensive response has been reported.

27

Ketamine, pancuronium and possibly halothane should be avoided. The use of adrenaline (epinephrine) with the local anaesthetic in a regional block may be inadvisable. Vasoconstrictors should not be sprayed into the nose as an adjunct to surgery or nasotracheal intubation. Directly acting vasopressors (e.g. metaraminol) are recommended for the treatment of hypotension.

MANIC DISORDERS

The clinical presentation of mania is one of hyperactivity and heightened mood. It may progress to hallucinations and delusions. It appears to be inherited in an autosomal dominant manner, and pathophysiological changes include abnormalities in central neurotransmitter regulation.

The routine treatment for manic disorders is lithium. Lithium has a very narrow therapeutic window. The therapeutic plasma level is 1–1.2 mmol l^{-1}, whereas toxicity appears when the level is over 2 mmol l^{-1}. Signs of lithium toxicity include muscle weakness, sedation, ataxia, hypotension and ECG changes. Hypothyroidism, polyuria and polydipsia may occur with long-term treatment. Plasma lithium concentration must be measured before anaesthesia to ensure that it is not in the toxic range. There may be a reduced requirement for general anaesthetics. The action of neuromuscular blocking agents is prolonged. Exercise care if a dose of a loop diuretic, such as furosemide (frusemide), is required as the plasma lithium concentration may be increased.

SCHIZOPHRENIA

Patients with schizophrenia may exhibit a wide variety of symptoms including hallucinations, withdrawal from society, flat affect and disinterest in personal appearance. A wide variety of drugs is used in the treatment of schizophrenia (e.g. phenothiazines, haloperidol and clozapine). These drugs possess a wide variety of side-effects, in particular extrapyramidal symptoms and signs, anticholinergic effects, sedation, dyskinesia and parkinsonian symptoms. Postural hypotension may be present and there may be an exaggerated response to hypotensive drugs (including anaesthetic agents), fluid loss and intermittent positive-pressure ventilation (IPPV).

BIBLIOGRAPHY

Anderson IM. The new antidepressants. Current Anaesthesia and Critical Care 1999; 10:32–39

Miller RD, Way WL, Eger EI. The effects of alpha-methyl-dopa, reserpine, guanethidine and iproniazid on minimum alveolar anesthetic requirement (MAC). Anesthesiology 1968; 29:1153–1158

Stack CJ, Rogers P, Linter SPK. Monoamine oxidase inhibitors and anaesthesia. British Journal of Anaesthesia 1988; 60:222–227

27

Substance abuse

B. J. Pollard

This may be defined as the self-administration of a substance that is not for normal medicinal purposes and that may lead to physical and/or psychological dependence. Physical dependence occurs when the presence of the substance is necessary for normal physiological well-being and when specific symptoms ('withdrawal') occur if the substance is not taken. Psychological dependence occurs when the substance produces a desire to repeat the experience again and again. Tolerance to a substance may develop such that increasing doses are required to produce the same effect. There is an association with hepatitis, AIDS, personality disorders, unwanted pregnancy and antisocial behaviour. Drug overdoses are common due to mistakes, the desire to try more, unexpected variation in strength, and mixing with other drugs or substances.

OPIOIDS

Opioids may be ingested by a number of routes including oral, intranasal and intravenous. They produce physical dependence. Tolerance also commonly develops and the addict needs an increased dose for the same 'high'. Tolerance does not develop when opioids are used for the management of acute pain. The effects seen in cases of overdose or acute administration include slow respirations, very small constricted pupils, impaired conscious level, dysarthria and slurred speech, and, later, coma and death. Fits are not common and suggest that the individual might have also ingested another substance. Pulmonary oedema may complicate an acute overdose. Opioid addicts have a higher incidence of anaemia, nutritional deficiencies, sepsis, phlebitis and cellulitis, and bacterial endocarditis.

ANAESTHESIA

Maintain opioid administration with a suitable opioid in a dose equivalent to the addict's routine daily requirement to prevent withdrawal symptoms. Methadone is useful. Avoid giving any opioid antagonists or agonist–antagonist agents. Cross-tolerance to other CNS depressants may be seen with an increase in the requirements for anaesthesia. The analgesic effect of entonox is reduced. Hypotension is common and should be treated with fluids in the first instance. If hypotension does not respond to fluids or a vasopressor, a dose of morphine has been reported to restore the blood pressure. For rehabilitated addicts, try to avoid drugs of the opioid family: use an inhalational agent combined with a regional block. Opioid addicts are usually difficult and manipulative. It may be difficult to determine whether postoperative pain requests for additional doses of opioid are genuine or not.

ALCOHOL

Excess ingestion of alcohol affects all age groups, including the elderly. It has been suggested that there may be a genetic predisposition to the development of alcoholism. A high index of suspicion should always be entertained when non-specific symptoms that do not fit any clear pattern are observed. Many of the central effects of alcohol appear to result from an action on the γ-aminobutyric acid (GABA) system. Alcohol increases the GABA-mediated increase in chloride conductance and is closely related to the action of benzodiazepines and barbiturates.

Withdrawal of alcohol produces a number of symptoms, which can occasionally be severe and life threatening (delirium tremens) (Box 27.6). Following longer-term chronic alcohol ingestion, cerebellar neurone loss may occur associated with vitamin B_1 deficiency (Wernicke's encephalopathy or Korsakoff's psychosis).

ANAESTHESIA

When the patient has acute alcohol intoxication it is wise to delay anaesthesia, if possible. If it is necessary to proceed, expect the requirements

27

27

BOX 27.6

Symptoms of acute alcohol withdrawal

- Tremor
- Hallucinations
- Agitation
- Confusion
- Tachycardia
- Hypertension
- Cardiac arrhythmias
- Nausea and vomiting
- Insomnia

Delirium tremens

- Hallucinations
- Tachycardia
- Hypertension
- Hyperthermia
- Convulsions

---

of anaesthetic and sedative agents to be reduced. The patient should be treated as at increased risk of pulmonary aspiration, and a rapid sequence induction performed. Hypoglycaemia may develop during the hangover phase following the acute period and blood glucose levels should be measured at regular intervals. The sedative and respiratory depressant effects of opioid administration may be potentiated.

In the chronic alcoholic patient, tolerance to anaesthetic agents is often present. In the later stages impaired hepatic function may lead to slower drug metabolism and reduced plasma protein concentrations, producing an exaggerated response to some agents. Hepatic cirrhosis and nutritional deficiencies may also be present. Regional techniques may prove attractive but care should be taken if any degree of alcohol-induced polyneuritis is present.

Disulfiram treatment potentiates benzodiazepines and other sedative agents. A reduced dose may be needed. In cases of hypotension, metaraminol may be preferable to ephedrine. Avoid alcohol-containing skin preparations and medications.

COCAINE

This highly addictive substance is often taken by smoking. It causes a profound 'high' and its central stimulatory effects are mediated through enhancement of adrenergic and dopaminergic pathways. It is metabolised by plasma cholinesterase and the risk of toxicity is increased

in patients with low plasma cholinesterase levels. Withdrawal causes fatigue, depression and increased appetite.

Acute administration can cause tachycardia, arrhythmias (including ventricular fibrillation), hypertension, coronary spasm, and myocardial ischaemia or infarction. Smoking cocaine may also cause lung damage, pulmonary oedema and atrophy of the nasal septum. Agitation, paranoid thoughts, hyperreflexia, hyperpyrexia and convulsions may also be seen.

ANAESTHESIA

If acutely intoxicated, there is a likelihood of arrhythmias and myocardial ischaemia. Requirements for anaesthetic agents may be increased. Hypertension is likely so it is wise to have a nitrate infusion ready. Avoid volatile agents, which can sensitise the myocardium to catecholamines, and the use of cocaine spray to the nose. Thrombocytopenia has been described, and so platelet count should be checked before considering a regional block.

BARBITURATES

These are not abused so much as was the case in the past due to stricter controls and less availability for medicinal use. Chronic abuse causes tolerance to sedative agents. The effects of acute ingestion include hypotension, hypothermia, ataxia and slurred speech. In higher doses or overdose, myocardial depression, coma and acute renal failure may be seen. Acute withdrawal may produce potentially life-threatening side-effects, including tachycardia, anxiety, tremor, hyperreflexia, hyperpyrexia, hypotension, convulsions and cardiovascular collapse.

ANAESTHESIA

Cross-tolerance to anaesthetic agents will be present, leading to the need for higher doses. Chronic induction of hepatic enzymes will alter the pharmacokinetics of a number of drugs including warfarin, digoxin and phenytoin.

BENZODIAZEPINES

Chronic benzodiazepine ingestion produces physical dependence. Tolerance also develops. Withdrawal symptoms are similar to those for barbiturates, but much less severe. Depression of respiration may occur with overdose but is much more likely if another substance (e.g. alcohol) has been taken in addition. Beware of the use of flumazenil in acute benzodiazepine overdose; convulsions may occur.

ANAESTHESIA

Cross-tolerance to anaesthetic agents occurs, leading to the need for higher doses. Induction of hepatic enzymes does not seem to be a feature of chronic benzodiazepine usage.

AMPHETAMINES

These drugs stimulate catecholamine release causing a heightened awareness and reduced need for sleep. Appetite is also suppressed, and amphetamines have been used in the past for this purpose. Tolerance develops rapidly, leading to an escalation of dose. Chronic amphetamine abuse leads to daytime somnolence, weight loss and malnutrition. In overdose anxiety, hyperreflexia, hyperactivity, tachycardia, hypertension, hyperthermia and convulsions may occur. Withdrawal leads to increased appetite, lethargy and depression.

ANAESTHESIA

A reduced requirement for anaesthetic agents may be seen in chronic amphetamine use. Profound hypotension on induction may be seen, which may not respond to ephedrine. Metaraminol is preferable. If acutely intoxicated, tachycardia, hypertension, hyperpyrexia and increased requirement for anaesthetic agents should be expected.

MARIJUANA

This agent is becoming more readily available and it is likely that its use may be legalised in some countries in the future. It is also increasingly being used for its medicinal purposes (antiemetic and claimed possible benefit in certain chronic neurological disorders). It is usually smoked and produces euphoria, drowsiness, tachycardia and postural hypotension. Long-term use may cause tar deposits in the lungs.

ANAESTHESIA

A reduced dose of anaesthetic agent may be required. Delayed recovery and respiratory depression are possible. There is otherwise little effect on anaesthesia.

BIBLIOGRAPHY

Giuffrida JG, Bizzarri DV, Saurec AC et al. Anesthetic management of drug abusers. Anesthesia and Analgesia 1970; 49:273–282

May JA, White HC, Leonard-White A, Warltier DC, Pagel PS. The patient recovering from alcohol or drug addiction: special issues for the anesthesiologist. Anesthesia and Analgesia 2001; 92:1601–1608

Lee PKY, Cho MH, Dobkin AB. Effects of alcoholism, morphinism and barbiturate resistance on induction and maintenance of general anesthesia. Canadian Anaesthetists Society Journal 1974; 11:366–371

27

Preoperative assessment of cardiovascular risk in non-cardiac surgery

S. Christian and J. M. Hull

Perioperative cardiac morbidity (PCM) is defined as the occurrence of myocardial infarction (MI), unstable angina, congestive cardiac failure, serious arrhythmia or cardiac death during the intraoperative, perioperative or postoperative period. In view of the stresses that anaesthesia and surgery impose on the body, it should be of no surprise that PCM is both a common and a major cause of death following these procedures.

The exact pathological mechanisms involved in perioperative MI are still not clear. In the usual setting of MI, rupture of a coronary artery atherosclerotic plaque causes platelet aggregation and subsequent thrombus formation. During perioperative MI, plaque rupture is seen in only 50% of cases. It is for this reason that many of these infarctions are thought to occur as a result of a prolonged imbalance between myocardial oxygen supply and demand in the presence of coronary artery disease (CAD). In postoperative surgical patients who suffer plaque rupture, it is thought that an increased heart rate and contractility, induced by high circulating levels of catecholamines, produce shear stresses on the atherosclerotic plaques, predisposing them to rupture. Both of these observations help explain why perioperative MIs frequently do not occur during surgery, but typically peak 1–3 days after operation.

History, examination and clinical investigations have been used for many years to identify individual patients at risk of suffering PCM, often in the context of risk indices. A score is assigned to a specific clinical variable, allowing a final total to stratify the patient's risk of suffering PCM. In 1977, Goldman designed a risk index score that assigned patients to four classes, from I (low risk) to IV (high risk). This risk index was modified in 1986 by Detsky, with the additional factors of unstable angina and remote MI, as well as the simplification of risk groups to three classes. Risk stratification is now used as a screening tool in order to decide which patients will benefit from further investigation of the cardiovascular system with advanced and more invasive investigations prior to surgery. Indeed, the whole focus of this process should be aimed at deciding on the optimal management of patients who are known to be at significant risk of PCM, instituting beneficial therapies (such as beta-blockade where indicated) in the perioperative period, and arranging a suitably safe environment for the patient after surgery (i.e. critical care bed).

PREOPERATIVE ASSESSMENT FOR CARDIOVASCULAR DISEASE

ROUTINE:
- Clinical history
- Physical examination
- Laboratory tests
- Chest radiography
- 12-lead ECG.

NON-ROUTINE:
- Exercise stress testing
- Ambulatory ECG
- Echocardiography
- Nuclear imaging
- Cardiac catheterisation.

PROPOSED PREOPERATIVE PREDICTORS OF PCM

AGE
Increasing chronological age is widely recognised as a major risk factor in the development of CAD and is associated with a reduction in the cardiac response to stress. Age has been reported to be a predictor of PCM only in the presence of other factors and hence may not be as important as overall physiological status.

CORONARY ARTERY DISEASE
Patients with a documented previous MI have a greater risk of perioperative infarction (5–8%). which is associated with a high mortal-

ity rate (36–70%). The incidence of reinfarction has also been shown to reduce, with increasing time, in the 6 months following MI. If, for clinical reasons, surgery cannot be delayed following a MI, the reinfarction rate has been shown to be significantly reduced with the use of advanced haemodynamic monitoring techniques.

Angina is usually associated with angiographically significant (> 70% stenosis) CAD. In these patients 75% of ischaemic episodes are painless ('silent ischaemia'). Most perioperative ischaemia is silent and is more common during the first 2 days after operation. Despite this, stable angina is considered to represent only an intermediate predictor of the risk for PCM. In contrast to this, patients with unstable coronary syndromes have a greatly increased risk of MI. These patients warrant urgent cardiological assessment, independent of their need for operation.

PREVIOUS CORONARY ARTERY BYPASS GRAFT (CABG)

When undergoing major surgery, patients who have undergone a CABG are known to have a lower mortality rate than patients treated with purely medical therapy. For this reason, the current advice from the American College of Cardiology (ACC) and the American Heart Association (AHA) is that patients who have remained symptom-free within 5 years of a CABG do not require further invasive tests for risk stratification. CABG does present its own risks of death, MI and stroke; therefore it should be performed only if the patient has symptoms or coronary artery anatomy that mandate CABG independent of planned non-cardiac surgery.

PERCUTANEOUS CORONARY INTERVENTION

There is little hard evidence to prove that preoperative percutaneous coronary intervention is beneficial in patients undergoing non-cardiac surgery. Indeed, in one study of patients undergoing non-cardiac surgery within 6 weeks of coronary artery stent placement, 20% died, 18% had a non-fatal MI and 28% suffered major bleeding. For these reasons it is suggested that percutaneous coronary interventions be performed purely on the grounds of clinical need, regardless of the patient's need for non-cardiac surgery.

CONGESTIVE CARDIAC FAILURE

Congestive cardiac failure (CCF) is associated with a poor prognosis in patients with CAD and is a predictor of cardiac death after acute MI. Although preoperative CCF is strongly predictive of PCM, the predictive value of specific signs seen in these patients is controversial.

HYPERTENSION

Hypertension is known to be a risk factor for the development of CAD, although mild to moderate hypertension (i.e. blood pressure < 110 mmHg) is not an independent risk factor for PCM. Secondary causes of hypertension should be sought in the preoperative period. It is important to continue antihypertensive drugs into the perioperative period to prevent 'rebound hypertension' associated with sudden discontinuation of these drugs.

DIABETES MELLITUS

Diabetes mellitus is strongly associated with CAD. Although it is only a modest independent predictor of PCM, diabetes mellitus presents diagnostic difficulties due to the high incidence of 'silent ischaemia' and 'silent MI'. Autonomic neuropathy caused by diabetes mellitus confers greater risks of intraoperative blood pressure instability.

DYSRHYTHMIAS

The cardiac dysrhythmias associated with an increased PCM are symptomatic ventricular dysrhythmias associated with an underlying cardiac problem (e.g. CAD, cardiomyopathy) or atrial fibrillation. High-grade conduction abnormalities, such as complete heart block, trifascicular block and bifascicular block, all carry significant mortality rates, independent of surgery.

PERIPHERAL VASCULAR DISEASE

Significant coronary artery stenosis is present in 14–78% of patients with peripheral vascular disease (PVD) regardless of their CAD symptoms. Patients with PVD can present difficulties in assessing the severity of CAD symptoms because their activities are limited by their PVD. Only 8% of patients with PVD have normal coronary angiograms. PVD patients undergoing vascular surgery have a high risk of PCM.

RENAL FAILURE

Chronic renal failure is an independent risk factor for PCM. Added to this, chronic renal failure is often associated with other risk factors for CAD (diabetes mellitus, hypertension).

VALVULAR HEART DISEASE

Patients with significant aortic stenosis have an increased incidence of sudden death due to the potential for a severe decrease in cardiac output. The 1994/1995 Confidential Enquiry into Perioperative Deaths recommended

27

preoperative cardiological assessment of the aortic valve in all patients with an ejection systolic murmur and evidence of left ventricular hypertrophy or myocardial ischaemia. The risks of PCM with other valvular lesions are less clearly defined; they are probably related to the severity of the valvular defect and the presence of other cardiac abnormalities.

CARDIOMYOPATHIES

Cardiomyopathies may cause an increased risk by decreasing ejection fraction and causing ventricular outlet obstruction. In addition to this, the cause of cardiomyopathy (e.g. alcohol, infiltration) may present a perioperative risk in its own right.

CIGARETTE SMOKING

Smokers are at a greatly increased risk of CAD; however, smoking has not be found to be an independent risk factor for PCM.

CHOLESTEROL

Although there is a direct relationship between serum cholesterol concentration and cardiovascular mortality, the risk of PCM is unknown.

DIAGNOSTIC TESTS

BIOCHEMICAL DATA

Biochemical tests are useful in determining a patient's baseline renal function, which may be important in those who have hypertension, diabetes mellitus or who may be taking angiotensin-converting enzyme (ACE) inhibitors. Serum potassium and magnesium levels should also be checked in patients who are taking diuretics or who have a cardiac dysrhythmia.

12-LEAD ECG

A routine ECG is frequently performed in patients as part of a preoperative screening process. Despite this, ECG has not been found helpful in predicting patients likely to suffer from PCM who have no cardiac risk factors. For these reasons, the suggested criteria for preoperative ECG are:
- Age over 50 years
- Risk factors for CAD
- Clinical history suggesting cardiac dysrhythmias, CCF or other cardiac disease.

Abnormalities seen on a 12-lead ECG that are associated with an increased risk of PCM are:
- Rhythm other than sinus
- ST–T-wave abnormalities
- Left ventricular hypertrophy
- Pathological Q waves
- Conduction abnormalities.

The predictive values of the above ECG findings remain controversial.

CHEST RADIOGRAPHY

Preoperative chest radiographs are useful to clarify clinical signs and confirm the position of implanted devices such as a pacemaker. In more than 70% of patients with CAD, cardiomegaly is associated with a low ejection fraction (< 40%) and may predict PCM.

EXERCISE STRESS TESTING

Exercise testing is used to produce an increase in heart rate to precipitate ECG evidence of myocardial ischaemia. Exercise testing also enables assessment of functional capacity. This form of testing has a sensitivity for detecting CAD of 68% and a specificity of 77%. A positive ischaemic response and low exercise tolerance have been shown to be predictors of PCM in non-cardiac surgery. The main advantages of exercise testing are that it is usually available locally and is relatively inexpensive. The disadvantages of the test relate to exclusion factors, which include an abnormal baseline ECG and an inability to exercise (e.g. PVD).

AMBULATORY ECG MONITORING

This test is successful in detecting silent MI. Some 18–40% of patients with or at risk of CAD have frequent ischaemic episodes (> 75% are 'silent'). The usefulness of ambulatory ECG monitoring in assessing preoperative patients has not been defined.

ECHOCARDIOGRAPHY

In the preoperative setting, echocardiography is used to assess valvular function, left ventricular function, the presence of left ventricular hypertrophy and the existence of pericardial effusions. Resting echo ejection fractions have not been found to correlate with PCM. Transthoracic echocardiography probably adds very little to the information acquired from routine clinical and electrocardiographic data in the majority of non-cardiac surgical patients.

Stress echocardiography involves imaging the heart at rest and under the influence of catecholamine stimulation, induced by either exercise or pharmacological agents (e.g. dobutamine). New areas of dyskinetic wall motion that develop during the test indicate the presence of myocardial ischaemia. Stress echocardiography has an excellent negative predictive value for PCM (93–100%) The test's relatively poor positive predictive value (7–30%) means that there is a high likelihood of a patient being subjected to further unnecessary evaluation prior to surgery. The other disadvantage is that local expertise, necessary for the test, may not be available.

RADIONUCLEOTIDE VENTRICULOGRAPHY

Multi-gated radionucleotide ventriculography (MUGA scanning) is a test aimed at determining left ventricular ejection fraction. An ejection fraction of less than 35%, as assessed by MUGA scanning, is associated with an increased risk of PCM. More recent studies have discovered that radionucleotide ventriculography adds very little to clinical assessment of patients and is probably not a cost-effective investigation.

THALLIUM SCINTIGRAPHY

During this investigation a radionucleotide agent is injected and then images of the myocardium are obtained in the presence and absence of a coronary vasodilator (e.g. dipyridamole, adenosine). This illustrates reversible perfusion defects and assesses left ventricular function. Patients who demonstrate reversible or fixed perfusion defects probably have CAD, one of the main risk factors for PCM. A large study in 1994 confirmed previous evidence that thallium redistribution is not associated with perioperative MI, prolonged ischaemia or other adverse myocardial events. For this reason thallium scintigraphy is not recommended as a routine test to assess preoperative patients.

CORONARY ANGIOGRAPHY

This test is considered to be the 'gold standard' to assess coronary anatomy. Both the ACA and AHA recommend coronary angiography to investigate patients deemed to be at high risk with non-invasive testing. Coronary angiography carries its own risks, so it is not indicated as a tool for stratifying PCM risk. Repeated coronary angiography is not indicated in patients who have had an adequate angiogram within the previous 2 years, with no worsening of symptoms.

SUMMARY

The most important predictors of PCM are recent MI, severe or unstable angina, current CCF and critical aortic stenosis. These are all factors that can be determined by clinical history, examination and simple routine investigations. The use of non-routine, advanced tests, such as stress echocardiography and coronary angiography, should be restricted to patients in whom the additional information provided by the test will alter the management of the patient.

BIBLIOGRAPHY

Detsky AS, Abrams HB, Forbath N et al. Cardiac assessment in patients undergoing non-cardiac surgery. A multifactorial clinical risk index. Archives of Internal Medicine 1986; 146:2131–2135

Goldman L, Cardera DL, Nussbaum SR et al. Multifactorial index of cardiac risk in non-cardiac surgical patients. New England Journal of Medicine 1977; 297:845–850

Grayburn PA, Hillis LD. Cardiac events in patients undergoing non-cardiac surgery: shifting the paradigm from non-invasive risk stratification to therapy. Annals of Internal Medicine 2003; 138:506–512

Hollenberg SM. Preoperative cardiac risk assessment. Chest 1999; 115:51S–57S

Juste RN, Lawson AD, Soni N. Minimising cardiac anaesthetic risk: the tortoise or the hare? Anaesthesia 1996; 51:255–262

Kelion AD, Banning AP. Is simple assessment adequate for cardiac risk stratification before non-cardiac surgery? Lancet 1999; 354:1837–1838

Mangano DT. Perioperative cardiac morbidity. Anesthesiology 1990; 70:153–184

Mangano DT. Assessment of the patient with cardiac disease. Anesthesiology 1999; 91:1521–1526

Nel L, Cone A. Cardiac assessment of patients undergoing non-cardiac surgery. In: Kaufman L, Ginsberg R, eds. Anaesthesia review, vol 16. London: Churchill Livingstone; 2001:29–51

27

Preoperative assessment of pulmonary risk

B. J. Pollard

The development of postoperative pulmonary complications is determined principally by a number of risk factors:

- The severity of pre-existing pulmonary disease
- The patient's general state of health
- The nature and extent of surgery
- The anaesthetic technique
- Preoperative and postoperative care.

It is difficult to assess the influence that individual variables may have on outcome, particularly with improvements in perioperative care, anaesthetic and surgical techniques, and in the health of the population as a whole. The risk from pre-existing pulmonary disease should be determined initially by history and examination. Additional risk factors (surgical, anaesthetic, age, etc.) can then be considered.

PRE-EXISTING PULMONARY DISEASE

HISTORY
Dyspnoea

Undue awareness of breathing or awareness of difficulty in breathing. Usually graded using Roizen's classification (Table 27.6). Dyspnoea at rest (grade IV) with low PaO_2 (< 7 kPa,

TABLE 27.6

Roizen's classification of dyspnoea

Grade	Findings
0	No dyspnoea while walking on the level at a normal pace
I	Able to walk as far as desired provided the person takes their time
II	Specific limitation – there is a need to stop and rest for a while after walking about 100–200 m
III	Dyspnoea on mild exertion – normal household tasks are limited by dyspnoea
IV	Dyspnoea at rest

55 mmHg) is associated with an increased likelihood of requiring assisted ventilation after abdominal surgery. The aetiology should be sought (e.g. asthma, chronic bronchitis, emphysema, fibrosing alveolitis). Hypoventilation due to failure of neural input or muscle weakness may not cause dyspnoea.

Cough
May indicate acute infection or, if productive of sputum on most days, suggests chronic bronchitis. Complications of excess sputum include airway plugging, atelectasis and respiratory infection. Loss of response to carbon dioxide and dependence on hypoxaemic respiratory drive need to be taken into account when planning the anaesthetic technique. Preoperative physiotherapy or bronchodilators may be required. Psychological preparation and training in breathing exercises can be invaluable. Sputum should be sent for culture.

Haemoptysis may be due to carcinoma, tuberculosis, pulmonary infarction or pneumonia, and must be distinguished from nasal bleeding.

Wheeze
May indicate asthma, chronic bronchitis, emphysema or acute foreign body inhalation. Asthma should be assessed by frequency of attacks, current drug therapy, and history of hospitalisation and ventilation. Steroid treatment contributes to muscle weakness and immune incompetence, both of which may result in prolonged ventilation and respiratory colonisation. Bronchospasm may occur with laryngoscopy, tracheal intubation and anaesthetic drugs that release histamine, particularly when given rapidly intravenously.

Other factors
Cardiovascular disease, drugs, allergies, smoking.

EXAMINATION
Observation:

- Rate and pattern of breathing
- Ease of talking

- Use of accessory muscles of respiration
- Nicotine staining of hands
- Finger clubbing (intrapulmonary shunting)
- Colour – cyanosis, anaemia
- Deformity – kyphoscoliosis
- Nutritional – obesity, malnutrition, muscle wasting.

Percussion:
- Pleural effusion
- Consolidation.

Auscultation:
- Reduced breath sounds
- Wheeze
- Bronchial breathing
- Pleural rub.

INVESTIGATION

Tests of pulmonary function are rarely abnormal in the absence of physical symptoms and signs. They should be used to quantify risk.

Chest radiography

Over 40 years of age, 4% of routine preoperative chest radiographs will detect an abnormality. The indications for preoperative chest radiography are:
- Symptoms or signs of active lung disease
- Patients with possible lung metastases
- Symptoms and signs of heart disease
- Recent immigrants from countries where tuberculosis is endemic and who have not had chest radiography in the previous year.

Emphysematous bullae increase the risk of pneumothorax with positive-pressure ventilation. Collapse, consolidation, pleural effusion and pneumothorax require preoperative treatment. Cardiomegaly and pulmonary oedema also indicate high risk and require specialist management. Unstable patients should be transferred to an ITU or HDU for appropriate monitoring in order to maximise physiological reserve before surgery.

Spirometry

Although peak flow, FEV_1 and vital capacity may be useful to follow the progression of pulmonary dysfunction, numerous studies have failed to demonstrate their predictive value for individual patient outcome. Even patients with a FEV_1 of less than 0.5 litres may cope without requiring postoperative ventilation.

Maximum breathing capacity (MBC), calculated as $FEV_1 \times 35$ or peak flow $\times 0.25$, may be used to assess respiratory reserve. MBC greater than 60 l min^{-1} is normal, and less than 25 l min^{-1} indicates severe pulmonary impairment.

Arterial blood gas tensions

A PaO_2 of less than 7.1 kPa, or less than 70% of normal for age, in combination with dyspnoea at rest, has been shown to predict dependence on postoperative respiratory support in patients undergoing upper abdominal surgery. PaO_2 may be used with a graph of isoshunt lines to assess pulmonary shunting and to estimate oxygen requirements.

However, $PaCO_2$ is of little predictive value for postoperative ventilation, although it may be useful to detect patients with a hypoxic respiratory drive in whom postoperative administration of oxygen will need careful monitoring. Detection of metabolic acidosis in the critically ill patient may indicate demands on respiratory work that cannot be met by spontaneous ventilation.

ADDITIONAL CONSIDERATIONS

SURGICAL FACTORS

Thoracic and upper abdominal surgery, by interfering with diaphragmatic movement, may both cause a reduction in functional residual capacity (FRC) after operation. In addition, as FRC falls below closing capacity, dependent airways close leading to increased V/Q mismatch, shunt and atelectasis. Pain and the supine position further contribute to a reduction in FRC.

ANAESTHETIC FACTORS

Anaesthesia causes a reduction in FRC and lung volume, leading to reduced compliance and increased shunting. Gas trapping of oxygen and nitrous oxide, which are soluble, may lead to alveolar collapse. General anaesthesia in excess of 2 h increases risk of atelectasis and infection. The incidence of pneumonia in one study was 40% in patients following thoracic or abdominal surgery lasting for more than 4 h (8% when less than 2 h).

Anaesthesia and surgery are associated with a reduced humoral immune response, impaired neutrophil chemotaxis and phagocytosis, and depressed mucociliary transport.

AGE

Muscle weakness, a stiff rib cage and loss of elastic recoil in the elderly results in airway closure at higher lung volumes. After approximately 45 years of age, closing capacity exceeds FRC when lying supine, which may contribute to risk of atelectasis. In one study the incidence of pneumonia following thoracic or abdominal surgery was 18% in patients aged

27

over 30 years, compared with 9% in those under 30 years.

NUTRITIONAL STATE

Obesity reduces chest compliance and FRC, and increases closing capacity. These are worsened by supine or head-down position. After operation, the semi-erect position is preferred in order to limit hypoxaemia. Epidural analgesia reduces pulmonary complications, but the benefit is less in the very obese patient. In those heavier than 115 kg, the incidence of postoperative pneumonia was reported to be doubled. Systemic illness, chronic disease and steroids cause muscle weakness, which may increase risk of pulmonary complications. Low serum albumin levels have been linked with an increased risk of postoperative pneumonia.

SMOKING

Smoking causes impaired mucociliary transport, reduced neutrophil activity, raised closing capacity and increased V/Q mismatch. The tracheobronchial tree is hyperactive and there is an increased risk of bronchospasm following airway manipulation. The risk of postoperative pneumonia is doubled in smokers. Carboxyhaemoglobin levels are reduced by stopping smoking for 12 h, but 6 weeks is required for maximum benefit.

SLEEP APNOEA SYNDROMES

Approximately 1 in 50 men develop obstructive sleep apnoea in the supine position, leading to hypoxaemia, hypercapnia and haemodynamic instability. Patients at risk may be identified by a history of snoring and daytime sleepiness. Sleep deprivation worsens the risk, as do hypnotic, analgesic and sedative drugs. Obstruction may occur following premedication, and airway maintenance may be difficult. Oxygen therapy alone may be inadequate, and nasal continuous positive airway pressure (CPAP) may be needed.

UPPER RESPIRATORY TRACT INFECTION

In a child with an upper respiratory tract infection (URTI) who receives a general anaesthetic, there is up to seven times the risk of a perioperative respiratory complication. Children under 1 year of age with an URTI should have elective surgery postponed. The risk increases if intubation is performed. In otherwise healthy children over 5 years and in adults, where there is no reduction in physical activity, no pyrexia and the chest examination is normal, there appears to be no increased risk from minor surgery of further respiratory complications. However, airways are often hyperactive with increased risk of bronchospasm, and lung defence mechanisms, particularly mucociliary clearance, may be impaired. For major surgery few data are available for the effect on pulmonary risk, but in combination with other risk factors a cautious approach is wise.

OTHER FACTORS

Other risk factors leading to respiratory failure should be identified. Prophylaxis may be needed for deep vein thrombosis leading to pulmonary embolus, particularly in the obese and patients with prolonged immobilisation. Preoperative hospitalisation of more than 2 days doubles the risk of postoperative pneumonia.

BIBLIOGRAPHY

Barrowcliffe MP, Jones JG. Respiratory function and the safety of anaesthesia. In: Taylor TH, Major E, eds. Hazards and complications of anaesthesia. Edinburgh: Churchill Livingstone; 1987:33–51

Garibaldi RA, Britt MR, Coleman ML, Reading JC, Page NL. Risk factors of postoperative pneumonia. American Journal of Medicine 1981; 70:677–680

Lawrence VA, Page CP, Harris GD. Preoperative spirometry before operations. A critical appraisal of its predictive value. Archives of Internal Medicine 1989; 149:280–283

Nunn JF. Applied respiratory physiology. 3rd edn. Oxford: Butterworths

Nunn JF, Milledge JS, Chen D, Dore C. Respiratory criteria of fitness for surgery and anaesthesia. Anaesthesia 1988; 43:543–551

27

Scoring systems relevant to anaesthesia

B. J. Pollard

Scoring systems measure case-mix, severity of illness, workload or cost. Their accuracy is assessed by the ability to predict a given outcome, such as death, disability or expenditure. Scoring systems are increasingly being used to correct for variations in case-mix in order to examine differences in outcome that may be attributable to different treatments or quality of care. Anaesthesia may need objective measures of case-mix relevant to anaesthetic practice, in order to explain variations in throughput and outcome that might be attributable to anaesthetic practice.

CLASSIFICATION

Scoring systems use physiological, clinical or anatomical variables, in varying combinations. Physiological methods are powerful and have been widely validated, but are sensitive to timing of data collection and to the effects of treatment. Methods using clinical variables (presence or absence of cancer, organ–system failures, symptoms) are often simple to apply and may be treatment independent, but require rigid definitions and may be unduly dependent on population characteristics. Anatomical methods are used mainly for trauma, but data can be acquired only once the full extent of injuries is known; these methods therefore tend to be applied retrospectively.

RISK PREDICTION IN ANAESTHESIA

Many intensive care scoring systems predict mortality with overall correct classification rates of 75–85%. The problem for anaesthesia is usually different: how to quantify the prior risk of a given procedure on a stable patient with limited physiological reserve.

There are two difficulties. First, reserve is not easy to measure because detection may require a standardised stress, and there are few equivalents to the cardiac treadmill for other organ systems. Second, the independent impact of surgical and anaesthetic skills on outcome must also be taken into account. These difficulties may explain the absence of an objectively derived, universally applicable, scoring system to determine anaesthetic risk. Important factors are given in Box 27.7.

BOX 27.7

Factors increasing anaesthetic risk

- Ischaemic heart disease
- Impaired myocardial function
- Pulmonary hypertension
- Obstructive airway disease
- Impaired renal function
- Co-morbidities
- ASA status IV–V
- Emergency surgery
- Complex surgery
- Male sex
- Increasing age
- Diabetes

TABLE 27.7

ASA classification of physical status

Grade	Findings
I	Healthy patient
II	Mild systemic disease, no functional limitations
III	Severe systemic disease with functional limitation
IV	Severe systemic disease that constantly threatens survival
V	Moribund, not expected to survive 24 h without surgery
E	Additional code for emergency surgery

27

SCORING SYSTEMS

ASA

The American Society of Anesthesiologists (ASA) classification (Table 27.7) originally consisted of six categories (subsequently reduced to five) which described physical status in order to facilitate charging for services, a concept now being reintroduced in the UK. Although its simplicity may explain its continuing use, there is considerable variability between different anaesthetists in assessments made using the ASA system. It does not correlate linearly with mortality, but it was not intended as a prognostic system, more as a method of finding a common language to describe complexity and potential therapeutic effort.

CARDIAC RISK INDEX (GOLDMAN)

The Cardiac Risk Index examined cardiovascular predictors retrospectively in over 1000 patients. It confirmed that ischaemic heart disease was a risk factor, but, despite the initial enthusiasm generated by what was then a novel approach, others have been unable to validate the index as a whole and it is now of historical interest rather than practical value.

POSSUM

This perioperative general surgical score uses multivariant analysis to identify 12 preoperative physiological variables and six grades of operative and diagnostic complexity to predict morbidity and mortality. POSSUM (Physiological and Operative Severity Score for the enUmeration of Mortality and morbidity) is probably too complex for routine use, but may have a role in audit or research projects. This type of approach needs development within single diagnostic categories in order to direct attention to those patients who might need postoperative HDU care.

PARSONNET SCORE

This is a good example of a well designed system for predicting risk in a single diagnostic category: adult patients undergoing cardiac surgery. It uses routine preoperative data and is easy to apply. It has two advantages; (1) 'noise' is reduced by examining a homogeneous patient group undergoing a standardised procedure, and (2) many of the variables are objective and verifiable (e.g. ejection fraction, blood pressure, intra-aortic balloon pump).

APACHE

The Acute Physiology And Chronic Health Evaluation (APACHE) method is one of the most widely used of all scoring systems for intensive care. The 34 variables and weights in the original version (APACHE I) were selected by clinical consensus, and then refined by statistical techniques to 12 physiological variables, with additional weighting for previous health related to urgency of admission, and age (APACHE II). The sum of the weighted values provides the score, which is converted to a risk of death using logistic regression for specific weighted diagnostic categories. Version III employs 17 physiological variables and has some improvement in predictive power over version II. The system uses the worst values recorded within the first 24 h of ITU admission. It is not designed to assess preoperative risk, but performs well when stratifying critically ill operative and non-operative patients with their greater range of physiological derangements.

EARLY WARNING SCORE (EWS)

This centres around the prediction of when a patient might be developing the need for HDU or ICU treatment rather than trying to rescue the situation once the patient is in trouble. Simple clinical observations are recorded and given a numerical score depending on how far they deviate from the normal range. If a predetermined threshold is exceeded, a referral is made to the critical care or medical emergency team. The system is essentially a tool to enable ward nursing staff to target appropriate help and treatment to sick patients by using a combination of their routine observations. The critical care or emergency medical team reviews the patient urgently The aim is to institute more invasive or specifically targeted treatment in order to reduce the subsequent need for ICU admission and improve outcome.

MORTALITY PROBABILITY MODEL (MPM)

The MPM employs binary variables, including emergency or previous ITU admission, age, coma, previous cardiorespiratory arrest, chronic renal failure, cancer, infection, systolic blood pressure, heart rate and surgery. It provides risk estimates at the time of ITU admission and, being treatment independent, can be used for prior stratification. It might therefore be of use for intensive care triage.

ORGAN–SYSTEM FAILURES SCORE

The advantage of simplicity is offset by the lack of formally agreed definitions, these being dependent on understanding the pathophysiology involved. The greater the number of organ–system failures and the longer their duration, the worse the outcome.

GLASGOW COMA SCALE (GCS)

This scale was developed to standardise terminology and facilitate communication in neurosurgical intensive care. It uses simple neurological responses to stratify patients who have been in a coma for 6 h or more from the time of head injury. Interobserver variation is low, and the system has been validated internationally for many thousands of patients. The scale has become converted to a score (3, worst; 15, best), thereby treating ordinal data as continuous data. This is not strictly valid; nevertheless, the system works. Care should be taken when the GCS is applied to patients with non-traumatic coma, as it was not designed for that purpose. As part of the APACHE system, it appears best to categorise the score, with values of 7 or less giving the worst outcome.

Alternatives to the GCS are required for small children and infants, and two based on the adult version have been described.

THERAPEUTIC INTERVENTION SCORING SYSTEM (TISS)

This system categorises therapeutic intensity or workload. A score of 1–4 points are awarded to each of 70 nursing and medical procedures. At the end of the patient's stay, all the daily TISS points are summed for the total score. TISS is used as a surrogate for measuring costs, and performs well for this purpose. Yearly recalibration is needed. Nurses can collect the data, but training is required to ensure consistency. In the UK one TISS point is worth approximately £30.

INJURY SEVERITY SCORE (ISS), TRAUMA SCORE (TS) AND TRISS

The ISS converts the gradings of the Abbreviated Injury Scale into a score by summing the squared values for each of six anatomical areas; this converts a quadratic relationship into one that is near-linear. It is calculated at death or discharge, in order to ensure accurate information. The revised form of the TS is a simple physiological system that sums coded values for three intervals of the GCS, and five intervals of systolic blood pressure and respiratory rate. Both systems perform well when used for outcome prediction of groups of patients. Combination of the two scores gives an anatomical and physiological index of severity of injury, the TRISS system, which is being used as the comparative index in the multiple trauma outcome study in the USA and the UK to examine the effect on mortality of differences in case-mix and quality of care.

27

BIBLIOGRAPHY

Baker SP, O'Neil B, Haddon W, Long W. The injury severity score: a method for describing patients with multiple injuries and evaluating emergency care. Journal of Trauma 1974; 14:187–196

Boyd CR, Tolson MA, Copes WS. Evaluating trauma care: the TRISS method. Journal of Trauma 1987; 27:370–378

Champion HR, Sacco WJ, Carnazzo AJ, Copes W, Fouty WJ. Trauma score. Critical Care Medicine 1981; 9:672–676

Dripps RD, Lamont A, Eckenhoff JE. The role of anaesthesia in surgical mortality. Journal of the American Medical Association 1961; 178:261

Farrow SC, Fowkes FGR, Lunn JN, Robertson IB, Sweetnam P. Epidemiology in anaesthesia: a method for predicting hospital mortality. European Journal of Anaesthesiology 1984; 1:77–84

Goldman L, Caldera DL, Nussbaum SR et al. Multifactorial index on cardiac risk in noncardiac surgical procedures. New England Journal of Medicine 1977; 297:845–850

Jennett B, Teasdale G, Braakman R, Minderhoud J, Knill-Jones R. Predicting outcome in individual patients after severe head injury. Lancet 1976; i:1031–1034

Knaus WA, Draper EA, Wagner DP et al. Prognosis in acute organ-system failure. Annals of Surgery 1985; 202:685–693

Knaus WA, Draper EA, Wagner DP, Zimmerman JE. APACHE II: a severity of disease classification system. Critical Care Medicine 1985; 10:818–829

Lemeshow S, Teres D, Klar J et al. Mortality probability models (MPM II) based on an international cohort of intensive care unit patients. Journal of the American Medical Association 1993; 270:2478–2486

Owens WD, Felts JA, Spitznagel EL Jr. ASA physical status classifications: a study of consistency of ratings. Anesthesiology 1978; 49:239–243

Parsonnet V, Dean D, Bernstein AD. A method of uniform stratification of risk for evaluating the results of surgery in acquired adult heart disease. Circulation 1989; 79:3–12

Pine RW, Wertz, Lennard ES et al. Determinants of organ malfunction or death in patients with intra-abdominal sepsis. Archives of Surgery 1983; 118:242–249

Subbe CP, Fruger M, Rutherford P, Gemmel L. Validation of a modified Early Warning Score in medical admissions. Quarterly Journal of Medicine 2001; 94:521–526

Teasdale G, Jennett B. Assessment of coma and impaired consciousness. A practical scale. Lancet 1974; ii:81–84

27

CROSS-REFERENCES

Preoperative assessment of cardiovascular risk
    Anaesthetic Factors 27: 634
Preoperative assessment of pulmonary risk
    Anaesthetic Factors 27: 638
Head Injury
    Patient Conditions 1: 15

28

AIRWAY
I. Calder

Hypoxaemia under anaesthesia

I. Calder

HYPOXAEMIA AND CIRCULATORY ARREST

Acute hypoxaemia will eventually cause circulatory arrest due to myocardial hypoxia. At some time around the point of arrest, irreversible cerebral damage occurs. The period of anoxia necessary to produce circulatory arrest will depend on cardiac health, the oxygen content of the body prior to the anoxic episode and the oxygen consumption. Anecdotal accounts suggest that complete airway obstruction for about 10 min will cause circulatory arrest in healthy adults.

BRADYCARDIA AND HYPOXAEMIC CARDIAC ARREST

Hypoxaemic cardiac arrest is invariably preceded by bradycardia. Hypoxaemia must be excluded before treating bradycardia with atropine.

CEREBRAL DAMAGE AND HYPOXAEMIA

For ethical reasons this topic is not well researched. The evidence is largely anecdotal.

ACUTE HYPOXAEMIA

This causes cerebral dysfunction (confusion), particularly in the elderly, but structural damage seems to be unusual, unless hypoxaemic circulatory arrest occurs. In one report, a volunteer was confused but still conscious, despite an oximeter reading of 37%.

CEREBRAL DAMAGE AND HYPOXAEMIC CIRCULATORY ARREST

Severe cerebral damage is invariable, but it is sometimes possible to restore circulatory function. Many survivors die later from the complications of coma.

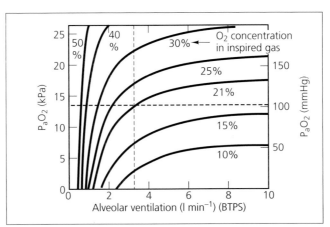

Fig. 28.1 Effect of ventilation on alveolar gas tensions (Pa_{O_2}, Fi_{O_2} and alveolar ventilation). BTPS, body temperature and pressure saturated. (From Benumof 1990, with permission.)

Note that at high levels of Fi_{O_2}, the critical level of ventilation is reduced, but when reached the Pa_{O_2} may fall suddenly. Pa_{O_2} depends on Fi_{O_2} and Pa_{CO_2}. The relationship is described by the 'alveolar air equation', which in its simplest form (applicable only to a patient breathing 100% oxygen) is:

$Palv_{O_2} = Pi_{O_2} - Pa_{CO_2}$

Corrections have to be introduced if there are other components to the inspired gas.

PROLONGED HYPOXAEMIA

This has been shown to cause structural cerebral damage (diminished finger-tapping ability) in mountain climbers. The subjects had a saturation of about 60% for many hours.

CAUSES OF HYPOXAEMIA UNDER ANAESTHESIA

- Equipment failure
- Hypoventilation
- 'Shunt'.

EQUIPMENT FAILURE

A rapid check of the equipment is always the first step, in particular the $F\text{iO}_2$ and the patency and correct connection of the anaesthetic circuit, and any artificial airway.

HYPOVENTILATION

Hypoventilation results from central or peripheral depression of ventilation and/or an obstructed airway.

The effect of hypoventilation on oxygen saturation is complex. Oxygen absorption depends more on the $F\text{iO}_2$ than on alveolar ventilation. At a given inspired oxygen concentration, reducing alveolar ventilation makes little difference to oxygenation, until a 'critical' level is reached (Fig. 28.1).

Apnoeic oxygenation

Provided the airway is at least partially open, passive entrainment of high oxygen concentrations can prevent desaturation during lengthy periods of apnoea, as the $Pa\text{CO}_2$ rises by only about 0.5 kPa min^{-1} (see 'alveolar air equation' in the legend to Fig. 28.1). Insufflation of oxygen into the mouths of apnoeic anaes-

thetised patients has been shown to prevent desaturation for 10 min (the study was terminated after 10 min for ethical reasons). Apnoeic oxygenation in one (brain-stem dead) patient prevented circulatory arrest for 3 h 20 min.

Practical points:
- Hypoxaemia due to hypoventilation will respond rapidly to an increase in $F\text{iO}_2$.
- $S\text{pO}_2$ readings are not a reliable guide to the adequacy of ventilation when the $F\text{iO}_2$ is high – *oximeters measure saturation not ventilation*.

'SHUNT'

The term 'shunt' is used here to mean failure of oxygenation of blood during passage through the pulmonary circulation ('venous admixture'). In most cases this is due to a ventilation–perfusion mismatch.

Some causes of 'shunt':
- General anaesthesia
- Intermittent positive-pressure ventilation (IPPV)
- Bronchial intubation
- Aspiration
- Embolus
- Oesophageal intubation
- Pulmonary oedema
- Malignant hyperthermia.

Reduced cardiac output and shunt

A reduced cardiac output may result in a low mixed venous oxygen content, because more oxygen is extracted in the tissues. In many circumstances increased venous admixture causes a decrease in shunt fraction, so that $Pa\text{O}_2$ is not decreased. However, anaesthesia may interfere with this useful adaptation, and desaturation

28

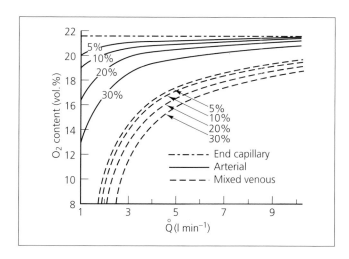

Fig. 28.2 Oxygen content, cardiac output and 'shunt'. At higher levels of shunt, a drop in cardiac output may be associated with a substantial fall in saturation. (From Kelman et al 1967, with permission.)

results. Reductions in cardiac output may result in areas of ventilated lung being under-perfused, and increases in output may improve the ventilation–perfusion profile. In any case, a fall in cardiac output will decrease the oxygen flux to the tissues (Oxygen flux = Oxygen content × Cardiac output) (Fig. 28.2). It is therefore necessary to ensure that cardiac ouput is adequate, particularly when the patient has pulmonary pathology.

Practical points:
• Hypoxaemia due to shunt may not respond to small increases in FiO_2.
• Hypoxaemia due to shunt will often respond to intravenous fluids, inotropes or positive end-expiratory pressure (PEEP).

PREOXYGENATION

Desaturation (SaO_2 less than 90%) is common during induction of (and emergence from) anaesthesia. This can be prevented by allowing the patient to breathe high concentrations of oxygen before induction and emergence. Farmery & Roe (1996) have developed a computer model, which predicts the effect on SaO_2 of increasing durations of apnoea occurring after breathing varying fractions of inspired oxygen. Their model predicts that the SaO_2 will decline to 60% after 9.9 min if the subject was breathing 100% oxygen before the apnoea, and in 2.8 min after breathing air.

Opinion is divided as to which patients should receive preoxygenation. A case can be made for preoxygenating all patients, because accurate identification of difficult mask ventilation remains elusive. About 3–5 min of ventilation is required to wash out the nitrogen in the lungs, blood and tissues. A non-rebreathing circuit must be used for this purpose, such as a Mapleson A circuit with a fresh gas flow of 8 l min^{-1}, and the efficacy of the system will be substantially reduced if there is any leak around the face-mask. The most efficient method of preoxygenation appears to be to allow the patient to take eight deep breaths of oxygen in 1 min. Less complete, but clinically

valuable, preoxygenation can be accomplished by applying a standard recovery pattern oxygen mask to all patients on arrival in the anaesthetic room.

PERIOPERATIVE HYPOXAEMIA

Desaturation (SpO_2 below 90%) is common for a week after surgery, particularly at night. Obesity is a risk factor for postoperative hypoxaemia. About 4% of the adult male population of the UK have a significant degree of obstructive sleep apnoea. The significance of minor hypoxaemia is unknown and treatment is difficult, because patient compliance with oxygen delivery systems is poor. Postoperative opiate analgesia causes episodes of upper airway obstruction and hypoxaemia. It has been shown that giving supplementary oxygen in the postoperative period often prevents hypoxaemia, despite the fact that airway obstruction still occurs. Additional oxygen has also been shown to be an effective treatment for postoperative nausea and vomiting.

MONITORING OXYGEN SATURATION

• Cyanosis is a difficult sign, especially in individuals with increased skin pigmentation. The surgical wound is the best site to observe.
• Pulse oximetry is regarded by most as a massive contribution to patient safety, despite the fact that it is not proven that patient outcome (in terms of death and cerebral damage) is improved.
• The accuracy of pulse oximeters is reduced by black and purple nail varnish and poor peripheral perfusion. For ethical reasons, instrument calibration at low saturations is impossible.
• It must be understood that a value of saturation gives little information about ventilation. A hypopnoeic patient exposed to a high FiO_2 may have a satisfactory saturation for a prolonged period.

28

BIBLIOGRAPHY

Baraka AS, Taha SK, Aouad MT, El-Khatib MF, Kawkabani N. Pre-oxygenation: comparison of maximal breathing and tidal volume breathing techniques. Anesthesiology 1999; 91:612–616

Benumof JL. Respiratory physiology and respiratory function during anaesthesia. In: Millar RD, ed. Anesthesia. 3rd edn. New York: Churchill Livingstone; 1990:504–549

Benumof JL. Preoxygenation. Best method for both efficacy and efficiency. Anesthesiology 1999; 91:603–605

Benumof JL. Obstructive sleep apnea in the adult obese patient: implications for airway management. Journal of Clinical Anesthesia 2001; 13:144–156

Farmery AD, Roe PG. A model to describe the rate of oxyhaemoglobin desaturation during apnoea. British Journal of Anaesthesia 1996; 76:284–291

John RE, Peacock JE. Limitations of pulse oximetry. Lancet 1993; 341:1092–1093

Kelman GR, Nunn JF, Prys Roberts C, Greenbaum R. The influence of cardiac output on arterial oxygenation: a theoretical study. British Journal of Anaesthesia 1967; 39:450–458

Moller JT, Johannessen NW, Espersen K et al. Randomized evaluation of pulse oximetry in 20 802 patients. Anesthesiology 1993; 78:436–445

Powell JF, Menon DK, Jones JG. The effects of hypoxaemia and recommendations for postoperative oxygen therapy. Anaesthesia 1996; 51:769–772

28

Death or brain damage due to upper airway problems

I. Calder

The true incidence of death or brain damage due to airway problems is not known. Statistics are hard to assemble; death due to airway problems may occur years after the event. Many incidents are followed by legal proceedings, usually civil but sometimes criminal. Most of our knowledge stems from the closed insurance claims analysis performed by the American Society of Anesthesiologists. The incidence appears to be decreasing; in two recent publications, airway deaths were matched by deaths due to complications of central venous cannulation. The majority of cases are due to repeated failed attempts to intubate, which result in difficult mask ventilation, oesophageal intubation and mucosal perforation with subsequent infection. A small number of deaths result from aspiration or airway obstruction due to laryngospasm, cervical haematomas or infections.

Causes:

- Equipment
- Failed intubation or ventilation
- Mucosal perforation
- Oesophageal intubation
- Upper airway obstruction
- Aspiration

EQUIPMENT

FAULTY EQUIPMENT
Leaks and misconnections in the anaesthetic equipment must be detected by rigorous pre-anaesthetic checks.

UNAVAILABLE EQUIPMENT
Never – except in bizarre, exceptional circumstances – induce general anaesthesia without access to:

- A source of oxygen
- A means of inflating the lungs
- Suction apparatus
- Muscle relaxant drugs
- Laryngoscope and tracheal tubes.

EXTREMELY DESIRABLE EQUIPMENT:
- Laryngeal mask airway
- Gum elastic bougie
- Oesophageal detector device
- Capnometer
- Oximeter
- Disconnection alarm.

FAILED INTUBATION OR VENTILATION

Repeated attempts at intubation can result in mask ventilation becoming impossible, so that repeated attempts to intubate should not be undertaken. The precise mechanism of the airway obstruction that occurs is not certain. It is likely to be a combination of tissue swelling due to trauma, inadequate depth of anaesthesia and paralysis, and operator fatigue.

MUCOSAL PERFORATION

Vigorous attempts to intubate can result in mucosal perforation, especially if stylets are used. Mediastinitis or deep cervical abscess may follow. If there is any possibility that a perforation has occurred, the anaesthetist must communicate this to the patient's postoperative staff. Symptoms and signs are more difficult to evaluate if a warning is withheld. Features include neck and chest pain, dysphagia, dyspnoea and fever. Early treatment with antibiotics, drainage and repair is vital; the mortality rate is high.

OESOPHAGEAL INTUBATION

Deaths from oesophageal intubation continue to occur. Experienced anaesthetists have nearly always experienced 'near misses'. Distraction of the anaesthetist by extraneous problems, and failure to consider the diagnosis after apparently easy laryngoscopy, account for some of the tragedies. Oesophageal intubation can be identified by:

- Auscultation of chest and abdomen
- Oesophageal detector device
- Expired air carbon dioxide monitoring.

It is vital to appreciate that no one method is completely reliable, and this includes capnometry. The term 'gold standard' has been applied to capnometry, implying that the method is completely reliable. This is far from the case. Remember that the presence of carbon dioxide in the expired air does not mean that a tube is definitely in the trachea (think of a trace from a laryngeal mask). Nor does the absence of carbon dioxide mean that the tube is definitely in the oesophagus (think of circulatory arrest). Circulatory arrest is a particular trap for the unwary: oesophageal intubations have not been recognised because anaesthetists ascribed the absence of carbon dioxide to the arrest.

The oesophageal detector device described by John Nunn (a self-inflating bulb such as a bladder wash-out bulb, which is attached to the tracheal tube and squeezed) provides rapid confirmation of tube position, without the need for inflation, and is cheap, portable, independent of power, light and cardiac output. The bulb of the oesophageal detector device may refill slowly in about 15% of cases, despite the tube being in the trachea. Inflation may be very slow, amounting to a false-positive finding in occasional obese and bronchospastic patients. A false-negative finding (bulb inflates, tube in oesophagus) has been reported after a patient's oesophagus had been inflated with oxygen for a considerable period.

If auscultation of the chest is used alone, about 25% of cases are missed, possibly because inflation of the stomach may cause quiet expiratory breath sounds. Auscultation becomes reliable if the upper abdomen is also auscultated.

Oesophageal intubation:

- Check every case
- Use more than one method for identification

UPPER AIRWAY OBSTRUCTION

Laryngospasm does kill. Fatalities have also resulted from pulmonary oedema following airway obstruction due to laryngospasm.

Postoperative nocturnal airway obstruction in patients with obstructive sleep apnoea is an increasing problem because of the prevalence of obesity. Opiate drugs will increase the tendency to obstruction, both while they are administered and for some nights after cessation of treatment, because of a rebound increase in rapid eye movement (REM) sleep. Patients known to suffer from obstructive sleep apnoea should be nursed in a HDU environment, and suspect cases and obese patients should receive nocturnal oxygen.

ASPIRATION

The incidence of aspiration pneumonitis is low (0.05% overall, 0.1% in emergencies); about 5% of patients die and 17% require mechanical ventilation. Aspiration causes desaturation. Patients without symptoms who have a normal saturation on air 2 h after apparent aspiration are unlikely to develop pulmonary sequelae.

Current guidelines for preanaesthetic eating and drinking suggest that solids and milk should be allowed until 6 h before anaesthesia, and water or juice until 2 h beforehand.

LONG-TERM BRAIN DAMAGE

The possibility that prion diseases might be transmitted by contamination of anaesthetic devices with tonsillar tissue has been raised. The risks are unknown, but are probably smaller than the risks of airway death or brain damage due to the substitution of 'disposable' equipment. Nevertheless, protein deposits can be found on reusable laryngeal masks, laryngoscopes and bougies.

28

BIBLIOGRAPHY

Andersen KH, Hald A. Assessing the position of the tracheal tube: the reliability of different methods. Anaesthesia 1989; 44:984–989

Caplan RA, Posner KL, Ward RJ, Cheney FW. Adverse respiratory events in anaesthesia: a closed claims analysis. Anesthesiology 1990; 72:828–833

Domino KB , Posner KL, Caplan RA et al. Airway injury during anesthesia: a closed claims analysis. Anesthesiology 1999; 91:1703–1711

Miler DM, Youkhana I, Karunaratne WU, Pearce A. Presence of protein deposits on 'cleaned' re-usable anaesthetic equipment. Anaesthesia 2001; 56:1069–1072

Newland MC, Ellis SJ, Lydiatt CA et al. Anesthetic-related cardiac arrest and its mortality: a report covering 72 959 anesthetics over 10 years from a US teaching hospital. Anesthesiology 2002; 97:108–115

Olsson GL, Hallen B, Hambraeus-Jonzon K. Aspiration during anaesthesia: a computer-aided study of 185 358 anaesthetics. Acta Anaesthesiologica Scandinavica 1986; 30:84–92

Sanehi O, Calder I. Capnography and the differentiation between tracheal and oesophageal intubation. Anaesthesia 1999; 54:604–605

Strunin L. How long should patients fast before surgery? Time for new guidelines. British Journal of Anaesthesia 1993; 70:1–4

Warner MA, Warner ME, Weber JG. Clinical significance of pulmonary aspiration during the perioperative period. Anesthesiology 1993; 78:56–62

Williamson JA, Webb RK, Szelely S, Gillies ER, Dreosti AV. The Australian incident monitoring study. Difficult intubation: an analysis of 2000 incident reports. Anaesthesia and Intensive Care 1993; 21:602–607

28

Effect of general anaesthesia on the airway and upper alimentary canal

I. Calder and R. Vanner

A 'submarine' analogy can be made regarding safety during anaesthesia – depth is safety. Most of the troublesome phenomena we experience, such as coughing, biting, breath-holding, laryngospasm and regurgitation, occur during light planes of anaesthesia.

EFFECT ON OROPHARYNGEAL AND GLOTTIC STRUCTURES

Induction of anaesthesia usually causes obstruction of the upper airway. Alterations in the tone of the skeletal muscles of the pharynx and neck are thought to be responsible. It has been shown that the soft palate, tongue and glottic opening may all impinge on the posterior pharyngeal wall when anaesthesia is induced. The glottic opening is similar to the tip of a Tuohy needle. This can be appreciated by examining a lateral cervical radiograph. It is easy to see how the glottis can obstruct against the posterior pharyngeal wall.

The standard manoeuvres employed to clear an obstructed airway are known as 'head tilt' and 'jaw thrust'. Head tilt stretches the anterior neck tissues, which lifts the glottic opening from the posterior pharyngeal wall. Jaw thrust has the same effect. Jaw thrust was described in 1874, whereas head tilt seems to have first been recommended in 1960.

It is sometimes easier to maintain a clear airway in the supine position, as opposed to the lateral 'coma' position often recommended for unconscious patients. It seems that a surface under the occiput allows more effective head extension. Continuous positive airway pressure (CPAP) is often effective in relieving airway obstruction, particularly in children.

RECOGNITION OF AN OBSTRUCTED AIRWAY

A *conscious patient* will complain bitterly of difficulty in breathing. The patient may be dys-phonic, aphonic, anxious, unwilling to be supine and, ultimately, exhausted. Patients' complaints have sometimes been ignored on the grounds that an oximeter showed near-normal readings.

A *spontaneously breathing patient* will generate large negative intrathoracic pressures (but not if there is also respiratory depression), which will cause:

- Noisy inspiration, due to turbulent gas flow – a completely obstructed airway is silent
- Tracheal tug, intercostal recession
- Paradoxical respiratory movements.

A *ventilated patient* will have high inflation pressures.

In both spontaneous and artificial ventilation:

- Carbon dioxide excretion will be impaired – capnometer traces will be flattened or absent; arterial blood gases may show a respiratory acidosis.
- Desaturation may be late and sudden, if the FiO_2 is high.
- Oximetry is not a good monitor of airway patency.

Signs of obstruction:

- Noise
- Tracheal tug
- Paradoxical movements
- Inflation pressure high
- Abnormal carbon dioxide trace

PULMONARY OEDEMA FOLLOWING RELIEF OF AIRWAY OBSTRUCTION

The large transpulmonary pressure gradients during obstruction may cause alveolar fluid collection. This presents as pulmonary oedema when the obstruction is relieved. Positive-pressure ventilation may be required. An adult respiratory distress syndrome (ARDS)-like picture may result.

28

GLOTTIC REFLEXES

The minimum alveolar concentration (MAC) for glottic stimulation is 30% higher than that for surgical incision. Tachycardia and hypertension follow laryngoscopy and intubation, unless adequate anaesthesia is given.

'LARYNGOSPASM'

Glottic closure reflexes are hyperexcitable during light anaesthesia. Laryngospasm may complicate induction of anaesthesia, surgical stimulation, extubation and recovery. It is probably the most frequent serious airway complication. The incidence is reduced if propofol is used for the induction of anaesthesia.

Desaturation can often be avoided by giving 100% oxygen. Deepening the level of anaesthesia with intravenous propofol (0.25 mg kg^{-1}) is usually effective. Muscle relaxants may be required to relieve laryngospasm, and suxamethonium remains popular for this indication because of its rapid onset. The intense stimulation caused by bilateral digital pressure in 'the laryngospasm notch' (the posterior temporomandibular joint) has been claimed to be an effective treatment for laryngospasm and breath-holding (Larson's manouevre).

OESOPHAGEAL SPHINCTER FUNCTION AND ANAESTHESIA

THE LOWER OESOPHAGEAL SPHINCTER

The intraluminal pressure at the gastro-oesophageal junction is 15–25 mmHg above gastric pressure, which normally prevents gastro-oesophageal reflux. The pressure is produced by smooth muscle cells of the lower oesophageal sphincter. Contraction of the surrounding skeletal muscle of the diaphragmatic crura increases the intraluminal pressure during inspiration, and also during straining. Straining does not cause gastro-oesophageal reflux in normal conscious patients. Reflux may occur spontaneously after a meal.

Reflux does not occur spontaneously during anaesthesia, but diaphragmatic tone decreases and thus its protective effect may be lost. Reflux is associated with hiccup, straining, deep inspiration with surgical stimulus, and bucking on the tracheal tube – all features of light anaesthesia.

A sudden, brief rise in lower oesophageal sphincter pressure is seen at the same time as the onset of fasciculation after suxamethonium, probably as a result of diaphragmatic contraction.

Intravenous atropine and other cholinergics may produce a decrease in lower oesophageal sphincter pressure sufficient to permit free reflux. Sphincter pressure is unaffected when atropine is combined with neostigmine.

Very small, and probably clinically insignificant, decreases in sphincter pressure are caused by intravenous and inhalational anaesthetic agents, the laryngeal mask airway and the lithotomy position.

The steep Trendelenburg position used during pelvic laparoscopy does not cause gastro-oesophageal reflux.

THE OESOPHAGUS

The oesophagus is a muscular tube about 25 cm in length, which begins at the caudal border of the cricoid cartilage and ends at the cardiac orifice of the stomach, usually about 1.5 cm below the diaphragm. The upper quarter is composed of skeletal muscle only, the lower third comprises smooth muscle only, and the middle is a mixture of the two types. The oesophagus can contain a large volume of fluid (up to 200 ml).

Refluxed gastric contents are cleared by oesophageal peristalsis, which is initiated by swallowing or local reflex.

Both general anaesthesia and intravenous atropine inhibit oesophageal motility. Oesophageal clearance may not occur despite gastro-oesophageal reflux during general anaesthesia. The refluxed contents will remain in the oesophagus, increasing the risk of regurgitation into the pharynx, until swallowing recommences as the patient awakes.

THE UPPER OESOPHAGEAL SPHINCTER

The upper sphincter is formed by the lamina of the cricoid cartilage anteriorly and the striated muscle cricopharyngeus posteriorly. Resting upper oesophageal sphincter pressure is about 40 mmHg. Relaxation of the upper oesophageal sphincter at induction of anaesthesia can precipitate regurgitation.

Both intravenous thiopental and suxamethonium decrease upper oesophageal sphincter pressure to less than 10 mmHg, a pressure low enough to allow regurgitation of oesophageal contents. The low upper oesophageal sphincter pressure caused by suxamethonium is not further reduced by laryngoscopy. With thiopental, the fall in sphincter pressure starts before loss of consciousness.

Intravenous induction with ketamine or inhalational induction with halothane main-

28

tains upper oesophageal sphincter pressure, in the absence of neuromuscular blockade. Upper oesophageal sphincter pressure may rise to over 100 mmHg during coughing and straining under light anaesthesia, and prevent regurgitation.

Intravenous benzodiazepines, such as midazolam, reduce upper sphincter pressure. They also depress laryngeal reflexes. Heavy sedation may allow aspiration.

There have been case reports of regurgitation during anaesthesia when a laryngeal mask has been in use. This is probably no more frequent than when an oral Guedel airway and face-mask are used.

BIBLIOGRAPHY

Chung DC, Rowbotham SJ. A very small dose of suxamethonium relieves laryngospasm. Anaesthesia 1993; 48:229–230

Drummond GB. Keep a clear airway (editorial). British Journal of Anaesthesia 1991; 66:153–156

Herrick IA, Mahendran B, Penny FJ. Postobstructive pulmonary edema following anesthesia. Journal of Clinical Anesthesia 1990; 2:116–120

Larsen CP. Laryngospasm – the best treatment. Anesthesiology 1998; 89:1293–1294

Nandi PR, Charlesworth CH, Taylor SJ, Nunn JF, Dore CJ. Effect of general anaesthesia on the pharynx. British Journal of Anaesthesia 1991; 66:157–162

Nawfal M, Baraka A. Propofol for relief of extubation laryngospasm. Anaesthesia 2002; 57:1036

Vanner RG. Oesophageal sphincter function. In: Prys-Roberts C, Brown BR, eds. International practice of anaesthesia. Oxford: Butterworth-Heinemann; 1996

28

Artificial airways

I. Calder

Artificial airways:

- Face-mask
- Oral and nasal airways
- Laryngeal mask
- Combitube
- Tracheal tube
- Cricothyroid cannula
- Tracheostomy

FACE-MASK

Designed to fit the face; many practitioners believe that edentulous patients should be encouraged to wear their dentures during anaesthesia, as a good fit is difficult if they are removed.

ORAL OR NASAL AIRWAY

The timing of airway insertion calls for judgement. An airway will often relieve an obstruction, but if the patient is too 'light', it may provoke coughing, breath-holding and laryngospasm.

A nasal airway should be used in patients with fragile teeth, crowns or bridges. Nasal airways should be avoided in patients with bleeding disorders.

LARYNGEAL MASK

For easy insertion of a laryngeal mask (LM) the patient must be deeply anaesthetised or paralysed. Propofol provides the best conditions for insertion. There is a small insertion failure rate. Positive-pressure ventilation can be performed. A bite block should be used and the device should be left in until the patient is awake. The LM is a very useful aid to fibreoptically guided intubation.

Further developments of the LM continue to appear, notably the intubating laryngeal mask, which allows blind placement of a tracheal tube, and the Pro-Seal, which provides a more effec-

tive laryngeal seal. LM 'lookalikes' have also emerged, although none seems to be superior.

COMBITUBE

This device has two lumens and two inflatable cuffs. It is easier to insert if a laryngoscope is used, and appears to be more traumatic than the LM. However, it allows higher inflation pressures and may be a more effective device in patients with restricted mouth opening and profuse intraoral bleeding.

TRACHEAL TUBE

INTUBATION

The glottic closure reflexes must be obtunded before a tracheal tube can be placed. This can be achieved with topical anaesthesia, deep general anaesthesia or muscle relaxant drugs.

The tracheal tube can be placed under direct vision, over a flexible fibreoptic endoscope or retrogradely over a guide passed from the trachea, either blind or by observation of transillumination from a lighted tip (Lightwand, Trachlite). Techniques that allow visualisation of the glottis are generally preferred in the belief that trauma to the glottis and pharynx is less likely to occur. The success rate that can be achieved by an experienced operator with the intubating laryngeal mask (ILMA) approaches that obtained with a Macintosh laryngoscope. However, the ILMA was less successful than the Trachlite in a study where the patients' heads were restrained in a neutral position.

Direct laryngoscopy

A 'line of vision' must be established from eye to glottis. This requires:

- Artificial *protrusion* of the mandible, tongue and hyoid bone with the blade of the laryngoscope. The pattern of blade designed by Robert Macintosh is almost universally employed in the UK. However,

28

there is renewed interest in straight laryngoscope blades, such as the pattern introduced by Henderson, because a line of vision can be established in cases resistant to the Macintosh.

- *Extension* at the craniocervical junction, combined with a slightly flexed cervical spine – the 'sniffing the morning air' position, described by Magill.

SIZE OF TUBE
It has been suggested that the cross-sectional area of the narrowest point of the glottic opening (true cords) corresponds to that of an 8.0-mm tracheal tube in men and a 7.0-mm tube in women. Smaller sizes can be used, as resistance to gas flow is clinically significant only below 6.0 mm. There is little to be gained and a price to be paid (insertion is more difficult and the incidence of sore throat is higher) when larger sizes are used.

TISSUE DAMAGE AND OROTRACHEAL INTUBATION
Sore throat and hoarseness are common, but should settle within 48 h. Persisting or severe symptoms require investigation. Haematoma of the cords is the commonest glottic complication. Cord palsy after intubation has been variously ascribed to recurrent laryngeal nerve damage and arytenoid dislocation. Paulsen and colleagues attempted to produce arytenoid dislocation in cadavers but were unsuccessful, although the joint could be damaged fairly reliably. They suggested that trauma to the joint produced a haemarthrosis, which resulted in fixation, and proposed the term 'post-intubation arytenoid dysfunction'.

Dental damage due to laryngoscopy usually affects the left upper first or second incisor. Displaced teeth should be replaced immediately or stored in milk. They should not be placed in water.

Perforation of the pharyngeal mucosa by stylets, bougies or tubes can cause mediastinitis or retropharyngeal abscess. Perforation has been recorded after blind oral suction, nasogastric tube insertion and Doppler probe insertion. The risk of mucosal perforation is the principal objection to blind techniques such as the ILMA.

ORAL OR NASAL TUBE?
Nasal tube – against:
- Mucosal damage is common, both in the nasal cavity and to the posterior pharyngeal wall. Death from pharyngeal abscess has been reported. Damage to, or even avulsion

of, the turbinates occurs. Much damage can be avoided by using a suction catheter or fibreoptic endoscope as an introducer.
- Severe bleeding may occur – bleeding disorders and infected blood represent contraindications. Mucosal engorgement in pregnant women at term is a relative contraindication.
- Closed base-of-skull fractures can be converted to open fractures by nasal intubation.
- Bacteraemia is common after nasal intubation (but not after insertion of nasal airways). Half of nasally intubated patients develop bacterial sinusitis if intubated for more than 4 days; nasogastric tubes are also associated with an increased incidence of sinusitis.

Nasal tubes – for:
- The nasal route is often necessary when direct laryngoscopy is difficult. The gag reflex is produced by contact with the tongue and the reflex is difficult to abolish with glossopharyngeal nerve blocks. Gagging can make awake fibreoptic intubation difficult so that the nasal route is usually easier.
- Intraoral surgery.
- A nasal tube is easier to fix and the patient cannot bite it. There are fewer episodes of accidental extubation and main bronchus intubation with a nasal tube. It is often claimed that a nasal tube is more comfortable for the patient.

Conclusion
Nasal tubes can cause serious morbidity and occasional mortality. The popularity of long-term nasal intubation has decreased, but it may be justified in situations in which accidental extubation might have serious consequences.

EXTUBATION
Desaturation is probably commoner at extubation than at any other time. Preoxygenation is recommended.

Direct laryngoscopy and suction should be performed prior to extubation, if possible. Blind suction of the pharynx may be traumatic; mucosal perforation and mediastinitis have been reported.

Laryngospasm, breath-holding and severe coughing may complicate extubation, unless the patient is wide awake (patient takes own tube out) or deeply anaesthetised (no reaction to laryngoscopy and suction). Problems arise when the level of anaesthesia is somewhere

28

between the two extremes. It may be necessary to deepen anaesthesia and/or reparalyse the patient.

An 'airway exchange catheter' may be useful in cases where reintubation may have to be performed. These hollow catheters allow oxygenation and are well tolerated by patients.

Deep anaesthesia extubation
The airway is inevitably unprotected and must be supported. However, recovery is usually smoother in terms of coughing and laryngospasm. Desaturation has been found to be less frequent than with extubation at light levels of anaesthesia. If the patient coughs when the cuff is deflated, the depth is usually insufficient.

Awake extubation
This is preferable if the patient has a difficult airway (see below).

CRICOTHYROID CANNULAE AND TRACHEOSTOMY

PERCUTANEOUS CRICOTHYROID MEMBRANE PUNCTURE
This can be life-saving in airway obstruction. More anaesthetists are familiar with the technique because of the popularity of percutaneous tracheostomy. It has been shown that it is very difficult to construct a system capable of delivering oxygen at a rate sufficient both to oxygenate and to ventilate a patient from scratch in an emergency. It is therefore necessary for a suitable system (which includes a Sanders injector) to be available at all times. Pulmonary barotrauma is a theoretical hazard if expiration is obstructed, but appears not to be a problem in practice, so that the insertion of a separate cannula to allow expiration is unnecessary.

Larger percutaneous cannulae, such as the Quicktrach (Dulker) with a 4.0-mm internal diameter, have the advantage that expiration should be relatively unobstructed and capnography can be used. They may also have a lower incidence of misplacement.

The condition(s) that made the intervention necessary may well make the insertion of a percutaneous device difficult.

TRACHEOSTOMY
Tracheostomies should be stitched in place as well as taped until a track has formed. Recannulation after accidental decannulation before a track has formed (about 10 days) is often unsuccessful.

Percutaneous dilatational (Ciaglia) tracheostomy has largely supplanted surgical tracheostomy in ITU patients. A fibreoptic laryngoscope or bronchoscope should be used to visualise needle and guidewire insertion. Emergency percutaneous tracheostomy has been reported, but surgical cricothyrotomy remains the technique generally regarded as the most likely to succeed in a dire emergency. A trial performed in cadavers between surgical and Seldinger technique cricothyrotomy showed that successful ventilation was achieved in only 70% of the surgical and 60% of the Seldinger technique cadavers (difference not statistically significant). The time to first ventilation was 102 ± 42 s and 100 ± 46 s for the surgical and Seldinger techniques. The conclusion was that both methods showed equally poor results.

BIBLIOGRAPHY

Agro F, Frass M, Benumof JL, Krafft P. Current status of the Combitube: a review of the literature. Journal of Clinical Anesthesiology 2002; 14:307–314

Bach A, Boehrer H, Schmidt H, Geiss HK. Nosocomial sinusitis in ventilated patients. Nasotracheal versus orotracheal intubation. Anaesthesia 1992; 47:335–339

Benumof JL, Scheller MS. The importance of transtracheal jet ventilation in the management of the difficult airway. Anesthesiology 1989; 72:828–833

Eisenburger P, Laczika K, List M et al. Comparison of conventional surgical versus Seldinger technique emergency cricothyrotomy performed by inexperienced clinicians. Anesthesiology 2000; 92:1845–1847

Ferson DZ, Rosenblatt WH, Johansen MJ, Osborn I, Ovassapian A. Use of the intubating LMA-Fastrach in 254 patients with difficult-to-manage airways. Anesthesiology 2001; 95:1175–1181

Hartley M, Vaughan RS. Problems associated with tracheal extubation. British Journal of Anaesthesia 1993; 71:561–568

Henderson JJ. The use of paraglossal straight blade laryngoscopy in difficult tracheal intubation. Anaesthesia 1997; 52:552–560

Inoue Y, Koga K, Shigematsu A. A comparison of two tracheal intubation techniques with Trachlight and Fastrach in patients with cervical spine disorders. Anesthesia and Analgesia 2002; 94:667–671

Koh KF, Hare JD, Calder I. Small tubes revisited. Anaesthesia 1998; 53:46–49

Paulsen FP, Rudert HH, Tillmann BN. New insights into the pathomechanism of postintubation arytenoid subluxation. Anesthesiology 1999; 91:659–666

Pennant JH, White PF. The laryngeal mask airway: its uses in anesthesiology. Anesthesiology 1993; 79:144–164

28

Difficult airway – overview

I. Calder

AIRWAY 'PLANS'

There is obvious merit in the practice of conducting a 'what if' exercise when formulating tactics to deal with the establishment of an anaesthetic airway. If 'plan A' fails, one should have 'plan B' ready. If a patient comes to harm, failure to construct such a template will attract criticism. If in doubt, ask for help. Additional assistance was found to be 'the most desired aid' in the Australian study of airway incidents. This includes surgical assistance, in case an elective or emergency tracheotomy is required.

CAUSES AND DEFINITIONS

A large number of conditions have been reported to cause difficulty with the airway during anaesthesia. From the point of view of the exam candidate, it is helpful to have an 'aetiological' framework to work with, whereas a 'practical' classification may be more useful in day to day practice. Totally satisfactory definitions are elusive because 'difficulty' is itself subjective, and a clinical situation is often a mixture of problems.

CAUSES – AETIOLOGICAL:
- Reflexes – laryngospasm, breath-holding, regurgitation
- Stiffness – arthritides, fixation devices, contractures, scleroderma
- Deformity – congenital and acquired
- Swelling – infections, tumours, trauma, anaphylaxis, acromegaly
- 'High tariff' patients – this factor encompasses patients who have features that complicate their management, either as a result of the problem itself or the effect of stress on the anaesthetist. Uncooperative patients are an example and 'precious' patients another. Difficulty with venous access or a 'full stomach' are further examples. The deleterious effect of excessive stress on performance was described in 1908 by Yerkes and Dodson.

CAUSES – PRACTICAL:
- Difficult mask anaesthesia or ventilation
- Difficult direct laryngoscopy
- Difficult intubation
- Aspiration risk.

28

Difficult airway – difficult mask anaesthesia or ventilation

I. Calder

Any patient whose lungs cannot be inflated with the aid of a mask is in immediate danger of death, unless a laryngeal mask, tracheal tube or tracheostomy cannula can be inserted promptly. In most cases the situation is alarming rather than impossible. Benumof's description of a spectrum of difficulty from easy to impossible, despite two operators (one squeezing the reservoir bag) and the insertion of oral and nasopharyngeal airways, is useful. The place of the laryngeal mask in this scheme has not yet been established. However, the author would certainly proceed to insertion of a laryngeal mask if mask ventilation proved impossible.

CAUSES

- No seal between face and mask (facial abnormalities). Reasons range from absence of teeth and beards to massive facial trauma.
- Reduced cross-sectional area of airway. Tissue swelling from infection, trauma, burns, tumour or oedema (cervical haematoma, anaphylaxis). Laryngospasm is the commonest cause.
- Standard airway-clearing manoeuvres not possible. Cervical rigidity or poor mouth opening and/or mandibular protrusion may make it impossible to counteract the effects of anaesthesia on airway patency. Patients in halo-body frames or with interdental wiring are obvious examples of this problem. Difficulty with mask ventilation has been

reported to occur in 1 : 7 difficult laryngoscopies, but complete failure is very rare (0.01–1 : 10 000).

PREDICTING DIFFICULT MASK VENTILATION

Cases with readily identifiable problems, such as facial injuries, can be predicted. However, serious difficulty is, fortunately, very rare in apparently normal people. It is therefore unlikely that a predictive method will be successful (see difficult direct laryngoscopy). Age over 55 years, a beard, a history of snoring, body mass index (BMI) > 26 and absence of teeth have been suggested as factors indicative of difficulty, but their positive predictive value is poor.

In general, a tracheal airway should be placed before induction of anaesthesia in patients in whom it might be difficult to perform positive-pressure ventilation with a mask.

BIBLIOGRAPHY

Benumof JL. The difficult airway: definition, recognition, and the ASA algorithm. In: Benumof JL, ed. Airway management – principles and practice. St Louis: Mosby; 1996:121

Langeron O, Masso E, Huraux C et al. Prediction of difficult mask ventilation. Anesthesiology 2000; 92:1229–1236

28

Difficult airway – difficult direct laryngoscopy

I. Calder

Definition:

'Difficult' direct laryngoscopy is generally regarded as Cormack and Lehane grades 3 and 4 (see Fig. 28.3). The division of grade 3 into 3a and 3b has been recommended, where 3b describes an epiglottis closely applied to the posterior pharyngeal wall.

INCIDENCE

Grade 3 glottic visibility occurs in only 1.5% of unselected patients. Grade 4 is rare; severe rheumatoid arthritis is the commonest cause.

CAUSES

Difficult laryngoscopy is caused by poor mouth opening and stiffness of the cervical spine, particularly the craniocervical junction. Swelling of the oropharyngeal tissues may also prevent vision.

Difficulty is rare in the young and healthy, whose joints are mobile.

Diseases regularly associated with difficulty include arthritis (particularly rheumatoid arthritis), oropharyngeal infections and tumours, ankylosing spondylitis, acromegaly and the Klippel–Feil abnormalities of the cervical spine. Iatrogenic causes include interdental wiring and cervical fixators.

PREDICTION

It is rare for a patient without a cause, such as the diseases already mentioned, to present severe problems. Various tests have been described (Mallampati, Patil) that appear to perform well when applied retrospectively to difficult patients. However, prospective trials have shown that the false-positive rate associated with prediction in a general population may be as high as 96%. It is also unfortunately the case

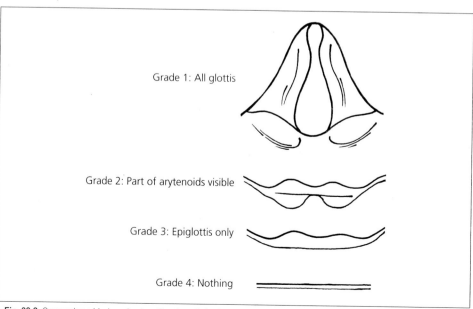

Grade 1: All glottis

Grade 2: Part of arytenoids visible

Grade 3: Epiglottis only

Grade 4: Nothing

Fig. 28.3 Cormack and Lehane's classification of glottic visibility.

that the available tests have sensitivities of about 50% (i.e. half the cases are missed).

Farmery has described one of the available tests (sternomental distance) as 'having an accuracy approaching worthlessness', and Yentis has indicated that routine testing may be a 'useless ritual'. The current position is somewhat difficult, as is the case in all programmes where symptomless populations are 'screened' for diseases such as cervical, breast or prostatic cancer. The screening may not be effective in reducing mortality and may actually increase morbidity, but practitioners may be criticised for not attempting to predict problems. Studies in the USA and Scandinavia have indicated that the majority of anaesthetists would proceed to an attempt to intubate with a Macintosh laryngoscope despite a history of difficult intubation (in the belief that they will do better). An isolated finding of an abnormal test is unlikely to change an anaesthetist's technique.

Expecting to be able to identify the rare difficult patient without predisposing cause is probably unrealistic. It is more important to be aware of the various methods of dealing with difficult laryngoscopy, and the dangers inherent in repeated attempts to intubate.

AVAILABLE TESTS

The examination described by Mallampati has a logical force; if pharyngeal visibility is good then it should only be improved with the aid of a laryngoscope. Unfortunately, poor grades (that is grade 3, which is the poorest grade used by Mallampati – there is no basis for using four grades) have been found to have poor sensitivity and positive predictive values in general surgical patients (approximately 50% and 10–25% respectively). Tests of cervical movement appear to be difficult to apply successfully, but the only series in which the Mallampati examination performed well was in a cervical spine disease population. The Mallampati appears to be as good as any test in patients with cervical spine problems, probably because craniocervical extension is required for normal mouth opening.

Mandibular protrusion can be assessed on an ABC basis: A, lower incisors in front; B, edge to edge; C, lower incisors cannot be brought forward to touch the upper incisors. Direct laryngoscopy is always difficult in patients with grade C protrusion, but this is a rare finding, largely confined to patients with rheumatoid arthritis.

THE 'ANTERIOR LARYNX'

This term is the predecessor of the Cormack and Lehane classification, and is now redundant.

MANAGEMENT OF DIFFICULT LARYNGOSCOPY

SEVERE DIFFICULTY EXPECTED

Awake fibreoptic intubation is the method of choice, and is acceptable to most patients. Fibreoptic laryngoscopy can be regarded as part of preoperative examination and should be presented to the patient in that manner. The cardiovascular stability associated with fibreoptic intubation under topical anaesthesia is an attractive feature of the technique.

Nasal intubation is frequently easier in this group of patients because of limited mouth opening and the poor 'angle of attack' with the oral route. Topical anaesthesia is more effective if glycopyrrolate is given to dry the mucosa. A vasoconstrictor should be applied to the nasal mucosa (xylometazoline or phenylephrine) before endoscopy. Lidocaine (lignocaine) is poorly absorbed from the nasopharynx; doses up to 10 mg kg^{-1} are acceptable. Lidocaine is irritant to the nasal and glottic mucosa. Initial application should be with a warm 1% solution or 2% gel; 10% lidocaine can then be applied to nasal and pharyngeal mucosa. The glottis is liberally sprayed with 4% lidocaine through the endoscope (about 6 ml). An alternative is to inject 4% lidocaine through the cricothyroid membrane. Coughing can be very vigorous, but will result in satisfactory anaesthesia. The glottis will not be anaesthetised if the patient does not cough.

It is foolish to attempt to pass a tube with an internal diameter greater than 7.0 mm over a fibreoptic endoscope. Flexible metal-reinforced tubes are recommended, and rotation of the tube as it is passed is helpful. The nasal tissues (or the shaft of the laryngeal mask) grip the tube and it is often necessary to apply several turns to the proximal end of the tube to produce one turn at the distal end. Severe laryngeal damage has been reported after awake fibreoptic intubation; the glottic reflexes must be obtunded, force not used, and multiple attempts not made. It is sensible to administer some sedation as the tube is passed, as the passage of the tube through the nose is unpleasant.

Retrograde intubation

This is an alternative when fibreoptic technology and skill is not available. An epidural catheter or J-tipped wire is passed through a Tuohy needle into the pharynx, recovered in the pharynx, and an introducer (a fibreoptic laryngoscope is ideal) or tracheal tube passed

28

over it. The cricotracheal membrane may be a better entrance site than the cricothyroid membrane (reduced incidence of bleeding and deeper penetration of the glottis by the tube).

Transtracheal jet ventilation
The insertion of a cricothyroid cannula (13 G) permits transtracheal jet ventilation. This means that the patient can be oxygenated, ventilated and anaesthetised while a definitive airway is established.

UNCOOPERATIVE, UNCONSCIOUS OR LESSER DEGREE OF EXPECTED DIFFICULTY
Such patients can be managed fibreoptically under general anaesthesia, or with a gum elastic bougie or laryngeal mask, as described below. The Trachlite is gaining in popularity.

'Taking over ventilation before paralysis' in suspected difficult laryngoscopy
This practice is designed to identify the 'can't ventilate, can't intubate' situation before the patient is rendered apnoeic by muscle relaxants. Goodwin and colleagues have shown that efficient ventilation can be established without muscle relaxation.

Use of suxamethonium in expected difficulty
The rationale here is that spontaneous ventilation may return before cardiac arrest if ventilation and intubation prove impossible. The practice is not 'evidence based', and some have expressed concern that critical desaturation will occur before the return of breathing, so that the technique may hold no real advantage over the use of long-acting relaxants.

UNEXPECTED DIFFICULTY
Gum-elastic bougie
This outstandingly useful item should always be ready for use. Henderson has pointed out that the term 'bougie' is actually inappropriate. The device is an introducer. Disposable, single-use tube introducers are much less effective than the classic gum-elastic model.
   Technique:
• Continue exposure of the glottis with laryngoscope throughout.
• Lubricate only the tip of the bougie. Pass the bougie, suitably bent, before loading a small (6.0–7.0-mm) tube.
• Lubricate the tip of the tube, and the bougie, as the tube enters the mouth.
• Rotate the tube 90° anticlockwise as it approaches the glottis.
• Remove bougie and laryngoscope. Apply oesophageal detector device.

Laryngeal mask
In some cases successful positioning of a laryngeal mask (LM) may be all that is required. The use of the LM as a fibreoptic intubation guide is especially useful after failed direct laryngoscopy. The device lifts the glottis out of the blood and secretions that tend to be present.

A fibreoptic laryngoscope is usually easy to pass into the trachea via a size 3 or 4 LM. A 6.0-mm tube is then rotated into the trachea. The only 6.0-mm tube of adequate length is the metal-reinforced tube manufactured by Mallinkrodt. This is a very successful technique. A size 5 LM allows the passage of a 7.0-mm tube, but 5 cm of the shaft of the LM must be cut off, because the tube will otherwise be too short. Alternatively, an 'Aintree' catheter can be passed over a fibreoptic laryngoscope and a tube rail-roaded over it after removal of the LM.

Blind nasal intubation
Skilful practitioners can achieve a remarkable degree of success. A combination of direct laryngoscopy and guiding a nasal tube towards the glottis with Magill's forceps is easier for most anaesthetists. Blind nasal intubation is a dying art due to the availability of flexible fibreoptic systems.

DIRECT LARYNGOSCOPY AND THE UNSTABLE CERVICAL SPINE
There is no evidence that direct laryngoscopy (and cricoid pressure) is more dangerous than any other method of intubation. Many patients with severe instability are in cervical fixation devices, which restrict mouth opening and cervical movements. In these circumstances, awake fibreoptic intubation is probably the method of choice.

BIBLIOGRAPHY

Benumof JL, Dagg R, Benumof R. Critical haemoglobin desaturation will occur before return to an unparalyzed state following 1 mg/kg intravenous succinylcholine. Anesthesiology 1997; 87:979–982

Calder I, Calder J, Crockard HA. Difficult direct laryngoscopy in patients with cervical spine disease. Anaesthesia 1995; 50:756–763

Goodwin MW, Pandit JJ, Hames K, Popat M, Yentis SM. The effect of neuromuscular blockade on the efficiency of mask ventilation of the lungs. Anaesthesia 2003; 58:60–63

Henderson JJ. The use of paraglossal straight blade laryngoscopy in difficult tracheal intubation. Anaesthesia 1997; 52:552–560

Henderson JJ. Development of the 'gum-elastic bougie'. Anaesthesia 2003; 58:103–104

Maktabi MA, Hoffman H, Funk G, From RP. Laryngeal trauma during awake fiberoptic intubation. Anesthesia and Analgesia 2002; 95:1112–1114

McCleod ADM, Calder I. Direct laryngoscopy and cervical cord damage – the legend lives on. British Journal of Anaesthesia 2000; 84:705–709

Nolan JP, Wilson ME. An evaluation of the gum elastic bougie. Intubation times and incidence of sore throat. Anaesthesia 1992; 47:878–881

Popat M. Practical fibreoptic intubation. Oxford: Butterworth-Heinemann; 2001

Sidhu VS, Whitehead EM, Ainsworth QP, Smith M, Calder I. A technique of awake fibreoptic intubation. Experience in patients with cervical spine disease. Anaesthesia 1993; 48:910–913

Silk JM, Hill HM, Calder I. Difficult intubation and the laryngeal mask. European Journal of Anaesthesiology. Supplement 1991; 4:47–51

Williamson JA, Webb RK, Szekely S, Gillies ERN, Dreosti AV. Difficult intubation: an analysis of 2000 incident reports. Anaesthesia and Intensive Care 1993; 21:602–667

Wilson ME. Predicting difficult intubation. British Journal of Anaesthesia 1993; 71:333–334

Yentis SM. Predicting difficult intubation – worthwhile exercise or pointless ritual? Anaesthesia 2002; 57:105–109

28

Difficult airway – difficult tracheal intubation

I. Calder

28

In day to day practice 'difficult intubation' tends to be synonymous with difficult laryngoscopy. Definitions of difficult intubation have suggested periods of time or number of attempts as measures of difficulty. Benumof has pointed out that this excludes the cases where difficulty is immediately obvious and the experienced anaesthetist does not persist. His definition of failure as 'failure despite an optimal best attempt' is sensible.

'True' difficult intubation could be said to be due to those, fortunately unusual, conditions that narrow the glottis or trachea, such as epiglottitis, abscess, tumour, airway burns and oedema due to cervical haematomas or anaphylaxis.

Stridor is the cardinal sign of a narrowed airway, and is said to occur at rest when the airway diameter is reduced to 4.0 mm. The diameter of the airway can be dangerously reduced without stridor being present. If the patient complains of difficulty in breathing, the situation is usually serious. Complaints of awakening at night with sensations of choking are characteristic of glottic obstruction. Patients with airway obstruction should be allowed to adopt their preferred position and interfered with as little possible. If the patient panics, the situation is likely to become truly dreadful.

Cervical haematomas (thyroid or anterior cervical surgery) produce oedema of the glottis and periglottic tissue. The swelling may be largely due to lymphatic obstruction and the haematoma may be small. The wound should be opened immediately to relieve lymphatic and venous obstruction.

Inhalation of nebulised adrenaline (epinephrine) (1 ml of 1 : 1000, in 10 ml saline) may buy some time. In cases of anaphylaxis, adrenaline (epinephrine) (0.5–1.0 ml of 1 : 10 000) should be given intravenously.

MANAGEMENT

This will depend entirely on the severity of the condition.

PATIENTS IN EXTREMIS (DETERIORATING CONSCIOUS LEVEL)

Emergency tracheotomy or cricothyrotomy will be required if direct laryngoscopy fails. In many cases a gum-elastic bougie can be passed and a 6.0–7.0-mm tube introduced over it.

LESS URGENT CASES

In such cases decision making is more complex.

Tracheostomy under local anaesthesia is often sensible, particularly if the condition is likely to persist.

Flexible fibreoptic laryngoscopy may be part of the diagnostic process in many cases. There is debate about the problems that can follow from attempts to provide topical anaesthesia – lidocaine (lignocaine) is irritant and has produced complete airway obstruction on at least one occasion. In some hands fibreoptic intubation may be successful, but it is not a technique for the inexperienced. In patients with very swollen necks it may be the only sensible option.

Inhalational induction with sevoflurane or halothane is the traditional method. Inhalational induction can succeed only if the airway is at least partially patent. Problems can arise with a prolonged excitement phase. Complete obstruction may occur. Judicious use of an intravenous agent, such as propofol, and application of CPAP may be helpful. Intravenous glycopyrrolate may reduce troublesome secretions.

SURGICAL ASSISTANCE

It is prudent to obtain surgical assistance if an emergency tracheostomy might be necessary.

ANTERIOR MEDIASTINAL MASSES

Obstruction of the trachea or main bronchus can occur during anaesthesia in symptomless patients. General anaesthesia should be avoided if possible. Flow–volume loops may predict airway obstruction – obstruction has occurred during both spontaneous and positive pressure ventilation.

EXTUBATION AFTER INTUBATION FOR AIRWAY OBSTRUCTION

The minimum period of intubation should probably be 24 h. Adequate sedation must be prescribed, to prevent accidental extubation. A small tube should have been passed, so that deflation of the cuff and blocking the tube can demonstrate a satisfactory airway.

BIBLIOGRAPHY

Crosby E, Reid D. Acute epiglottitis in the adult: is intubation mandatory? Canadian Journal of Anaesthesia 1991; 38:914–919

Mason RA, Fielder CP. The obstructed airway in head and neck surgery. Anaesthesia 1999; 54:625–628

Neuman GG, Weingarten AE, Abramowitz RM et al. The anesthetic management of a patient with an anterior mediastinal mass. Anesthesiology 1984; 60:144–147

Sparks CJ. Ludwig's angina causing respiratory arrest in the Solomon Islands. Anaesthesia and Intensive Care 1993; 21:460–463

28

Difficult airway – aspiration risk

R. Vanner

Patients at risk include those with:
- Full stomach
- Gastro-oesophageal reflux
- Oesophageal pathology
- Last half of pregnancy
- Hiccups, straining or coughing during light anaesthesia.

PROPHYLACTIC DRUGS

Decreasing the volume of gastric contents reduces the chance of regurgitation. Raising the gastric pH may limit lung damage if aspiration does occur. Oral ranitidine and sodium citrate are commonly used. Soluble paracetamol is also an effective antacid.

OPTIONS FOR ANAESTHESIA

- Regional anaesthesia with an awake patient
- Awake fibreoptic intubation before induction of general anaesthesia
- Intubation after rapid sequence intravenous induction with preoxygenation and cricoid pressure
- Intubation after induction in the left lateral head-down position.

Pulmonary aspiration has been reported with all the options mentioned above.

STOMACH TUBES

Patients with bowel obstruction, peritonitis or diabetic ketoacidosis should always have nasogastric tube drainage before surgery, which should be aspirated before induction of anaesthesia. A Salem sump tube with two lumens is the most efficient.

A recent meal may be difficult to aspirate through a tube, and inducing emesis is probably the only way to empty the stomach, albeit unreliably. It is unwise to induce emesis in a patient with a reduced conscious level.

The nasogastric tube, open to the atmosphere, should be left in place during induction of anaesthesia. A nasogastric tube does not interfere with oesophageal sphincter function or cricoid pressure.

The stomach should be decompressed with a large-bore orogastric tube before extubation.

CRICOID PRESSURE

- A pillow should be placed under the occiput, not the shoulders.
- A properly trained assistant is mandatory.
- A bimanual technique is preferred by some – the neck support prevents the head from flexing on the neck – although others prefer the single-handed technique that leaves the assistant's other hand free to help with intubation. The bimanual technique is used if a fractured cervical spine is suspected and another assistant is needed.
- The nasogastric tube should be left in place, but it must be open to vent gas or liquid.
- Cricoid pressure should be applied to the awake patient with a force of 10 N (1 kg), after preoxygenation but before intravenous induction.
- If retching occurs after intravenous induction, the cricoid pressure should be released because oesophageal rupture may occur.
- Cricoid pressure should be increased to a force of 30 N (3 kg) after loss of consciousness and before the onset of suxamethonium fasciculations.
- The assistant should practise the correct application of force on a weighing scale.
- Sellick originally described a three-fingered technique, with the main force applied by the index finger; others have recommended two fingers.
- The assistant should try to keep the larynx in the midline. This may not be possible

and passing a bougie in the midline may not find the larynx.

- Cricoid pressure should not be released until tracheal intubation is confirmed. Cricoid pressure should be released if the anaesthetist cannot ventilate the lungs following a failed intubation.

FAILED INTUBATION IN THE PATIENT WITH A FULL STOMACH

Repeated unsuccessful attempts at intubation can cause airway obstruction; a 'mature' anaesthetist will admit failure early. If a gum-elastic bougie cannot be passed within 1 min, serious consideration should be given to abandoning intubation attempts.

Failure occurs most commonly in obstetric practice (1 in 200–300 obstetrical cases, 1 in 2000 general surgical patients). The drill below refers to obstetric patients, but is applicable to all. The patient has already had preoxygenation, cricoid pressure followed by intravenous induction and suxamethonium.

'Failed intubation' drill:

- Inform surgeon and call for senior anaesthetic help
- Maintain cricoid pressure and keep patient in supine wedged position
- Insert an oral airway and ventilate with 100% oxygen
- Continue to mask-ventilate until spontaneous ventilation starts, then turn patient into the left lateral position, remove the pillow and then release cricoid pressure
- If mask ventilation is not possible, try the following:
  —insert a laryngeal mask; remove mask if no success
  —cricothyroid puncture

BIBLIOGRAPHY

Vanner RG, Asai T. Safe use of cricoid pressure. Anaesthesia 1999; 54:1–3

28

Paediatric airway

R. Bingham

The infant airway is smaller and anatomically distinct from that of the adult. The tongue is relatively large and forms a seal with the palate. Infants are obligatory nose breathers when breathing quietly, and airway obstruction at oropharyngeal level is likely when pharyngeal muscle tone is reduced.

The external nares are the narrowest part of the airway and contribute up to 30% of the total airway resistance. Any additional obstruction at this point (e.g. nasogastric tube) may significantly increase the work of breathing.

The larynx is more cephalad and anterior than in adulthood; the epiglottis is long, floppy and U-shaped in cross-section. Intubation with a curved blade laryngoscope is difficult as the epiglottis cannot easily be lifted from above. It is easier to view the vocal cords with a straight blade used to lift the epiglottis from underneath.

The larynx itself is cone shaped. The narrowest part is at the level of the cricoid cartilage (the cricoid ring) and is circular in cross-section. A plain, uncuffed tube will form an effective seal at this point to facilitate IPPV.

The resistance to gas flow through a tube is inversely related to the fourth power of the radius. As a result, mucosal oedema results in large changes in airway resistance. Partial airway obstruction is therefore common in infants with upper airway inflammation (e.g. following extubation or in laryngotracheobronchitis). Stridor occurs because of turbulent flow during inspiration. Wheezing occurs when the intrathoracic airways collapse during expiration; intrathoracic airway obstruction therefore results in an expiratory noise.

Oxygen consumption in the infant is approximately double that of an adult and there is a reduced reserve of oxygen within the lungs. Should a problem with oxygenation occur, the onset of hypoxaemia is far more rapid.

AIRWAY MAINTENANCE

During induction, children are predisposed to upper airway obstruction. Simple airway manoeuvres may be used to overcome this.

HEAD TILT/CHIN LIFT:
- No pillow – a protuberant occiput generates cervical spine flexion
- Gentle extension of the head at the atlanto-occipital joint
- Do not compress the soft tissues under the jaw as this may push the tongue base upwards and backwards and further obstruct the airway
- Pressure is exerted on the bony mandible only.

If this fails to clear the airway, there are further options (see below).

JAW THRUST MANOEUVRE
This is more efficient than the head tilt/chin lift, but requires two hands.

OROPHARYNGEAL OR NASOPHARYNGEAL AIRWAY:
- Oral airways may cause laryngospasm or retching.
- Sizes range from 000 to 4 – estimate size by comparison to child's face; it should extend from the lips to the angle of the jaw.
- Nasal airways are better tolerated in conscious or semiconscious children; the correct diameter is the same as that for an orotracheal tube.

CONTINUOUS POSITIVE AIRWAY PRESSURE (CPAP):
- CPAP provides a pneumatic splint, which distends the structures of the oropharynx.
- CPAP is best provided with a T-piece circuit and partial obstruction of the reservoir bag outlet.

LARYNGEAL MASK (LM):
- Particularly useful in anatomical deformities associated with an anterior larynx (e.g. Pierre Robin syndrome)
- Insertion more difficult than in adults, as the angle between the palate and posterior pharynx is more acute. Solutions include:
  —inserting the device upside down initially and then rotating it

—partial inflation
—guiding it round the posterior pharynx with a finger.

INTUBATION WITH STRAIGHT-BLADE LARYNGOSCOPE

This is most useful in neonates and small infants. One of two techniques is employed:
• The epiglottis is visualised; the laryngoscope is then slid underneath it and the tip of the blade lifted so that the glottis is exposed.
• The laryngoscope blade is deliberately advanced into the oesophagus and then, with the tip lifted anteriorly, it is withdrawn slowly until the larynx drops into view.
Both techniques bring the blade in contact with the epiglottis. There is therefore intense vagal stimulation; atropine premedication is advantageous.

In order to avoid damage to the cricoid region, it is essential to choose an uncuffed tube of the correct diameter. Tubes a half-size smaller and larger than the estimated correct size should also be available. Once the tube is in place there should be a small air leak at an inflation pressure of 29–30 cmH$_2$O, but none during normal ventilation. If the correct size of tube is chosen (Table 28.1) there is no danger from aspiration of gastric contents, and a pharyngeal pack is unnecessary.

The length of the tube is crucial in small infants. Problems with calculating this can be avoided by:
• The use of uncut tubes
• Passing 3 cm of tube through the glottis
• Careful checking for air entry into both lungs.
This system has the additional advantage that connectors for the breathing circuit, capnograph, humidifier, etc. are distanced from the child's face.

Firm fixation of the tube is vital. Most people use a system based on adhesive tape

TABLE 28.1

Paediatric tracheal tube sizes

Age	Tube size (internal diameter) (mm)
Newborn	3.0
6 months	3.5
1 year	4.0
> 1 year	(Age/4) + 4

fixed to the face and then wrapped around the tube. Extra security can be obtained by the application of a sticky substance such as tincture of benzoin.

For long-term intubation, nasal intubation is more secure than oral. It also reduces movement of the tube in the larynx and simplifies mouth care. There is a low incidence of complications when this method is used in children.

Regular saline instillation and suction is important, as small tubes easily become obstructed by inspissated mucus.

DIFFICULT PAEDIATRIC LARYNGOSCOPY AND INTUBATION

This problem is less common than in adults. It is usually associated with:
• Obvious deformity of the child's head or neck
• Mandibular hypoplasia (e.g. Pierre Robin or Treacher Collins syndrome) or space-occupying lesions within the oropharynx (e.g. cystic hygroma, haemangioma).
The technique used will depend on the presence or absence of airway obstruction, the site of the anatomical problem and the age of the child.

DIFFICULT LARYNGOSCOPY WITHOUT AIRWAY OBSTRUCTION
Intubation is usually performed under general anaesthesia as:
• Awake intubation is physically possible in neonates only in the first few days of life
• Fibreoptic laryngoscopy under topical anaesthesia may be possible, but it may be difficult to obtain full cooperation.
The anaesthetic technique usually involves spontaneous respiration although, in the absence of obstruction, a muscle relaxant may be used. It is prudent to check that manual ventilation is possible before instituting paralysis.

A variety of options may be used for the intubation itself.

Gum-elastic bougie
Most difficult paediatric intubations can be accomplished by conventional laryngoscopy using this device. Occasionally, a two-operator technique may be useful: one operator manipulates the laryngoscope and brings the larynx into view by pressing on the neck, while the second performs the intubation itself.

Fibreoptic laryngoscope
A 2.5-mm internal diameter tracheal tube can pass over the smallest fibreoptic laryngoscope

(although difficult to control). Larger sizes (3.8 mm outer diameter) can be used in the same way as in adults.

The technique is as follows:
- Anaesthesia is maintained via the nasal airway.
- A two-person technique has been suggested for the smaller scope:
  —The first operator guides the tip as close to the larynx as possible using a conventional laryngoscope and Magill's forceps.
  —The second operator monitors the advance into the larynx through the fibrescope itself.

Laryngeal mask

A plain 5.0-mm internal diameter tracheal tube can be passed through the size 2 mask or a 6.0-mm one through the size 2.5 mask. The tube can be advanced blindly, but as the epiglottis may be down-folded in children it is better to pass the tube under direct vision over a fibre-optic laryngoscope. The LM can then either be left in place or removed carefully. A further alternative for intubation with smaller tubes is to advance a Seldinger wire into the larynx through the fibreoptic scope and thread a stiff airway exchange catheter over this. The LM can then be removed and the tube railroaded over the catheter. In all these manoeuvres it is important to practise them in advance so that the sequence of events is familiar to all the participants.

DIFFICULT LARYNGOSCOPY ACCOMPANIED BY UPPER AIRWAY OBSTRUCTION

The management of this difficult problem will depend on the site and nature of the obstruction and the age of the child.

Supraglottic obstruction

Awake intubation may be possible. This may be achieved with either a conventional laryngoscope in the newborn or with a fibreoptic scope under topical anaesthesia in the cooperative older child.

GENERAL ANAESTHESIA

General anaesthesia may be preferable because coughing or straining associated with laryngeal stimulation in an awake patient may precipitate complete airway obstruction (particularly likely in infective conditions such as acute epiglottitis): Provision for instituting a surgical airway should be available.
- Spontaneous respiration must be maintained, usually with halothane or sevoflurane in oxygen.
- The delivery of CPAP with a T-piece circuit and a well-fitting mask is an essential part of the technique.
- If airway obstruction is severe, it may take a long time to reach a depth of anaesthesia sufficient to permit laryngoscopy.
- In laryngeal or tracheal obstruction, the intubation itself is usually accomplished with a conventional laryngoscope and a bougie.

For the initial control of the airway, intubation is usually oral. If long-term intubation is required, this may be changed electively for a nasal tube. To prevent accidental extubation, meticulous sedation is required. This is usually accomplished with a combination of a continuous intravenous morphine infusion and either intravenous benzodiazepines or nasogastric chloral hydrate. Neuromuscular paralysis should be avoided, if at all possible, because, although accidental extubation is less likely, the consequences should it occur would be catastrophic.

28

BIBLIOGRAPHY

Biack AE, Hatch DJ, Nauth-Misir N. Complications of nasotracheal intubation in neonates, infants and children: a review of 4 years' experience in a children's hospital. British Journal of Anaesthesia 1990; 65:461–467

Chadd GD, Crane DL, Phillips RM, Tunell WP. Extubation and reintubation guided by the laryngeal mask in a child with the Pierre Robin syndrome. Anesthesiology 1992; 76:640–641

Dubreuil M, Ecoffey C. Laryngeal mask guided tracheal intubation in paediatric anaesthesia. Paediatric Anaesthesia 1992; 2:344

Markakis DA, Sayson SC, Schreiner MS. Insertion of the laryngeal mask airway in awake infants with the Robin sequence. Anesthesia and Analgesia 1992; 75:822–824

Russell SH, Hirsch NP. Simultaneous use of two laryngoscopes. Anaesthesia 1993; 48:918

Ward CF. Pediatric head and neck syndromes In: Katz RL, Steward DJ, eds. Anaesthesia and uncommon pediatric conditions. Philadelphia: WB Saunders; 1987:238–271

White AP, Billingham IM. Laryngeal mask guided tracheal intubation in paediatric anaesthesia. Paediatric Anaesthesia 1992; 2:265

Wilson I G. The laryngeal mask airway in paediatric practice. British Journal of Anaesthesia 1993; 70: 124–125

Zideman D, Bingham R, Beattie T et al. Guidelines for paediatric life support. A statement by the Paediatric Life Support Working Party of the European Resuscitation Council. Resuscitation 1994; 27:91–105

28

29

EQUIPMENT AND MONITORING
N. I. Newton

The anaesthetic machine

N. I. Newton

Prior to the introduction of the continuous-flow anaesthetic machine (the 'Boyle's machine') the concentration of anaesthetic inhaled by a patient was dependent on many factors that were variable and difficult to quantify. Observation of the patient's response to the anaesthetic was often the only means by which the concentration of anaesthetic being administered was assessed.

The essential element of the anaesthetic machine is that it enables known concentrations of anaesthetic gases and vapours to be delivered accurately. This is achieved by controlling the way in which the supplies of oxygen and nitrous oxide are mixed; the resultant carrier gas is then passed through calibrated vaporisers where an accurate percentage of volatile anaesthetic agent is taken up and subsequently delivered to the patient.

Following the demise of explosive or inflammable anaesthetic agents such as cyclopropane and ether, the basic pneumatic anaesthetic machine has developed into the electronically integrated 'anaesthetic workstation'.

The anaesthetic workstation may have an electronically controlled ventilator as well as integral output monitoring devices and associated alarms. Furthermore, the workstation typically incorporates integrated patient monitors, providing a sophisticated comprehensive platform for the safe administration of anaesthesia.

The basic anaesthetic machine comprises several elements, as described below.

CYLINDERS

See Table 29.1.
- Cylinder valves should be opened slowly and closed without using undue force. Never use oil or grease, as spontaneous combustion may occur in the presence of oxygen.
- The pin index system ensures that the correct cylinder is fitted.
- Cylinders are connected at their respective yokes via Bodok seals.
- Free-standing cylinders should be properly secured at all times to prevent any risk of their falling over and being damaged.

PIPELINES

- Each 'complete hose assembly' is permanently attached via a non-interchangeable screw-thread (NIST) connector at the machine end, and has a Schraeder male probe at the distal end to insert into the gas supply at the wall or pendant.
- Pipeline gases are supplied at the anaesthetic machine working pressure of 400 kPa via flow restrictors.
- Backflow check valves on the anaesthetic machine prevent gases escaping from the empty cylinder yoke when a cylinder is changed or from the pipelines when these are not plugged into the gas terminal outlets.

TABLE 29.1

Gas cylinders used with the Anaesthetic machine

Gas	Cylinder pressure (× 100 kPa)	Critical temperature (°C)
Oxygen	135	– 119
Nitrous oxide[a]	44	36.5
Medical air	137	– 141
Carbon dioxide[a]	49	31

[a]These gases liquefy under pressure at room temperature; the cylinder pressure does not therefore reflect the state of filling.

PRESSURE GAUGES

- Aneroid 'Bourdon gauges' monitor high gas pressures in cylinders and pipelines.
- Pressures are displayed as kPa × 100.

PRESSURE REGULATORS

- Reduce cylinder pressures to safe working levels (just below 400 kPa).
- Maintain a constant flow despite changes in supply pressure.
- Are required for all gases where the supply pressure exceeds 1000 kPa (i.e. not needed for pipeline supplies).

FLOW CONTROL VALVES

- Manually operated fine-adjustment needle valves that control the flow rates of the carrier gases and the oxygen concentration of the gas mixture.
- Note that the oxygen control knob has distinctive shape to avoid confusion and is always on the left (in the UK).

FLOW METERS

- Enable flows of individual gases to be visualised and measured.
- Rotameter bobbins rotate to avoid sticking.
- Tubes must be vertical.

VAPORISERS

- Plenum vaporisers have a vaporising chamber and bypass channel.
- Control knob alters the 'splitting ratio', thereby determining the percentage of carrier gas that becomes fully saturated.
- Vaporisers are compensated for temperature and flow rate.
- Modern vaporisers can be removed from the machine by means of the 'Selectatec'-type mechanism on the backbar. Leaks may occur when the vaporiser is not seated properly; this must be checked each time the vaporiser is replaced.

PRESSURE RELIEF VALVE

- Protects the machine from high pressure due to obstruction at common gas outlet or breathing system.
- Typically opens when the pressure exceeds approximately 35 kPa.

OXYGEN FAILURE

ALARMS:

- Primary audible oxygen alarm powered by oxygen as it fails. Alarm sounds when the oxygen supply pressure falls below 200 kPa (half normal pressure), giving a whistle lasting a minimum of 7 s.
- Secondary alarms may operate to give a more persistent warning, for instance a siren driven by nitrous oxide being vented.

PROTECTION DEVICES:

- Ensures other gases are cut off when oxygen fails.
- May open the breathing system to atmosphere, allowing a non-paralysed patient to breathe air.

OXYGEN FLUSH

- Bypasses all vaporisers.
- Supplies 35–75 litres of oxygen per minute.
- Ideally self-closing, but may have facility to be locked on (risk of awareness or barotrauma if unnoticed).

COMMON GAS OUTLET

- Final pathway for gases to leave anaesthetic machine
- Male 22-mm taper, female 15-mm taper
- Cardiff swivel allows breathing system to swing into best position – beware possible interaction between breathing system and oxygen flush.

BREATHING SYSTEM

- Connects the patient to the common gas outlet.
- Integral pressure-limiting valve commonly employed to protect the patient (opens at 60–80 cmH$_2$O).

VENTILATOR

Most anaesthetic machines are equipped with an automatic ventilator.

ANAESTHETIC GAS SCAVENGING SYSTEM

- Normally an active system using assisted flow
- Levels of nitrous oxide in operating theatre can be kept below 100 p.p.m. with effective scavenging
- Such levels are achievable by:
  —scavenging at all times

29

—avoiding leaving gases flowing when the patient is not connected to machine

—care in filling vaporisers will reduce contamination from volatile agents.

OTHER

In the sophisticated anaesthetic workstation, it may not always be possible to identify the individual components listed above. It is important to obtain specific training before using such equipment.

A backup system to allow maintenance of anaesthesia (e.g. intravenous anaesthetic agent) as well as an independent means of ventilation with oxygen must always be present in case of unexpected workstation failure where the cause is not obvious.

Electrically powered anaesthetic workstations should always be plugged directly into a wall-mounted mains socket, and never via a multisocket extension lead.

Where auxiliary mains plugs are provided on the machine, the anaesthetist must take direct responsibility to ensure that only appropriate devices with the correct current rating are plugged in. Multisocket extension leads must never be plugged into the anaesthetic machine auxiliary sockets, as there may be no control over what they are used for.

BIBLIOGRAPHY

British Standards Institution. European Standard BS EN 740. Anaesthetic workstations and their modules – particular requirements. British Standards Institution; London: 1998

International Standard IEC 60601–2–13. Medical electrical equipment–part 2–13: Particular requirements for the safety and essential performance of anaesthetic systems. British Standards Institution; London: 2003

Moyle JTB, Davey A, Ward CS, eds. Wards Anaesthetic Equipment, 4th edn. Elsevier Health Sciences; 1998

29

Breathing systems

D. M. Miller

Breathing systems deliver anaesthetic gas mixtures from an anaesthetic workstation to the patient. They may be classified (Table 29.2) according to their configuration and functional performance related to fresh gas flow (FGF) requirements (Miller 1995a). The non-absorber bidirectional flow systems include those labelled by Mapleson from A to F (Miller 1988). The reservoir in this classification refers to the site where bidirectional flow and storage of gases occur (see Fig. 29.1). The reservoir may be situated either in the exhaust limb in efferent reservoir systems (D, E, F), the supply limb in afferent reservoir systems (A), or at the junction of the supply and exhaust limb in junctional reservoir systems (B, C).

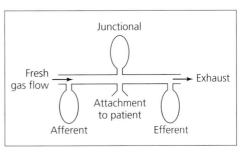

Fig. 29.1 The reservoir is where storage of gases occurs. It may be situated in the exhaust limb in efferent reservoir systems (Mapleson D, E, F), in the supply limb in afferent reservoir systems (Mapleson A) or at the junction of the supply and exhaust limb in junctional reservoir systems (Mapleson B, C).

TABLE 29.2

Classification of breathing systems

29

Classification	System	Fresh gas flow required[a]	
		Spontaneous	Controlled
Carbon dioxide absorption			
Unidirectional flow			
Circle systems	Various[b]	NA	NA
Bidirectional flow			
To and fro	Waters' canister	NA	NA
Non-absorber			
Unidirectional flow			
Non-rebreathing valves	Ambu E, Ruben, Fink	1	1
Bidirectional flow			
Efferent reservoir	Ayre's T-piece, Jackson–Rees[c], Bain	2	1
Junctional reservoir	Mapleson B, C	1.5	1.5
Afferent reservoir	Magill, Lack	0.7	2
Displacement afferent reservoir	Enclosed afferent[d], Maxima[e]	0.7	0.7

[a]Relates to minimal fresh gas flow units in multiples of resting minute ventilation of an anaesthetised patient (approximately 70 ml kg⁻¹ min⁻¹) for both spontaneous respiration and controlled ventilation. NA, not applicable.
[b]Eger & Ethans (1968).
[c]Willis et al (1975).
[d]Miller & Miller (1988).
[e]Miller (1995b).

CARBON DIOXIDE ABSORPTION SYSTEMS

- Soda lime – 94% $Ca(OH)_2$, 5% NaOH, 1% KOH with silicates to make granules
- Baralyme – 80% $Ca(OH)_2$, 20% $Ba(OH)_2$
- Amsorb – $CaCl_2$, $Ca(OH)_2$
- Moisture required for efficient absorption, to prevent carbon monoxide and substance A formation with volatile agents. Baralyme worse than Soda lime, and Amsorb the safest.
- Indicators that change colour when absorbent is exhausted.

WATERS' CANISTER (BIDIRECTIONAL FLOW)

Obsolete because: it is cumbersome, dead-space increases as granules nearest the patient become exhausted and channelling occurs.

CIRCLE SYSTEM (UNIDIRECTIONAL FLOW):

- Carbon dioxide absorption eliminates the carbon dioxide accumulation effect of rebreathing, making FGF requirements less critical.
- Lowering FGF increases the economy of the system. However, the lower the FGF, the less correlation between the composition of the gases being delivered to the circle and the gases being inhaled by the patient.
- The lower the FGF entering the circle, the longer the time constants and the less control there is over the concentrations within the circuit. Time constant = Volume of circle/(FGF – uptake).
- In the absence of monitoring, low-flow circle system anaesthesia is associated with a dangerous risk that a hypoxic mixture may be delivered. In addition there may be inadvertent wrong dosage of inhalational agents, rebreathing due to unrecognised exhaustion of carbon dioxide absorbent and impaired control of the anaesthetic procedure.

Monitoring minimises these risks:
- Essential monitoring of gases within the circle must include: (1) oxygen concentration, (2) volatile anaesthetic monitor, (3) capnography and (4) circulating gas volume (rising bellows ventilator is the simplest).
- With monitoring, minimal flows (< 1 l min^{-1}) can be used even for short

cases. The use of newer rapid-acting insoluble agents (e.g. sevoflurane and desflurane) makes it possible to start with low flows of 2–3 l min^{-1}, and to reduce to minimal flows within 2–3 min if high concentrations of nitrous oxide are not required. To achieve adequate concentrations of volatile agent quickly, high vaporiser settings are required initially.
- Because of the low agent uptake with desflurane, and to a lesser degree with sevoflurane, the inspired concentration will be close to the delivered value even at low flow rates down to 1 l min^{-1}.
- If the benefit of nitrous oxide is required, denitrogenation by preoxygenation before induction should be performed.

Humidity control:
- Minimum concentration of 20 mg l^{-1} H_2O (saturation at ambient temperature of about 22°C) should be employed during long-term anaesthesia. (Fully saturated gas contains 44 mg l^{-1} H_2O at 37°C).
- To achieve adequate humidity for the patient with low flows can take much longer than 1 h
- Improved humidity may be achieved by (1) using an HME filter, (2) lagging the inspiratory tubing, (3) heating the inspiratory line (Drager Cicero machine), (4) circulating the flow of gases rapidly (Physioflex circulates gas at 70 l min^{-1}).

Extraneous substance accumulation:
- Carbon monoxide leading to carboxyhaemoglobin accumulation is usually less than 0.1% per hour. Beware low flows with smokers (flush regularly – at least once an hour).
- Methane, acetone, ethanol, hydrogen, substance A – not really a problem in practice.

NON-ABSORBER BREATHING SYSTEMS

NON-REBREATHING VALVE SYSTEMS (UNIDIRECTIONAL FLOW)

Requires the fresh gas flow to match the patient's minute ventilation exactly. Too high a flow may result in the valve jamming in inspiration, causing barotrauma, hypoventilation and falling cardiac output. For this reason continual attention is required – therefore not really practical.

29

RESERVOIR SYSTEMS (BIDIRECTIONAL FLOW)
Efferent reservoir systems (Willis et al 1975, Miller 1998)

Bain system

Advantages:
- Minimal deadspace, so may be used for children and adults
- Simple interchange between spontaneous and controlled ventilation
- Useful for limited access to head and neck
- Efficient in controlled ventilation
- Scavenging convenient.

Disadvantages:
- Inefficient in use of FGF in spontaneous ventilation
- Inner tube disconnection risk resulting in very large deadspace.

Jackson–Rees system

Advantages:
- Minimal deadspace, so may be used for children
- Reservoir bag close at hand for monitoring respiration and controlling ventilation with simple interchange between spontaneous and controlled ventilation.

Disadvantages:
- Large deadspace with face-mask unless special mask flushing characteristics included
- Scavenging difficult
- Inefficient in use of FGF in spontaneous ventilation.

Junctional reservoir systems

Mapleson C or B systems

Advantages:
- Reservoir bag close at hand for monitoring respiration and controlling ventilation with simple interchange between spontaneous and controlled ventilation.

Disadvantages:
- Intermediate efficiency in all modes of ventilation.

Afferent reservoir systems

Magill and Lack system

Advantages:
- Maximal efficiency in spontaneous ventilation
- Good heat and moisture exchange.

Disadvantages:
- Very inefficient in controlled ventilation
- Cannot be used with a ventilator
- Magill has inconvenient (for scavenging and adjustment) valve situated close to the patient.

Displacement afferent reservoir systems
Maxima system (Miller 1995b), Carden system (Carden & Nelsen 1972) (MIE Carden ventilator; Fletcher et al 1983), Ohmeda enclosed afferent reservoir system

Advantages:
- Maximal efficiency in spontaneous ventilation (Miller 1995b)
- Maximal efficiency in controlled ventilation (Miller 1995b)
- Convenient interchange between modes of ventilation
- Satisfactory humidity even without HME
- Easy scavenging
- Zero deadspace – suitable for neonates to adults (Miller 1998)
- Face-mask flushing characteristics (Miller 1998)
- No moving parts
- Cardiac output estimation with carbon dioxide monitor (Miller & Wessels 1997).

Disadvantages:
- Difficult to understand how it works.

Combination systems
Humphrey ADE (Humphrey 1983) and others combine the advantages of efferent and afferent reservoir systems.

29

BIBLIOGRAPHY

Carden E, Nelsen D. A new highly efficient circuit for paediatric anaesthesia. Canadian Anaesthetic Society Journal 1972; 19:572–582

Eger EI, Ethans CT. Effects of inflow, overflow and valve placement on economy of the circle system. Anesthesiology 1968; 29:93–100

Fletcher IR, Carden E, Healy TEJ, Poole TR. The MIE Carden ventilator. Anaesthesia 1983; 38:1082–1089

Humphrey D. A new anaesthetic breathing system combining Mapleson A, D and E principles. Anaesthesia 1983; 38:361–372

Miller DM. Breathing systems for use in anaesthesia. Evaluation using a physical lung model. British Journal of Anaesthesia 1988; 60:555–564

Miller DM. Breathing systems reclassified. Anaesthesia and Intensive Care 1995a; 23:281–283

Miller DM. An enclosed efferent afferent reservoir system: the Maxima. Anaesthesia and Intensive Care 1995b; 23:284–301

Miller DM. Paediatric breathing systems: their use and misuse in South Africa. South African Journal of Anaesthesiology and Analgesia 1998; 4:28–34

Miller DM, Miller JC. Enclosed afferent reservoir breathing systems. British Journal of Anaesthesia 1988; 60:469–475

Miller DM, Wessels JA.. A simple method for the continuous non-invasive estimate of cardiac output using the Maxima breathing system. A pilot study. Anaesthesia and Intensive Care 1997; 25:23–28

Willis BA, Pender JW, Mapleson WW. Rebreathing in a T-piece: volunteer and theoretical studies of the Jackson–Rees modification of Ayre's T-piece during spontaneous respiration. British Journal of Anaesthesia 1975; 47:1239–1245

29

Monitoring

M. J. Jordan and R. Langford

MONITORING STANDARDS

ASA STANDARDS FOR BASIC ANAESTHETIC MONITORING 1986 (AMENDED 1998):
- Standard I – Continuous presence of anaesthetist
- Standard II – Monitoring of oxygenation, ventilation, circulation and temperature
- F_iO_2 by oxygen analyser with low concentration alarm in use
- Blood oxygenation, by quantitative method (e.g. pulse oximetry)
- Ventilation by capnography; spirometry encouraged
- Tracheal tube and laryngeal mask position by F_eCO_2
- IPPV circuit integrity by audible ventilator disconnection alarm
- ECG by continuous display
- Arterial blood pressure, heart rate measured at least every 5 min
- Continual monitoring of circulation, for example by pulse or arterial trace
- Temperature measurement available and used when clinically significant change expected.

AAGBI STANDARDS 1988 (REVISED 2000):
- Continuous presence of anaesthetist
- Monitoring of equipment
  —F_iO_2 by oxygen analyser
  —Leak or disconnection by capnography and IPPV overpressure by airway pressure alarm
  —Vapour concentration by vapour analyser
- Monitoring of patient – induction:
  —pulse oximeter, non-invasive blood pressure, ECG and capnography mandatory; nerve stimulator and temperature monitoring must be available.
- Monitoring of patient – maintenance:
  —as for induction, with addition of vapour analyser.

- Monitoring of patient – recovery:
  —pulse oximetry, non-invasive blood pressure mandatory
  —ECG, nerve stimulator, temperature measurement and capnography must be available.
- Regional techniques and sedation:
  —pulse oximetry, non-invasive blood pressure, ECG mandatory.
- Transfer:
  —SpO_2, ECG and arterial pressure mandatory; invasive arterial pressure should be considered
  —IPPV airway pressure, tidal volume and $F_E^1CO_2$.

GAS MONITORING

F_iO_2:
- Simple oxygen analysers should be placed in the inspiratory limb of breathing system.
- Pressurisation will cause overreading of analysers calibrated at atmospheric pressure.
- Multigas analysers using slow-response technology for oxygen analysis (e.g. fuel cell) may give value intermediate between F_iO_2 and F_EO_2 when sampling at tracheal tube.

$F_E^1CO_2$:
- Persisting $F_iO_2 - F_EO_2$ difference greater than 5% may indicate hypoventilation or low cardiac output state
- $F_E^1CO_2$ is useful in monitoring nitrogen and nitrous oxide washout.

$F_E^1CO_2$
Sudden falls in F_eCO_2 are suggestive of disconnection, air embolism or fall in cardiac output.
P_ECO_2 will also underestimate $PaCO_2$ in:
- Significant intrapulmonary or extrapulmonary shunting
- Respiratory rates too high for accurate analysis

29

- Tidal volumes too low for accurate sampling
- Dilution of sample by fresh gas, for example in the Bain system.

NITROUS OXIDE AND VOLATILE AGENTS:

- Analysers requiring selection of agent in use introduce serious errors if this is incorrect, when nitrous oxide compensation is not appropriate or when mixtures of volatile agents are used.
- End-tidal volatile agent concentrations will overestimate arterial concentrations in presence of high A–a gradients.

NITROGEN

Sudden rises in $F_E^1N_2$ in absence of inspired nitrogen are indicative of air embolism.

RESPIRATORY MECHANICS

- Pulmonary compliance monitoring, for example with pressure–volume or flow–volume loops, is particularly useful in:
- Patients prone to bronchospasm
- Laparoscopic or thoracoscopic surgery
- Surgery in proximity of tracheal tube.

BODY TEMPERATURE

- Oesophageal temperature correlates best with blood (core) temperature.
- Nasopharyngeal or tympanic membrane temperature reflects brain temperature.
- Infrared-type ear thermometers correlate poorly with core temperature.
- Rectal temperature lags behind core temperature in the adult.

OXYGEN SATURATION BY PULSE OXIMETRY (Sp_{O_2})

- *In vivo* spectrophotometric measurement of haemoglobin oxygen saturation by a probe, usually located on a finger or the ear lobes (less reliable).
- Fails in low perfusion states (cold, hypovolaemia, low cardiac output), or with movement or shivering
- Erroneous results if incorrectly positioned, nail varnish not removed, or in presence of carboxyhaemoglobin or methaemoglobin
- Ideally, pulse waveform should be displayed or discernible to confirm signal strength

- Peripheral Sp_{O_2} may lag 30–45 s behind central Sp_{O_2}
- Administration of high inspired oxygen may initially maintain oxygen saturation, even when ventilation is inadequate.

ELECTROCARDIOGRAPHY

Continuous observation of:
- Rate, rhythm (including ectopics) and conduction
- Myocardial ischaemia identified from single lead (e.g. CM5) ST segment depression, or with greater sensitivity by computer-analysed multilead system
- Electrolyte status:
  —peaked T waves (hyperkalaemia)
  —prolonged QT (hypocalcaemia).

SYSTEMIC BLOOD PRESSURE

NON-INVASIVE BLOOD PRESSURE

The automated oscillometric technique is now the commonest.
  Accuracy is mainly dependent on:
- Correct cuff size – width 20% greater than arm diameter, or one-third of arm circumference
- Correct application – loose wrapping results in falsely high readings.

Regular calibration of aneroid sphygmo-manometers is required.

INVASIVE BLOOD PRESSURE

A mechanoelectrical transducer produces small changes in voltage or resistance proportional to pressure waves transmitted from a vessel though fluid-filled tubing.
  To obtain an optimally damped, accurate waveform:
- The connecting tubing should be 60–120 cm in length, 1.5–3.0 mm in internal diameter, and made with rigid walls.
- Eliminate any air bubbles in the system.
- Use 4 ml h^{-1} continuous flush to prevent thrombotic occlusion.

Precautions:
- Use a 20 g cannula to avoid arterial occlusion or damage.
- Avoid accidental intra-arterial injection by using colour-coded taps.
- Display waveform to prevent blood loss from disconnection.

CENTRAL VENOUS PRESSURE

Central venous pressure (CVP) is measured via a jugular, subclavian or long brachial venous cannula to indicate right atrial pressure (Table 29.3).

TABLE 29.3

Complications in measuring CVP and their avoidance

Complication	Avoidance
Air embolism	Head-down tilt during insertion Use Luer–Lok connections
Sepsis	Aseptic insertion; minimise number of injections into tubing
Pneumothorax or haemothorax	

PULMONARY ARTERY AND CAPILLARY WEDGE PRESSURES

Measured via balloon-tipped floatation-directed catheter. Facilitates measurement of cardiac output and (by balloon occlusion of pulmonary artery) left atrial pressure.

Indications:
• Ejection fraction < 40%
• Left ventricular failure or hypertrophy
• Cardiac output studies.

Complications:
• Dysrhythmias
• Sepsis
• Pulmonary infarction
• Haemorrhage.

TRANSOESOPHAGEAL ECHOCARDIOGRAPHY

Modern instruments allow multiplane imaging of heart and colour Doppler visualisation of blood flow. Conventional transthoracic echocardiography can be difficult in ventilated patients.

Particularly useful in cardiac surgery, allowing monitoring of left ventricular function, regional ventricular wall motion abnormalities (suggestive of ischaemia), detection of air or clot emboli, and assessment of valve or septal repairs and prosthetic valve function.

NEUROMUSCULAR FUNCTION

The muscular response to a supramaximal electrical stimulation of a peripheral motor nerve is measured by eye, feel, force transducer or electromyography.
• A train of four (TOF) stimuli (at 2 Hz, 10 s apart) indicates the degree of neuromuscular blockade.
• TOF count (number of twitches seen):
  —satisfactory blockade if 0–2 twitches detectable
  —TOF ratio (fourth twitch force as a fraction of the first) is useful for monitoring recovery from blockade.
• Tetanic stimulation (50 or 100 Hz for 5 s) in the presence of partial non-depolarising blockade results in 'fade' (failure to sustain muscular contraction) and 'post-tetanic facilitation' of force from a single stimulus.

DEPTH OF ANAESTHESIA MONITORING

ELECTROENCEPHALOGRAPHIC (EEG) MONITORING

EEG is a low-amplitude (microvoltage) signal, requiring low impedance electrodes and care to avoid interference artefacts, especially in the electrically 'noisy' environment of the operating theatre. Systems are now available to monitor depth of anaesthesia, but they do not measure arousability and are poorly predictive of response to surgical stimulus.

The proprietary bispectral index (BIS) algorithm utilises both bispectral analysis and weighted use of frequency and amplitude measures to compute a single number indicative of the depth of anaesthesia. The EEG is collected via forehead electrodes.

AUDITORY EVOKED RESPONSES (AER)

Averaged, summated AER waveforms permit measurement of the time delay (latency) to the appearance of specific identified peaks or troughs. Such latency measurements may also be used to generate a numerical output as a measure of depth of anaesthesia.

29

BIBLIOGRAPHY

Association of Anaesthetists of Great Britain and Ireland. Recommendations for standards of monitoring during Anaesthesia and Recovery 3. London: AAGBI; 2000

Pre-use check procedures for anaesthetic machines

P. J. Bickford-Smith

All anaesthetic gas machines must be checked systematically before use. A check should be performed by the anaesthetist at the beginning of each list.

If there is a change of anaesthetist during the list, the checked status of the machine must be agreed at handover.

PERFORMING A PRE-USE CHECK PROCEDURE

The most serious deficiency in an anaesthetic machine is the failure to deliver adequate supplies of oxygen. Modern machines are fitted with at least two safety devices to prevent the delivery of a hypoxic gas mixture:

- A primary oxygen-supply-failure protection device (with an audible alarm)
- A secondary gas cut-off device, to prevent the common gas outlet from delivering a hypoxic gas mixture.

NB: The sounds of electronic oxygen failure alarms may be difficult to distinguish from other machine-generated alarm signals and warrant familiarisation (Andrzejowski & Freeman 2002).

In 2001, the Medical Devices Agency and the Department of Health directed that 'all anaesthetic machines capable of delivering hypoxic gas mixtures must have a (mechanical) hypoxic guard or use an oxygen analyser with audible alarms to warn of the delivery of hypoxic gas mixtures'.

In line with recommendations from the Royal College of Anaesthetists (2001), the majority of new machines within the UK are fitted with a 'minimum ratio' device, which actively reduces the proportion of non-respirable gases to guarantee adequate oxygen delivery. The minimum ratio device may or may not be linked to an oxygen analyser. If not, the relative flows of oxygen to non-respirable gas are controlled either by a mechanical link between the respective flow control valves or via a differential gas pressure detector. In the absence of an oxygen analyser, neither system can identify a crossed gas pipeline or a misfilled (e.g. with non-respirable gas) oxygen cylinder.

The correct function of the minimum ratio device must be tested with an oxygen analyser calibrated in room air (21% oxygen) and 100% oxygen (from a separate source, such as a wall flowmeter). Integral oxygen analysers can be used if the sampling point can be placed at the common gas outlet.

All oxygen analysers and many of the alarm systems on modern machines require a supply of electricity, as do patient monitors, syringe drivers and Tec 6 vaporisers. These impose a requirement for a large number of mains power outlets. Up to four auxiliary power outlets may be found on the back of anaesthetic machines. These are commonly protected by a circuit breaker or fuse with a low power rating ($\leq$ 2 A), suitable only for the devices noted above. Overload of the power outlets may be averted by never connecting inappropriate high-load devices (> 250–500 W), such as patient-warming or blood-warming devices, to these sockets. A failure of the electricity supply to a machine may precipitate discontinuation of all gas flow. The ready availability of a manual means of assisting ventilation, for instance a self-inflating bag, should be integrated within the systematic check.

A systematic check procedure ensures the provision and correct function of:

- The supply of medical gases, primarily oxygen
- The supply of mains and battery electricity
- Vaporisers for volatile anaesthetic agents
- Breathing system(s) – tubing, bags, valves
- Ventilator(s)
- Suction apparatus
- Sundry apparatus (e.g. airway maintenance and intubation equipment).

29

MEDICAL GAS SUPPLY CHECK

Some (AAGBI 1997, Cartwright 2000) now consider routine testing of the integrity of compressed gas supply via pipelines unnecessary. However, such a test must be performed whenever a new pipeline installation is being used for the first time or after major (including work on the services) refurbishment of an operating theatre facility has been undertaken. In addition, a formal check should be made whenever an anaesthetic machine has been moved from one location to another, including the 'first time in service' use.

The increasing use of total intravenous anaesthesia (TIVA) has led to a lessening of the perceived need for cylinders other than oxygen or air being specified and fitted on to anaesthetic machines. A check of the reserve oxygen cylinder(s) must remain standard practice.

STEP 1:
- Disconnect all gas pipelines, turn off all cylinders and vaporisers.
- Remove all unwanted cylinders and blank off empty yokes with blanking plugs.
- Connect (calibrated) oxygen analyser to common gas outlet.
- Turn on (mains) electrical supply to machine.
- Turn on gas supply master switch (if fitted; see note in step 6).
- Open all gas-flow-control valves.

STEP 2:
- Turn oxygen cylinder on and check that the pressure rises on the relevant gauge to above half full; bobbin rises in oxygen flowmeter only. Adjust flow to 5 l min^{-1}.
- Watch analyser concentration rise towards 100%.
- Turn nitrous oxide cylinder on and check the relevant gauge pressure shows full; check that nitrous oxide bobbin rises. Adjust flow to 5 l min^{-1} (check that the oxygen bobbin has remained at 5 l min^{-1}).

STEP 3:
- Turn oxygen cylinder off; press emergency oxygen button.
- Watch the cylinder pressure fall, the oxygen bobbin fall, and the audible oxygen failure alarm sound (check that visual indicator, if present, changes from green to red) and that gas flow from common gas outlet ceases.

STEP 4:
- Connect the oxygen pipeline and perform a 'tug' test: the audible alarm should stop, the visual indicator (if present) should change from red to green, and the gas flow should recommence at the common gas outlet.
- Watch the oxygen bobbin rise to 5 l min^{-1} and the pipeline pressure gauge rise to 400 kPa.

STEP 5:
- Turn the nitrous oxide cylinder off; connect the nitrous oxide pipeline and perform a 'tug' test.
- Watch the nitrous oxide bobbin rise to 5 l min^{-1}; the pipeline pressure gauge rises to 400 kPa.

STEP 6:
- Attempt to turn off the oxygen flow control valve and see whether the oxygen bobbin falls to zero or remains at around 250 ml min^{-1}.
  NB: If the nitrous oxide bobbin also falls and the oxygen analyser reading remains above 21%, the machine is fitted with a minimum ratio antihypoxic device.
- Turn gas control master switch to 'off' to discontinue the basal oxygen flow.
  NB: The flow of oxygen may not stop for some minutes.

STEP 7:
- Repeat steps 2–4 for any other cylinders of gas.
- If there is no gas control master switch, turn off all flow control valves individually.

ELECTRICITY SUPPLY

- Check that the anaesthetic machine is connected directly to a mains supply (never via an extension lead or multisocket extension) and switched on, and that mains indicator light(s) and battery charging light(s), if present, are illuminated (Newton 2002).
- Check which systems (ventilator, oxygen supply) still operate when the mains supply is disconnected.
- Identify display and check status of back-up battery.
- Check auxiliary 240-V power sockets on anaesthetic machine – unplug any devices not directly related to the functioning of the machine or its associated monitors.

29

Reconnect unplugged devices to another 13-A supply (e.g. wall or pendant socket) (Chawla & Newton 2002).

VAPORISERS

- Detachable vaporisers must be locked on to the backbar and appear to be level.
- Check mains supply and status indicator lights on desflurane vaporisers.
- Check the orientation of any flexible inflow or outflow pipes.
- Check the fluid level – at 'full' or significantly above 'empty'.
- Check that filling port cap or valve control is tightly closed.
- Turn on oxygen flow to 5 l min^{-1}, switch vaporiser to full scale, briefly (maximum 2 s) occlude the common gas outlet, and look for any fluid leakage.
- Turn vaporiser off; then turn oxygen flow off.

VENTILATOR

- Check configuration and correct operation.
- Check for presence of a self-inflating bag – for manual assistance of ventilation.
- Check for presence and function of a disconnection alarm.
- Set controls for next patient.

BREATHING SYSTEM CHECK

This check should include all components – masks, tracheal tubes, catheter mounts.
- Check the overall configuration, especially coaxial tubes and circle absorber systems.
- Check reservoir bag and expiratory valve – presence and function.
- Check tightness (push and twist) of all tubing connectors.
- Make a visual inspection for bore patency – to exclude foreign bodies within the breathing system.
- Flush system with oxygen when fully assembled.
- Leak test – occlude patient-end, close expiratory valve, fit a manometer into the circuit with a T-piece adjacent to the bag.

- Distend bag to 20–35 mmHg using the oxygen flush button – pressure should remain unchanged after 1 min.

GAS SCAVENGING

- Check integrity of pathways (lack of obstructions or kinks, connector integrity) of exhaust gas pipes from airway pressure limiting (APL) valve(s) to the active gas scavenging system (AGSS) collecting vessel.
- Check indicator float movement within transparent window of AGSS collecting vessel, if present. If no movement, or absence of transmitted sound from vacuum pump, check AGSS terminal connection and that AGSS pump is switched on (usually via a wall-mounted switch or indicator within each theatre or theatre suite).

SUCTION

- Adequate suction of – 60 kPa or less, achieved after ≤ 5 s when the patient-end of tubing is occluded
- Check all components securely assembled.

SUNDRIES

- Two laryngoscopes – check bulbs and operation of light when blade opened for use
- Appropriate sizes of oropharyngeal or laryngeal mask airways
- Face-masks – check adequate pressure in pneumatic seal.

FAULTS DETECTED DURING CHECK – ACTION

- Correct fault if possible (e.g. calibrate monitor).
- Note minor faults in the logbook, including date of detection and your name.
- Major fault (e.g. persistent large gas leak) – remove equipment from service and attach label indicating date fault detected and type of fault, and stating that machine must not be used.
- Inform theatre staff and service engineer. If patient care was compromised, complete a critical incident report.

29

BIBLIOGRAPHY

Andrzejowski J, Freeman R. Oxygen failure on modern anaesthetic machines. Anaesthesia 2002; 57:931–932

Association of Anaesthetists of Great Britain and Ireland. Checklist for anaesthetic apparatus 3. London: AAGBI; 2003

Cartwright DP. Limitations of the current checklist for anaesthetic machines. Anaesthesia 2000; 55:298

Chawla AV, Newton NI. Machines and monitor failure from electrical overload. Anaesthesia 2002; 57:1134–1136

Chief Medical Officer, Chief Executive of the Medical Devices Agency. Joint letter to chief executives, NHS Trusts. 24/10/01 MDA CEL 2001 (03).

Medical Devices Agency. Anaesthetic machines: prevention of hypoxic gas mixtures. MDA SN2001 (15). London: MDA; 2001

Newton N. Anaesthesia workstations and the checklist. Anaesthesia News 2002; 183:17

Royal College of Anaesthetists. Safety notice on prevention of hypoxic gas mixtures. Royal College of Anaesthetists Bulletin 2001; July:354

29

Ventilators

A. C. Pearce

The correct term is 'ventilatory breathing system'. This comprises:
- Ventilator
- Breathing system attached to patient.

FUNCTIONAL CLASSIFICATION

INSPIRATORY PHASE GAS CONTROL:
- Volume – a preset volume is delivered
- Pressure – a preset pressure is not exceeded.

CYCLING (INSPIRATION–EXPIRATION):
- Time
- Pressure
- Volume
- Flow.

INSPIRATORY FLOW CHARACTERISTICS:
- Flow generator – the inspiratory flow pattern predetermined by ventilator settings
- Pressure generator – the inspiratory pressure applied to the patient's airway is determined by ventilator settings.

THREE COMMON TYPES OF VENTILATOR

VOLUME PRESET, TIME CYCLED, FLOW GENERATOR:
- Includes virtually all adult ITU machines and many adult anaesthetic ventilators.
- Delivery of a preset tidal volume is maintained despite changes in lung compliance.
- Inflation pressure depends on lung compliance and is limited by a safety blow-off valve (usually 60 cmH$_2$O).
- Cycles from inspiration to expiration at the end of a preset time.
- Powerful machines powered by a high-pressure driving gas (400 kPa) or substantial electric motors.

- Examples include Servovent, Cape, Oxford, Nuffield 200 with adult valve.

PRESSURE PRESET, TIME CYCLED, FLOW GENERATOR:
- Common arrangement in paediatric ventilators.
- Set airway pressure (usually 15–20 cmH$_2$O) not exceeded during inspiration.
- Cycles to expiration at the end of a set time, even if the desired inflation pressure is not reached.
- Inspiratory flow rate must be set at high enough level to reach desired pressure in the time allowed for inspiration.
- Tidal volume delivered is affected by changes in lung compliance.
- Compensates to a degree for leaks (e.g. uncuffed paediatric tracheal tube or laryngeal mask).
- Examples include paediatric Babylog, Sechrist, Nuffield 200 with paediatric valve.

TIME CYCLED, PRESSURE GENERATOR:
- Weighted bellows apply constant set pressure during inspiration.
- Inspiratory flow is high initially and then declines – characteristic of a pressure generator.
- Delivered tidal volume will depend on pressure in the bellows and lung compliance.
- Possible to set a desired tidal volume only if there is sufficient weight on bellows.
- Examples include East-Radcliffe, Manley Blease.

OTHER VENTILATORS

Ventilators can also be classified by how they work. The commonest types used in operating theatres are:
- Minute volume dividers – these use the power of the fresh gas flow from the anaesthetic machine and divide the

delivered minute volume into preset tidal volumes.

- T-tube occluders – these occlude intermittently the expiratory limb of a T-piece; the constant gas flow into the circuit then inflates the patient's lungs.
- Bag squeezers – these compress a bellows in the breathing circuit, usually by means of high-pressure gas or an electric motor.
- Intermittent blowers – these are powered by a high-pressure driving gas which enters the breathing circuit in controlled 'bursts'.

CHECKING AND SETTING

Checking and setting the ventilatory breathing system before use is vital:

- Connect to electricity supply, high-pressure gas, low-pressure gas, etc.
- Set tidal volume to 10–15 ml kg^{-1} or inflation pressure to 20 cmH$_2$O.
- Set respiratory rate to 10–16 breaths per min.
- Set I : E ratio to 1 : 2 or 1 : 3, with an inspiratory time of not less than 1 s.
- Switch on and see whether pressure develops in the circuit.
- Check that the pressure relief valve is functioning at correct value.
- Check that gas monitoring is present and working.
- Check that airway pressure monitor is working.
- Check manual mode functioning, if fitted.
- Check that the emergency air intake is patent, if appropriate.

MODES OF VENTILATION

Sophisticated ventilators may function in a number of modes, some providing mandatory ventilation and others providing some form of respiratory support when triggered by the patient. Triggered modes can be used safely only when there are spontaneous patient breaths.

- CMV – controlled mandatory ventilation in which a preset minute volume is delivered, usually to a paralysed or apnoeic patient.
- SIMV – synchronised intermittent mandatory ventilation in which a preset minute volume is set, but the ventilator is able to adjust the timing of mandatory breaths to coordinate with any spontaneous

breathing by the patient. This helps to reduce the tendency for a patient to 'fight' against the ventilator.

- Triggering indicates the ability of the ventilator to detect the initiation of a spontaneous breath by the patient, usually by detecting a set negative pressure in the breathing system. The patient triggers the onset of the inspiratory phase.
- Pressure support is one commonly used mode in which the patient triggers the inspiratory phase. The clinician-adjusted level of pressure support (often 5–20 cmH$_2$O) determines the degree of respiratory support provided by the ventilator. Often the inspiratory phase during pressure support is terminated when the inspiratory flow rate decreases below a critical value.
- SIMV with pressure support indicates a mode in which a mandatory number of breaths is delivered, coordinated as far as possible with any spontaneous breaths, with spontaneous breaths being supported by the ventilator.
- PEEP – positive end-expiratory pressure during controlled ventilation.
- CPAP – continuous positive airway pressure during spontaneous respiration.

THE IDEAL VENTILATORY BREATHING SYSTEM

The ideal ventilatory breathing system should have the following characteristics:

- Wide range of tidal volumes and respiratory rates to encompass paediatric and adult use
- Pressure- or volume-controlled mode
- Adjustable inspiratory/expiratory timing (I/E ratio)
- Airway pressure display, with alarm limits
- Expired minute volume display, with alarm limits
- Adjustable, monitored, inspired oxygen concentration
- Provision of PEEP and CPAP
- Sophisticated ventilatory modes – SIMV, pressure support, mandatory minute volume (MMV), triggering
- Humidification
- Adjustable inspiratory waveforms
- Adjustable pressure relief valve
- Facility for drug administration into breathing system – nitric oxide, inhaled bronchodilator.

29

BIBLIOGRAPHY

Moyle JTB, Davey A, Ward CS, eds. Ward's Anaesthetic Equipment. 4th edn. Elsevier Health Sciences; 1998

Ehrenwerth J, Eisenkraft JB. Anesthesia equipment, principles and applications. London: Mosby; 1993

Hayes B. Ventilators: a current assessment. Recent Advances in Anaesthesia and Analgesia. 1993; 18:83–102

Pinnock C, Lin T, Smith T, eds. Fundamentals of Anaesthesia 2nd edn. Chapter 3: Anaesthetic Equipment. Greenwich Medical Media; 2003

Aitkenhead AR, Rowbotham DJ, Smith G, eds. Textbook of Anaesthesia 4th edn. Chapter 32, Anaesthetic Apparatus. Churchill Livingston, London; 2001

29

30

TECHNIQUES
B. Al-Shaikh

Awake or blind nasal intubation

O. Duff and B. Al-Shaikh

Blind nasotracheal intubation is a useful technique in the anaesthetist's armamentarium when dealing with patients with a difficult airway. It is used for intubating spontaneously breathing patients with or without sedation, or even under general anaesthesia. This method has the advantage of being independent from visualisation of the glottis and has a good chance of success in a variety of patients of different ages and body sizes, in both elective and selected emergency situations. Unfortunately, in approximately 20% of patients it can cause upper airway bleeding that is very uncomfortable, and may compromise subsequent fibreoptic efforts. When available, intubation using a fibreoptic bronchoscope should be the technique of choice.

Indications (similar to fibreoptically assisted intubation)

- Difficult laryngoscopy due to inability to open mouth, mandibular agenesis, buck teeth
- History and/or anticipated difficulty with other techniques of intubation
- Severe risk of aspiration
- Inability to apply a face-mask
- Cervical injuries limiting neck movement
- Severe risk of haemodynamic or respiratory instability on induction of general anaesthesia or paralysis

Contraindications

- Airway tumour, abscess or trauma
- Recent nasal surgery
- Coagulopathy
- Basal skull fracture and unstable mid-face injuries

SEDATION

It is essential that the patient cooperates with the technique and is able to speak and respond to commands. The provision of suitable sedation to the patient may improve the chances of

a successful intubation. This can easily be achieved using intravenous propofol by target-controlled infusion (TCI): $0.5-1$ μg ml^{-1} target plasma concentration combined with opioids (e.g. fentanyl), which offer analgesia. Benzodiazepines such as midazolam can be used as alternatives when titrated carefully.

AIRWAY ANAESTHESIA

Local anaesthesia of the airway is used in awake sedated patients. Careful explanation is given to the patient before sedation and local anaesthetic administration. The airway can be anaesthetised as a whole using nebulised local anaesthetic and/or in stages. Nebulised lidocaine (lignocaine) 4% (4–10 ml) can be used, and acts within 10 min. The effect of local anaesthesia may worsen the upper airway obstruction. In patients with a full stomach, local anaesthesia should not extend beyond the glottis.

- An anticholinergic antisialagogue agent is given (e.g. glycopyrrolate 0.2 mg) intravenously to reduce secretions and improve the contact of topical anaesthesia.
- *Nose* – In addition to the local anaesthetic, the nasal mucosa should be gently prepared with a vasoconstrictor to reduce bleeding and oedema. Phenylephrine 1%, xylometazoline (Otrivine) or cocaine 4% can be used. Full effectiveness requires application for 2–5 min with a duration of action of 30–45 min.
- *Mouth, pharynx and larynx* – Tetracaine (amethocaine) lozenges in addition to nebulised lidocaine (lignocaine) can be used. The superior laryngeal nerves can be blocked bilaterally; 3 ml 2% lidocaine is injected inferomedial to the greater cornu of the hyoid on both sides, providing a 20–30-min block.
- *Trachea* – The mucosa below the larynx is best blocked by a midline transtracheal injection of local anaesthetic through the

30

cricothyroid membrane; 3 ml 2–4% lidocaine (lignocaine) is injected using a 23-G needle with its bevel directed downwards. On penetration of the trachea, the patient exhales as deeply as possible so that the subsequent deep inspiration (and cough) will result in maximal distribution of lidocaine.

INTUBATION

The patient is positioned with the neck flexed and the head extended at the atlantoaxial joint (sniffing position) if the cervical spine is stable. A prewarmed, well lubricated, curved, nasal tracheal tube (7.0–7.5 mm internal diameter) is gently passed perpendicularly through the more patent nostril into the hypopharynx. With the other nostril and the mouth occluded, the tube is advanced in midline, listening for the breath sounds. The tube is passed into the larynx during inspiration. Monitoring the carbon dioxide concentration in the exhaled air can be used to monitor the progress and to confirm tube position. The tube is advanced until one of the positions shown in Table 30.1 is reached.

Movement of the breathing system reservoir bag, condensation on the tracheal tube or catheter mount, and audiocapnography can provide further confirmation of the position of the tube.

BIBLIOGRAPHY

Latto IP. Management of difficult intubation. In: Latto IP, Vaughan RS, eds. Difficulties in tracheal intubation. 2nd edn. London: WB Saunders; 1997:140–143

Murrin KR. Awake intubation. In: Latto IP, Vaughan RS, eds. Difficulties in tracheal intubation. 2nd edn. London: WB Saunders; 1997:161–171

Stone DJ, Gal TJ. Airway management. In: Miller RD, ed. Anesthesia. 4th edn. Edinburgh: Churchill Livingstone; 1994:1423–1426

TABLE 30.1

Tube placement

Position	Confirmation	Response
Trachea	Breath sounds continue through tube with its advance; coughing through tube	Secure tube, auscultate bilaterally, confirm $EtCO_2$
Anterior larynx	Breath sounds continue through tube, but unable to advance further; coughing mostly through tube	Slightly withdraw and re-advance tube while patient's head and neck are gradually flexed
Left or right piriform fossa	No breath sounds, tube unable to advance, no cough; tube may be palpable on one side of neck	Slightly withdraw until breath sounds through tube resume; slowly rotate (back toward midline) and re-advance
Oesophagus	No breath sounds, tube continues to advance; no cough	Withdraw tube until breath sounds through tube resume, then (separately or together): • *Extend* patient's head and re-advance • *Inflate cuff* (e.g. 15 ml air) so directing the tip anteriorly, advance until resistance is felt; maintain some advancing pressure on tube while cuff is slowly deflated • Apply posterior pressure on the larynx and re-advance tube

30

Epidural and spinal anaesthesia

U. Akhigbe and B. Al-Shaikh

30

INDICATIONS

- *Surgery* – Axial blocks can be used alone for surgery below the level of T6, when it may be preferable if there is a risk of aspiration, difficult intubation, or where respiratory function may be further compromised. Compared with general anaesthesia, postoperative mortality and morbidity rates are reduced, with increased mental alertness and responsiveness. The latter is of a particular importance in pregnant women.
- *After surgery* – In addition to the superior analgesia, there is a significant reduction in the incidence of respiratory depression, pneumonia, deep venous thrombosis (DVT), pulmonary embolus and ileus, leading to a shorter hospital stay.
- *Pre-emptive analgesia* – This has been shown in animal studies, but not in human surgery. However, it has been shown that its use can influence the development of chronic pain syndromes after surgery.
- *Modification of the perioperative stress response* – Axial blockade reduces the hormonal and metabolic response to surgery. This may be of benefit in the management of high-risk surgical patients.

CONTRAINDICATIONS

- Patient refusal
- Coagulopathy or full therapeutic anticoagulation
- Sepsis at site
- Hypovolaemia
- Anaphylaxis to drugs used
- Fixed cardiac output
- Raised intracranial pressure (ICP).

DIFFERENTIAL BLOCKADE

Small-diameter fibres (sensory and autonomic) are more easily blocked than large motor fibres because local anaesthetic penetrates them more easily. Thus autonomic function, temperature and pain sensation are lost before loss of motor function. The concentration of local anaesthetic agent used similarly influences the type of block produced. Low concentrations produce analgesia with minimal motor blockade. High concentrations produce profound motor blockade in addition to analgesia. Sympathetic block is usually two levels above the sensory block, which in turn is two levels higher than the motor block.

CONTROVERSIES

EPIDURAL HAEMATOMA:

- *Antiplatelet agents* (e.g. aspirin and non-steroidal anti-inflammatory drugs (NSAIDs) – Use of these drugs does not appear to be associated with an increased risk of epidural haematoma formation.
- *Low-dose heparin and low-molecular-weight heparin (LMWH)* – In the absence of other risk factors, there is no evidence of an increased risk. The risk of a haematoma formation is 1 in 150 000 following an epidural block and 1 in 220 000 following a spinal block. To reduce risk, block should be sited at least 4 h after low-dose heparin and 12 h after LMWH. A similar guideline applies to removal of an epidural catheter.
- *Low platelet count* – Although a count of less than $100 \times 10^9\,l^{-1}$ is generally regarded as a contraindication to an epidural, thromboelastographic findings have been normal, with counts as low as $50 \times 10^9\,l^{-1}$.
- *Temporary intraoperative anticoagulation* – This is safe as long as the anticoagulation is delayed for 1 h after siting the block and the epidural catheter is removed only once clotting has returned to normal.

SERIOUS LONG-TERM NEUROLOGICAL SEQUELAE

These appear to be extremely rare. Possible causes include trauma, infection, chemical irritation, compression and ischaemia of the spinal cord.

PRE-EXISTING NEUROLOGICAL DEFICIT

Although this is not a specific contraindication, a detailed history, clinical examination, documentation and counselling are essential.

PRE-EXISTING SYSTEMIC INFECTION

There is an increased risk of meningitis and epidural abscess following an axial block. The risk may be reduced with prophylactic antibiotics.

EPIDURAL AND SPINAL OPIOIDS

Opioids provide analgesia by binding to receptors in the dorsal horn of the spinal cord. They lack sensory, motor or autonomic effects and have a synergistic effect when used with local anaesthetic. Highly lipid-soluble drugs such as fentanyl or sufentanil may also have some systemic action. Opioids containing preservative are neurotoxic and should be avoided. Commonly used opioids include fentanyl, sufentanil, diamorphine, morphine and pethidine.

SIDE-EFFECTS

Side-effects may occur with any opioids or when given by either route, but tend to be more common following morphine and intrathecal administration. Naloxone is effective in the treatment.

Pruritus

This is the most common side-effect; it is often minor but may be severe in 1% of patients. It is often localised to the head, face, neck or upper chest, but may occasionally be generalised. Incidence is unrelated to dose. Pruritus is thought to result from interaction of opiate with opioid receptors in the trigeminal nucleus or nerve root.

Nausea and vomiting

May result from interaction with opioid receptors in the area postrema. The incidence (30%) is higher in females and is similar with opioids given parenterally.

Urinary retention

This is not dose related and is thought to result from binding with opioid receptors in the sacral spinal cord, inhibiting parasympathetic outflow with relaxation of detrusor muscle.

Respiratory depression

The incidence of respiratory depression requiring intervention is 1%, similar to that for par-

enteral opioids. Respiratory depression may present within minutes or after several hours. Early respiratory depression results from systemic absorption and is commonly associated with highly lipid-soluble drugs. Late respiratory depression results from cephalad migration and interaction with opioid receptors in the medullary centre, and is more commonly associated with water-soluble drugs such as morphine. The risk is increased in the elderly, children, with concomitant use of parenteral opioids or respiratory depressant drugs, and in those with pre-existing respiratory impairment.

Other

Other reported, rare, side-effects include muscle rigidity, sexual dysfunction, reduced gastric emptying, hair loss, water retention and reactivation of herpes simplex labialis virus.

EPIDURAL ANAESTHESIA

Anatomy:

- The epidural space lies between the dural sac and the periosteum lining the vertebral bodies, extending from the foramen magnum to the sacral hiatus.
- Anteriorly it is bounded by the posterior longitudinal ligament, posteriorly by the ligamentum flavum, and laterally by the vertebral pedicles and intervertebral foramina.
- It communicates freely with the paravertebral space via the intervertebral foramina.
- It contains nerve roots, venous plexi, fat and lymphatics.

Technique:

- Access can be gained through the ligamentum flavum via a median or paramedian approach with a loss of resistance technique using saline or air, or through the sacrococcygeal membrane as a caudal block.
- The lumbar or low thoracic regions are commonly used in adults, and the caudal route is most common in children.
- Local anaesthetic solution injected into the epidural space acts on nerve roots or the spinal cord.
- As epidural local anaesthetic provides segmental analgesia, it should be sited at the level where anaesthesia is required. Epidural opioids act at spinal cord level, so the site of insertion is less important.
- The incidence of dural tap is 1–3%, but is dependent on the experience of the operator and patient anatomy.

30

Advantages:
- Level of block can be controlled with titrated doses of local anaesthetic and site of epidural cannulation
- Greater cardiovascular stability due to slow onset of block and the ability to titrate local anaesthetic via an epidural catheter
- Block can be extended via an epidural catheter.

Disadvantages:
- Slow onset
- Use of large volume of local anaesthetic increases the risk of toxicity
- Risk of catheter migration or fragmentation
- Risk of dural puncture with postdural puncture headache
- Subjective endpoint may result in higher failure rate.

SPINAL ANAESTHESIA
Anatomy:
- Cerebrospinal fluid is located within the subarachnoid space.
- The spinal cord ends at the lower border of L1 in adults and L3 in children. Lumbar puncture above these levels increases the risk of spinal cord damage and should therefore be avoided.

Technique:
- A line joining the upper part of the iliac crests is at L4 or the L4–L5 interspace and serves as a useful landmark for lumbar puncture.
- Dural puncture may be done via a median or paramedian approach. The spinal needle passes through skin, subcutaneous tissue, supraspinous ligament, interspinous ligament, ligamentum flavum, epidural space, dura and into the subarachnoid space where CSF is obtained.
- Local anaesthetic solution injected mixes with the CSF and act on nerve roots and dorsal root ganglia.
- The extent of the block obtained is determined mainly by the baricity of the local anaesthetic agent, position of the patient, and the concentration and volume of local anaesthetic injected.
- Hyperbaric solutions such as heavy bupivacaine, which contains 8% glucose, have a higher specific gravity in comparison to CSF and therefore tend to move downwards following injection. A small volume (1 ml) of hyperbaric solution injected in the sitting position and the patient left sitting for at least 5 min

produces a 'saddle' block suitable for perineal operations. A unilateral block may similarly be produced with hyperbaric solution in the lateral position, but the block becomes bilateral when the patient is turned supine.
- Hypobaric solutions such as plain bupivacaine have a lower specific gravity than CSF and tend to rise following injection, therefore producing an unpredictable level of block.
- The density and duration of the block is influenced by the dose, while the height of the block is also influenced by the volume and the speed of injection. Large volumes of concentrated solutions produce motor blockade over a large area, whereas low doses block sensory and sympathetic fibres with preservation of motor function.

Advantages:
- Clear endpoint of technique, thus low failure rate
- Rapid onset of block
- Use of a small non-toxic dose of local anaesthetic
- Rapid sacral block
- Posture with heavy bupivacaine produces a reliable low haemodynamically stable block
- Good muscle relaxation.

Disadvantages:
- Difficulty in controlling height of block above T10
- Greater haemodynamic instability resulting from higher denser block
- Risk of postdural puncture headache
- Single-shot technique limits the ability to extend anaesthesia or analgesia during surgery.

Postdural puncture headache
The incidence is increased in young patients, females, obstetric patients, with a larger size of spinal needle and with the use of cutting (Quincke) rather than pencil-point (Whiteacre or Sprotte) needles. An incidence of 1% is reported with the use of 26- or 27-G spinal needles, compared with 15% and 75% with 20- and 16-G needles respectively.

Spinal catheters
These are introduced into the CSF through spinal needles, providing flexibility as anaesthesia can be extended with titrated boluses of local anaesthetic. Their use has been limited by a high incidence of postdural headache, risk of infection and reports of cauda equina syn-

drome following continuous spinal anaesthesia. The introduction of a 32-G microcatheter may reduce the incidence of headache, although difficulty may be experienced on advancing the catheter.

COMBINED SPINAL–EPIDURAL ANAESTHESIA

This offers greater flexibility, the spinal block providing rapid onset while the epidural catheter can be used to extend the block.

- *Single-space technique* – The epidural space is located with a Tuohy needle and a long spinal needle is passed through it into the CSF. The spinal needle is withdrawn following injection, and a catheter is passed into the epidural space. The risk of the epidural catheter migrating through the hole made in the dura into the CSF is low, as very small gauge spinal needles (e.g. 26 G) are used.
- *Double-space technique* – Spinal injection is performed and an epidural catheter is inserted in an intervertebral space above.

BIBLIOGRAPHY

Chaney MA. Side effects of intrathecal and epidural opioids. Canadian Journal of Anaesthesia 1995; 42:891–903

De Tommaso O, Caporuscio A, Tagariello V. Neurological complications following central neuraxial blocks: are there predictive factors? European Journal of Anaesthesiology 2002; 19:705–716

Horlocker TT, Wedel DJ, Schroeder DR et al. Preoperative antiplatelet therapy does not increase the risk of spinal haematoma associated with regional anaesthesia. Anesthesia and Analgesia 1995; 80:303–309

Tyagi A, Bhattacharya A. Central neuraxial blocks and anticoagulation: a review of current trends. European Journal of Anaesthesiology 2002; 19:317–329

30

Closed-circle anaesthesia

J. R. Shelgaonkar and B. Al-Shaikh

The introduction of the expensive, newly developed, inhalational anaesthetic agents with low blood solubility and the increased awareness of the pollution produced by the inhalational agents have renewed interest in low-flow and closed-circle anaesthesia. It is so named because its components are arranged in a circular manner. It prevents the rebreathing of CO_2 but allows rebreathing of other gases and vapours. It consists of:

- Fresh gas flow (FGF) source
- Inspiratory and expiratory unidirectional valves
- Inspiratory and expiratory corrugated tubing
- Y-piece connector
- Airway pressure limiting (APL) valve
- Reservoir bag
- Carbon dioxide absorber.

DEFINITIONS

CLOSED-CIRCLE ANAESTHESIA

The FGF is just sufficient to replace the volume of gas and vapour taken up by the patient. No gas leaves via the APL valve, and the exhaled gases are rebreathed after carbon dioxide is absorbed. Significant leaks from the breathing system are eliminated. In practice, this is possible only if the gases sampled by the gas analyser are returned back to the system.

LOW-FLOW ANAESTHESIA

The FGF is less than the patient's alveolar ventilation (usually below 1.5 l min^{-1}). Excess gases leave the system via the APL valve.

PRINCIPLES

High FGF is needed in the initial period to denitrogenate the circle system and the functional residual capacity (FRC). This is important to avoid the build-up of unacceptable levels of nitrogen in the system. In closed-circle anaesthesia, a high FGF is needed for up to 15 min. In low-flow anaesthesia, a high FGF of up to 6 min is required.

Wash-in and wash-out curves for changes in vapour concentration within the closed system are exponential. The time constant is the duration needed to reach 63% of the intended FGF concentration in the system:

Time constant for circle =
Volume of circle system/FGF

So, the time constant is dependent on the volume of the system and FGF, and can be between 1 and 2 min. Three time constants are required for 95% equilibration of FGF with circle gases.

To calculate the dose of an anaesthetic agent required, we need to know:
- Minimum alveolar concentration (MAC)
- The amount of vapour needed to achieve this within the system and lungs
- The amount of vapour required for uptake into the circulation
- The amount required for uptake into the tissues.

The amount of anaesthetic vapour required to achieve the target anaesthetic concen-tration in the breathing system and the lungs depends on the volume of the system and lungs. This is known as the 'ventilation priming dose':

Ventilation priming dose =
Target concentration ×
(Volume of system + Volume of lungs)

This volume of system and FRC provides a large reservoir, within which the anaesthetic gases are diluted at the beginning of anaesthesia.

Component	Volume (ml)
Absorber (2 kg)	2000
Breathing tubing (1 m)	1000
FRC	3000

30

Ventilation priming dose
= 1.3 MAC × (Volume of circuit +
    Volume of lungs)/100
= millilitres of anaesthetic vapour.

MINIMUM ALVEOLAR CONCENTRATION

MAC is a measure of dose (ED_{50}) necessary to immobilise 50% of the patients when exposed to a noxious stimulus. The ED_{95} dose of a volatile agent is achieved at concentrations of 1.3 MAC and higher:

Agent	MAC (%)	1.3 MAC
Halothane	0.75	> 0.95
Enflurane	1.7	> 2.26
Isoflurane	1.2	> 1.5
Sevoflurane	2.0	> 2.6
Desflurane	6.1	> 8.1

UPTAKE AND ELIMINATION OF GASES AND VAPOURS

UPTAKE OF INHALATIONAL AGENT
The uptake into the circulation and tissues can be calculated using Lowe's formula:

$$V an \text{ (arterial prime) (ml min}^{-1}) = f\,MAC \times \lambda_{B/G} \times Q \times t^{-1/2}$$

where f MAC is the target concentration (1.3 MAC), $\lambda_{B/G}$ is the blood/gas solubility coefficient of the agent, Q is cardiac output and t is the time constant.

This arterial prime dose equilibrates initially with the blood. Due to the continuous uptake of agent into the tissues, further anaesthetic agent is required to provide for this uptake into the tissues.

Tissue uptake
The amount of the anaesthetic agent taken up by tissues decreases with time. This affects the rate of uptake of the agent into the circulation, which decreases inversely with the square root of elapsed time.

The amount of anaesthetic vapour uptake in first minute (Table 30.2).

UPTAKE OF OXYGEN
Oxygen uptake during anaesthesia is generally lowered by 10–30%. This is due the metabolic depression caused by the anaesthetic agents leading to decreased consumption. This uptake is almost stable throughout the entire duration of anaesthesia. For clinical purposes, oxygen consumption can easily be estimated as:

$$V O_2 \text{ (ml min}^{-1}) = 3.5 \times \text{Bodyweight (kg)}$$

UPTAKE OF NITROUS OXIDE
The uptake of nitrous oxide, like that of volatile anaesthetics, follows a power function. As it is not metabolised, its uptake is determined solely by the alveolar–arterial partial pressure difference. This is high at the beginning of anaesthesia but reduces with time as the tissues become progressively more saturated with nitrous oxide. The uptake of nitrous oxide by a normal adult patient can be roughly estimated by:

$$V N_2O \text{ (ml min}^{-1}) = 1000 \times t^{1/2}$$

Time (min)	N₂O uptake (ml min⁻¹)
1	1000
25	200
50	140
> 120	90

CARBON DIOXIDE OUTPUT
Carbon dioxide output can be estimated by:

$$V CO_2 \text{ (ml min}^{-1}) = 3 \times \text{Bodyweight}$$

However, during anaesthesia, output is lowered by the effects of anaesthetic agent on metabolism. For example, during deep inhalational anaesthesia with sevoflurane or isoflurane, the

30

TABLE 30.2

Anaesthetic vapour uptake in first minute

	Halothane	Enflurane	Isoflurane	Sevoflurane	Desflurane
MAC (% v/v)	0.75	1.68	1.2	2.1	6.1
$\lambda_{B/G}$	2.3	1.8	1.4	0.65	0.42
Uptake in first minute (ml min⁻¹)	69	121	67.2	54.6	120

output of carbon dioxide in a 70-kg patient will typically be around 150 ml min^{-1}.

ELIMINATION OF INHALATIONAL AGENTS

To lower the inhalational agent concentration rapidly, the vaporiser is set at zero and the FGF is increased. Leaving a low FGF leads to a slow decrease in the agent's concentration as the vapour must leave the system through the APL valve, and during low-flow anaesthesia very little vapour is actually vented. The lower the solubility of the anaesthetic agent used, the more rapidly the concentration decreases.

PRACTICAL PRINCIPLES

- In closed-circle anaesthesia, the initial period of high FGF is needed to denitrogenate the circle system and FRC. This is important to avoid the build-up of an unacceptable level of nitrogen in the system.
- A 70-kg adult has approximately 2500–3000 ml nitrogen, of which 1300 ml is dissolved in the body (450 ml in the blood and 850 ml in the fat). The remaining 1200–1700 ml is contained in the FRC.
- With a high initial FGF of 10 l min^{-1}, more than 95% of nitrogen is usually washed out of the FRC and circle in 5 min. Thereafter, nitrogen build-up occurs slowly due to release by tissues.
- If no nitrous oxide is used during anaesthesia, it is not necessary to eliminate nitrogen. A short period of high flow is needed to prime the system and the patient with the inhalational agent.
- Soda lime is capable of absorbing 25 litres carbon dioxide per 100 g. However, in practice, small canisters containing 500 g soda lime appear exhausted with a carbon dioxide load of 10–12 litres per 100 g, and jumbo absorbers containing 2 kg soda lime appear exhausted with a carbon dioxide load of 17 litres per 100 g.
- For closed circuit and low-flow anaesthesia, it is necessary to use a ventilator with the bellows rising during exhalation as it will collapse if there is leak in the system. With the descending type of bellows, any leak in the circuit or bellows may lead to entrainment of driving gas.
- Side-stream gas or vapour monitors remove between 150 and 200 ml min^{-1} of gases from the breathing system for analysis. The sample can either be returned to the system or discarded.

- The absorber granules, usually soda lime, are consumed more rapidly the lower the FGF used. This is because most of the exhaled gases pass through the absorber with very little being discarded through the APL valve.
- Carbon dioxide absorption by the soda lime or baralyme is an exothermic reaction resulting in water vapour formation. The humidity generated by the reaction makes the use of a heat and moisture exchanger unnecessary.

DEGRADATION OF INHALATIONAL AGENTS BY CARBON DIOXIDE ABSORBER

COMPOUND A

Sevoflurane is partly degraded by soda lime, forming a vinyl ether (compound A), which is nephrotoxic in rats. The amount produced is proportional to the sevoflurane concentration and the temperature of the absorber. The latter is higher with lower FGF. Sevoflurane use in humans is safe, although it is advisable that it should not be used with a FGF of less than 1.5 l min^{-1} for more than 3–4 h.

CARBON MONOXIDE

Desflurane and enflurane react with totally dry soda lime or baralyme to produce carbon monoxide. Carbon monoxide is produced when the absorber has been flushed with dry fresh gas for a considerable period of time without being attached to a patient before the agent is used (i.e. dry absorber). Humidity prevents its production.

The new carbon dioxide absorbant, Amsorb, does not contain strong base (sodium and potassium hydroxide) and does not produce compound A or carbon monoxide when used with sevoflurane or desflurane.

MONITORING

- Inspired oxygen
- End-tidal carbon dioxide
- End-tidal nitrous oxide
- End-tidal agent
- End-tidal volume
- End-tidal nitrogen
- Other standard monitoring.

ANAESTHETIC TECHNIQUE

- Intravenous access and monitoring.
- Intravenous or inhalational induction.

- Maintenance of airway with laryngeal mask or tracheal tube.
- High FGF for first three time constants – depends on the volume of the circle system in use and FGF.
- High initial flows are essential for removal of nitrogen and to provide sufficient anaesthetic agent during a period of high uptake.
- Close the circuit.
- Adjust oxygen flow to the calculated oxygen consumption.
- Maintain desired end-tidal anaesthetic concentration by adjusting vaporiser dial setting.
- Adjust oxygen and nitrous oxide flow rates to maintain required oxygen concentration.
- Adjust ventilatory settings to maintain appropriate carbon dioxide level.
- Intermittently increase the FGF:
  —to remove accumulated nitrogen, and
  —to remove other undesired gases, or
  —to change depth of anaesthesia rapidly.

- At the end of anaesthesia switch off anaesthetic gases and increase oxygen flow to begin rapid washout of anaesthetic agents.

BIBLIOGRAPHY

Baum JA, Aitkenhead AR. Low flow anaesthesia. Anaesthesia 1995; 50:37–42

Baxter AD. Low and minimal flow inhalation anaesthesia. Canadian Journal of Anaesthesia 1995; 44:643–652

Mapleson WW. The theoretical ideal fresh-gas flow sequence at the start of low-flow anaesthesia. Anaesthesia 1998; 53:264–272

White DC. Closed and low flow system anaesthesia. Current Anaesthesia and Critical Care 1992; 3:98–107

30

Induced hypotension during anaesthesia

S. Polhill and B. Al-Shaikh

Induced hypotension is usually defined as deliberate and controlled reduction of mean arterial blood pressure (MAP) by at least 20% of the baseline during anaesthesia. It is usually used to decrease blood loss during surgery. A balance between patient safety and improved surgical field with reduced blood loss, and thus reduced blood transfusion requirement, must be attained.

The technique has a reported morbidity rate of 3.3% and a mortality rate of 0.2–0.6%.

An understanding of the physiological factors that control perfusion of the vital organs is essential. Autoregulation can maintain blood flow at a MAP as low as 50–55 mmHg. In hypertensive patients, higher ranges are required.

Hypotension increases ventilation–perfusion mismatch, leading to an increased physiological deadspace.

Bleeding during operation can be:

- *Arterial* – Bleeding is dependent on MAP, which is the major factor in bleeding during surgery. It is dependent on the cardiac output and peripheral resistance. It is also dependent on the vertical height of the surgical site from the aortic root. For each 10-cm elevation, MAP is decreased by 7.5 mmHg.
- *Capillary* – Bleeding that is dependent on the local blood flow in the capillary bed.
- *Venous* – Bleeding that is related to the posture and venous tone.

From Box 30.1, it can be predicted that a reduction in both arterial and venous pressures at the operative site is required to achieve the desired effect.

GENERAL PRINCIPLES

- Administer a smooth anaesthetic with adequate analgesia.
- Ensure a patent airway with good oxygenation and prevent carbon dioxide retention.

BOX 30.1

Indications and contraindications to induced hypotension

Indications

- To reduce excessive blood loss (e.g. major orthopaedic procedures)
- To reduce the risk of vessel rupture (e.g. intracranial aneurysms, aortic dissection, arteriovenous malformations)
- To minimise the need for homologous blood transfusion and its complications
- To improve the surgical field (e.g. plastic, maxillofacial and ENT surgery)

Contraindications

- Cardiovascular instability, hypovolaemia, anaemia
- Severe peripheral or cerebral vascular disease
- Untreated hypertension
- Severe renal, hepatic or respiratory disease
- Diabetes mellitus and glaucoma
- Pregnancy

- Avoid factors that might lead to excessive catecholamine release.
- If the patient is intubated, avoid straining and coughing on the tracheal tube.
- Intermittent positive-pressure ventilation can be used to reduce venous return, cardiac output and blood pressure, and to induce hyperventilation and hypocapnia.
- Adequate premedication is given to reduce circulating levels of catecholamines, avoiding atropine.
- Use an inspired oxygen concentration of 50% or more.

HYPOTENSIVE AGENTS

Reduction of blood pressure can be achieved via various sites of action:

- *Baroreceptor* sensitivity to decreased blood pressure can be reduced by the inhalational agents, such as isoflurane, so reducing the reflex tachycardia.
- *The vasomotor centre* in the CNS is depressed by general anaesthesia, so reducing the sympathetic tone and blood pressure.
- *Preganglionic sympathetic nerves* (from spinal cord levels T1–L2) can be blocked by spinal or extradural analgesia. Vasodilatation of both resistance and capacitance vessels can be achieved.
- *Sympathetic ganglia* can be blocked using ganglion blockers such as trimetaphan or pentolinium. Compensatory tachycardia, tachyphylaxis and histamine release may be encountered with ganglion blockers. Currently, ganglion blockers are not widely used.
- *α-Adrenergic blockers* cause vasodilatation. Phentolamine (5–10 mg i.v.) can be used with a duration of 20–40 min, but there is a reflex tachycardia.
- *β-Adrenergic blockers* decrease heart rate and myocardial contractility. Selective ß₁ blockers are used, such as metoprolol (up to 5 mg i.v.). Esmolol is also suitable and has a rapid onset (1–2 min) and offset (half-life approximately 9 min) and can be given as a slow intravenous bolus of 0.5–2.0 mg kg^{-1} or as an infusion of 25–500 μg kg^{-1} min^{-1}. Owing to its severe cardiac depressant effect, esmolol should not be given as the sole hypotensive agent. Labetalol has α- as well as ß-blocking action. Its ß-blocking action is greater than its α blockade, so preventing the reflex tachycardia due to the α blockade. Labetalol can be given as a bolus of 5–10 mg or by infusion. It has a half-life of about 4 h.
- *Vessel wall* – where the drugs have a direct vasodilating effect. Some drugs act predominantly on the resistance vessels and some on the capacitance vessels:
  —*Sodium nitroprusside (SNP)* is a powerful vasodilator with rapid onset (30 s) and offset (3 min), mainly affecting the resistance vessels. The solution, when prepared, has to be protected from light. Associated problems are reflex tachycardia, increased cerebral blood flow (CBF), rebound hypertension and cyanide toxicity. The maximum safe total dose is 1.5 mg kg^{-1} and an infusion rate of 0.25–1.5 μg kg^{-1} min^{-1}. For prolonged use in the ITU, red cell cyanide levels should be measured.

—*Hydralazine* acts mainly on the resistance vessels, with a duration of action of up to 45 min.
—*Isoflurane* is a powerful vasodilator, mainly on the resistance vessels, with reduced reflex tachycardia and little effect on CBF. Similar results can be achieved with sevoflurane and desflurane.
—*Adenosine* acts on the resistance vessels with a similar degree of hypotension as SNP, but with a more rapid recovery and no rebound hypertension. Problems associated with adenosine are increased CBF and coronary steal effect. Adenosine should be given via a central venous catheter as partial breakdown occurs with peripheral administration.
—*Glyceryl trinitrate (GTN)* acts mainly on the venous system, with a consequent reduction in right atrial filling pressure. The systolic pressure is reduced only moderately, while the diastolic pressure is largely maintained and the coronary vasculature is dilated. Coronary perfusion pressure is therefore maintained or enhanced, making GTN of particular use in treating hypertension associated with cardiac surgery. Problems include raised ICP, reflex tachycardia and resistance to its hypotensive effects. GTN is absorbed into plastics and polypropylene, so a glass syringe and pump should be used.

Prostaglandin E₁ and calcium channel blockers, such as nicardipine, have been used to induce hypotension but are not widely used.

MONITORING

- ECG – ST depression and ectopics indicate inadequate myocardial perfusion.
- Blood pressure – beat-to-beat measurement using an arterial line, with a transducer at the level of the head if in the head-up position. An arterial line also allows for intermittent sampling for blood gas analysis.
- Oxygen saturation – low pressure may lead to loss of signal.
- EtCO₂ – look for hypoventilation and air embolism.
- Blood loss – careful observation is required, as normal compensatory mechanisms to hypovolaemia are lost.
- Temperature – heat is lost more rapidly from dilated skin vessels.
- Bladder catheter to measure urine output should be used in lengthy cases.

30

- Central venous pressure is measured if large fluid losses are anticipated.
- Bispectral index analysis to monitor electrical activity in the brain.
- Biochemistry such as serum electrolyte levels, blood gases and haematocrit.

—myocardial infarction, cardiac failure, cardiac arrest.
- Air embolism in the head-up position
- Increased risk of skin ischaemia and pressure sores.

RECOVERY

- Maintain a clear airway and give oxygen.
- Take care with posture.
- Blood pressure should return to the preoperative level before the patient is discharged to the ward.

COMPLICATIONS

- Inadequate hypotension
- Reactionary haemorrhage, haematoma and DVT
- Excessive hypotension leading to:
  —cerebral ischaemia, thrombosis, oedema
  —acute renal failure

BIBLIOGRAPHY

Boldt J, Weber A, Mailer K et al. Acute normovolaemic haemoglobin vs controlled hypotension for reducing the use of allogenic blood in patients undergoing radical prostatectomy. British Journal of Anaesthesia 1999; 82:170–174

Moss E. Cerebral blood flow during induced hypotension. British Journal of Anaesthesia 1995; 74:635–637

Williams-Russo P, Sharrock NE, Mattis S et al. Randomized trial of hypotensive epidural anesthesia in older adults. Anesthesiology 1999; 91:926–935

Regional anaesthesia techniques

B. Al-Shaikh

In recent years the use of regional anaesthesia has increased, mainly due to the widespread use of nerve stimulators, specially designed regional anaesthesia insulated needles and also a better understanding of the pharmacology of local anaesthetics. Regional anaesthetic techniques are used to block individual nerve(s) or plexuses. Spinal and epidural blocks are discussed in the section above on Epidural and spinal anaesthesia

INDICATIONS

- As the sole anaesthetic technique
- With sedation or general anaesthesia
- To provide analgesia (e.g. postoperative, following fractures).

CONTRAINDICATIONS

ABSOLUTE:
- Patient refusal
- Infection at the site of needle insertion
- Allergy to local anaesthetics – rare with the amides, common with the esters.

RELATIVE:
- Coagulopathy
- Pre-existent unstable neurological deficit
- Lack of patient cooperation.

PREOPERATIVE PREPARATION

- Full patient assessment is carried out with a clear explanation of the procedure, after effects and possible side-effects.
- Adequate resuscitation facilities must be available because of the risk of local anaesthetic toxicity leading to convulsions or cardiac arrhythmias.
- In the event of failure of the local anaesthetic technique, conversion to a general anaesthetic may be required. The patient should therefore be starved,

consented and prepared as for general anaesthesia.

- Intravenous access must be established and monitoring (e.g. ECG, blood pressure, SpO_2) should be connected.
- As there is no need to elicit paraesthesia when nerve stimulators are used, if combined with general anaesthesia, the local anaesthetic block can be done either before or after the induction of general anaesthesia. However, it is advisable to do the block before general anaesthesia is induced to reduce the risk of undetected direct trauma to the nerve tissues.
- Accurate positioning of the patient.
- The site of the block is cleaned. A sterile approach using gloves and no-touch technique is used. For the inexperienced, it is preferable to err on the side of caution and use gowns and drapes.
- Sound knowledge of the potential side-effects of the blocks is essential; for example, interscalene blocks have an almost 100% incidence of phrenic nerve palsy on the affected side. Thus, bilateral interscalene blocks are contraindicated.

NERVE BLOCK NEEDLES

- Short, bevelled (e.g. 45°), blunt needles with a side port for injecting the local anaesthetic solution are used. The bluntness gives a better feedback feel as the needle passes through the different layers of tissues, and minimises the potential trauma to the nerve tissues.
- Most of the needles are insulated with a Teflon coat, leaving an exposed tip. The electric current passes through to the tip only, allowing easier identification of the nerve(s) or plexus.
- 22-G needles are optimal for the vast majority of blocks. The length can vary (e.g. 50, 100 and 150 mm) depending on the depth of the nerve or plexus.

30

- The immobile needle technique is used when large volumes of local anaesthetic solutions are injected for major nerve and plexus blocks. One operator maintains the needle in position, while the second operator, after aspiration, injects the local anaesthetic solution through the side port. This technique reduces the possibility of accidental misplacement and intravascular injection.
- A catheter can be left *in situ*, and boluses or a continuous infusion of local anaesthetic solution used to prolong the duration of the block.

NERVE STIMULATORS

- These battery-operated stimulators are designed to produce visible muscular contractions at a predetermined current and voltage once a nerve plexus or peripheral nerve(s) has been located. Use of a nerve stimulator can increase the success rate of nerve blocks. Nerve stimulators have a linear and constant output.
- The stimulator consists of two leads: one is connected to an ECG skin electrode and the other to the locating needle. The polarities of the leads are clearly indicated and colour coded, with the negative lead being attached to the needle. Less current is needed if the needle is connected to the negative lead.
- A small current (0.25–0.5 mA) is used to stimulate the nerve fibres, causing the motor fibres to contract with a frequency of 1–2 Hz. The stimulus has a short duration (1–2 ms) to generate painless motor contraction. The low currents used stimulate the larger A-α motor fibres more than C pain fibres.
- An initially high current (e.g. 3–5 mA) is used until nerve stimulation is noticed. The current is then reduced until maximal

stimulation is obtained with minimal output (e.g. 0.5 mA), indicating that the tip of the needle is very close to the nerve.
- The stimulation is markedly reduced after only a small volume (about 2 ml) of local anaesthetic solution has been injected. This is due to displacement of the nerve from needle tip.
- Use of the nerve stimulator is not an excuse for not having a sound knowledge of the anatomy required to perform a block.

LOCAL ANAESTHETIC DRUGS

The choice of local anaesthetic drugs depends on:
- Speed of onset
- Potency
- Duration of action
- Sensory–motor differentiation
- Potential toxicity.

Lidocaine (lignocaine), prilocaine, ropivacaine, bupivacaine, *levo*-bupivacaine and etidocaine are some of the amide local anaesthetics that are currently available (Table 30.3):
- Lidocaine and bupivacaine have been used extensively in various regional blocks.
- Prilocaine is the agent of choice for intravenous regional anaesthesia (IVRA). Its metabolite *o*-toluidine may cause methaemoglobinaemia. Methaemoglobinaemia appears as cyanosis when 1.5 g 100 ml^{-1} haemoglobin is in the reduced state. This is rapidly reversed with the intravenous injection of 1 mg kg^{-1} methylthioninium (methylene blue).
- Levo-bupivacaine is a single $S(-)$-isomer of bupivacaine with a similar clinical profile but less systemic toxicity.
- Ropivacaine has better sensory–motor differentiation than bupivacaine, mainly affecting the sensory fibres. This makes it ideal for postoperative analgesia.

TABLE 30.3

Local anaesthetic drugs

	Onset	Duration	Relative potency	Toxicity
Lidocaine	Fast	++	++	++
Prilocaine	Fast	++	++	+
Bupivacaine	Moderate	+++	++++	+++
Levo-bupivacaine	Moderate	+++	++++	++
Ropivacaine	Moderate	+++	++++	++
Etidocaine	Fast	++++	+++	+++

30

- Etidocaine has a rapid onset and very prolonged duration of action. The motor fibres are mainly affected.

VASOCONSTRICTORS

These are added to the local anaesthetic solution to induce vasoconstriction at the site of injection, so slowing the rate of absorption and thus prolonging the duration of action and reducing systemic toxicity. Vasoconstrictors are absolutely contraindicated in blocks near end-arteries, such as ring blocks and penile blocks, and in IVRA due to the risk of ischaemia.

Adrenaline (epinephrine) in a 1 : 200 000 concentration is used. This low concentration is to reduce the systemic side-effects of adrenaline, which are particularly undesirable in patients with cardiovascular disease. If given intravenously, 15 μg adrenaline (3 ml 1 : 200 000) will increase the heart rate by at least 30% within 1 min. 1 : 200 000 adrenaline is useful in combination with lidocaine (lignocaine), reducing the peak concentration in the blood and causing a 50% decrease in the peak plasma concentration when used for subcutaneous infiltration, but a 20–30% decrease when used for intercostal or brachial plexus blocks. Adrenaline (epinephrine) decreases the blood concentration of bupivacaine significantly less than that of lidocaine (lignocaine), so that it is not usually worth using bupivacaine with adrenaline.

Felypressin is a vasoconstrictor with less systemic side-effects than epinephrine. It is mainly used in dental and ENT surgery.

BIBLIOGRAPHY

Fanelli G, Casati A, Garancini P, Torri G. Nerve stimulator and multiple injection technique for upper and lower limb blockade: failure rate, patient acceptance, and neurologic complications. Study Group on Regional Anesthesia. Anesthesia and Analgesia 1999; 88:847–852

McClure JH. Ropivacaine. British Journal of Anaesthesia 1996; 76:300–309

Pither C, Ford D, Raj P. Peripheral nerve stimulation with insulated and uninsulated needles: efficacy of characteristics. Regional Anesthesia 1984; 9:73–77

Pither CE, Raj PP, Ford DJ. The use of peripheral nerve stimulators for regional anesthesia: a review of experimental characteristics. Regional Anesthesia 1985; 10:49–58

Urmey WF, Talts KH, Sharrock N. One hundred percent incidence of hemidiaphragmatic paresis associated with interscalene brachial plexus anesthesia as diagnosed by ultrasonography. Anesthesia and Analgesia 1991; 72:498–503

30

One-lung anaesthesia

A. Addei and S. Stacey

One-lung anaesthesia involves the complete functional separation of the two lungs and is often the most important anaesthetic consideration for patients undergoing thoracic surgery.

INDICATIONS

ABSOLUTE:

- To prevent contamination of one lung by pus, secretions or blood from the contralateral lung.
- To control the distribution of ventilation between the two lungs in the presence of, for example, bronchopleural fistula, ruptured bulla or surgical opening of major airway.
- Bronchopulmonary lavage, for instance for alveolar proteinosis.

RELATIVE:

- To facilitate surgical exposure, for example in oesophageal surgery, descending thoracic aneurysm, thoracic spinal surgery. Many thoracic procedures can be accomplished with a normal tracheal tube.

TECHNIQUES OF LUNG SEPARATION

- Double-lumen tube, such as Robertshaw (red rubber), Bronchocath (PVC) – allows rapid transition between one- and two-lung ventilation; either lung can be suctioned and continuous positive airway pressure (CPAP) can be applied to the non-ventilated lung.
- Bronchial blockers (e.g. Cook Arndt Endobronchial blocker, Univent tube) – cannot ventilate distal to the blocker.
- Uncut tracheal tube – can be advanced into the relevant main bronchus; not ideal, but useful in an emergency.

PHYSIOLOGICAL EFFECTS OF THE LATERAL DECUBITUS POSITION

Owing to the combined effects of general anaesthesia, positive-pressure ventilation and the lateral decubitus position and open chest during thoracotomy, there will be considerable V/Q mismatch.

During thoracotomy, the compliance of the dependent lung is reduced and the upper lung is therefore ventilated preferentially. The effect of gravity on the low-pressure pulmonary circulation increases blood flow to the lower lung. With the onset of one-lung ventilation, the preferential distribution of ventilation to the upper lung is eliminated completely. Perfusion to this lung continues, resulting in increased shunting. At this stage the dependent lung receives the entire minute volume and a high proportion (about 60%) of the cardiac output.

Hypoxic pulmonary vasoconstriction increases the pulmonary vascular resistance of the collapsed lung. However, its effects, and the effects of anaesthetic agents on it, are usually of little clinical importance in routine thoracic practice.

PREOPERATIVE ASSESSMENT AND INVESTIGATIONS

- Full blood count; urea and electrolytes (e.g. reduced Na^+ in patients with syndrome of inappropriate antidiuretic hormone secretion – SIADH)
- Chest radiography – it is important to assess the anatomy of the airways to see whether endobronchial intubation is possible. Often, computed tomography of the thorax is also available
- Arterial blood gases
- Pulmonary function tests
- ECG.

30

PERIOPERATIVE MANAGEMENT

MONITORING:
- ECG
- Sao_2
- Fio_2, $Etco_2$, end-tidal for agent
- Airway inflation pressure, flow–volume loops are also useful
- Blood pressure – ideally measured via arterial cannulation on the dependent side, which also allows for sampling for arterial blood gas analysis
- Fluid balance and blood loss
- Core temperature
- Central venous pressure
- Nerve stimulator to assess neuromuscular function
- Central venous cannulation should ideally be performed on the same side as the thoracotomy to minimise the risk of pneumothorax to the dependent lung.

ANAESTHETIC TECHNIQUE:
- Premedication is by no means mandatory and the type, if any, will depend largely on the patient and the mode of postoperative analgesia chosen.
- Give general anaesthesia – total intravenous anaesthesia (TIVA) or inhalational agent – with muscle relaxation and controlled ventilation, usually through a double-lumen tube.

DOUBLE-LUMEN TUBES

Robertshaw double-lumen endobronchial tubes are available in three sizes (small, medium and large). The PVC derivative (Bronchocath) is more malleable, but also more likely to migrate peroperatively and to suffer cuff damage by teeth during insertion. The PVC tubes are available in a wide range of right and left sizes: Ch 41, 39, 37, 35, (32 and 28 left only). Care must be taken not to overdistend the bronchial cuff, as bronchial rupture may be catastrophic.

The right main bronchus gives rise to the right upper lobe bronchus after 2.5 cm. Right-sided endobronchial tube placement should be avoided where possible because of the high risk of right upper lobe occlusion.

The correct positioning of a double-lumen tube is traditionally confirmed by observation of chest expansion and auscultation while each lumen in turn is occluded. However, reliance on clinical signs alone will miss a significant number of malpositioned tubes. The National Confidential Enquiry into Perioperative Deaths (1998) highlighted the morbidity and mortality associated with malpositioned double-lumen tubes. The use of a flexible fibreoptic broncho-scope allows direct visual confirmation of tube position and is now the method of choice.

ARTERIAL HYPOXAEMIA

This is one of the most important problems encountered during one-lung anaesthesia. The elimination of carbon dioxide during one-lung ventilation is not a problem if the minute volume is maintained at the amount previously delivered to the two lungs. Two-lung anaes-thesia should be maintained for as long as possible.

MANAGEMENT OF HYPOXAEMIA DURING ONE-LUNG VENTILATION
- Increase inspired oxygen up to 100%.
- Check position of double-lumen tube with fibreoptic bronchoscope. Suctioning of secretions may be required.
- Ensure adequate blood pressure and cardiac output.
- Maintain positive end-expiratory pressure (PEEP) of 5–10 cmH$_2$O to the dependent lung to decrease atelectasis and increase functional residual capacity. Excessive PEEP increases pulmonary vascular resistance and may increase shunting.
- Maintain CPAP of 5–10 cmH$_2$O with 100% oxygen to the non-ventilated lung to facilitate oxygen uptake in this lung while not adversely affecting the surgical condition.
- Abandon one-lung ventilation and intermittently ventilate the collapsed lung after warning the surgeon.
- Early clamping of the appropriate pulmonary artery will stop the shunt.

POSTOPERATIVE PERIOD

Adequate pain relief, physiotherapy and high-dependency care are important factors for reducing the incidence of postoperative com-plications and hospital stay.

30

BIBLIOGRAPHY

Eastwood J, Mahajan R. One-lung anaesthesia. British Journal of Anaesthesia CEPD Reviews 2002; 2:83–87

Gothard JW. Thoracic anaesthesia. Baillière's Clinical Anaesthesiology, vol 1. London: Baillière Tindall; 1987.

Gothard JWW, Branthwaite MA. Anaesthesia for thoracic surgery. Oxford: Blackwell Scientific

Pennefather SH, Russell GN. Placement of double lumen tubes – time to shed light on an old problem (editorial). British Journal of Anaesthesia 2000; 84:308–311

Sherry K. Management of patients undergoing oesophagectomy. In: Gray AJG, Hoile RW, Ingram GS, Sherry KM, eds. The Rrport of the National Confidential Enquiry into Perioperative Deaths 1996/1997. London: NCEPOD; 1998:57–61

Vaughan RS. Double-lumen tubes (editorial). British Journal of Anaesthesia 1993; 70:497–498

30

Prolonged anaesthesia

U. Akhigbe and B. Al-Shaikh

Various problems are associated with prolonged anaesthesia. Adequate preparation, good management and close attention to detail may reduce the associated risks. Prolonged anaesthesia contributes to perioperative complications, which in turn may lead to delayed hospital discharge.

PROBLEMS ASSOCIATED WITH PROLONGED ANAESTHESIA

- Accumulation of anaesthetic agents leading to delayed emergence. This depends on the drug's total tissue uptake, which is related to drug solubility and the average concentration used.
- Potential toxicity of administered agents:
  —*Inhalational agents* – degradation of inhalational agents by carbon dioxide absorber may lead to accumulation of toxins. Sevoflurane is partly degraded by soda lime, forming a vinyl ether (compound A) that is nephrotoxic in rats. Although problems have not been noted in clinical practice, the United States Food and Drug Administration recommends the use of sevoflurane with a fresh gas flow rate of at least 2 l min^{-1} for procedures lasting more than 1 h. Inorganic fluoride production due to the hepatic metabolism of sevoflurane and enflurane may be nephrotoxic in patients with chronic renal impairment.
  —*Nitrous oxide* – prolonged exposure may result in acute vitamin B$_{12}$ deficiency with megaloblastic anaemia and neurological deficit. Nitrous oxide oxidises cobalamin, which inactivates methionine synthetase resulting in decreased methionine production. Toxic manifestations may occur in susceptible individuals after shorter exposures. Risk of nitrous oxide toxicity is increased in pernicious anaemia, exposure to DNA synthesis inhibitors (e.g. methotrexate),

pre-existing bone marrow depression, folate deficiency, diseases of the ileum and malabsorption (e.g. Crohn's disease). Nitrous oxide also causes expansion of air spaces (e.g. pneumothorax).
- Impairment of gas exchange and respiratory mechanics secondary to dependent atelectasis.
- Problems with accurate management of fluid and electrolyte balance.
- Hypothermia leading to increased wound infection, surgical bleeding, impaired immune function and increased incidence of myocardial infarction and malignant arrhythmias.
- Prolonged immobility can lead to:
  —increased risk of DVT
  —nerve damage and pressure sores
  —rhabdomyolysis
  —corneal damage if eyes are left open.
- Postoperative delirium.
- Immunosuppression and increased susceptibility to infection.
- Increased opportunity for human error due to fatigue.

PREPARATION

- Staffing level, patient supports and padding for pressure areas.
- Adequate scavenging – recommended maximum accepted concentrations over an 8-h time-weighted period in the UK are:
  —100 parts per million (p.p.m.) for nitrous oxide
  —50 p.p.m. for enflurane and isoflurane
  —10 p.p.m. for halothane.
- Low-flow circuit system.
- Maintenance of body temperature (appropriate selection of theatre temperature, forced air warmer, warming blanket, fluid warmers, humidification of inspired gases, clothing and limb wrapping, hat). Forced air warmers have been found to

30

be the most effective, even when applied to a limited surface area of body.

MONITORING

- ECG
- Sao_2
- Direct blood pressure
- Core and skin temperature
- Blood loss
- Bispectral index analysis
- Tracheal tube cuff pressure
- Peripheral nerve stimulator
- Blood gases (temperature corrected), electrolytes, glucose, coagulation
- Pressure–volume loop and lung compliance
- Inspiratory and expired concentration of oxygen, nitrous oxide, anaesthetic vapour and carbon dioxide concentration
- Fluid balance – central venous pressure, hourly urine output via urinary catheter.

ANAESTHETIC TECHNIQUE

The technique chosen is dependent on the operation proposed, anticipated blood loss and the chronic health status of the patient. Controlled ventilation provides the ability to manipulate oxygenation and carbon dioxide. There have been case reports of healthy patients having prolonged surgery on the extremities breathing spontaneously via a laryngeal mask for 8 h with no adverse effect. Regional anaesthesia may be used as the sole anaesthetic technique for surgery on the lower extremities, but the prolonged immobilisation often necessitates light general anaesthesia or sedation for patient comfort.

- Consider using an oxygen–air technique, omitting nitrous oxide with minimal FiO$_2$ to

achieve an acceptable oxygen saturation or tension.

- Consider TIVA or TCI.
- Give muscle relaxants by infusion (e.g. atracurium) with guidance from train-of-four.
- Use a high-volume low-pressure cuff with regular tracheal tube suctioning.
- Pay careful attention to body positioning with frequent repositioning of the head.
- Cover exposed body surfaces.
- Eye protection – lubrication, tapes, padding or eye shields.
- DVT prophylaxis – thromboembolism deterrent (TED) stockings, heparin and mechanical calf compression.
- Use a team of staff to avoid fatigue.

POSTOPERATIVE CARE

Consider:
- ITU or HDU stay for continued ventilation until warm and stable; awaken slowly
- Regular physiotherapy
- Maintenance of DVT prophylaxis
- Ensure adequate fluid input and output.

BIBLIOGRAPHY

Brimacombe J, Shorney N. The laryngeal mask airway and prolonged balanced regional anaesthesia. Canadian Journal of Anaesthesia 1993; 40:360–364

Girgis Y, Broome IJ. Monitoring failure and awareness hazard during prolonged surgery. Anaesthesia 1997; 52:504–505

Higuchi H, Sumikura H, Sumita S et al. Renal function in patients with high serum fluoride concentration after prolonged sevoflurane anesthesia. Anesthesiology 1995; 83:449–458

30

Total intravenous anaesthesia

B. Al-Shaikh

TIVA is a technique whereby general anaesthesia is induced and maintained using one (or more) drugs administered intravenously. A continuous intravenous infusion is usually used. Inhalational anaesthetic agents are not used.

CHARACTERISTICS OF THE IDEAL AGENT

- Soluble in water and stable for the duration of the infusion with no deterioration on exposure to light
- Long shelf-life
- No absorption into plastic
- Induces anaesthesia in one arm–brain circulation time
- Analgesic properties
- No side-effects on injection – pain, thrombophlebitis, anaphylactic or anaphylactoid reactions
- Not irritant if injected extravascularly
- No adverse effects on major organ systems
- No epileptiform movements
- No major interaction with other anaesthetic drugs
- Rapid metabolism and elimination, through different pathways to ameliorate accumulation of drug or metabolites
- Rapid recovery without hangover or nausea.

Both hypnosis and analgesia can be achieved using an intravenous technique. At present, propofol is the hypnotic of choice for TIVA. Analgesia can be achieved using the newer synthetic short-acting opioids, such as alfentanil and the μ-opioid receptor agonist remifentanil. More recently, target-controlled infusion (TCI) has been widely used, although TIVA can also be achieved using intermittent bolus injection or manual infusion techniques.

TIVA must achieve the following goals: smooth induction, reliable and titratable maintenance, and rapid emergence. Achieving these has been possible with TCI.

TARGET-CONTROLLED INFUSION

Sophisticated TCI syringe drivers incorporating real-time pharmacokinetic models, such as the Diprifusor, that deliver the appropriate dose of the drug to achieve and maintain the requested target concentration are used. For this to be achieved, the appropriate infusion rates required to produce the target concentration are calculated continuously by the microprocessor within the syringe driver. Anaesthesia is induced by the syringe driver infusing propofol very rapidly, which is equivalent to a slow bolus. This is followed by a progressively decreasing infusion rate. To increase the target plasma concentration further, the syringe driver delivers another bolus to achieve the desired concentration and then maintains that. To decrease the target plasma concentration, the syringe driver stops infusing until the microprocessor calculates that the new target has been achieved and then maintains it. The predicted concentration in the brain, which is displayed on the syringe driver, increases much slower than that in the plasma. Rapid infusion rates of propofol achieve unconsciousness sooner, but increase the incidence of cardiovascular and respiratory depression.

With the Diprifusor, the anaesthetist enters the age and weight of the patient and selects the desired target plasma concentration. Prefilled 50-ml syringes with propofol in a 1% or 2% concentration are used. Propofol TCI allows easy control and rapid change of the propofol plasma concentration. In adults under the age of 55 years, a target propofol concentration of 4–8 μg ml^{-1} is usually adequate for the induction of anaesthesia. Induction is smooth and usually takes 60–120 s. Co-administering an analgesic, anaesthesia can be maintained using propofol concentrations of 3–6 μg ml^{-1}. Lower target concentrations are used in elderly patients, reducing the risks of side-effects. Currently, propofol TCI is not licensed for children under the age of 16 years, because of their different pharmacokinetic profile.

30

MANUAL INFUSION TECHNIQUE

This can be achieved by a bolus dose for induction using a syringe driver with a rapid bolus facility. Anaesthesia is maintained using a step-down sequence of infusion rates. A popular method is to administer propofol 10 mg kg^{-1} h^{-1} for 10 min, 8 mg kg^{-1} h^{-1} for 10 min, and 6 mg kg^{-1} h^{-1} thereafter. Another method is to administer a constant maintenance infusion rate of about 6 mg kg^{-1} h^{-1}. The plasma propofol concentration might be low initially with the constant infusion rate technique.

The manually intermittent technique leads to wide variations and fluctuations in plasma concentrations and anaesthetic effects.

The majority of anaesthetists prefer to use the TCI system, owing to its simplicity and reliability.

ANALGESIA

As propofol has no analgesic properties, TIVA is generally achieved by combining a propofol infusion with a regional local anaesthetic block or supplemental opioids.

The shorter-acting opioids are often suggested as an ideal complement to propofol. Of these, alfentanil and remifentanil are widely used. Remifentanil has a unique metabolic and pharmacokinetic profile. It undergoes rapid methyl esterase hydrolysis by tissues and plasma esterases (not plasma cholinesterases) to relatively inactive metabolites. Its effect is terminated by rapid metabolic clearance rather than redistribution (elimination half-time 10 min), resulting in rapid reduction in plasma concentration even after prolonged infusion. The time required for the drug concentration to fall by 50% is always the same (about 2 min). This is independent of age, weight, sex, or hepatic and renal function (context insensitive), making remifentanil ideal for a continuous intravenous technique. As a rule, it is preferable to maintain the opioid infusion within the steep section of the dose–response curve and to adjust anaesthetic depth by altering propofol infusion.

When propofol and alfentanil are administered together, alfentanil can increase the concentration of propofol by 20% because of its effect on clearance and redistribution. Alfentanil concentration can be increased by propofol, possibly due to the inhibition of oxidative phosphorylation of alfentanil via cytochrome P$_{450}$. Similar interaction can happen with other opioids.

The addition of nitrous oxide decreases hypnotic requirements during TIVA; 67% nitrous oxide decreases propofol requirements by about 25%.

Propofol is cleared from the body mainly by metabolism. It has been successfully used in patients with liver cirrhosis, and the pharmacokinetics are not significantly affected by the disease. The pharmacokinetics of propofol may be influenced by age. Values for clearance and plasma concentration on awakening are higher in children than in adults. Children require significantly higher doses of propofol than adults do.

The rapid recovery from propofol is due to its short distribution phase, high clearance rate and short elimination half-life.

DOSE–RESPONSE RELATIONSHIP

To compare TIVA with inhalational anaesthesia, CP50$_m$, similar to the MAC, is the measured plasma concentration required to prevent 50% of patients from responding to painful stimuli.

The bispectral index analysis (BIS) has been shown to be a reliable tool to monitor the effect of the drugs on the brain during TIVA.

USES OF TIVA

TIVA has been used successfully in a wide range of operations, including cardiac and intracranial procedures (propofol increases cerebral compliance). TIVA is potentially useful when inhalational anaesthesia is difficult or contraindicated, for instance in rigid bronchoscopy or malignant hyperthermia susceptibility. TCI has also been successfully used for sedation in a variety of procedures.

ADVANTAGES OF TIVA

- Avoiding the use of nitrous oxide with its effect on air emboli and pneumothoraces, bone marrow suppression
- Elimination of volatile agents and their possible toxicity to the liver and kidney, and their effect on the uterus
- Elimination of the need for accurately calibrated vaporisers
- Superior quality recovery with less hangover
- Propofol is a powerful antiemetic.

DISADVANTAGES

- Pharmacokinetic and pharmacodynamic variability of response to the injected drug

- Variations in the haemodynamic state of the patient
- Propofol may be associated with bradycardia and convulsions.

BIBLIOGRAPHY

Campbell L, Engbers FH, Kenny GNC. Total intravenous anaesthesia. CPD Anaesthesia 2001; 3:109–119

Petrie J, Glass P. Intravenous anaesthetics. Current Opinion in Anaesthesiology 2001; 14:393–397

30

31

MANAGEMENT PROBLEMS
B. J. Pollard

31

Allergic reaction

T. Strang and D. O'Connor

Allergic reactions are unpredictable life-threatening events. Prompt recognition and treatment are essential. The incidence of anaphylaxis is between 1 : 4500 and 1 : 20 000 anaesthetics. The estimated mortality rate is 5%.

When associated with anaesthesia, the causative agents are commonly:

- Neuromuscular blockers, especially suxamethonium (50–70%)
- Latex (notably risen in recent years) (> 10%)
- Antibiotics
- Induction agents
- Colloids
- Opioids
- Radiocontrast media.

PATHOPHYSIOLOGY

Anaphylactic and anaphylactoid reactions are clinically indistinguishable (Fig. 31.1). The terms refer to the triggering pathway responsible for the final common endpoint, i.e. the release of potent circulating inflammatory mediators from degranulated mast cells.

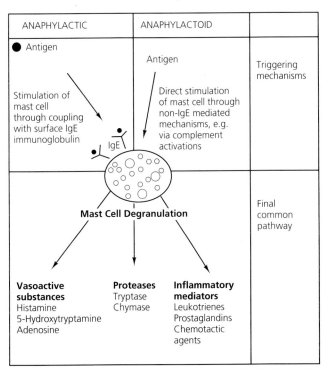

ANAPHYLACTIC	ANAPHYLACTOID	
● Antigen	Antigen	Triggering mechanisms
Stimulation of mast cell through coupling with surface IgE immunoglobulin	Direct stimulation of mast cell through non-IgE mediated mechanisms, e.g. via complement activations	
Mast Cell Degranulation		Final common pathway
Vasoactive substances Histamine 5-Hydroxytryptamine Adenosine	**Proteases** Tryptase Chymase **Inflammatory mediators** Leukotrienes Prostaglandins Chemotactic agents	

Fig. 31.1 Immune mechanisms of anaphylactic and anaphylactoid reactions. The 'antigen' refers to the drug or substance responsible for activating the triggering mechanism. In some cases, for example penicillin, binding to a hapten (carrier protein) is necessary prior to coupling with surface membrane IgE antibody.

31

Anaphylactic reactions involve cross-linking of two adjacent IgE antigen-specific antibodies to the mast cell surface, causing a type I hypersensitivity reaction.

Reactions caused by any other triggering pathways are, therefore, anaphylactoid, as in anaesthetic drug mixtures causing 'aggregate anaphylaxis'.

In many cases, previous sensitisation to the antigen or similar compound cannot be demonstrated.

SIGNIFICANT CLINICAL FEATURES

When associated with anaesthesia, symptoms often occur rapidly but may not manifest until after 30 min in the case of anaphylaxis to latex.
- Profound hypotension or cardiac arrest may be seen in up to 88% of cases.
- Hypoxia:
  —inability to ventilate
  —bronchospasm
  —laryngeal oedema.
- Urticarial or erythematous rashes feature more prominently in the out-of-hospital setting.

PRIMARY TREATMENT (AS ADVISED BY THE AAGBI):

- Discontinue administration of suspected agent.
- Maintain airway. Give 100% oxygen.
- Elevate legs to increase venous return.
- Give adrenaline (epinephrine):
  —intravenously, 1 ml of 1 : 10 000 (0.1 mg) over 1 min, repeat as necessary (note mini-jet syringes are latex free), *or*
  —intramuscularly, 1 ml of 1 : 1000 (1 mg) repeated as necessary every 10 min.
- Start intravenous fluid resuscitation with colloid or crystalloid.

SECONDARY TREATMENT

- Chlorpheniramine 10–20 mg i.v.
- Hydrocortisone 100–300 mg i.v.
- Adrenaline (epinephrine) infusion 0.05–0.1 $\mu g\ kg^{-1}\ min^{-1}$ (i.e. 10–20 ml h^{-1} of 1 mg in 50 ml solution for a 70-kg person)
- Consider sodium bicarbonate
- Consider bronchodilators (aminophylline, salbutamol)
- Airway evaluation (before extubation).

FURTHER INVESTIGATION

- Investigations should not be undertaken at the expense of resuscitation.
- Detailed written record of events is important in establishing the diagnosis.
- Approximately 1 h after onset take 10 ml venous blood and store at − 20°C. Released mast cell tryptase indicates that a reaction has taken place: raised for up to 6 h after cell degranulation in 70% of cases.
- The anaesthetist is responsible for providing advice to the patient and for ensuring appropriate follow-up takes place.
- Seek advice from a specialist in allergy and clinical immunology as further investigation is required.
- See useful addresses for Committee on Safety of Medicines (CSM), Medic-Alert and Immunology Society websites.
- Commonly, skin prick tests are performed with a range of drugs at concentrations of 1 in 10–1000 several weeks after the acute episode and after discontinuation of antihistamines (false negatives occur).
- Radio-allergosorbent (RAST) tests are available for suxamethonium, latex and penicillins. A morphine-based solid immunoassay has been developed to act as a highly sensitive generic marker for non-depolarising muscle relaxant allergy. As yet, screening is not advised by the AABGI.

LATEX ALLERGY

There has been an increasing incidence of latex allergy over the past 20 years especially in certain population groups with previous repeated exposure to latex:
- Spina bifida (60% – repeated urethral catheterisation)
- History of numerous surgical procedures
- Gynaecological procedures
- Healthcare workers (10%)
- General population (0.7%).

HISTORY OF LATEX ALLERGY:
- Reactivity to party balloons, barrier contraceptives, dentist's gloves
- Cross-reactivity to certain foods – banana, kiwi, chestnut, avocado
- Positive investigation – serological tests, skin prick, intradermal.

Sensitivity to latex may vary from contact dermatitis to anaphylaxis. Anaphylaxis may occur via any route but is more likely after intravenous or direct mucosal exposure.

MANAGEMENT OF THE PATIENT WITH LATEX ALLERGY

- Provision of a latex-free environment is the most important management strategy.
- Preoperative immunological testing may be helpful in selected cases but false negatives occur.
- Consider premedication with chlorpheniramine, ranitidine, hydrocortisone.
- Put the patient first on the morning operating list to minimise exposure to airborne antigens.
- Communicate risks to other anaesthetic, nursing and surgical staff.
- Check that *all* equipment is latex free, especially gloves (all staff), face-masks, reservoir bag, syringes and drip injection ports.
- Departments should have a management protocol and a designated box of latex-free equipment available (for suggested contents see Dakin & Yentis 1998, Farley & Jones 2002)
- Monitor after operation for up to 1 h for delayed reactions
- Vigilance and full resuscitation resources are essential.

BIBLIOGRAPHY

Association of Anaesthetists of Great Britain and Ireland and British Society of Allergy and Clinical Immunology. Suspected anaphylactic reactions associated with anaesthesia. Revised edn. London: AAGBI; 1995

Clarke RSJ, Watkins J. Drugs responsible for anaphylactic reactions in anaesthesia in the United Kingdom. Annales Françaises d'Anesthesie et de Réamination 1993; 12:105–108

Dakin MJ, Yentis SM. Latex allergy: a strategy for management. Anaesthesia 1998; 53:774–781

Farley CA, Jones HM. Latex allergy. British Journal of Anaesthesia CEPD Reviews 2002; 2(1)

Fisher M. Anaphylaxis to anaesthetic drugs: aetiology, recognition and management. Current Anaesthesia and Critical Care 1991; 2:182–186

Lieberman P. Anaphylactic reactions during surgical and medical procedures. Journal of Allergy and Clinical Immunology 2002; 110:S64–S69

Poley GE Jr, Slater JE. Latex allergy. Journal of Allergy and Clinical Immunology 2000; 105:1054–1062

USEFUL WEBSITES

British Society of Allergy and Clinical Immunology: http://www.bsaci.org/

Committee on Safety of Medicines (CSM). Yellow Card scheme. Online. Available: http://www.mca.gov.uk

Medic-Alert Foundation: http://www.medicalert.org.uk

31

Amniotic fluid embolism

M. Alveraz and E. L. Horsman

Amniotic fluid embolism (AFE) is the syndrome that occurs when amniotic fluid gains entry into the maternal circulation. It may be the composition of the amniotic fluid that determines the severity of the pathological events comprising the syndrome. The syndrome has similarities to anaphylaxis and septic shock, and the same mediators may be involved. Interestingly, in primate models clear autologous amniotic fluid had no clinical effect when injected into the maternal circulation (Adamsons et al 1971).

AFE has a quoted mortality rate of between 61% and 86%, and in the Triennial United Kingdom Maternal Mortality Reports was the third most common cause of maternal death in 1994–1996 and the fifth commonest cause in 1997–1999. Relying only on mortality statistics and case reports, the true incidence is unknown with estimates ranging from 1 in 8000 to 1 in 80 000. When clinical criteria as well as autopsy proof was used, more than 10% of maternal mortality in the USA was due to this condition. National registers, such as those kept by Clark in the USA and Tufnell in the UK, should more lead to more accurate statistics in the future.

AFE occurs most commonly during labour, but has been associated with the list of events shown in Box 31.1.

BOX 31.1

Aetiological factors in AFE

- Dilatation and curettage
- Termination of pregnancy
- Intra-amniotic saline
- Amniocentesis
- Amniotomy
- Induction of labour
- Insertion of prostaglandin gel
- Lower uterine segment, cervical and vaginal tears
- Caesarean section
- Uterine rupture

Morgan, in his 1979 review of AFE, effectively refuted the association between AFE and tumultuous labour, oxytocin augmentation of labour, traumatic delivery, large babies and fetal death preceding AFE. Recently it has been suggested that amniotic fluid containing meconium and the presence of a male fetus influence the severity of the response to AFE.

CLINICAL PRESENTATION

The three main maternal features of AFE are:
- Cardiorespiratory problems
- Convulsions
- Haematological problems.

These may be accompanied by fetal distress.

CARDIORESPIRATORY PROBLEMS

The classical presentation is at or around delivery with the symptoms and signs of severe cardiorespiratory collapse (Box 31.2). From case reports where patients have survived long enough to have a pulmonary flotation catheter inserted, the picture has been one of left ventricular heart failure with raised left ventricular end-diastolic pressure (LVEDP) and increased pulmonary capillary wedge pressure (PCWP). These measurements validate the clinical and radiographic picture of pulmonary oedema, which occurs in many of the 50–75% of patients who survive the initial cardiopulmonary collapse. Whether, as previously thought, severe intrapulmonary shunting, pulmonary hypertension and right heart failure precede, or even precipitate, the documented left heart failure is unproven. There is evidence of release of a potent vasoconstrictor in AFE, which may be responsible for pulmonary, coronary and, perhaps, systemic vasoconstriction. It has been suggested that endothelin may be the vasoconstrictor.

CONVULSIONS

Convulsions due to cerebral hypoxaemia or hypotension may delay the diagnosis of AFE because of confusion with eclampsia.

BOX 31.2

Cardiorespiratory symptoms and signs

- Dyspnoea
- Hypoxia
- Hypotension
- Convulsions
- Bronchospasm
- Arrhythmias
- Cardiac arrest
- Fetal bradycardia

HAEMATOLOGICAL PROBLEMS

Coagulopathy accompanying cardiorespiratory collapse, following cardiorespiratory collapse or occurring without cardiorespiratory symptoms or signs, is the other main feature of AFE. The coagulopathy may be obvious as severe vaginal haemorrhage or as severe haemorrhage during caesarean section, and may be compounded by uterine atony. Activation of the extrinsic pathway of the clotting cascade by fetal antigens or trophoblastic tissue exerting a thromboplastin-like effect is possibly the trigger. Occasionally, AFE has to be included in the differential diagnosis when abnormal bleeding occurs from wounds or intravenous access sites without preceding evidence of AFE. In 40% of patients with AFE there is evidence of coagulopathy, and this should be anticipated if the diagnosis of AFE has been made.

TREATMENT

CARDIAC ARREST

Commence the cardiac arrest algorithm with lateral tilt where appropriate.

HYPOXIA OR HYPOTENSION WITHOUT CARDIAC ARREST:

- Avoid aortocaval compression by lateral tilt where appropriate.
- Administer 100% oxygen; where appropriate intubate and ventilate.
- Site a large-bore cannula. If the patient is hypotensive give colloid rapidly and inotropes (dopamine) and/or vasoconstrictors (phenylephrine) as indicated depending on availability.
- Undertake full monitoring including, if possible, an arterial line
- Site a central venous pressure cannula or pulmonary flotation catheter if available.

- Manipulate fluids and cardiovascular drugs according to haemodynamic measurements including diuretics if there is evidence of pulmonary oedema.
- Deliver the fetus if still *in utero*. Although a 79% fetal survival rate has been reported, the survival rate of a neurologically intact infant is around 39%.
- Transfer to the ITU.

COAGULOPATHY:

- Take blood for a full coagulation screen, including platelets.
- Inform the haematology laboratory of the problem.
- Give fresh frozen plasma, platelets, cryoprecipitate and concentrated red cells, depending on clotting results and blood loss. Haematological advice should be sought before the use of serine protease inhibitors or heparin.
- Give oxytocics if uterine atony is present, syntocinon intravenously, ergometrine intravenously, or prostaglandin $E_1\alpha$ by intramuscular or intrauterine injection.

OTHER REPORTED TREATMENTS:

- Cardiopulmonary bypass and pulmonary thrombectomy
- Nitric oxide and inhaled aerosol prostacyclin to treat refractory hypoxaemia
- Extracorporeal membrane oxygenation and intra-aortic balloon counterpulsation.

CONFIRMATION OF DIAGNOSIS

ANTEMORTEM LABORATORY DIAGNOSIS OF AFE

In 1947, Gross & Benz reported that centrifuged blood obtained from the right heart of patients with AFE showed three strata rather than two, and that this was pathognomic of AFE. They also advocated looking at sections of smears of this 'flocculent' layer for mucus and squames. In 1985, Masson & Ruggieri described a new diagnostic application of the pulmonary artery catheter to obtain microvascular blood and demonstrated the presence of fetal squames in suspected AFE. However, Clark et al (1986) advocated caution when they showed that squames could be demonstrated in both pregnant and non-pregnant patients. Meticulous technique using the correct stain and evidence of other amniotic fluid debris such as mucin, hair and fat droplets should be obtained to validate the

31

diagnosis of AFE. More recently, two studies by the Japanese workers Kanayama et al (1992) and Kobayashi et al (1993) described an estimation of plasma zinc co-proporphyrin, a component of meconium, and a monoclonal antibody technique to detect mucin-like glycoproteins in maternal serum. A significantly raised concentration of such antigens was found in four patients with symptoms suggestive of AFE.

POST-MORTEM DIAGNOSIS OF AFE

The presence of amniotic fluid debris, squames, lanugo hair and mucin on sectioning of lung specimens is the cornerstone of the diagnosis of AFE.

DIFFERENTIAL DIAGNOSIS

See Box 31.3.

BOX 31.3

Differential diagnosis of AFE

- Local anaesthetic toxicity
- Transfusion reaction
- Other emboli
- Septic shock
- Myocardial infarction
- Anaphylaxis
- Eclampsia
- Placental abruption
- Uterine rupture

31

BIBLIOGRAPHY

Adamsons K, Mueller-Heubach E, Myer RE. The innocuousness of amniotic fluid infusion in the pregnant rhesus monkey. American Journal of Obstetrics and Gynecology 1971; 109:977–984

Clark SL. New concepts of amniotic fluid embolism: a review. Obstetrical and Gynaecological Survey 1990; 45:360–368

Clark SL, Pavlova Z, Greenspoon J. Squamous cells in the maternal pulmonary circulation. American Journal of Obstetrics and Gynecology 1986; 154:104–106

Clark SL, Hankins GDV, Dudley DA, Dildy GA, Porter TF. Amniotic fluid embolism: analysis of the national registry. American Journal of Obstetrics and Gynecology 1995; 172:1158–1169

Davies S. Amniotic fluid embolism: a review of the literature. Canadian Journal of Anesthesia 2001; 48:88–98

Gross P, Benz EJ. Pulmonary embolism by amniotic fluid. Surgery, Gynecology and Obstetrics 1947; 85:315–320

Kanayama N, Ohi H, Tereo T. Determining zinc coproporphyrin in maternal plasma—a new method for diagnosing amniotic fluid embolism. Clinical Chemistry 1992; 38:526–529

Kobayashi H, Yamazaki T, Naruse H, Sumimoto K, Horiuchi K, Terao T. A simple non-invasive sensitive method for diagnosis of amniotic fluid embolism by monoclonal antibody TKH-2. American Journal of Obstetrics and Gynecology 1993; 168:848–853

Masson RG, Ruggieri J. Pulmonary microvascular cytology. A new diagnostic application of the pulmonary artery catheter. Chest 1985; 88:908–914

Morgan M. Amniotic fluid embolism. Anaesthesia 1979; 34:20–32

Tuffnell DJ, Johnson H. Amniotic fluid embolism: the UK register. Symposium on Obstetrics and Gynaecology. Hospital Medicine 2000; 61(8):532–534

Awareness

C. J. D. Pomfrett

DEFINITION

- The patient remembers part or all of the anaesthetic or surgical procedure.
- Recall of specific words or sounds in the operating room will distinguish awareness from hallucination or dreaming.
- A low incidence of awareness may be accompanied by unbearable pain and give rise to postoperative psychological trauma, and litigation.
- Recall may be explicit, when the patient is capable of speaking of the event, or implicit, where subconscious learning during anaesthesia surfaces as a behavioural change, sometimes after a considerable time delay. Implicit recall may be studied by means of postoperative hypnosis of the patient, or recall of key words or phrases.

RECOLLECTION

Events recalled may be many if the patient is aware (Table 31.1). Auditory stimuli are most

TABLE 31.1

Events recalled under anaesthesia

Event	%	Sample size
Sounds	89	23
Paralysis	85	22
Visual perception	39	10
Intubation or tube	7	27
Anxiety or panic	92	24
Helplessness	46	12
Sequelae	69	18

From Moerman et al (1993).

frequently recalled, especially negative comments regarding the patient's condition or appearance.

INCIDENCE

It is interesting to note that the incidence of awareness under anaesthesia has decreased over the past 30 years (Table 31.2). Estimates

TABLE 31.2

Incidence of awareness

Year of study	Awareness (%)	Dreaming (%)	Sample size
Structured interview (Liu et al 1991)			
1960	1.2	3	656
1971	1.6	26	120
1973	1.5	–	200
1975	0.8	7.7	490
1990	0.2	0.9	1000
No structured interview			
1983	13	–	91 (caesarean)
1984	11	–	37 (casualty)
1986	8	11	36 (caesarean)
1988	0	19	120 (paediatric)
1990	0	3	200 (caesarean)

31

vary, depending on the anaesthetic procedure and nature of postoperative interview.

Even with an incidence of 0.2%, 1 in 500 patients will be aware. It is not possible to determine the reason for this change. A number of factors are likely to be involved, including improved anaesthetic agents, improved monitoring and fear of litigation.

IDENTIFICATION

- Increased blood pressure, heart rate, sweating, tear formation
- Advanced monitoring, such as electroencephalography (EEG)-based technology (e.g. BIS™)
- Structured postoperative interview, avoiding leading questions
- The hand-written anaesthetic record is limited as a method of determining why awareness and recall have occurred (Moerman et al 1993).

SEQUELAE

- Sleep disturbances, such as nightmares
- Flashbacks
- Anxiety, possibly bordering on psychosis
- Increased fear of anaesthesia.

CAUSES

INDUCTION:

- Intubation immediately after induction with an intravenous agent (i.e. too early) may lead to awareness of intubation.
- Any delay before intubation (e.g. waiting for the relaxant to take effect, problems with intubation) may mean that the action of the intravenous induction agent will be wearing off.

BETWEEN INDUCTION AND SURGERY

Any delay between induction and transfer to the operating room may allow the blood concentration of the intravenous agent to decay before an inhalational agent has reached anaesthetic levels, leading to awareness of incision.

DURING SURGERY:

- Anaesthetic machine maintained incorrectly
- Low minute-volume settings on some electrically driven ventilators may lead to dilution of the anaesthetic with air, leading to awareness during surgery
- Oxygen bypass tap left on
- Exhausted vaporizer
- Failure to eliminate air from a closed circuit
- Exhausted, disconnected or malfunctioning syringe driver.

PREVENTION

- Know exactly how your anaesthetic machine and associated equipment work and check it all before use.
- Periodically check vaporiser levels and use an agent meter.
- Flush circles with a high flow for the first 5 min.
- Use a commercial depth-of-anaesthesia monitor, especially if the patient has a history of possible past awareness.
- Remember that patients differ considerably in their anaesthetic requirements.

TREATMENT

- Postoperative interview
- Referral for counselling.

BIBLIOGRAPHY

Couture LJ, Edmonds HL. Monitoring responsiveness during anaesthesia. Baillière's Clinical Anaesthesiology 1989; 3:547–558

Liu WHD, Thorp TAS, Graham SG, Aitkenhead AR. Incidence of awareness with recall during general anaesthesia. Anaesthesia 1991; 46:435–437

Moerman N, Bonke B, Oosting J. Awareness and recall during general anaesthesia. Anesthesiology 1993; 79:454–464

Blood transfusion

N. M. Tierney

Amongst other reasons, the advent of human immunodeficiency virus (HIV) has led to a more critical approach to the use of blood and blood products. Two-thirds of all transfusions are given during the perioperative period.

INDICATIONS FOR TRANSFUSION

- Blood:
  —treatment of acute life-threatening and ongoing blood loss
  —restoration of oxygen-carrying capacity.
- Platelets:
  —evidence of a clinical coagulopathy
  —thrombocytopenia
  —platelet dysfunction.
- Fresh frozen plasma (FFP):
  —demonstrable deficiency of coagulation factors.

Blood transfusion remains the treatment of choice where there is severe blood loss, such as major trauma, ruptured aortic aneurysm. In the extreme situation, group O Rhesus-negative packed cells or type-specific blood may be given. As a result, haemolysis will occur in 3% of these 'transfusion episodes'.

There is evidence that the treatment of continuing blood loss with coagulation factors and platelets leads to no reduction in blood loss. There is, however, evidence that in large-volume blood transfusion continuing blood loss is exacerbated by hypotension, acidosis and hypothermia.

RISKS OF TRANSFUSION

The overall morbidity of blood transfusion is 1 in 30 transfusion episodes. There are risks associated with all homologous transfusions.

IMMUNOLOGICAL:
- Red cell antigen
  —haemolysis
  —immediate (ABO)
  —delayed (non-ABO)
  —alloimmunisation

- White cell antigen
- Platelet antigen
- Plasma protein.

TRANSMITTED INFECTION:
- Risk is less than 1 in 1000
- Hepatitis types A, B, non-A/non-B, C
- HIV-1, HIV-2
- Cytomegalovirus
- Bacterial contamination.

IMMUNOSUPPRESSIVE EFFECTS:
- Increased transplant survival
- Increased incidence of recurrence of colorectal carcinoma
- Increased incidence of postoperative sepsis.

ABO incompatibility can be severe. It may be produced by only 30 ml of transfused blood. More than half of these events are due to clerical error. Their incidence is between 1 in 10 000 and 1 in 100 000. Of these, death from disseminated intravascular coagulation (DIC) occurs in 1 in 1000.

Blood can be demonstrated to reduce the immune competence of the recipient, and immunological mechanisms have been discovered that can explain these phenomena. No causal relationship has yet been proved, however.

There are particular problems associated with large-volume transfusion (more than one circulating volume):
- Fluid overload
- Dilutional thrombocytopenia.

and further problems where blood is given at a rate greater than 90 ml min^{-1}:
- Hyperkalaemia
- Hypothermia
- Hypocalcaemia.

METHODS FOR REDUCING EXPOSURE TO HOMOLOGOUS BLOOD

- Intraoperative haemodilution
- Intraoperative controlled hypotension

31

- Autologous transfusion
- Intraoperative blood salvage
- Use of synthetic oxygen transport media.
- Positioning of patient to reduce surgical bleeding
- Pharmacological approaches:
  —recombinant erythropoietin
  —recombinant activated factor VII
  —aprotinin
  —tranexamic acid
  —desmopressin.

Intraoperative haemodilution represents the most widely available technique for avoiding homologous blood transfusion and its attendant problems. It is based on the premise that, while maintaining normovolaemia, the maximum oxygen delivery (Do_2) rises to 110% of normal at a haematocrit of 30% (Fig. 31.2). This effect relies on a reduction in blood viscosity. The increase in Do_2 occurs without an increase in energy consumption. On the other hand, a haematocrit of 30% or less has been found to give an unacceptable risk of coronary ischaemia in patients with pre-existing ischaemic heart disease. In addition, it has been demonstrated that patients over 60 years of age are unable to increase their cardiac output to compensate for a haematocrit of less than 30% without an unacceptable rise in oxygen consumption.

Erythropoietin may be used to increase preoperative haemoglobin concentration, and possibly increase the yield of autologous blood donation. Stroma-free haemoglobin and perfluorochemicals remain a potential (but currently unavailable) method for avoiding homologous blood.

Recombinant factor VII was originally used in haemophilia where antibodies to factors VIII and IX were present. It has been shown to reduce perioperative blood loss and eliminate the need for transfusion in major surgery. It may prove useful in major trauma and DIC in future, and is undergoing trials.

- No clinical trials exist concerning the effects of moderate anaemia (6–9 g dl⁻¹) in the perioperative period.
- In the absence of coexisting disease, a postoperative haemoglobin level of 8–9 g dl⁻¹ may be acceptable in reducing exposure to homologous blood.
- Any decision regarding the patient's preoperative haemoglobin level should be linked to the potential surgical blood loss.
- In patients over 60 years, those with coexisting medical disease and those with ischaemic heart disease, a haemoglobin level no lower than 10 g dl⁻¹ should be sought prior to operation.
- The decision to transfuse should always be made on an individual patient basis.

BIBLIOGRAPHY

Association of Anaesthetists of Great Britain and Ireland. Blood transfusion and the anaesthetist. London: AAGBI; 2001

Crosby ET. Perioperative haemotherapy. I. Indications for blood component transfusion. Canadian Journal of Anaesthesia 1992; 39:695–707

Crosby ET. Perioperative haemotherapy. II. Risks and complications of blood transfusion. Canadian Journal of Anaesthesia 1992; 39:822–837

Friederich PW, Henny CP, Messelink EJ et al. Effect of recombinant activated factor VII on perioperative blood loss in patients undergoing retropubic prostatectomy: double-blind placebo-controlled randomised trial. Lancet 2003; 361:201–205

Kovesi T, Rouston D. Pharmacological approaches to reducing allogenic blood exposure. Vox Sang 2003; 84:2–10

Nicholls MD. Transfusion: morbidity and mortality. Anaesthesia and Intensive Care 1993; 21:15–19

Ong SM, Taylor GJ. Can knee position save blood following total knee replacement? Knee 2003; 10:81–85

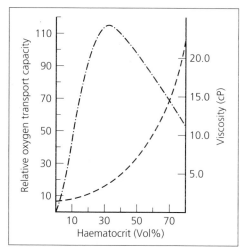

Fig. 31.2 Influence of the haemocrit on viscosity [-----] and relative oxygen transport capacity [-•-•-•-].

Cardiopulmonary resuscitation

K. A. Bruce

MECHANISMS OF CARDIORESPIRATORY ARREST

Cardiorespiratory arrest results from either primary cardiac or respiratory arrest. Cardiac arrest may be:
- Primary – due to dysrhythmia or severe myocardial failure
- Secondary – due to hypoxaemia (respiratory arrest), electrolyte imbalance, etc.

There are three fundamental 'rhythms' of cardiac arrest:
- Ventricular fibrillation (VF), or pulseless ventricular tachycardia (VT)
- Asystole, or extreme bradycardia
- Pulseless electrical activity (PEA) – previously referred to as electromechanical dissociation (EMD).

FACTORS AFFECTING SURVIVAL

Survival is most likely when:
- The rhythm is VF or VT
- The arrest is witnessed
- Basic life support is started immediately
- Defibrillation and advanced life support are given early.

BASIC LIFE SUPPORT

All medical, nursing and other hospital staff, as well as the general public, should be able to perform basic life support (BLS). The BLS algorithm is shown in Figure 31.3.

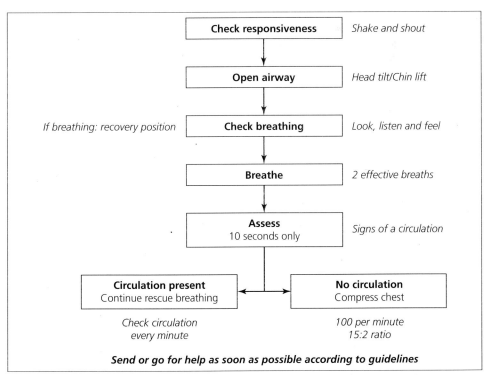

Fig. 31.3 The basic life support (BLS) algorithm.

IMPORTANT POINTS:

- Check that there is no danger to yourself or to the casualty before starting resuscitation.
- If the casualty is unresponsive, first shout for help, then check airway and breathing.
- Airway foreign bodies may be removed under direct vision, or by finger sweeps, back blows or abdominal thrusts.
- If breathing is absent, summon for advanced life support (ALS) personnel before starting BLS. Administer two effective ventilations and then assess for a circulation, taking up to 10 s to do so. If the central circulation is absent, commence cardiopulmonary resuscitation (CPR). Survival is very unlikely without ALS and defibrillation.
- The ratio of chest compressions to ventilation should be 15:2.
- Ventilation can be performed either by mouth-to-mouth techniques or by means of airway adjuncts (pocket masks or bag–valve–mask systems).
- Be aware of the possibility of neck trauma before considering extending the neck in order to open the airway.
- Lifting the jaw anteriorly (jaw thrust) may be required to open the airway.
- The techniques of artificial ventilation and external chest compressions cannot be learnt from a book but only from a properly supervised training session.

ADVANCED LIFE SUPPORT

All medical staff and appropriate senior nursing and paramedical staff should be capable of performing ALS. The ALS algorithm is shown in Figure 31.4. All persons who may be called upon to perform ALS should be familiar with this algorithm. Regular refresher courses are recommended.

IMPORTANT POINTS:

- A precordial thump may restore a cardiac rhythm. It is recommended in witnessed arrest situations where a defibrillator is not immediately available.
- Defibrillation is the only cure for VF or VT, but must be given as soon as possible. Up to three shocks should be given initially at 200, 200 and 360 J (or the biphasic equivalent). Give the first three shocks without pausing for CPR unless the charging time is very slow. If necessary, 1 min of CPR should then be provided before further defibrillation shocks are

given. Adrenaline (epinephrine) (1 mg) should be given every 3 min. Advanced airway interventions (intubation or the insertion of a laryngeal mask or Combitube) should be considered. Once the airway is secured, chest compressions may be continued uninterrupted at a rate of 100 per min. Ventilations should continue at 12 per min. If VF or VT persists after 1 min of CPR further shocks at 360 J (or biphasic equivalent) should be delivered without delay.

- VF may masquerade as asystole on the ECG, so check leads, connections and gain. If in any doubt, defibrillate up to three times. (Automatic external defibrillators (AEDs) may not allow this.)
- Adrenaline (epinephrine) is given to improve cerebral and cerebral blood flow, not to terminate VF or asystole.
- Atropine may be considered in asystole and PEA (where the rate is less than 60 per min).
- Amiodarone may be considered in refractory VF or VT (where the rhythm does not respond to the first three initial shocks).
- Sodium bicarbonate is no longer recommended at an early stage, as it may worsen intracellular acidosis. It may be given for severe metabolic acidosis later in the process of resuscitation, preferably guided by arterial blood gases.
- PEA is usually secondary, and CPR is unlikely to be successful unless the cause is treated.
- In PEA, calcium chloride may be useful in hypocalcaemia, hyperkalaemia, or after use of calcium channel blockers.
- Drugs are best given through a central line. Central line insertion during CPR is hazardous if done by the inexperienced. If intravenous access is not possible, the endotracheal route is an alternative for adrenaline (epinephrine) and atropine, using two to three times the intravenous dose. Intracardiac injection of drugs is not recommended.

POSTRESUSCITATION CARE

The patient should be nursed in an ITU or HDU following successful resuscitation. The following points should be considered.

HISTORY:

- Previous medical history
- Events preceding the arrest
- Cause of the arrest.

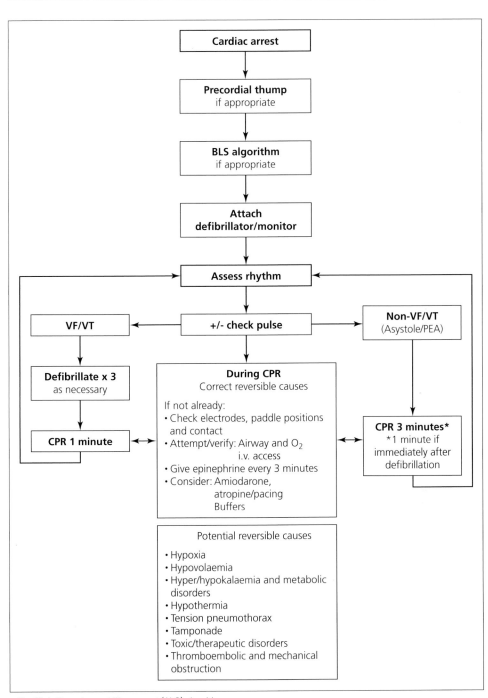

Fig. 31.4 The advanced life support (ALS) algorithm.

31

EXAMINATION:
- Respiratory:
  —endotracheal tube position
  —pneumothorax
  —fractured ribs or sternum.
- Cardiovascular:
  —pulse
  —blood pressure
  —adequacy of perfusion

—jugular venous pressure
—urine output.
- Neurological:
  —Glasgow Coma Score
  —pupil size and reactivity
  —neurological deficit.

INVESTIGATIONS:
- Arterial blood gases
- Chest radiography
- 12-lead ECG
- Urea and electrolytes
- Consider invasive haemodynamic monitoring.

TREATMENT:
- Oxygen, according to arterial blood gases
- Continued ventilation
- Analgesia
- Antiarrhythmics
- Inotropes and/or vasodilators
- Specific organ system support (e.g. renal support).

PAEDIATRIC RESUSCITATION

The principles of CPR in children are similar to those in adults, but the following differences apply.

CAUSES OF ARREST:
- Asystole or severe bradycardia are the commonest dysrhythmias. They may be secondary to hypoxaemia or circulatory failure, and may be cured by BLS and oxygenation.
- Cardiac arrest may be due to sudden infant death syndrome, airway obstruction (foreign bodies, epiglottitis or croup), near-drowning, asthma, trauma or severe infection.

AIRWAY AND VENTILATION:
- Mouth to nose-and-mouth ventilation may be needed – remember the smaller tidal volumes required.
- The Heimlich manoeuvre, finger sweeps and incisional cricothyrotomy are contraindicated in younger children. Back blows, chest thrusts and needle cricothyrotomy are alternatives.
- Endotracheal tube sizes (Table 31.3):
  — internal diameter = $(4 + Age/4)$
  — length = $(12 + Age/2)$.
  — alternatively, choose the same diameter as the child's little finger or nostril.
- Uncuffed tracheal tubes should be used in children. Over the age of about 12 years, cuffed tubes may be used, depending on the size and maturity of the child.

EXTERNAL CHEST COMPRESSIONS
The compression rate should be 100 per min. Remember to use less force.

DEFIBRILLATION
The initial charge is 2 J kg^{-1}, increasing to 4 J kg^{-1} if necessary.

TABLE 31.3

Paediatric tracheal tube sizes

Age (years)	Approximate weight (kg)	Tracheal tube Internal diameter (mm)	Length (cm)
3 months	5	3.0–3.5	10
6 months	6–7	3.5	12
9 months	8–9	4.0	12
1	10	4.0–4.5	13
2	12	4.5–5.0	14
3	14	5.0	14
4	16	5.5	15
5	18	5.5	15
6	20	6.0	16
8	25	6.5	17
10	30	7.0	18
12[a]	40	7.0–7.5	18–20

[a]Cuffed tubes may be used in children over the age of about 12 years.

DRUG DOSES

In children, drugs may be given by either the intravenous or the intraosseous routes.

- Adrenaline (epinephrine): 10–100 μg kg^{-1}
- Amiodarone: 5 mg kg^{-1}
- Atropine 0.02 mg kg^{-1} (minimum 0.1 mg, maximum 0.6 mg)
- Lidocaine (lignocaine): 0.1 ml kg^{-1} of 1% lidocaine
- Calcium: 0.1 ml kg^{-1} of 10% calcium chloride
- Sodium bicarbonate: 1 mmol kg^{-1}.

BIBLIOGRAPHY

Advanced Life Support Group. Advanced paediatric life support – the practical approach. 3rd edn. London: BMJ; 2001

International Liaison Committee on Resuscitation (ILCOR) Guidelines 2000 for cardiopulmonary resuscitation and emergency care – an international consensus on science. Resuscitation 2000; 46(1–3):1–448

Resuscitation Council (UK). Advanced life support course provider manual. London: Resuscitation Council (UK); 2000

31

Complications of positioning under anaesthesia

N. M. Tierney

Inappropriate handling of the unconscious or partially paralysed patient carries a risk of serious morbidity and even fatality. Knowledge of the reported complications together with a high standard of care and patient monitoring are necessary to reduce the risk.

Commonest causes of complications

- Accidental trauma
- External pressure
- Extreme passive movement
- Physiological trespass

PREOPERATIVE ASSESSMENT

Check for:
- Head and neck mobility in patients where neck rotation is anticipated, for example for ENT or neurosurgical procedures, and in all cases of rheumatoid or ankylosing arthritis
- Brachial neurovascular symptoms if the patient's arms are to be positioned above their head
- Symptoms of ulnar nerve entrapment syndrome
- Active and passive range of limb movement in elderly or arthritic patients where the anticipated position may cause problems
- Arterial pressure changes or symptoms of supine hypotension in pregnant patients.

DANGERS OF THE POSITIONING PROCESS AND PATIENT TRANSFER

Skilled and motivated assistants are critically important in delivering adequate patient care. Complications may result from the following.

FAILURE TO SUPPORT THE HEAD ADEQUATELY:
- Sliding patients from trolley to operating table and back, and the use of 'operating trolleys', have probably reduced risk. An example would be the consequences of previously lifting a patient where a pillow concealed the patient's head being unsupported by the absent stretcher canvas causing whiplash injury to the neck.
- Uncoordinated movement of assistants when turning the patient may damage the neck.

FALLS FROM THE OPERATING TABLE OR TROLLEY:
- Failure to apply brakes on transfer trolley allows the patient to fall between the operating table and the trolley.
- Problems may occur more frequently at the conclusion of procedures when staff are potentially tired and less vigilant.
- Failure to raise the side guard-rails on narrow transfer trolleys.

FAILURE TO PREVENT LOCALISED DAMAGE:
- Intraoperative movement during eye surgery leading to damage and resultant blindness.
- Fingers can be amputated by hinged sections of the operating table.
- Careless sliding of patients can cause skin abrasions that may be the focus for development of pressure sores. Risk factors for the formation of pressure sores have been identified for critically ill patients.
- Accidental traction on infusion lines, drainage tubes and urethral catheters can cause internal damage.
- The 'perineal post' of the orthopaedic traction table can cause genital damage and pudendal nerve trauma.

WELL RECOGNISED PROBLEMS ASSOCIATED WITH SPECIFIC POSITIONS

THE SUPINE POSITION
Pressure necrosis of skin and mucosa:
- Occipital – may be associated with alopecia

- Sacral – coincident thermal damage is most often a risk with the use of circulating water warmers and perhaps in poor peripheral perfusion states.
- Heels – a special and serious risk in diabetic patients.
- The laryngeal mask airway has a good track record with regard to theoretical risk of mucosal compression and resultant ischaemia.

Nerve compression problems:
- The supraorbital nerve may be compressed by airway tubing.
- Brachial plexus neurapraxia can result from faulty arm board positioning.
- The radial nerve can be trapped against a head-screen support.
- The ulnar nerve may be damaged against the edge of the mattress. More commonly this injury has no demonstrable cause according to the American Society of Anesthesiologists Closed Claims Project (http://www.asaclosedclaims.org).

THE LITHOTOMY POSITION
Nervous system complications:
- Straight-leg sling systems may cause sciatic and femoral nerve problems.
- The common peroneal nerve may be trapped against the head of the fibula.
- The saphenous nerve may be trapped against the supporting posts.
- In extreme flexion of the thighs, the femoral nerve can be kinked around the inguinal ligament.

Lower-limb compartment syndrome
This appears to result from a combination of reduced perfusion pressure (arterial pressure – intramuscular pressure) due to prolonged elevation of the lower limbs during various forms of surgery with or without superadded pressure on calf muscles from leg supports.

Skeletal damage:
- Ligamentous damage of the hip and knee joints ensue if passive movement exceeds the normal active range.
- Sacroiliac joint strain is a risk if the legs are not raised symmetrically.

Physiological risks:
- The extent of surgically induced hypovolaemia may be masked by intraoperative autotransfusion from the legs, which is lost when the patient is returned to supine.

- Increased intra-abdominal pressure enhances the possibility of gastric regurgitation – general anaesthesia should never be induced in this position.

THE LATERAL POSITION
Stability of position is essential. This is best achieved through the use of an evacuatable mattress.

Pressure problems:
- The skin covering the iliac crest is at risk.
- The underlying sciatic nerve is at risk in emaciated patients.
- The underlying common peroneal nerve is vulnerable around the neck of the fibula.
- The weight of the upper body may be taken by a support between the lateral thorax and the operating table. This relieves pressure from the point of the shoulder, protecting the underlying brachial plexus and obviating any risk of the 'crush syndrome' in the deltoid muscle.

THE SITTING POSITION
Physiological problems:
- Venous air embolism – the classical risk
- Postural hypotension – can be exacerbated by bradycardia or surgical hypovolaemia.

Nervous system complications:
- Quadriplegia has been reported following head flexion and cervical spine rotation.
- Brachial plexus damage may occur if the arms are not properly supported.

THE PRONE POSITION
- Very simple surgical procedures can be performed with the patient supported by a pillow beneath the chest and another beneath the pelvis. More complex procedures, such as spinal axis surgery, usually require that the groins and abdomen are completely free of external pressure.
- The Mohammedan prayer position should never be used – lower-limb congestion can cause myoglobinuria and acute renal failure (Fig. 31.5).
- Methods used to support the pelvis under the iliac crests are satisfactory only if the props are positioned so that the patient is unable to slip sideways (Fig. 31.6). If this does occur, occlusion of one femoral neurovascular bundle is unavoidable, and back-pressure transmitted to the epidural veins may cause troublesome surgical haemorrhage.

31

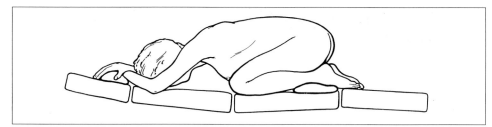

Fig. 31.5 The Mohammedan prayer position. This position should never be used.

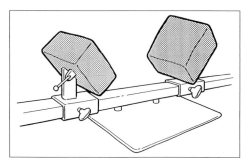

Fig. 31.6 Positioning of props to support the pelvis under the iliac crests.

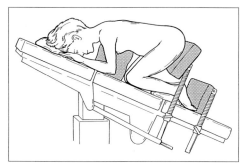

Fig. 31.7 The safest position (Tarlov) for all lower thoracic and lumbar disc surgery.

- The position originally described by Tarlov is the safest and most satisfactory for all lower thoracic and lumbar disc surgery (Fig. 31.7). In some patients it can be used for operations on the cervical and upper thoracic spine. Although inferior vena cava pressures are known to be around 0–3 cmH$_2$O, venous air embolism is a very rare complication of surgery in this position.

OTHER DANGERS

DANGERS RESULTING FROM THE METHOD OF PRONE POSITIONING:

- Pressure necrosis of weight-bearing skin areas.

- Patients with previous coronary artery bypass graft surgery are at risk of graft occlusion.
- Neurapraxia, both brachial and axillary, can occur if the arms are positioned above the head.
- Blindness from external orbital pressure.

DANGERS ARISING FROM THE OPERATION BEING PERFORMED

Damage to underlying abdominal major vessels or bowel perforation are well recorded when discectomy is being performed. Serious, hidden, intraperitoneal haemorrhage can rapidly cause acute hypovolaemic shock. Abandoning surgery and resuscitation in the supine position is the only action likely to avert disaster.

COMPLICATIONS OF ANAESTHESIA

The correct placement and securing of a non-kinking tracheal tube is the cornerstone of anaesthetic technique. Obesity and respiratory disease may necessitate the alternative use of the lateral position.

VENOUS AIR EMBOLISM

This can be caused by any open vein or sinus above heart level.
- Inability of the vein to collapse:
  —Intracranial venous sinuses and emissary veins
  —Self-retaining surgical retractors
  —Tracks formed around indwelling catheters (e.g. central venous pressure catheter).
- The level of venous pressure at the site:
  —Posture and positioning are important
  —Raising the adult patient's head to +25° lowers intracranial venous sinus pressure to zero, and at +90° produces a negative pressure of -12 ± 3 cmH$_2$O
  —Spontaneous ventilation causing negative intrathoracic pressure potentiates negative pressure at the operating site

—In the prone position, the suction effect of a pendulous abdomen can potentiate negative venous pressure within the epidural veins.

INCIDENCE:

- Posterior fossa surgery in the sitting position
- Head and neck surgery in the supine head-up position
- Caesarean section
- Intrauterine manipulations in the lithotomy position
- Major reconstructive spinal surgery in the prone position.

SUMMARY

- Look after the neck.
- Do not drop the patient.
- Avoid pressure on:
  —major blood vessels
  —main nerve trunks.
- Do not strain arthritic joints or cause pressure sores.

BIBLIOGRAPHY

Anderton JM. The prone position for the surgical patient: historical review of the principles and hazards. British Journal of Anaesthesia 1991; 67:452–463

Connor H. Iatrogenic injuries in theatre. British Medical Journal 1992; 305:956

Gild WM, Posner KL, Caplan RA, Cheney FW. Eye injuries associated with anaesthesia. A closed claims analysis. Anesthesiology 1994; 81:273–274

Iwabuchi T, Sobata E, Susuki M, Susuki S, Yamashita M. Dural sinus pressure as related to neurosurgical positions. Neurosurgery 1983; 12:203–207

McKinney B, Grigg R. Epiglottitis after anaesthesia with a laryngeal mask. Anaesthesia and Intensive Care 1995; 23:618–619

Theaker C, Mannam M, Ives N, Soni N. Risk factors for pressure sores in the critically ill. Anaesthesia 2000; 55:221–224

Vartikar JV, Johnson MD, Datta S. Precordial Doppler monitoring and pulse oximetry during caesarean section delivery: detection of venous air embolism. Regional Anaesthesia 1989; 14:145–148

Young JVI. The role of the evacuatable mattress. In: Anderton JM, Keen RI, Neave R, eds. Positioning the surgical patient. London: Butterworths; 1988:90

31

Failure to breathe or wake up after surgery

J. Barrie

NORMAL RESTORATION OF BREATHING

All anaesthetic agents and opioids are respiratory depressants and may cause apnoea. Failure to breathe after surgery may also follow the use of intraoperative muscular relaxation. There may be more than one cause operating simultaneously, and these causes may be cumulative.

FAILURE TO BREATHE AFTER SURGERY

CAUSES
Non-depolarising agents:
- Inadequate antagonism of neuromuscular block. The effects of non-depolarising muscle relaxants are usually antagonised with neostigmine ($50\ \mu g\ kg^{-1}$) (together with atropine ($20\ \mu g\ kg^{-1}$) or glycopyrrolate ($10\ \mu g\ kg^{-1}$), and this should have been given before 'failure to breathe' is noted.
- Concomitant drugs which themselves depress neuromuscular function or potentiate a neuromuscular blocking agent, e.g.:
  —aminoglycoside antibiotics
  —verapamil
  —phenytoin
  —ciclosporin A.
- Cholinergic crisis secondary to excessive neostigmine (rare).

Depolarising agents:
- Pseudocholinesterase deficiency – genetic or acquired
- Dual block – type II block.

Other factors:
- Respiratory depressants
- Opioids
- Volatile anaesthetic agents
- Benzodiazepines
- Pain, especially if thoracic or abdominal in origin

- Hypocapnia
- Severe hypercapnia
- Hypothermia, especially in children
- Metabolic disturbance
- Acidosis
- Hypokalaemia
- Hypomagnesaemia
- Coexisting neuromuscular disease
- Intraoperative cerebral event.

MANAGEMENT
The patient may be pink and display an acceptable $S\text{p}O_2$.
- Ensure the patient's safety.
- Ensure that the airway is protected and that adequate ventilation is maintained, by hand if necessary.
- If the patient is conscious, reassure them and consider sedation.
- Monitor vital signs:
  —ECG
  —$S\text{p}O_2$
  —non-invasive blood pressure
  —$Et\text{CO}_2$, if possible.
- Determine cause:
  —monitor neuromuscular function
  —review doses of other agents that have been given
  —check whether all anaesthetic agents are turned off
  —consider the patient's metabolic status
  —take temperature.
- If residual paralysis is present and the post-tetanic count is 12 or more, give a further dose of neostigmine and an anticholinergic (up to $100\ \mu g\ kg^{-1}$ total dose of neostigmine).
- If excessive narcotic is present, give increments of 0.1 mg naloxone
- If central respiratory depression is present, consider titrated doses of doxapram (1–$1.5\ mg\ kg^{-1}$ over 30 s).
- If excessive benzodiazepines have been used, give flumazenil ($200\ \mu g$

over 15 s, then 100 μg every 60 s, as required).
- Control pain with local techniques or carefully titrated doses of opioids.
- Optimise the patient's metabolic condition.
- If ventilation is still not adequate, transfer patient to the ITU.

NORMAL AWAKENING

Awakening occurs when the concentration of anaesthetic agent in the brain falls to a level insufficient to maintain unconsciousness. This occurs due to the redistribution (usually) or metabolism of intravenous agents and the elimination of volatile agents. It is therefore a passive process, with specific antagonists existing only for opioids and benzodiazepines.

FAILURE TO WAKE UP

CAUSES
There may be more than one reason present, and effects are cumulative:
- Overdose (absolute or relative) of anaesthetic agent, premedication (including benzodiazepines) or opioid
- Hypothermia, particularly in children
- Hypercapnia
- Severe hypothyroidism
- Severe liver disease, in which anaesthesia may precipitate encephalopathy
- Cerebral hypoxia.

MANAGEMENT:
- Ensure the patient's safety.
- Ensure the airway is protected and ventilation is adequate.
- Continue monitoring:
  —ECG
  —non-invasive blood pressure
  —Spo_2.
- Assess cause:
  —arterial blood gas analysis
  —core temperature
  —coexisting disease.
- Treat any treatable causes:
  —correct any abnormalities in acid–base status
  —rewarm if necessary
  —administer a cautious dose of antagonists, if appropriate.
- Wait.
- Consider transfer to the ITU if awakening continues to be delayed.

The only cause of prolonged (hours or days) failure to recover from anaesthesia is a cardiorespiratory or cerebrovascular disaster with cerebral hypoxia. Thankfully, this is rare.

BIBLIOGRAPHY

Morris RW. Desaturation. Baillière's Clinical Anaesthesiology 1993; 7:215–235

Ward DS, Temp JA. The role of hypoxia in the control of breathing. In: Kauffman L, ed. Anaesthesia review, vol 8. London: Churchill Livingstone; 1991:89–102

31

Fat embolism

R. M. Slater

DEFINITION

Fat embolism is defined as the presence of fat globules within the lung parenchyma or peripheral microcirculation. The fat embolism syndrome (FES) is defined as fat in the circulation associated with a clinical pattern of symptoms and signs. It is most commonly associated with:

- Fractures of long bones and pelvis
- Prosthetic joint replacement
- Liposuction
- Bone marrow harvest or transplant
- Acute pancreatitis
- Hepatic necrosis and fatty liver
- Acute sickle cell crisis (bone marrow necrosis)
- Altitude illness
- Following extracorporeal circulation.

Three clinical forms of FES are described.

SUBCLINICAL FES

Seen in more than 50% of patients with long-bone fractures. Mild hypoxaemia and minor haematological abnormalities develop up to 3 days after injury.

NON-FULMINANT (SUBACUTE) FES

Seen in 1–5% of major trauma patients. Onset delayed by 12–36 h after injury. Classical syndrome of hypoxaemia and respiratory failure, petechial rash, fever, tachycardia, neurological symptoms and associated haematological abnormalities. A partial or incomplete picture is the commonest presentation.

FULMINANT FES

Sudden onset, within a few hours of injury. Pulmonary and systemic embolisation of fat, right ventricular failure and cardiovascular collapse. This can occur during surgery. Progresses rapidly, often with a fatal outcome.

PATHOPHYSIOLOGY

Fat emboli are thought to originate from exposed marrow at the site of injury. Fat globules enter the circulation, facilitated by movement of the fracture site. Subsequent pulmonary and neurological damage is thought to be due partly to vascular occlusion and partly to local effects of free fatty acids released from fat emboli. Respiratory insufficiency results from emboli entering the venous circulation and lodging in the pulmonary circulation. Cerebral involvement and petechial rash result from fat emboli entering the arterial circulation, either via the pulmonary alveolar capillaries or via precapillary pulmonary shunts that have opened as a result of pulmonary hypertension.

DIAGNOSIS

RESPIRATORY INSUFFICIENCY:

- Occurs in 75% of patients with FES
- Dyspnoea, tachypnoea and hypoxaemia associated with fine inspiratory crackles on auscultation, 12–36 h after injury
- Chest radiograph is normal at first, then shows bilateral fluffy shadowing
- In 10% of cases respiratory failure develops and progresses to the adult respiratory distress syndrome.

CEREBRAL FEATURES

Neurological signs exist in up to 80% of patients with FES, and may precede respiratory signs. Encephalopathy produces drowsiness, confusion and/or coma. A subgroup develops focal neurological signs such as decerebrate posturing, hemiparesis or tonic–clonic seizures. The severe neurological symptoms of FES usually resolve. Computed tomography (CT) may show generalised cerebral oedema or high-density spots, but is non-specific and usually unhelpful. Magnetic resonance imaging (MRI) may detect specific lesions in the presence of a normal CT scan.

DERMATOLOGICAL FEATURES:

These occur in 60% of cases.

A petechial rash develops within 36 h of the event. Found in the conjunctiva, oral mucous membrane, neck and axilla. This distribution may be explained by fat droplets accumulating in the aortic arch prior to embolisation to non-dependent skin via the subclavian and carotid vessels. Factors contributing to the rash may be stasis, loss of clotting factors and platelets, and endothelial damage from free fatty acids leading to rupture of thin-walled capillaries. It is self-limiting, usually resolving within 7 days.

OTHER FEATURES:
- Pyrexia and tachycardia are common non-specific findings.
- ECG may show signs of right ventricular strain.
- Retinal haemorrhages and exudates can occur.
- Renal emboli may result in oliguria, lipuria, proteinuria or haematuria; these changes are short-lived and unrelated to any subsequent renal impairment.
- Jaundice is rare and self-limiting.

LABORATORY FINDINGS:
- Fall in haemoglobin level, thrombocytopenia (platelet count $< 150 \times 10^9 \ l^{-1}$) and other coagulation abnormalities.
- Blood and urine may show fat globules (non-specific signs). Fat macroglobulinaemia and raised levels of free fatty acids (FFAs) and triglycerides in serum. High FFA levels may result in hypocalcaemia due to the affinity of FFAs for calcium.

OTHER INVESTIGATIONS
A pulmonary artery catheter may be useful in detecting a rise in mean pulmonary artery pressure or in sampling pulmonary artery blood for fat.

Bronchoscopy and bronchoalveolar lavage (BAL) in trauma patients have been used to provide samples containing macrophages, which act as lung scavengers and may contain fat in FES. This has shown promise as a method for diagnosing FES in the first 24 h.

MANAGEMENT

- Treatment is non-specific and supportive.
- Early resuscitation and stabilisation to minimise the stress response and hypovolaemia.
- Maintain adequate oxygenation and ventilation.
- Indications for respiratory support:
  —sustained $SaO_2 < 90\%$ and $PaO_2 < 8$ kPa on oxygen
  —respiratory rate > 35 breaths per min.

- Early immobilisation of fractures – pulmonary complications are increased where fixation is delayed for more than 24 h. External fixation or plating produces less lung injury than intramedullary fixation.
- Avoid hypovolaemia – increases the mortality rate.
- Use of human albumin solution – thought to bind FFAs.
- Adequate analgesia.

SPECIFIC THERAPIES:
A number of specific therapies have been tried:
- Corticosteroids (methylprednisolone) have been shown to have beneficial effects in some series, although the optimal timing and dosages are unclear.
- Heparin is known to clear lipaemic serum by stimulating lipase activity, and has been suggested for treatment of FES. However, this may increase FFA activity and produce unwanted bleeding in patients with multiple trauma.
- Alcohol decreases serum lipase activity.
- Aspirin has been recommended as a prophylactic agent as it blocks the production of thromboxane, which occurs in animal models of FES.

OUTCOME

The overall mortality rate of FES is 5–15%. The condition is usually self-limiting with adequate supportive therapy. Long-term morbidity is related to focal neurological lesions.

31

BIBLIOGRAPHY

Bannier B, Poirier T, Viaud JY, Laurens E, Turbide A. Fat embolism: diagnostic interest of the bronchoalveolar lavage. Intensive Care Medicine 1992; 18:59–60

Gurd AR. Fat embolism, an aid to diagnosis. Journal of Bone and Joint Surgery 1970; 52B:732–737

Mellor A, Soni N. Fat embolism. Anaesthesia 2001; 56:145–154

Robert JH, Hoffmeyer P, Broquet PE, Cerutti P, Vasey H. Fat embolism syndrome. Orthopaedic Review 1993; 22:567–571

Van Besouw JP, Hinds CJ. Fat embolism syndrome. British Journal of Hospital Medicine 1989; 42:304–311

Fluid and electrolyte balance

S. Varley

Disease processes can impair the complex homeostatic mechanisms that safeguard the *milieu intérieur*. It is important to ensure that the stable chemical environment upon which normal cellular function depends is maintained during the perioperative period.

PHYSIOLOGY

Body water content varies with age and sex as a percentage of bodyweight (Table 31.4).

Approximately two-thirds of the total body water (TBW) is intracellular fluid (ICF) and one-third is extracellular fluid (ECF). The ECF is further subdivided into interstitial fluid (ISF) and plasma.

The TBW and electrolytes in a 70-kg man are distributed between the various compartments as shown in Table 31.5.

OSMOTIC ACTIVITY

Water moves between compartments from areas of low solute concentration to areas of high concentration by osmosis. The number of osmotically active particles in solution is expressed in osmol (Osm). Osmolarity is the number of particles per litre of solvent (Osm l^{-1}), and osmolality is the number of particles per kilogram of solvent (Osm kg^{-1}).

The density of water is 1 kg l^{-1}; osmolality and osmolarity are therefore equivalent in the body.

Osmolality can be estimated by adding the concentrations of osmotically active particles within compartments. ECF osmolality is usually calculated by adding the plasma concentrations (mmol l^{-1}) of sodium, potassium, chloride, urea and glucose. An alternative, commonly used, rule of thumb is to add twice the sodium plus urea plus glucose.

Osmotic pressure is calculated by multiplying osmolalities by 19.3 to give pressures (mmHg). Thus, ICF has an osmolality of 281 mOsm l^{-1} and an osmotic pressure of 5430 mmHg, but plasma has an osmolality of 281 mOsm l^{-1} but an osmotic pressure of 5453 mmHg. This difference of 23 mmHg is due to the presence of plasma proteins.

THE FATE OF INTRAVENOUS FLUIDS

The redistribution of infused fluid within the body will depend on its composition relative

TABLE 31.4

Body water composition in health as a percentage of TBW

	TBW	ICF (%)	ECF (%)
Neonate	75	40	35
Infant	70	40	30
Adult male	60	40	20
Adult female	55	35	20
Elderly female	45	30	15

TABLE 31.5

Distribution of water and electrolytes in a normal 70-kg man

	ICF	ECF	
		ISF	Plasma
% of TBW	40	16	4
Volume (litres)	28	11	3
Ions (mmol l^{-1}):			
Na$^+$	10	140	140
K$^+$	150	4	4
Ca^{2+}	–	2.5	2.5
Mg^{2+}	26	1.5	1.5
Cl$^-$	–	114	114
HCO$_3^-$	10	25	25
HPO$_4^{2-}$	38	1	1
SO$_4^{2-}$	–	0.5	0.5
Prot$^-$	74	2	16

31

TABLE 31.6

Approximate fractional distribution of infusions within compartments[a]

	ICF	ECF	
		ISF	Plasma
Saline (0.9%)	0	4/5	1/5
Dextrose (5%)	2/3	1/4	1/12

[a]These values demonstrate why large volumes of crystalloids are required to expand plasma volume. Replacement of a given blood loss requires three times the volume as saline (0.9%) or nine times the volume as dextrose (5%).

to that of each compartment, as shown in Table 31.6. Salt solutions are excluded from the ICF by the cell membrane Na^+/K^+ pump. Dextrose (5%) behaves like water and is distributed throughout the TBW.

NORMAL REQUIREMENTS

WATER

A normothermic 70-kg man with a normal metabolic rate loses approximately 2500 ml of water per day (urine 1500 ml, faeces 100 ml, sweat 500 ml, lungs 400 ml). Water is gained from ingested fluid (1300 ml), food (800 ml) and metabolism (400 ml). Maintenance requirements are therefore approximately 1.25–1.5 ml kg^{-1} h^{-1} for adult surgical patients.

SODIUM

Loss in faeces and sweat is about 10 mmol daily, renal excretion being dependent mainly on dietary intake. Average requirements are 1 mmol kg^{-1} day^{-1}. This could be provided by:

- 2500 ml of 4% dextrose/0.18% saline over 24 h
- 2000 ml of 5% dextrose and 500 ml of 0.9% saline over 24 h.

POTASSIUM

Loss is via the same routes as sodium, but renal retention is less efficient. The average requirement is 1 mmol kg^{-1} day^{-1}. This should be added to the infusion regimen.

PERIOPERATIVE FLUID MANAGEMENT

The fluid status of a patient undergoing surgery will depend on the presenting complaint, the previous health of the individual and whether surgery is elective or urgent. Fluid and electrolyte depletion is a common problem faced by the anaesthetist.

The history and examination will point to decreased intake or increased loss:

- Note the duration of preoperative fasting
- Patients at the extremes of age are less likely to maintain fluid balance during illness
- Note the presence of diarrhoea and vomiting
- Pyrexia – insensible loss increases by 10% for each 1°C rise in body temperature
- Acute abdomen – large volumes of fluid may be sequestered in the abdomen.

ASSESSMENT OF THE DEFICIT IN TBW

- Up to 5%:
  —dry mucous membranes
  —skin turgor almost normal
  —normal sensorium.
- Up to 10%:
  —drowsiness
  —decreased skin turgor
  —decreased intraocular pressure
  —increased heart rate and respiratory rate
  —oliguria
  —sunken fontanelle in infants.
- Up to 15%:
  —stuporose
  —parched mouth
  —sunken eyes
  —fast and thready pulse
  —respiratory distress
  —hypotension
  —extreme oliguria.

INVESTIGATIONS

History and examination are the key to good assessment, although simple blood tests supply additional information:

- Look for increased levels of urea or creatinine
- Look for raised haematocrit
- Check plasma levels of sodium and potassium.

PREOPERATIVE REQUIREMENTS

In general, healthy patients undergoing elective minor surgery do not need perioperative fluid replacement unless they are unable to drink normally in the early postoperative period. In other patients the following deficits should be considered.

PREOPERATIVE FASTING

If there has been a fluid restriction of 1.5 ml kg^{-1} h^{-1}, replace with dextrose (4%)/saline (0.18%) or similar.

31

ABNORMAL LOSSES

This is common in surgical patients. Replacement is based on an estimate of the composition and volume of loss. Losses from the gut are particularly important and, although the compositions of the various gastrointestinal secretions differ, they are adequately replaced with equal volumes of saline (0.9%) and potassium chloride (10–20 mmol l^{-1}).

SEVERE HYPOVOLAEMIA WITH SIGNS OF SHOCK

Give colloid (10 ml kg^{-1}) as a bolus, with additional fluid given according to the patient's response.

INTRAOPERATIVE REQUIREMENTS

MAINTENANCE

Give dextrose (4%, 1.5 ml kg^{-1} h^{-1}) with saline (0.18%).

LOSSES FROM SKIN, LUNGS, ABDOMINAL CAVITY AND THIRD SPACE SEQUESTRATION

These losses can be replaced with 2–10 ml kg^{-1} h^{-1} of balanced salt solution. This should be judged according to the patient response: heart rate, blood pressure, tissue perfusion and urine output (not less than 0.5 ml kg^{-1} h^{-1}). Central venous pressure (CVP) monitoring may be necessary.

BLOOD LOSS

Consider transfusion when 10% of estimated blood volume has been lost (Table 31.7). Give blood when 15% or more has been lost. Take into account both preoperative and intraoperative haemorrhage.

POSTOPERATIVE REQUIREMENTS

MAINTENANCE:

- 1.5 ml kg^{-1} h^{-1} of 4% dextrose with 0.18% saline
- Replace any further blood losses.

TABLE 31.7

Estimated blood volumes

	Volume (ml kg^{-1})
Infant	90
Child	80
Adult male	70
Adult female	60

Opinions about the electrolyte requirements of postoperative patients differ widely in clinical practice. Although the stress response to surgery increases renal excretion of potassium, tissue trauma and catabolism release intracellular potassium, thus maintaining plasma levels. Potassium is not required for the first 24–48 h in most patients. Whatever fluid composition is chosen, all fluid replacement should be regularly reviewed according to the patient's response: heart rate, blood pressure, respiratory rate, tissue perfusion, plasma electrolytes, urine output (at least 0.5 ml kg^{-1} h^{-1}) and CVP (if a central line is *in situ*).

BIBLIOGRAPHY

Ganong WF. Review of medical physiology. 13th edn. California: Lange Medical Publications; 1985

Guyton AC. Textbook of medical physiology. 6th edn. Philadelphia: WB Saunders; 1981

Shearer ES, Hunter JM. Perioperative fluid and electrolyte balance. Current Anaesthesia and Critical Care 1992; 3:71–77

CROSS-REFERENCES

Water and electrolyte disturbances
    Patient Conditions 27: 624

31

Intraoperative arrhythmias

N. P. C. Randall

More than 60% of patients experience some form of arrhythmia in the perioperative period. The majority are benign. This must not, however, obscure the association of rhythm disturbance with potential serious adverse outcomes. The significance of the arrhythmia has to be evaluated in the context of:

- Preoperative coexisting medical problems and drug treatment
- The surgical condition
- The operative procedure
- Anaesthetic drugs and technique
- Haemodynamic effect of the arrhythmias, and the risk of progression to a more serious arrhythmia.

For example, in a fit patient having a halothane anaesthetic for minor surgery, a nodal rhythm producing little fall in blood pressure can be observed and is unlikely to require treatment. The same rhythm in a patient with aortic stenosis, or in a fit patient about to have squint surgery, is likely to require intervention.

BOX 31.4

Preoperative conditions associated with arrhythmia

- Ischaemic heart disease
- Pre-existing arrhythmias
- Hypertension
- Congestive heart failure
- Electrolyte disorders
- Valvular heart disease
- Medications:
  —β_2 agonists
  —theophylline
  —tricyclic antidepressants
- Less common causes:
  —thyrotoxicosis
  —cardiomyopathy (including alcoholic)
  —myocarditis
  —trauma – myocardial and intracranial
  —connective tissue disorders
  —drug and solvent abuse

PREOPERATIVE EVALUATION

Conditions associated with arrhythmias are given in Box 31.4.

The following symptoms and signs may indicate an arrhythmia:

- Paroxysmal dyspnoea
- Palpitations
- Dizziness
- Syncope.

Physical examination and a 12-lead ECG with rhythm strip may help little, and further evaluation requires 24-h ECG monitoring. The diagnosis and management of arrhythmias can be complex, particularly with the pro-arrhythmic potential of antiarrhythmic drugs. A cardiological opinion may be required.

HYPOKALAEMIA

Hypokalaemia is a common electrolyte disturbance. It prolongs repolarisation non-uniformly, which predisposes to arrhythmias. While a serum potassium level as low as 3.0 mmol l^{-1} is usually acceptable, this may not be so in the presence of other risk factors (e.g. digoxin). The effect of ventilation should be remembered. A pH change of 0.1 will change the serum potassium level by 1.0 mmol l^{-1} in the opposite direction.

HYPERKALAEMIA, HYPOMAGNESAEMIA AND HYPERCALCAEMIA

These changes can all provoke arrhythmias. In contrast, extremes of sodium concentration seem to have little effect.

MONITORING

V1 is the lead of choice for rhythm monitoring. In a three-lead system, MCL I or II is best.

31

BOX 31.5

Anaesthetic factors

- Hypotension or hypertension (e.g. inadequate anaesthesia)
- Oxygenation
- Carbon dioxide
- Laryngoscopy
- Drugs:
  —volatile anaesthetic agents
  —suxamethonium
  —pancuronium
  —central venous pressure lines (microshock hazard)

BOX 31.6

Surgical factors

- Catecholamines:
  —endogenous, from any surgical stimulus
  —exogenous – topical or infiltrated adrenaline (epinephrine)
- Autonomic stimulation
  —peritoneal and visceral traction
  —peritoneal insufflation
  —trigeminovagal reflexes – most notably the oculocardiac reflex, but seen throughout the trigeminal nerve distribution
  —laryngoscopy, bronchoscopy, oesophagoscopy
  —carotid artery and thyroid surgery
- Direct stimulation of the heart during cardiac or thoracic surgery
- Embolism
  —thrombus
  —fat
  —bone cement
  —air
  —carbon dioxide
  —amniotic fluid
- Other
  —aortic cross-clamping
  —limb reperfusion
  —glycine intoxication

INTRAOPERATIVE FACTORS

Certain anaesthetic and surgical interventions may specifically induce arrhythmias. The development of arrhythmias, however, may indicate an adverse change to myocardial oxygen balance.

ANAESTHETIC FACTORS

See Box 31.5.

The relationship between volatile agents and arrhythmias involves effects on:

- Duration of the action potential
- Automaticity
- Calcium flux
- Interactions with adrenaline (epinephrine)
- Myocardial oxygen balance.

Atrioventricular conduction is prolonged (least with isoflurane and sevoflurane). The direct volatile agent effect of decreased automaticity is countered by the potentiation of catecholamine arrhythmias. The significance of coronary steal in clinical practice is doubted.

SURGICAL FACTORS

See Box 31.6.

ASSESSMENT

During operation, more than one factor is likely to be contributing to a new arrhythmia.

- Identify the rhythm and evaluate its significance.
- Identify and remove any precipitating factors, which includes optimising myocardial oxygen balance.
- Only when the arrhythmia persists should specific treatment be given.

MANAGEMENT

The same management can be used for intraoperative dysrhythmias as is used for awake patients.

- Correct factors that may be contributing to the development of an arrhythmia, such as hypoxia, hypercapnia, hypokalaemia, hypomagnesaemia, inadequate anaesthesia.
- Treat the whole patient and not just the ECG.
- If the circulation is inadequate, external cardiac massage will be needed.
- Synchronised cardioversion is often a more attractive treatment option in the already anaesthetised patient.
- Consider an antiarrhythmic drug.

The negative inotropic effect of many antiarrhythmic drugs should be remembered. Adenosine is a useful agent for supraventricular tachycardias. Its value in slowing supraventricular tachycardia but not ventricular tachycardia (Box 31.7) is particularly valuable during operation when a 12-lead ECG is difficult to record. Adenosine will also be effective in Wolff–Parkinson–White tachycardia. Alternatively, dis-

opyramide or propranolol may be used, but verapamil and digoxin are contraindicated.

BOX 31.7

Distinguishing broad complex tachycardias

Supraventricular tachycardia (SVT)

- No axis change and same pattern of bundle
  branch block as pre-SVT ECG
- Conforms to right or left bundle branch
  block pattern
- Dominant R in V1 and Q in V6

Ventricular tachycardia (VT)

- Axis change from previous ECG
- Deep S wave in V6
- Fusion beats
- Capture beats

[a]Haemodynamic stability is not a distinguishing factor.
VT is much commoner than broad complex SVT,
especially if a previous ECG shows narrow complexes.

BIBLIOGRAPHY

Atlee JL, Bosnjck ZJ. Mechanisms for cardiac
dysrhythmias during anaesthesia. Anesthesiology
1990; 72:347–374

Singh BN, Opie LH, Marcus Fl. Antiarrhythmic agents.
In: Opie LH, ed. Drugs for the heart. 3rd edn.
Philadelphia: WB Saunders; 1991: ch 8

31

Intraoperative bronchospasm

J. Hammond

31

GENERAL FEATURES

- Lower airway obstruction due to bronchiolar constriction, characterised by an expiratory wheeze and raised airway pressures
- Potentially fatal complication
- Rare in comparison to upper airway obstruction and occlusion of breathing circuit, both of which should be excluded before the diagnosis of bronchospasm is made.

INCIDENCE

Asthma, coronary artery disease, smoking and respiratory infection are recognised as risk factors. A majority of cases, however, including those leading to adverse outcomes (brain damage, death), will occur in patients with no such factors.

One study revealed an overall incidence of 1.7 per 1000 anaesthetics, with a higher incidence at ages 0–9 years (4.0 per 1000) and 50–69 years (1.8 per 1000). These subgroups were analysed according to a number of variables (Table 31.8).

TABLE 31.8

Incidence of bronchospasm

Age group (years)	Studied variable	Incidence of bronchospasm (per 1000 cases)
0–9	Organic heart disease	15.3
	Abnormal ECG	24.3
	Respiratory infection	41.1
	Obstructive lung disease	21.9
	Tracheal intubation	9.1
50–69	Previous myocardial infarction	5.4
	Obstructive lung disease	7.7

Interestingly, cardiac disease is associated with an increased frequency of bronchospasm. This may be due to abnormal cardiopulmonary reflexes.

CAUSES

AIRWAY INSTRUMENTATION:
- Instrumentation and irritation of the airway may produce reflex bronchospasm.
- Tracheal intubation is the commonest trigger.
- Carinal stimulation, for example by a tracheal tube or suction catheter, is another common trigger.
- More likely under light anaesthesia.

SURGICAL STIMULATION:
- Nociception may trigger reflex bronchoconstriction.
- Patients undergoing upper abdominal, anal and cervical procedures are more prone to this reflex.
- Inadequate anaesthesia may be a predisposing factor.

BRONCHIAL ASPIRATION:
- May present with unilateral bronchospasm
- Could account for the higher incidence in children and during abdominal surgery.

ANAPHYLACTIC AND ANAPHYLACTOID REACTIONS
Bronchospasm is the first sign in 25% of reactions and the sole feature in 8%.

DRUGS
Various agents may predispose to bronchospasm:
- Beta-blockers – inhibition of β_2-mediated bronchodilatation
- Neostigmine – muscarinic effect if inadequately blocked by anticholinergic drugs

- Non-steroidal anti-inflammatory durgs (NSAIDs) – contraindicated in patients with aspirin-induced asthma (beware the 'aspirin triad' of asthma, nasal polyps and aspirin intolerance)
- Overall it has been estimated that 1 in 10 adult asthmatics will react adversely to various drugs.

REGIONAL TECHNIQUES

These are not devoid of risk. Psychological factors may trigger spasm in asthmatics.

Reports of bronchospasm occurring during spinal and epidural anaesthesia exist. These were attributed to a fall in circulating catecholamine levels due to block of sympathetic outflow to the adrenals (T10–L1).

CLINICAL FEATURES

SPONTANEOUS VENTILATION:
- Laboured respiration
- Intercostal recession
- Expiratory wheeze.

Intermittent positive-pressure ventilation:
- Increased airway pressure
- Decreased compliance.

Depending on the severity, ventilation and oxygenation become increasingly difficult.

Air trapping occurs with hyperinflation of the chest.

Acute pulmonary hypertension and reduced venous return due to increased intrathoracic pressure result in a fall in cardiac output in the severest cases.

Pneumothorax due to barotrauma may complicate the picture at any time. Suspect pneumothorax if there is a sudden deterioration.

MANAGEMENT

The action to be taken depends on the severity of the bronchospasm and the availability of equipment and agents. The majority of cases occur as a reflex response to airway instrumentation or surgery, and are relatively mild. They are managed simply by interrupting the operation temporarily and deepening anaesthesia. Further methods are indicated if there is an inadequate response.

GENERAL MANAGEMENT

It is vital to exclude a number of important differential diagnoses (Table 31.9).

TABLE 31.9

Differential diagnosis of bronchospasm

Diagnosis	Notes
Upper airway obstruction	Chin lift, jaw thrust, insert airway
Obstructed laryngeal mask	Reposition – if in doubt, remove
Obstructed tracheal tube	Verify patency – pass suction catheter, pass bronchoscope. If in doubt, remove
Breathing circuit malfunction	Check equipment
Breathing circuit obstruction	Check equipment
Tension pneumothorax	Airway pressure, auscultate chest
Oesophageal intubation	Observe capnograph trace

DRUG THERAPY
Volatile agents:
- All are effective bronchodilators.
- Many cases respond to an increase in the inspired concentration.
- Isoflurane is the least arrhythmogenic and is the agent of choice if using adrenaline (epinephrine).

β_2-Adrenoreceptor agonists:
- Salbutamol
  —250 μg i.v. (4 μg kg^{-1})
  —intravenous infusion (5–20 μg min^{-1})
  —nebulise in circuit (2.5–5 mg).
- Terbutaline (250–500 μg i.v.).

Aminophylline:
- No additional bronchodilatation if volatile agents used
- Inferior to β_2-adrenoreceptor agonists
- Administer 5 mg kg^{-1} slowly intravenously.

Corticosteroids:
- Of benefit in acute bronchospasm
- Mechanism of action is unclear, but there is evidence that they are beneficial in the acute situation
- Single dose of hydrocortisone (200–500 mg i.v.) or methylprednisolone (1 g i.v.).

Adrenaline (epinephrine):
- First-line agent in severe reactions and in anaphylaxis
- Give 3–5 ml of 1 : 10 000 intravenously.

31

Ketamine:
- Powerful bronchodilator
- Consider if there is a poor response to other agents.

VENTILATORY CONSIDERATIONS

Aim to reduce any risk of barotrauma and maintain oxygenation:
- Give 100% oxygen.
- Use a low frequency of ventilation with a long expiratory time; this minimises pulmonary distension.
- Use low tidal volumes to limit airway pressures.

A degree of hypercapnia is acceptable, provided that oxygenation is maintained. The minute volume can be increased as the bronchospasm resolves.

'Educated hand' manual ventilation may produce better oxygenation with higher minute volumes and lower airway pressures than with mechanical ventilation.

In the most severe cases, expiration due to passive recoil of lung and thorax cannot occur – conventional ventilation is impossible. Manual deflation of the chest may buy time:

- Inflate with 100% oxygen
- Disconnect tracheal tube
- Squeeze lateral aspects of chest for 10–15 s
- Repeat this cycle.

Worst-case scenario: catastrophic bronchospasm with the risk of severe barotrauma; cardiac arrest is imminent. Consider cardiopulmonary bypass, if available.

BIBLIOGRAPHY

Entrup MH, Davis FG. Perioperative complications of anaesthesia. Surgical Clinics of North America 1991; 71:1151–1173

Olsson GL. Bronchospasm during anaesthesia. A computer-aided incidence study of 136 929 patients. Acta Anaesthesiologica Scandinavica 1987; 31:244–252

CROSS-REFERENCES

Asthma
    Patient Conditions 3: 86

31

Intraoperative cyanosis

I. Banks

Cyanosis is a clinical sign. It results from the dark blue coloration of reduced haemoglobin (Gk. *kyanos*, blue). It occurs when the capillary concentration of reduced haemoglobin is greater than 5 g dl^{-1}.

Clinically there are two types of cyanosis:

- *Central* – results from imperfect oxygenation of blood in the general systemic circulation
- *Peripheral* – results from extraction of oxygen from blood in peripheries where blood flow is very sluggish (e.g. extreme cold). Any patient who is centrally cyanosed will also be peripherally cyanosed. However, a patient can be peripherally cyanosed without being centrally cyanosed.

Cyanosis results from:

- Hypoxic hypoxia – inadequate oxygenation
- Stagnant hypoxia – inadequate circulation.

NB: It is possible to be hypoxic without being cyanosed (e.g. anaemic hypoxia, carbon monoxide poisoning). The terms 'hypoxia' and 'cyanosis' are therefore not synonymous.

PREOPERATIVE CAUSES

- *Pulmonary disease* – severe chronic obstructive airway disease, lung collapse, trauma, restrictive lung disease, extreme obesity (pickwickian syndrome)
- *Ventilatory inadequacy* – drugs, airway obstruction, neurological problems
- *Cardiac problems* – severe cardiac failure, right-to-left shunt (congenital cyanotic heart disease, Eisenmenger's syndrome).

INTRAOPERATIVE CAUSES

RESPIRATORY:

- Inadequate inspired fraction of oxygen (hypoxic mixture).
- Airway obstruction – foreign body, forgotten throat pack, tongue against posterior pharyngeal wall, incorrectly placed laryngeal mask, laryngospasm, tracheal tube obstruction or kinking.
- Incorrect positioning of tracheal tube; oesophageal intubation, inadvertent endobronchial intubation.
- Inadequate ventilation:
  —spontaneous ventilation – depressant drugs such as opioids, anaesthetic agents
  —mechanical ventilation – disconnection of breathing system, incorrect ventilator settings, ventilator failure.
- Pulmonary problems – bronchospasm, collapse, pneumothorax, haemothorax, pre-existing lung disease, inhalation of gastric contents.
- Intentional one-lung ventilation.

CARDIOVASCULAR:

- Cardiac arrest
- Cardiac failure – from intraoperative fluid overload, myocardial infarction
- Embolism – pulmonary, air, carbon dioxide, amniotic fluid, fat
- Cardiac tamponade
- Tension pneumothorax
- Severe hypovolaemia
- Increased right-to-left shunt after reduction of systemic vascular resistance (Fallot's tetralogy).

OTHER CAUSES:

- Methaemoglobinaemia
- Transfusion reaction.

POSTOPERATIVE CAUSES

Almost all the above can also cause postoperative cyanosis. Other postoperative causes include:

- Inadequate inspired fraction of oxygen – diffusion hypoxia after use of nitrous oxide (NB: increased oxygen demand after surgery).
- Airway obstruction – forgotten throat pack, blood clot, tongue against posterior pharyngeal wall, laryngospasm

31

- Inadequate ventilation – residual depressant effect of anaesthetic drugs or opioids, inadequate reversal of neuromuscular blocking agents, pain, tight dressings, intraoperative intracerebral event, hypothermia.

DETECTION OF CYANOSIS

Patient observation may be difficult when the patient is completely draped, the lights are turned off, or the patient has dark skin. As cyanosis is a clinical sign, this is the only method of detecting cyanosis. Note that pulse oximetry will measure the percentage saturation of haemoglobin, which is helpful in the detection of hypoxia, but does not detect cyanosis itself.

TREATMENT OF THE CYANOSED PATIENT

- Administer a high concentration (ideally 100%) of oxygen and simultaneously assess airway patency. If obstructed, consider manipulations of airway, such as jaw thrust, airway insertion, possibility of foreign body, laryngospasm.

- Assess ventilation (hand ventilation may aid assessment, as may auscultation):
  —If chest is not moving, consider disconnection of breathing system, bronchospasm, apnoea secondary to drug administration, tracheal tube incorrectly positioned, tracheal tube blocked or kinked, ventilator failure
  —If chest movement is unilateral, consider endobronchial intubation, pneumothorax, lung collapse.
- Assess cardiovascular status.
- Further treatment depends on the underlying cause.

BIBLIOGRAPHY

Ganong WF. Review of medical physiology. 14th edn. California: Lange Medical Publications; 1989

CROSS-REFERENCES

Adult congenital heart disease
    Patient Conditions 4: 112
Children with CHD
    Patient Conditions 4: 126
Tetralogy of Fallot
    Patient Conditions 4: 144

31

Intraoperative hypertension

M. J. Jones

Intraoperative hypertension is a common complication during anaesthesia. Whether it is ultimately harmful to the patient depends on its degree, cause and duration, and on the condition of the patient. These factors also govern how actively it is treated.

Definitions

- An increase in blood pressure over 15% of the patient's baseline (the baseline is determined by a series of recordings).
- Systolic blood pressure > 160 mmHg and/or diastolic blood pressure > 95 mmHg.

HAEMODYNAMICS

$$MAP = SVR \times CO$$

where MAP is mean arterial blood pressure, SVR is systemic vascular resistance and CO is cardiac output.

The commonest cause of an increase in MAP is a raised SVR due to vasoconstriction. From the equation it can be seen that a raised blood pressure does not imply a raised CO. Indeed, the increased afterload due to vasoconstriction often causes a reduced CO.

COMPLICATIONS

CARDIOVASCULAR

Hypertension may precipitate myocardial ischaemia (especially subendocardial), infarction or failure.

HAEMORRHAGE

At operation site or from existing aneurysms.

NEUROLOGICAL

Cerebral encephalopathy, oedema or haemorrhage.

RENAL

Severe hypertension may precipitate acute renal failure.

MANAGEMENT

If severe and life-threatening, aggressive immediate therapy is warranted (e.g. MAP > 150 mmHg with signs of myocardial ischaemia). Confirmation of the diagnosis may require a trial of therapy. If there is no definite diagnosis, non-specific therapy is instituted.

INADEQUATE ANAESTHESIA OR ANALGESIA

This is the commonest cause. It usually accompanies a change in level of stimulation (e.g. movement of tracheal tube) or a waning of drug effect. It is usually associated with tachycardia (bradycardia if vagal tone increased), lacrimation, tachypnoea, movement or laryngospasm.

Treatment:
- Increase anaesthesia and/or analgesia (e.g. remifentanil)
- Consider reducing stimulation.

ANXIETY DURING LOCAL ANAESTHETIC TECHNIQUES

Reassure the patient and give sedation, if necessary.

INADEQUATE VENTILATION

Carbon dioxide retention causes catecholamine release.

Treatment:
- Check equipment and correct fault
- Optimise airway and ventilation
- Institute intermittent positive-pressure ventilation (IPPV).

OMISSION OF REGULAR ANTIHYPERTENSIVE MEDICINE

This may cause rebound hypertension (particularly clonidine).

31

TREATMENT

Assess preoperative therapy and administer appropriate drug, or use non-specific therapy.

DRUG INTERACTION

For example, monoamine oxygenase inhibitors + vasopressors or opioids (especially pethidine).

Treatment
May require drug therapy (e.g. beta-blockers or sodium nitroprusside).

DRUGS GIVEN BY SURGEON (FOR HAEMOSTASIS)

For example, adrenaline (epinephrine) infiltration.

Treatment
Beta-blockers.

DRUG ERROR OR SIDE-EFFECT

The wrong drug, dose or mode of administration (e.g. giving vasoactive drugs in variable carrier infusion). Ketamine, ergotamine, desflurane anaesthesia (greater than 1.0 MAC) etc. may cause hypertension.

Treatment:
- Careful handling and labelling of all drugs
- Use dedicated intravenous lines or locate connection close to patient to reduce risk of variable administration rate.

ARTEFACT

This may be due to the use of a blood pressure cuff of the wrong size, resonance in the arterial catheter or an incorrect zero point.

Treatment:
- Use appropriate cuff
- Calibrate arterial line and compare to cuff blood pressure
- Use correct tubing or clamping device
- Check zero point.

TOURNIQUET PAIN

Slow onset, often after 1 h. Bilateral tourniquets with exsanguination may cause sufficient fluid shift to increase blood pressure.

Treatment:
- Consult with surgeon
- May need drug therapy.

PRE-ECLAMPSIA

Treatment is with a non-specific hypotensive agent.

PHAEOCHROMOCYTOMA

This is a rare but important cause. Undiagnosed phaeochromocytoma is associated with a high perioperative mortality rate (approx. 50%).

Treatment:
- If suspected, a small bolus dose of phentolamine (2.5–5 mg) usually gives a significant fall in blood pressure (if systolic blood pressure falls more than 35 mmHg, phaeochromocytoma is likely)
- Give alpha-blockers in addition to beta-blockade (beta-blockade alone may worsen vasoconstriction).
- Remifentanil may be useful.

RARER CAUSES:
- Fluid overload
- Aortic cross-clamping
- Hyperthyroid storm
- Malignant hyperthermia
- Raised intracranial pressure
- Interference with carotid body or brainstem or spinal cord
- Bladder distension (especially postoperative)
- Alcohol or addictive drug withdrawal
- Autonomic hyperreflexia.

NON-SPECIFIC TREATMENT

If the cause of hypertension cannot be removed or diagnosed, the following may be useful.

VASODILATORS:
- Anaesthetic agents (e.g. isoflurane, sevoflurane, propofol) – easy to control.
- Hydralazine – arteriolar dilator, peak action after about 20 min following 5–10 mg i.v.
- Glyceryl trinitrate – arterial and venous dilator; dose $10–200\ \mu g\ min^{-1}$
- Nifedipine – sublingual or intranasal; onset 1–5 min after a 10-mg dose
- Labetalol – combined alpha- and beta-blockade; dose 5–20 mg i.v.
- Sodium nitroprusside – arteriolar dilator; very rapid response; administer by continuous intravenous infusion ($0.5\ mg\ kg^{-1}\ min^{-1}$ starting dose); larger doses may cause cyanide poisoning.

BETA-BLOCKERS:
- Propranolol – non-selective; dose 0.5–1 mg i.v.
- Esmolol – rapid onset; short half-life (9 min); $500\ \mu g\ kg^{-1}$ loading dose; $50–780\ \mu g\ kg^{-1}\ min^{-1}$ infusion
- Metoprolol – cardioselective (β_1); 5–15 mg i.v.

31

ALPHA-BLOCKERS

Phentolamine (0.2–2 mg i.v.).

REMIFENTANIL

The potent short-acting analgesic effect is proving very useful for the intraoperative control of blood pressure.

GANGLIONIC BLOCKERS

Trimetaphan (1–5 mg i.v.).

POSTOPERATIVE CARE

- Continue to monitor patient
- Provide adequate analgesia
- Consider face-mask oxygen (reduce myocardial ischaemia)
- May need continuing therapy
- May need investigations to exclude complications (e.g. myocardial infarction) or to identify cause of hypertension.

31

Intraoperative hypotension

B. J. Pollard

31

Mild falls in blood pressure commonly occur under anaesthesia and these are usually insignificant for the patient. When does a mild fall in blood pressure become a significant fall, however? That principally depends on the pre-operative blood pressure and medical condition (e.g. is the patient hypertensive?), the extent of the fall and the duration of the hypotension. Full monitoring of patients gives essential guidance. Development of atrial or ventricular ectopic beats and ST segment depression are two vital signs of inadequate myocardial perfusion. Increased ventilation–perfusion mismatch secondary to reduced pulmonary blood flow may produce a fall in SaO_2. In awake patients, nausea and dizziness are common symptoms of excessive hypotension. The lower limit of cerebral, renal and hepatic arterial autoregulation occurs at a mean arterial pressure of around 60 mmHg in a normal patient.

$$MAP = CO \times SVR$$
$$CO = HR \times SV$$

where MAP is mean arterial pressure, HR is heart rate, CO is cardiac output, SV is stroke volume and SVR is systemic vascular resistance.

Stroke volume depends on:

- Venous return
- Duration of ventricular diastole (which is affected by heart rate and rhythm)
- Cardiac contractility
- Correct functioning of heart valves and atria
- Afterload (SVR).

Heart rate depends on:

- Cardiac rhythm (sinus or other rhythm)
- The balance between opposing parasympathetic (vagal) and sympathetic tone.

SVR is determined by:

- Sympathetic vasoconstrictor tone
- Brainstem vasomotor outflow
- Exogenous sympathomimetic agents.

GRAVITY

MAP is reduced by 2 mmHg for every 2.5 cm of vertical height above the heart.

In an upright posture, cerebral perfusion pressure is 40 mmHg lower than the MAP measured at heart level.

Venous return, and therefore cardiac output, fall with the head-up position.

The beneficial effects on cerebral perfusion pressure, cardiac output and MAP of putting a patient in a head-down position, as an immediate treatment for excessive hypotension, should therefore be immediately apparent.

BARORECEPTOR COMPENSATION

Baroreceptors within the carotid sinus relay impulses via the ninth cranial nerve to the brainstem. A reduced discharge in response to hypotension disinhibits the vasomotor centre, resulting in a compensatory tachycardia and vasoconstriction. The Valsalva manoeuvre can be used to test the integrity of this reflex.

CAUSES OF HYPOTENSION UNDER GENERAL ANAESTHESIA

CARDIOVASCULAR DISEASE:

- Ischaemic heart disease with diminished cardiac contractility, including recent myocardial infarction and unstable angina
- Valvular heart disease – mitral or aortic stenosis and incompetence
- Heart failure, including cor pulmonale
- Dysrhythmias – rapid atrial fibrillation, third-degree heart block
- Hypertension, especially if untreated or poorly controlled
- Other – cardiomyopathy, myocarditis, constrictive pericarditis, myocardial contusion, tamponade, congenital cardiac anomalies, aortic coarctation.

CARDIOVASCULAR MEDICATION

Especially beta-blockers, but also angiotensin-converting enzyme (ACE) inhibitors, nitrates, calcium antagonists, α_1 antagonists (e.g. prazosin) and centrally acting α_2 agonists such as methyldopa and clonidine.

AUTONOMIC NEUROPATHY:

- Diabetes mellitus (both insulin and non-insulin dependent); incidence and severity increase with duration of diabetes
- Spinal cord injury and post-cerebrovascular accident states
- Parkinson's disease (in advanced cases)
- Guillain–Barré syndrome
- HIV or AIDS
- Amyloidosis
- Familial dysautonomia (Riley–Day syndrome)
- Shy–Drager syndrome.

INDUCTION AGENTS

These cause a dose-related fall in blood pressure due to a complex combination of effects involving vasodilatation, myocardial depression, altered baroreceptor reflex and bradycardia. Ketamine is an exception because of its central sympathomimetic action.

VOLATILE AGENTS

All volatile agents produce a dose-related fall in blood pressure due to a combination of vasodilatation, myocardial depression and impaired baroreceptor response. Myocardial depression and vagal stimulation resulting in bradycardia are features of halothane and higher doses of enflurane. Isoflurane at 1 MAC produces peripheral vasodilatation.

MUSCLE RELAXANTS

Any hypotensive effect is principally secondary to histamine release. This may occur with higher doses and rapid administration of atracurium or mivacurium.

OPIOIDS AND ANTIEMETICS

Opioids, especially morphine, may precipitate histamine release and hence vasodilatation. Bradycardia may also occur with larger doses of opioids. The butyrophenones and phenothiazines are weak α_1 antagonists.

DRUGS USED TO INDUCE HYPOTENSION DURING ANAESTHESIA

Interventions include sympathetic ganglion blockade (trimetaphan) and direct vasodilatation using glyceryl trinitrate or sodium nitroprusside. Labetalol may also be used and produces both α_1 and β blockade.

IPPV

The increased intrathoracic pressure that occurs with IPPV decreases venous return and consequently cardiac output. The effect is exacerbated with the application of positive end-expiratory pressure (PEEP). The baroreceptor response, although often partly obtunded under general anaesthesia, usually compensates for IPPV. However, this is not necessarily so in the presence of hypovolaemia, severe cardiac disease or autonomic neuropathy.

REGIONAL ANAESTHESIA

Epidural and spinal anaesthesia produce blockade of sympathetic as well as nociceptive fibres. The resulting vasodilatation reduces both venous return (and, therefore, cardiac output) and SVR. The height of the sympathectomy depends upon the site and dose used. Although reflex vasoconstriction occurs above the upper level of the block, blood pressure usually falls. With higher blocks (T4 and above) the cardiac sympathetics are obtunded reducing the compensatory tachycardia. In obstetric cases, aortocaval compression must be prevented as this further embarrasses venous return and in combination with epidural or spinal anaesthesia may produce profound hypotension.

SURGICAL CAUSES

These include use of a head-up position, blood loss, aortic cross-clamping and use of lower-limb tourniquets. Ischaemic tissues become maximally vasodilated. Release of the cross-clamp or tourniquet results in an acute fall in SVR and blood pressure. Inadvertent excessive intra-abdominal pressure during laparoscopic surgery may cause hypotension due to impaired venous return.

HYPOVOLAEMIA

Hypovolaemia is revealed under anaesthesia and the result is hypotension. Examples include dehydration from inadequate fluid intake, vomiting and diarrhoea; bowel preparation with a powerful cathartic; haematemesis, melaena, small bowel obstruction or acute inflammatory bowel disease; trauma and burns. Additional causes include metabolic disorders such as diabetic ketoacidosis, hypercalcaemia, diabetes insipidus and high-output renal failure.

ANAPHYLAXIS

This may result in the massive outpouring of inflammatory mediators, in particular histamine, which cause extreme vasodilatation and cardiovascular collapse. In addition to resuscitation, adrenaline (epinephrine) is the specific treatment. Pulmonary embolus (from a deep vein thrombosis), fat globules (from long-bone fractures), air bubbles (head and neck operations)

31

or carbon dioxide emboli (laparoscopic surgery) may also reduce cardiac output. Hypotension is accompanied by desaturation and alveolar hypocapnoea.

INTRAOPERATIVE MYOCARDIAL INFARCTION

This is strongly associated with pre-existing cardiac disease and is accompanied by ECG ischaemic changes.

TREATMENT OF INTRAOPERATIVE HYPOTENSION

First, remove the precipitating cause if possible; for example, correct hypovolaemia, increase cardiac output and SVR.

PRACTICAL POINTS

Manoeuvres to increase both cardiac output and SVR are most effective:

- Increase F_{IO_2} to maintain S_{aO_2}
- Place patient in head-down position
- Administer a rapid intravenous infusion (colloid gives a faster response than crystalloid)
- Vasopressors – ephedrine (mixed α and β_1 effects), methoxamine or phenylephrine (both α_1 agonists)
- If necessary, give an inotrope plus a vasoconstrictor; for example, dobutamine and noradrenaline (norepinephrine) together.

CROSS-REFERENCES

Induced hypotension
     Anaesthetic Factors 30: 704
Epidural and spinal anaesthesia
     Anaesthetic Factors 30: 696

31

Local anaesthetic toxicity

V. G. Venkatesan and I. McConachie

Considering the large numbers of local anaesthetics administered, the frequency of toxic reactions is very small. Here we concentrate on CNS and cardiac toxicity as manifestations of local anaesthetic toxicity. Causes of such toxicity are related to elevated plasma drug levels. This is due to:

- Accidental (or misinformed) overdosage
- Inadvertent intravenous injection.

There is a general relationship between plasma levels of local anaesthetics and symptoms and signs of toxicity (Table 31.10).

Initial excitation is due to selective inhibition of inhibitory pathways in the CNS. With increasing blood levels there is an inhibition of both inhibitory and facilitatory pathways, leading to generalised CNS depression.

However, although a general relationship between blood levels and toxicity exists, the rate of injection (if intravenous) or uptake also influences the chance of toxicity; for example, a faster rate of injection produces signs of toxicity at lower venous plasma levels.

METHODS OF REDUCING PLASMA LEVELS

Uptake is highest with concentrated solutions:

- Saturation of local binding sites
- Greater intrinsic vasodilating effects.

Uptake is highest from vascular sites, such as the epidural and intercostal spaces, and lowest from subcutaneous tissues.

The principal technique for minimising plasma levels is to reduce vascular uptake by the addition of adrenaline (epinephrine).

PHARMACOLOGY OF LOCAL ANAESTHETIC TOXICITY

- Potency varies directly with lipid solubility.
- Cardiac depression and CNS excitability vary directly with potency.

The mechanism for cardiac depression is unclear, but some experiments suggest that it may be related to decreased intracellular calcium concentration. In addition, at high plasma levels there will be generalised vasodilatation compounding the vascular collapse.

The relative potencies of bupivacaine and lidocaine (lignocaine) are about 4 : 1, which is similar to their relative CNS toxicities. Both the blood levels required for cardiac toxicity and the ratio of the doses required for cardiac toxicity, compared with doses required for CNS toxicity, suggest that bupivacaine is considerably more cardiotoxic than lidocaine, ropivacaine or levobupivacaine.

INFLUENCE OF ACIDOSIS

- The convulsive threshold is decreased.
- An increase in $PaCO_2$ leads to an increase in coronary blood flow, thus allowing more drug to enter the brain.
- A decrease in intracellular pH will increase the amount of ionised drug; this limits diffusion and prevents drug leaving the cell.

31

TABLE 31.10

Effect of increasing plasma drug levels

Symptom or sign	Drug level
Tingling in tongue and perioral region	. Low
Dizziness	↓
Blurred vision	↓
Tinnitus	↓
Twitching and signs of CNS excitation	Intermediate
Loss of consciousness	↓
Convulsions	↓
Deep coma	↓
Respiratory and cardiac arrest	High

- Decreased plasma protein binding results in more free drug.

Thus acidosis increases the chances of developing CNS toxicity and also prolongs the toxicity.

CLINICAL ASPECTS OF LOCAL ANAESTHETIC TOXICITY

SENSIBLE PRECAUTIONS:

- All resuscitation facilities and drugs must be available.
- Access to circulation should be secured before initiation of procedure.
- Trained assistance should be available.
- Maintain dialogue with patient during performance of block.

PREVENTION

- Careful technique
- Aspirate before injection and intermittently aspirate during prolonged injection if large volumes are used
- Choice of drug – for example, do not use bupivacaine for intravenous regional anaesthesia.

Ester local anaesthetics are metabolised by plasma cholinesterase. Thus, if toxic plasma levels are achieved, the toxic reaction should be short lived (except in the rare case of atypical cholinesterase).

TREATMENT

MINOR REACTIONS:

- Stop injection
- Observe patient.

MAJOR REACTIONS

Resuscitate according to standard guidelines.

CONVULSIONS

Convulsing patients rapidly become hypoxic and acidotic. Prompt treatment is therefore crucial.

- Convulsions should be quickly terminated with appropriate drugs such as benzodiazepines or thiopental.
- Suxamethonium may be required if the convulsions are severe or resistant to treatment, or if intubation is required.

CARDIAC DEPRESSION:

- Give oxygen – this is of prime importance
- Fluids
- Inotropes and vasopressors

- Defibrillation, if required
- Aggressive reversal of acidosis with bicarbonate is warranted, according to blood gas analysis
- If cardiac arrest supervenes, give CPR
- Prolonged CPR and resuscitation may be required.

LIDOCAINE (LIGNOCAINE)

- Is a potent antiarrhythmic agent.
- Arrhythmias are uncommon after overdosage.
- At high plasma levels, decreased cardiac conduction may be seen.

BUPIVACAINE

- The S isomer of bupivacaine is less toxic than the R isomer of bupivacaine.
- May potentiate arrhythmias.
- Exact mechanism is unknown.
- Markedly depresses the rapid phase of depolarisation of the cardiac action potential and prolongs the refractory period.
- May cause one-way block leading to re-entrant arrhythmias.
- Ventricular fibrillation is common in severe toxicity.
- Pregnant women are more sensitive to cardiotoxicity.
- Bupivacaine seems to be significantly associated with cardiac toxicity compared with other local anaesthetics. CPR is very difficult in bupivacaine-induced cardiotoxicity because the drug binds to cardiac muscle (exacerbated by acidosis).

ROPIVACAINE

This is a new amide drug intermediate in structure and potency to mepivacaine and bupivacaine. It is represented as the S isomer rather than a racemic mixture.

- Aggressive CPR may be successful with ropivacaine cardiotoxicity.
- Larger doses are required to produce early features of CNS toxicity and cardiotoxicity.
- Animal studies show similar cardiotoxicity profile in both pregnant and non-pregnant states.
- Produces greater differential block, with the motor block being less intense and of shorter duration.

LEVOBUPIVACAINE

- Single S isomer of bupivacaine.
- Long acting.

- Intermediate toxicity.
- Human volunteer studies suggest lesser cardiac depression with smaller changes in the indices of cardiac contractility compared with bupivacaine.
- Human studies also suggest lesser CNS depression compared with bupivacaine.
- Lethal dose is higher than that of bupivacaine.

BIBLIOGRAPHY

Gristwood RW. Cardiac and CNS toxicity of levobupivacaine. Drug Safety 2002; 25:153–163

Moore DC. Administer oxygen first in the treatment of local anaesthesia induced convulsions. Anesthesiology 1980; 53:346–347

Scott DB. Maximum recommended doses of local anaesthetic drugs. British Journal of Anaesthesia 1989; 63:373–374

Richards A, McConachie I. The pharmacology of local anaesthetic drugs. Current Anaesthesia and Critical Care 1995; 6:41–47

Whiteside JB, Wildsmith JAW. Developments in local anaesthetic drugs. British Journal of Anaesthesia 2001; 87:27–35

31

Malignant hyperthermia: clinical presentation

P. M. Hopkins

31

Due to the reduction in major morbidity and mortality rates from other causes, malignant hyperthermia (MH) is now one of the major potential anaesthetic hazards for the otherwise healthy individual. This is despite the mortality rate for MH declining from above 70% before 1980 to below 4% over the past 5 years. It is argued by some that, with the use of modern monitoring equipment and the mandatory availability of intravenous dantrolene, the mortality rate from MH should be zero.

The key to prevention of death from a MH reaction undoubtedly is recognition by the attending anaesthetist of the early signs of the reaction followed by an appropriate therapeutic response. It is interesting to note that the rapid decline in mortality in the UK began before the introduction of intravenous dantrolene; this is attributed to increasing awareness of the condition amongst UK anaesthetists.

MH is now known to be a genetically heterogeneous disorder. More than 30 different mutations of the major gene implicated in MH susceptibility ($RYR1$ – the sarcoplasmic reticulum calcium release channel gene) have been reported, but in many MH families the precise molecular defect is yet to be determined. The result of each defect is, however, the same and that is to produce an uncontrollable rise in intracellular calcium ion concentration in skeletal muscle cells in the presence of the triggering drugs (any potent inhalation anaesthetic drug or suxamethonium). This increase in myoplasmic calcium ion concentration is sufficient to explain all the clinical and biochemical features of MH, knowledge of which is crucial if an anaesthetist is to have the best chance of successfully managing a MH reaction.

The nature and course of MH reactions show considerable variation. The components of a reaction can be crudely divided into metabolic and muscle activity, both of which lead to rhabdomyolysis. The balance and severity of metabolic and muscle activity components generally vary according to which triggering drugs have been used. This is assumed to be a reflection of the dynamics of the rise in intracellular calcium ion concentration.

THE RESPONSE TO SUXAMETHONIUM

Suxamethonium is thought to produce a rapid and marked rise in intracellular calcium concentration, but its duration of effect is limited. The predominant feature is thus increased muscle activity, evident as rigidity. This muscle rigidity is sometimes generalised, but may be limited to the jaw muscles (masseter muscle spasm is discussed in more detail in a separate section). Because of the limited duration of effect of suxamethonium, homeostatic mechanisms restore the intracellular calcium towards resting levels, usually within 10 min. The muscle activity leads to extrusion of potassium ions, creatine kinase and myoglobin. The hyperkalaemia due to suxamethonium alone usually is not life threatening (unlike with the muscular dystrophies where suxamethonium can cause grossly increased serum potassium concentration), but the myoglobinaemia may be sufficient to cause acute renal failure. Indeed, postoperative renal failure has been the only presenting feature in some MH-susceptible patients. Serum creatine kinase is an indicator of the degree of muscle damage, reaching a maximum (often > 20 000 units) after about 24 h. Although metabolic processes will have been stimulated, the duration of the stimulus is so short that the resulting clinical features are mild and usually not noticed.

THE RESPONSE TO POTENT INHALATION ANAESTHETICS

The nature of the response to potent inhalation anaesthetics suggests that they cause a steadily increasing intracellular calcium ion concentration. Calcium, at concentrations lower than those required to activate the contractile apparatus, has other important intracellular functions. One of these is the regulation of the phosphorylation, and hence the activity, of various enzymes, including rate-limiting enzymes of the glycolytic pathway. During a gradually increasing intracellular calcium ion concentration, the first detectable features result from this metabolic stimulation: the earliest clinical signs are caused by increased carbon dioxide and lactate production. In the spontaneously breathing patient there will be an increasing respiratory rate, and where a circle system is in use the soda lime will be rapidly exhausted. Whatever mode of ventilation and breathing system is being used, the increased carbon dioxide production will be detected as an increasing end-tidal partial pressure of carbon dioxide by capnography. Either simultaneously with, or shortly after, the hypercapnoea, a tachycardia develops secondary to the effects of acidaemia on the cardiovascular regulatory centre of the midbrain. By the same mechanism there is a tendency for the blood pressure to rise, although in some cases the blood pressure falls, presumably due to a predominant effect of local metabolites on the vascular smooth muscle. As well as an increase in lactate and carbon dioxide as byproducts of metabolism, there is an increase in oxygen consumption that may lead to a fall in the saturation of haemoglobin with oxygen, detectable with pulse oximetry. Arterial blood gases taken at this stage will show acidaemia, hypercarbia, a base deficit and, usually, mild hypoxaemia.

The term malignant hyperthermia was originally coined because the most obvious clinical feature was that the patient would become excessively hot and then invariably died. This was, of course, at a time when monitoring during routine anaesthesia was purely clinical. We now know that hyperthermia resulting from the hypermetabolic state is a relatively late manifestation and, whereas during the 1970s and early 1980s monitoring of body temperature was advised for every anaesthetic, capnography has now superseded it. However, when some doubt exists as to whether some metabolic signs are due to MH, the finding of a rapidly rising body temperature is very persuasive, although, as indicated above, in some cases there is a delay before the rate of temperature rise becomes remarkable.

It is commonly considered that there is a stage of a MH reaction beyond which death is almost inevitable; this is likely to relate to the integrity of the mitochondria. In the early stages of the reaction, the mitochondrion responds to the increased production of pyruvate by increasing its utilisation to produce more ATP. This is important in limiting the intracellular calcium ion concentration as ATP is required for the normal functioning of two of the most important mechanisms for removing calcium from the myoplasm: the calcium pumps of the sarcolemma and the sarcoplasmic reticulum. The mitochondria themselves, however, also sequester calcium ions, the rate being entirely dependent on the myoplasmic calcium ion concentration. In the presence of continued release or influx of calcium into the myoplasm, the intramitochondrial calcium ion concentration will continue to increase until the accumulated calcium disrupts the mitochondria. A situation is thus reached where glycolysis is stimulated and the only route for further metabolism of pyruvate is to lactate. Simultaneously, there is a rapid decline in ATP production, leading to a reduced rate of calcium removal from the myoplasm, and hence setting up a vicious cycle. It is at this stage that muscle rigidity will become apparent. Muscle rigidity itself restricts microvascular perfusion of the tissue, in which case dantrolene administered intravenously will not reach its site of action. The perfusion of the muscle will also be compromised as muscles swell within their fascial compartments as a result of the oedema associated with mitochondrial failure and cell death.

Calcium ions also stimulate activity of some intracellular phospholipases, leading to increased turnover of sarcolemmal phospholipid. Under these circumstances, maintenance of the integrity of the sarcolemma is an ATP-dependent process, and when the demand for ATP exceeds the supply the membrane permeability increases. This will result in increased leakage of calcium into the cell and also leakage out of intracellular constituents such as potassium ions, creatine kinase and myoglobin. The resulting hyperkalaemia at this stage may be sufficient to cause cardiac arrest while, if the acute reaction is survived, the myoglobinaemia can result in renal failure.

A further feature of an advanced MH reaction is disseminated intravascular coagulation (DIC). Heat itself and/or procoagulant proteins that leak from dying muscle cells can cause DIC.

The response to the potent inhalation anaesthetics tends to be more rapid following suxamethonium, with some florid reactions

31

occurring within 15 min. In the laboratory setting, halothane certainly seems to be the most potent trigger of the potent inhalation anaesthetics, but clinical responses to enflurane, isoflurane and sevoflurane can be indistinguishable from those caused by halothane. Cases of human MH have been triggered by desflurane, but these are too few to comment on this drug's comparative potency or efficacy as a trigger of MH.

BIBLIOGRAPHY

Hopkins PM. Malignant hyperthermia: advances in clinical management and diagnosis. British Journal of Anaesthesia 2000; 85:118–128

CROSS-REFERENCES

Malignant hyperthermia
    Patient Conditions 2: 75

31

Masseter muscle spasm

P. M. Hopkins

The major problem with masseter muscle spasm (MMS) is in defining what it means. The first common usage of the term arose when malignant hyperthermia (MH) reactions subsequently occurred in patients whose mouths had been difficult to open following the use of suxamethonium. This association was apparent in 70% of patients given suxamethonium who went on to develop MH. Awareness of this association between MMS and MH led to the referral of many patients who developed MMS for investigation of their MH status. Of those with MMS as the only abnormal feature, 28% have proven to be susceptible to MH. The proportion rises to 57% if there were accompanying metabolic features, or to 76% if the MMS was followed by other features of muscle damage, such as myoglobinuria or severe incapacity from muscle pains. From this experience, which is similar amongst MH investigation centres, it seemed clear that patients developing MMS were at high risk from MH until proven otherwise. However, at that stage there was no definition of what was meant by MMS.

The situation really started to become confusing in the late 1980s with the publication of studies in which the tension developed by the jaw muscles following suxamethonium was found to rise in virtually all children and in a large proportion of adults. The unfortunate outcome of these studies was that some interpreted the results as meaning that most patients develop MMS following suxamethonium. The next stage in this trail of false logic was to extrapolate this interpretation for comparison with the incidence of MH in patients referred because of MMS. The result of this erroneous comparison could only be that the incidence of MH in the population was much higher than previously thought, or that the *in vitro* contracture tests used for MH diagnosis had a very high false-positive response rate.

A more consistent explanation can be realised by examining how patients came to be investigated for their MH status following an episode of 'MMS'. These cases were not those in which there was a measured increase in jaw muscle tension; rather they were cases in which the attending anaesthetist experienced a clinical problem in opening the mouth in order to achieve tracheal intubation. Prior to the publications by van der Spek et al (1987) and Leary & Ellis (1990), the commonly encountered mild and transient resistance to mouth opening following injection of suxamethonium was probably attributed to a failure of relaxation rather than to muscle tension development. The cases referred for MH investigation were therefore outside the normal experience of the attending anaesthetist in terms of the severity and duration of the difficulty in mouth opening.

The term MMS is therefore of practical and clinical significance only if its use is restricted to severe and, perhaps more importantly, the prolonged (more than 2 min) episodes of resistance to mouth opening following suxamethonium administration.

Another misleading feature of the relationship between MMS and MH is the lack of metabolic response following MMS. This is a reflection of the disproportionate effect of suxamethonium as a MH-triggering drug in terms of the balance between increased muscle activity and increased metabolic activity (see previous section on Malignant hyperthermia: clinical presentation). Also, a metabolic response may not be observed even if the anaesthetic is continued with volatile drugs, as we know that patients susceptible to MH do not have a reaction with every exposure to triggering drugs. The reasons for this are not clear.

MANAGEMENT OF MMS

IMMEDIATE

The patient who has been given suxamethonium will obviously be paralysed, so the first priority is ventilation of the lungs. Fortunately, upper airway muscle tone seems to

31

be maintained, thereby making ventilation with a face-mask via the nose a viable proposition.

DIFFERENTIAL DIAGNOSIS

Establish that the correct dose of suxamethonium has been given, intravenously; check the ampoule, syringe and injection site. It is, however, unusual for mouth opening to be a major problem even when no neuromuscular blocking drug has been given, unless the dose of induction agent was also inadequate; this would, of course, occur if a cannula had become dislodged from its intravenous site during induction.

FURTHER ANAESTHETIC MANAGEMENT

This will depend on the urgency of the operation and the feasibility of continuing non-urgent surgery without the use of volatile anaesthetic drugs. If the operation is not urgent and continuation with a volatile-free technique is potentially compromising, the patient should be allowed to wake up. Should the operation need to proceed, ventilation should continue via the face-mask until the spasm has eased, when a non-depolarising neuromuscular blocker can be given and intubation subsequently achieved. Anaesthesia should be maintained with intravenous drugs.

RECORDING OF DIAGNOSTIC PREDICTORS

Although the patient who develops MMS must be considered to be potentially susceptible to MH until proven otherwise, evidence of metabolic stimulation and other indicators of increased muscle activity increase the likelihood of MH. Therefore, the patient should be observed immediately for the presence of generalised muscle rigidity, and the duration of MMS should be recorded. An accurate chart of heart rate, blood pressure, pulse oximetry, capnography and central temperature readings should be made. Blood for arterial blood gas and serum potassium analysis should be sent. In the postoperative period, the first voided urine should be analysed for the presence of myoglobin and the serum level of creatine kinase should be estimated at 12 and 24 h.

FURTHER INVESTIGATIONS

The patient should be referred for determination of their MH status by muscle biopsy and *in vitro* contracture testing. They should he advised that they and all members of the family should be treated as potentially susceptible to MH until proven otherwise. In the interim, the reactor should undergo EMG studies to exclude congenital myotonia, some variants of which can be asymptomatic.

BIBLIOGRAPHY

Christian AS, Halsall PJ, Ellis FR. Is there a relationship between masseter muscle spasm and malignant hyperthermia? British Journal of Anaesthesia 1989; 62:540–544

Leary NP, Ellis FR. Masseteric muscle spasm as a normal response to suxamethonium. British Journal of Anaesthesia 1990; 64:488–492

van der Spek AFL, Fang WB, Ashton-Miller JA, Stohler S, Coulson DS, Schork MA. The effect of succinylcholine on mouth opening. Anesthesiology 1987; 67:459–465

CROSS-REFERENCES

31

Neuroleptic malignant syndrome

B. J. Pollard

Neuroleptic malignant syndrome (NMS) was first described in 1960 by Delay. It is a potentially fatal condition caused either by treatment with dopamine receptor antagonists or by withdrawal of dopamine receptor agonists.

PATHOGENESIS

CENTRAL MECHANISMS
There is acute dopaminergic transmission block in the:
- Nigrostriatum – producing rigidity
- Hypothalamus – producing hyperthermia
- Corticolimbic system – producing an altered mental state.

PERIPHERAL MECHANISMS
The clinical similarities between NMS and malignant hyperthermia (MH) suggest a common pathophysiological element. *In vitro* halothane–caffeine contracture tests carried out on patients with NMS and MH have not, however, supported any intracellular association between the two syndromes.

The pathophysiological mechanism underlying the skeletal muscle rigidity in NMS is controversial. The current view leans towards this being central in origin. This is supported by the observation that neuromuscular block-ing drugs produce flaccid paralysis in NMS, whereas in MH they have no effect.

EXCITATORY AMINO ACIDS
There is now believed to be a relative glutaminergic transmission excess as a consequence of a dopaminergic block, and it may be that drugs that antagonise glutamate have beneficial effects (see below).

INCIDENCE

Approximately 0.5–1%.

CLINICAL FEATURES AND DIAGNOSIS

NMS develops over a period of 24–72 h following exposure to neuroleptic agents. This exposure may have been over a period of days or months, and may even follow a low dose of a neuroleptic agent. The features may continue for up to 10 days, even after stopping the triggering agent. (See Box 31.8.)

MORTALITY

Rates of 8–30% are frequently quoted, but the number of deaths has declined since 1984 (less than 11% at present versus 25% before 1984). These values are apparently independent of the use of dopamine agonists and dantrolene.

Death from NMS is due to:
- Respiratory failure (commonest cause)
- Renal failure secondary to myoglobinuria (a strong predictor of mortality, representing a risk of 50%)
- Cardiac arrest.

Other complications are outlined in Box 31.9.

31

BOX 31.8

Criteria for diagnosis of NMS

Major criteria

- Fever
- Rigidity
- Raised serum creatine kinase level[a]

Minor criteria

- Tachycardia
- Raised blood pressure
- Tachypnoea
- Altered consciousness level
- Sweating

[a]May be mildly or grossly raised. No specific laboratory markers exist.

BOX 31.9

Complications

Respiratory

- Secondary infection
- Aspiration pneumonia

Cardiovascular

- Arrhythmias
- Pulmonary embolism

Musculoskeletal

- Peripheral neuropathy
- Rhabdomyolysis → myoglobinuria

DIFFERENTIAL DIAGNOSIS

Early diagnosis and distinction from other conditions presenting in a similar fashion is crucial in order to prevent fatalities.

NMS VERSUS FATAL CATATONIA

Rigidity is intermittent in fatal catatonia. Fatal catatonia demonstrates severe psychotic excitement in the early stages.

MH VERSUS NMS

Compared with MH, NMS demonstrates:
- Slow onset
- Rigidity of central origin (controversial)
- Latency of effect with dantrolene
- Uneventful anaesthesia with MH-triggering agents
- Lack of familial tendency (MH is autosomal dominant).

DRUGS OF ABUSE

Ethanol withdrawal, sedative hypnotic withdrawal, cocaine and amphetamine intoxication or monoamine oxidase overdoses must be excluded before NMS is diagnosed. Some of these agents may also release central serotonin, resulting in the central serotonin syndrome.

NEUROLEPTIC HEAT-STROKE

Flaccid muscle tone is the major distinguishing feature.

MANAGEMENT

NON-SPECIFIC THERAPY:
- Withdrawal of trigger agent
- Basic resuscitation measures
- Cooling.

SPECIFIC THERAPY
Dopamine agonists

Bromocriptine has reduced death rates to below 8%. Amantadine has reduced death rates to below 6%.

Dantrolene and bromocriptine

Dantrolene has reduce the death rate to below 9%. It may, however, cause hepatic damage (altered liver enzymes are already present in NMS). The success of dantrolene supports the 'muscle hypothesis', but the time to clinical effect is slow (several days).

Bromocriptine may be the type of choice in patients with NMS associated with hepatic dysfunction.

The relative reduction in death rate holds up at all the levels of syndrome severity in both dantrolene and bromocriptine groups.

Anticholinergic agents

These drugs are best avoided when rigidity is associated with pyrexia.

Glutamate antagonists

Amantadine and memantine are antagonists at the N-methyl-D-aspartate (NMDA) type of glutamate receptor. They:
- Restore the balance between glutaminergic and dopaminergic systems when dopaminergic transmission has been antagonised by neuroleptic drugs
- Exhibit hypothermic and central muscle relaxant properties.

These drugs could therefore be effective in the reversal of NMS.

ELECTROCONVULSIVE THERAPY (ECT)

This is controversial and may only be treating early psychosis following neuroleptic withdrawal, rather than NMS.

RE-EXPOSURE TO TRIGGER AGENT

Withdrawal of a neuroleptic agent, when treatment is required for severely psychotic patients, is obviously hazardous.

The mortality rate following reintroduction is variable (17–87%) and may be reduced by:
- Low-potency neuroleptic agents
- Lowest possible dose of neuroleptic agent
- Monitoring of creatine kinase levels.

ANAESTHESIA

Anaesthetists need to be aware of this syndrome in the context of anaesthesia for ECT. It is important to note that the technique of anaesthesia must not aggravate the muscle disorder or produce the complications of NMS.

It is advisable to avoid suxamethonium in the presence of active muscle disease, as it may release potassium into the circulation and cause rhabdomyolysis. Propofol is best avoided in ECT as it shortens the duration of seizures and increase the frequency of treatment.

MAIN POINTS

- The pathogenesis of NMS is still not fully understood.
- Early diagnosis is crucial.
- Differential diagnosis remains problematical in the absence of suitable animal models and biological markers for NMS.
- Anaesthesia for patients with NMS may continue safely in presence of MH trigger agents.
- The cornerstones of management are withdrawal of the trigger agent and supportive therapy; pharmacological therapy is merely adjunctive.
- Reintroduction of NMS trigger agents is possible, but must be done cautiously.

BIBLIOGRAPHY

Adnet PJ, Krivosic-Horber RM, Adamantidis MM et al. The association between the neuroleptic malignant syndrome and malignant hyperthermia. Acta Anaesthesiologica Scandinavica 1989; 33:676–680

Anderson WH. Lethal catatonia and the neuroleptic syndrome. Critical Care Medicine 1991; 19:1333–1334

Dickey W. The neuroleptic malignant syndrome (review). Progress in Neurobiology 1991; 36:425–436

Hard C. Neuroleptic malignant syndrome versus malignant hypothermia (letter; comment). American Journal of Medicine 1991; 91:322–323

Weller M, Kornhuber J. A rationale for NMDA receptor antagonist therapy of the neuroleptic malignant syndrome (review). Medical Hypotheses 1992; 38:329–333

CROSS-REFERENCES

ECT
    Anaesthetic Factors 26: 600
Malignant hyperthermia: clinical presentation
    Anaesthetic Factors 31: 764

31

Pacing and anaesthesia

A. Vohra

PATIENT CHARACTERISTICS

Most patients have a history of heart disease:
- Ischaemia
- Cardiomyopathy
- Idiopathic
- Congenital
- Following cardiac surgery.
  There may be other associated conditions:
- Peripheral vascular disease
- Diabetes
- Hypertension.

PREOPERATIVE EVALUATION

HISTORY:
- Surgical operation, especially site
- Assessment of cardiac disease.

It is wise to refer the patient to the cardiology department to check the pacemaker function and determine any unusual features of the patient or the pacemaker.

NB: These patients cannot undergo magnetic resonance imaging (MRI).

PACEMAKER FUNCTION:
- Reason for insertion.
- Type of pacemaker:
  —demand (synchronous)
  —fixed (asynchronous)
  —automated implantable cardioverter–defibrillator (AICD).
- When inserted – possibility of electrode displacement if within 4 weeks; possibility of battery failure if a long time ago.
- History of vertigo or syncope – possible battery failure.
- Irregular heart rate – possible competition with intrinsic heart rate.

ECG:
- May indicate ischaemia or previous myocardial infarction
- Confirm pacing capture (if pacing rate > intrinsic rate)

- No intrinsic rhythm (patient is pacemaker dependent)
- Only intrinsic rhythm seen – test pacemaker function by converting it to fixed mode with magnet.

CHEST RADIOGRAPHY:
- Usual assessment of heart size and lung fields
- Continuity of pacing leads; distal tips within cardiac cavity (especially in patients with chest trauma).

SERUM POTASSIUM
If high, pacing threshold is increased.

ACID–BASE BALANCE
Changes may affect pacing threshold.

ADDITIONAL PREPARATION

An AICD should be switched off before surgery. External pads should be attached to these patients.

MAGNET
This is used to convert the pacemaker to a fixed rate if necessary. Not to be used routinely.

CHRONOTROPIC DRUGS:
- Atropine (0.5–3.0 mg) – may not be effective
- Isoprenaline (10–100-μg bolus, or 1–10 μg min^{-1} infusion). NB: isoprenaline may decrease SVR
- Ephedrine (3–30 mg) – α and β effects
- Adrenaline (epinephrine) (1 : 200 000; 0.5–1-ml boluses).

DIATHERMY:
Problems:
- Inhibition of pacemaker
- Reprogramming of pacemaker
- Permanent damage to pulse generator
- Induction of ventricular fibrillation – by energy travelling down the leads to the heart

- Rise in capture threshold due to endocardial burns.

Precautions:
- Plate and current direction as far away from chest as possible
- No diathermy within 25 cm of pacing box
- Bipolar is safer than unipolar mode.

Transurethral resection of the prostate (TURP):
- Cutting mode can interfere – use short bursts
- Coagulation mode should not interfere
- Ask surgeon to use short bursts
- May need to convert pacing state to fixed mode if diathermy around chest
- There is a possibility of phantom reprogramming due to electromagnetic induction.

PERIOPERATIVE MANAGEMENT

PREMEDICATION
Not essential. An opioid or benzodiazepine is suitable.

MONITORING:
- Routine minimal monitoring, especially peripheral pulse to confirm cardiac output.
- Invasive monitoring if indicated for operation.
- Caution: possibility of entanglement with pacing wires if inserting central venous or pulmonary artery catheters. These should be considered only if absolutely necessary.
- Nerve stimulators can interfere with pacing – caution needed when using for brachial plexus blocks.

ANAESTHETIC TECHNIQUE:
- Consider local anaesthesia.
- Vasodilatation may be poorly tolerated with fixed heart rates.
- Volatile anaesthetics may increase atrioventricular delay and pacing threshold; avoid halothane.
- Total intravenous anaesthesia may be preferable.
- Caution with suxamethonium:
  —Acute release of potassium may increase pacing threshold
  —Myopotentials during fasciculation may be abnormally sensed.
- Avoid underhydration.

BIBLIOGRAPHY

Bloomfield P, Bowler GMR. Anaesthetic management of the patient with a permanent pacemaker. Anaesthesia 1989; 44:42–46

Shapiro WA, Roizen MT, Singleton MA, Morady F, Bainton C R, Gaynor RL. Intraoperative pacemaker complications. Anesthesiology 1985; 63:319–322

Zaidan JR. Pacemakers. Anesthesiology 1984; 60:319–334

31

Postoperative oliguria

P. Nightingale and M. Venning

DEFINITION

After operation the metabolic response to surgery produces sodium retention and decreased free water clearance so that a reduction in urine output is common.

The mean postoperative solute load is 600 (range 450–750) mosmol per day; this will be increased by intravenous electrolyte solutions. The maximum renal concentrating ability is 1200 mosmol per kg water, so the minimum urine volume required is:

600 mosmol daily/1200 mosmol per kg $H_2O = 0.5$ kg H_2O daily ≈ 220 ml h^{-1}

Oliguria is conveniently defined as a urine output greater than 20 ml h^{-1} for two consecutive hours.

PATHOPHYSIOLOGY

Postoperative oliguria may simply reflect the normal neuroendocrine response to trauma but often implies one or, more commonly, a number of the following factors:

REDUCED RENAL BLOOD FLOW:
- Hypovolaemia
- Poor cardiac output
- Hypotension – beware diabetes and myeloma
- Pre-existing renal damage
- Renal vascular disease – beware ACE inhibitors
- Renal vasoconstriction – beware NSAIDs
- Liver failure (hepatorenal syndrome)
- Sepsis

INTRINSIC RENAL DAMAGE:
- Hypoxia
  —from pre-renal causes
  —renal vein thrombosis
- Nephrotoxins
  —aminoglycosides
  —amphotericin
  —chemotherapeutic agents
  —NSAIDs
  —radiocontrast media – beware diabetes, myeloma, low cardiac output
- Tissue injury
  —pancreatitis
  —haemoglobinuria
  —myoglobinuria
  —tumour lysis (uric acid, xanthine, phosphate
- Inflammatory nephritides
  —glomerulonephritis
  —interstitial nephritis, including drug induced
  —polyarteritis
- Myeloma
- Sepsis

OBSTRUCTION TO FLOW:
- Renal or ureteric
  —calculi
  —clots
  —necrotic papillae
- Pelvic surgery
- Raised intra-abdominal pressure
- Prostate enlargement
- Bladder neck obstruction
- Blocked drainage system

A combination of reduced renal blood flow and previous intrinsic renal damage frequently presents as acute tubular necrosis.

Oliguria is most commonly due to renal hypoperfusion and only rarely from withdrawal of diuretic therapy. Total anuria is usually mechanical in origin but rarely may be due to renal artery occlusion or embolism; beware the patient with a single kidney.

Renal hypoperfusion may not produce oliguria if the ability to concentrate is poor:
- Prior renal disease
- Diuretic therapy
- The elderly
- Sickle cell disease.

31

INITIAL ASSESSMENT

HISTORY

Although a single causative factor that is extremely severe can cause acute renal failure, normally there are a number of predisposing factors (Box 31.10).

Check anaesthetic and other charts for episodes of tachycardia and/or hypotension. From estimates of fluid loss, assess whether adequate volumes of appropriate fluids have been given.

EXAMINATION

Physical examination and chest radiography alone are unreliable in assessing the haemodynamic and volume status in the seriously ill patient, where cardiac filling pressures often bear little relation to blood volume.

Note any of the following:
- Cardiorespiratory:
  —tachypnoea
  —tachycardia
  —jugular venous pressure
  —hypotension (check for postural drop)
  —third heart sound
  —absent peripheral pulses or vascular bruits
  —sacral or peripheral oedema
  —cool peripheries
  —reduced skin turgor (assess on forehead or neck).
- Abdominal:
  —tense abdomen
  —palpable bladder
  —obstructed drainage system.
- Evidence of infection or systemic disease:
  —pyrexia
  —sputum production
  —cloudy urine
  —soft tissue infection
  —vasculitic or drug rash
  —bruising
  —systemic emboli
  —muscle damage
  —ischaemic tissues
  —compartment syndrome.

INVESTIGATIONS

Consider investigations that will aid diagnosis and monitoring.

Exclude obstruction if the cause of oliguria is not immediately obvious.
- Ultrasonography to assess:
  —hydronephrosis or thrombosis of renal veins
  —bladder size and catheter location.
- Doppler studies may be helpful in some patients.
- Abdominal radiography (KUB) for:
  —calculi in ureter and kidney
  —aortoiliac calcification or nephrocalcinosis.
- Sepsis screen:
  —chest radiography
  —blood cultures
  —sputum culture
  —mid-stream sample of urine (MSSU).

BLOOD TESTS
- Arterial blood gases and lactate
- Full biochemical profile including electrolytes, urea, creatinine, blood sugar, bicarbonate, calcium, phosphate, liver function tests and C-reactive protein (CRP)

BOX 31.10

Factors associated with acute renal failure

Patient factors

- Advanced age
- Aortic surgery
- Atherosclerosis (especially aortic)
- Cardiac surgery
- Chronic renal disease
- Cirrhosis
- Diabetes
- Heart failure
- Hepatobiliary surgery or jaundice
- Hypertension
- Myeloma
- Nephrotoxic drugs
- Pre-eclampsia or eclampsia
- Sepsis

Perioperative factors

- Hypotension
- Arrhythmias
- Hypovolaemia
  —diuretic therapy
  —preoperative starvation
  —gastric aspiration or vomiting
  —third-space losses (e.g. ileus, obstruction, peritoneal exudate)
  —diarrhoea or bowel preparation
  —prolonged tissue exposure or surgical oedema
  —blood loss
- Hypoxia
- Tissue damage or inflammation
  —ischaemia and reperfusion
  —major burns
  —multiple fractures or muscle damage
  —pancreatitis
- Haemolysis (e.g. transfusion reactions)
- Specific surgical complications (e.g. pericardial tamponade)

31

- Osmolality
- Haemoglobin, platelets, white blood count including eosinophils
- Coagulation studies
- Amylase
- Creatinine kinase, myoglobin, uric acid
- Estimate creatinine concentration clearance as plasma creatinine concentration may not reflect glomerular filtration rate (GFR), especially in the elderly with little muscle mass. This can be done by means of a 2-h urine collection.
- Lactate dehydrogenase (LDH), haptoglobin, and direct and indirect bilirubin if haemolysis is suspected
- Immunoglobulins and electrophoresis to exclude myeloma
- Isotope investigations, angiography and renal biopsy may be indicated occasionally.

URINE CHEMISTRY
- Sodium, urea and creatinine
- Osmolality
- Urinalysis
- Blood, protein and myoglobin
- Microscopy to detect crystals and casts in the urine and to assess red cell morphology:
  —hyaline and granular casts suggest underperfusion or chronic renal damage
  —tubular casts suggest acute intrinsic renal injury
  —dysmorphic red cells and casts suggest glomerulonephritis
  —white cell casts suggest pyelonephritis or possible interstitial nephritis.

URINARY INDICES
These are relatively imprecise and become inaccurate after administration of mannitol and loop diuretics. Urinary osmolality and sodium concentration are insensitive discriminators between pre-renal azotaemia and acute renal failure.

The fractional excretion of sodium (FE_{Na}) is a more accurate guide to renal integrity:

$$FE_{Na} = (U_{Na}/P_{Na}) \div U_{Cr}/P_{Cr}$$

where U_{Na} and U_{Cr} are urinary concentrations of sodium and creatinine, and P_{Na} and P_{Cr} are the respective plasma concentrations.

Table 31.11 shows some common urinary indices.

TABLE 31.11

Common urinary indices

	Underperfusion	Intrinsic renal failure
U/P osmolality	> 1.5	< 1.1
U/P creatinine	> 40	< 20
U/P urea	> 20	< 10
U_{Na} (mmol l^{-1})	< 20	> 40
FE_{Na} (%)	< 1	> 3

MANAGEMENT

- Catheterise the bladder when convenient.
- Maintain adequate oxygenation and ventilation.
- Maintain intravascular volume but restrict fluids if oliguric acute renal failure is established and the patient is euvolaemic. Consider invasive monitoring early in high-risk groups.
- Assess fluid deficits and correct accordingly. Postoperative patients have an impaired ability to excrete a water-load, so avoid excessive dextrose administration.
- Maintain an adequate mean arterial blood pressure (a normal blood pressure of 120/80 mmHg equates to a mean arterial pressure of 93 mmHg).
- Initially, aim for a mean arterial pressure of 60–80 mmHg, *or higher if previously hypertensive or with widespread peripheral vascular disease.*
- Induce a diuresis of at least 30 ml h^{-1}; maintaining urine volume will make fluid management easier:
  —mannitol 20 g (200 ml of 10% solution)
  —furosemide (frusemide) bolus up to 250 mg, then infuse at 5–100 mg h^{-1}
  —dopamine 200 mg in 50 ml at 3 ml $h^{-1} \approx$ 3 μg kg^{-1} min^{-1} in a 70-kg patient (note that dopamine will not prevent acute renal failure).
- In myoglobinuria (also with haemolysis or tumour lysis syndrome) alkalinise the urine (pH > 7) with intravenous sodium bicarbonate and/or acetazolamide (up to 250 mg four times daily, although higher doses may cause confusion).
- For urate nephropathy, add allopurinol (200 mg three times daily).

BIBLIOGRAPHY

Baek S-M, Makabali GG, Bryan-Brown CW, Kusek JM, Shoemaker WC. Plasma expansion in surgical patients with high central venous pressure (CVP); the relationship of blood volume to hematocrit, CVP, pulmonary wedge pressure, and cardiorespiratory changes. Surgery 1975; 78:304–315

Bellomo R, Chapman M, Finfer S, Hickling K, Myburgh J. Low-dose dopamine in patients with early renal dysfunction: a placebo-controlled randomised trial. Australian and New Zealand Intensive Care Society (ANZICS) Clinical Trials Group. Lancet 2000; 356:2139–2143

Bersten AD, Holt AW. Vasoactive drugs and the importance of renal perfusion pressure. New Horizons 1995; 3:650–661

Connors AF, McCaffree DR, Gray B. Evaluation of right-heart catheterization in the critically ill patient without acute myocardial infarction. New England Journal of Medicine 1983; 308:263–267

Le Gall JR, Klar J, Lemeshow S et al. The Logistic Organ Dysfunction system. A new way to assess organ dysfunction in the intensive care unit. ICU Scoring Group. Journal of the American Medical Association 1996; 276:802–810

Sladen RN, Endo E, Harrison T. Two-hour versus 22-hour creatinine clearance in critically ill patients. Anesthesiology 1987; 67:1013–1016

Star RA. Treatment of acute renal failure. Kidney International 1998; 54:1817–1831

31

Postoperative pain management

D. O'Malley and A. Leonard

Good postoperative pain management is not only a humanitarian obligation, but clinically it can reduce morbidity and result in earlier mobilisation and a shortened hospital stay. It has even been suggested to record pain scores as 'the fifth vital sign'.

PREOPERATIVE CONSIDERATIONS

During the preoperative assessment, the anaesthetist should consider the provision of adequate postoperative pain relief and factors that might affect it, including:

• Available resources
• Pain characteristics:
  —site and origin
  —intensity
  —expected duration
• Patient's previous experience with pain relief
• Underlying medical conditions and current drug therapy
• Special needs – joint mobilisation, deep breathing, coughing, ambulation, etc.
• Risk : benefit ratio
• A pain assessment tool and the patient's understanding of this
• Interdisciplinary and patient communication – knowledge of the proposed analgesic strategy.

MEASUREMENT OF ACUTE PAIN

In order to treat pain and to evaluate analgesia effectively, it is necessary to be able to assess the pain.

A number of different methods are available, but a simple pain scoring system, such as a verbal rating scale with measures between 0 and 10 (0, no pain; 10, the worst possible pain) given by the patient both at rest and on movement is easy and quick to use.

A simple word descriptor scale (mild, moderate, severe) is better than no tool for patients with limited understanding.

MANAGEMENT OPTIONS

The management of an individual patient can include one or more of a number of options. A pre-emptive approach may prevent central sensitisation and reduce postoperative analgesic needs, if analgesia is used before the painful stimulus is applied. The provision of 'balanced analgesia' using a combination of techniques can provide optimal pain relief with the minimum of side-effects.

NSAIDs

• Useful for the management of mild to moderate postoperative pain
• Particularly useful for outpatient surgery, dental surgery and following a variety of orthopaedic procedures
• Can be used in conjunction with opioids for moderate to severe pain
• Consider prescribing regularly, not 'as required'
• Available in oral, rectal and parenteral preparations.

CONTRAINDICATIONS

There are a number of situations where NSAIDs are not recommended. Contraindications include:

• Coagulopathies
• Risk of bleeding
• History of gastrointestinal bleeding or ulceration
• Poor renal function
• Elderly, dehydrated patients
• Caution with asthmatic patients.

The newer cyclo-oxygenase (cox-2) selective inhibitors, may be safer to use where there is a potential for bleeding, but current evidence does not support their safety in other high risk applications.

OPIOID ANALGESICS

These comprise the cornerstone of postoperative pain management.

Moderate to severe pain should normally be treated initially with an opioid analgesic.

When used in conjunction with NSAIDs, and paracetamol, there are significant opioid dose-sparing effects which can be useful in reducing opioid side-effects.

INTRAMUSCULAR OR SUBCUTANEOUS INJECTIONS

Analgesia can be provided using this method of intermittent injections. Opioid administration relying on the patient's demands for analgesia 'as needed' ('PRN') however, produces delays in administration and intervals of inadequate pain control. If this method is to be used, choose an appropriate drug, dose and interval of administration, and consider using an intramuscular algorithm (Fig. 31.8), which can provide more effective administration.

INTRAVENOUS INJECTIONS

Intravenous administration is the route of choice after major surgery. This route is suitable for bolus administration, patient-controlled analgesia (PCA) and continuous infusion. Consider giving a loading dose to achieve minimum effective analgesic concentration. Table 31.12 provides simple guidelines for the loading doses for the most commonly used drugs.

CONTINUOUS INFUSIONS

This is a relatively simple technique, but is rather inflexible and requires careful monitoring. It can lead to side-effects, including sedation, and should be considered only for patients nursed in high-dependency areas.

PATIENT-CONTROLLED ANALGESIA

The opioid requirements of individual patients can vary by up to 400%. PCA allows self-administration of small boluses of opioid as required. The bolus dose is set and the minimum length of time between boluses programmed (lockout interval). One standard programme can encompass the needs of most patients; for example, for morphine a 1-mg bolus and a 5-min lockout is suitable. A 4-h dose limit is not normally recommended.

This approach is based on a negative feedback loop. When pain is reduced there will be no further demand for analgesia until the pain returns. Patients thus titrate the analgesia to their own needs within safe clinical parameters. Newer techniques include PCA administered intranasally or transdermally.

ORAL ANALGESIA

Oral administration of drugs is convenient and inexpensive. It is appropriate as soon as the patient can tolerate oral intake. Consider giving drugs regularly rather than 'as required'. There are a variety of oral analgesics available that are suitable for use in the postoperative period. Many combination analgesics are available, most of which consist of one or more of the following.

PARACETAMOL

This is a very useful analgesic and antipyretic. It may be used in conjunction with opioids when NSAIDs are contraindicated. It is available in oral and suppository form. An intravenous preparation, propacetamol, is available in Europe and may become available in the UK in the foreseeable future.

CODEINE

This is a naturally occurring, weak opioid. The usual adult dose is 30–60 mg every 4 h. The small amount (8–10 mg) found in proprietary combination analgesics probably has little effect. Constipation is a dose-related side-effect that may limit its usefulness.

DEXTROPROPOXYPHENE

This opioid is of similar potency to codeine and is often combined with paracetamol in a dose of 65 mg dextropropoxyphene with 500 mg paracetamol (coproxamol).

DIHYDROCODEINE

This semisynthetic derivative of codeine is about one-third more potent than codeine. It may cause confusion in the elderly.

TRAMADOL

This synthetic analogue of codeine has a dual mode of action: a low affinity for opioid receptors and neuronal uptake of 5-hydroxytryptamine (5-HT) and noradrenaline (norepinephrine). It is used for moderate to severe pain. The dose range is 50–100 mg four times a day and its oral bioavailability is

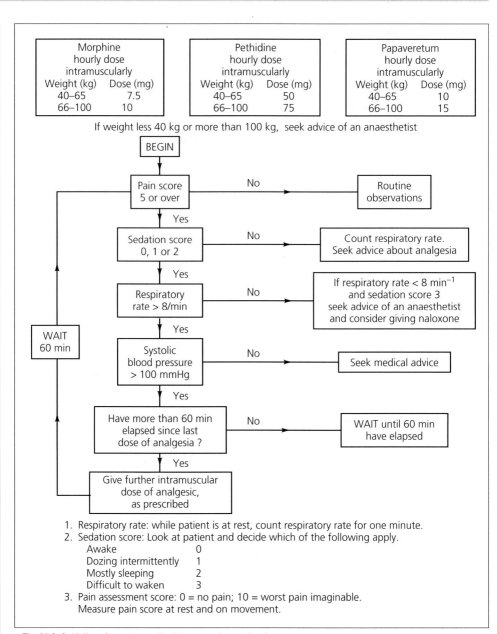

Fig. 31.8 Guidelines for postoperative intramuscular analgesia.

good. It is less constipating than codeine, but its tendency to cause nausea and confusion limits its usefulness.

ORAL MORPHINE

Many preparations exist, but short-acting formulations (Oramorph, Sevredol) are indicated for moderate to severe pain. They are particularly useful for patients who are discontinuing PCA or epidural techniques, and whose pain is still quite strong ('bridging the gap'). The dose should be titrated in increments of 10 mg to

effect. Renal patients who are sensitive to the effects of morphine-6-glucuronide may tolerate hydromorphone (Palladone) as an alternative, in 1.3-mg increments.

LOCAL ANAESTHETICS

A variety of neural blockade techniques may be continued into the postoperative period and can result in effective safe analgesia. Bupivacaine is often used for regional anaesthesia.

TABLE 31.12

Dosing data for opioid analgesics[a]

| Drug | Approximate equi-analgesic dose [mg] | | Recommended starting dose (adults > 50 kg bodyweight) | | Loading dose [mg kg⁻¹ i.v.] | Maintenance dose [mg kg⁻¹ h⁻¹ i.v.] |
	Oral	Parenteral	Oral	Parenteral		
Opioid agonists						
Morphine	30 (3–4 hourly)	10 (3–4 hourly)	30 (3–4 hourly)	10 (3–4 hourly)	0.15	0.01–0.04
Diamorphine	Not used	5 (3–4 hourly)	Not used	5 (3–4 hourly)	0.075	0.005–0.02
Codeine	130 (3–4 hourly)	75 (3–4 hourly)	60 (3–4 hourly)	60 (2 hourly i.m. or s.c.)		
Pethidine	300 (2–3 hourly)	100 (3 hourly)	Not recommended	100 (3 hourly)	1.5–2.0	0.3–0.6
Oxycodone	30 (3 hourly)	Not available	10 (3–4 hourly)	Not available		
Methadone	20 (6 hourly)	10 (6–8 hourly)	20 (6–8 hourly)	10 (6–8 hourly)	0.15	Unsuitable
Opioid agonist–antagonists and partial agonists						
Buprenorphine	Not available	0.3–0.4 (6–8 hourly)	Not available	0.4 (6–8 hourly)	0.004	0.002

[a]Published tables vary in the suggested doses that are equi-analgesic to morphine. Clinical response is the criterion that must be applied for each patient; titration to clinical response is necessary.

31

Levobupivacaine and ropivacaine are L-isomer preparations similar to bupivacaine, and these are thought to be less cardiotoxic and neurotoxic in higher doses. Commonly used techniques include:

- Local wound infiltration
- Interscalene brachial plexus anaesthesia for shoulder surgery
- Sciatic and femoral nerve blocks for ankle and foot surgery
- Intercostal blocks for thoracic and upper abdominal surgery
- A catheter in the intrapleural space can produce analgesia with little or no evidence of sensory block following a number of procedures, in particular renal surgery, cholecystectomy and unilateral breast surgery
- Local anaesthetic infusions into the femoral sheath, lumbar plexus and sciatic nerve have been used to maintain analgesia and sympathetic blockade after a variety of procedures; these may be particularly useful in patients in whom spinal or epidural blockade is contraindicated.

SPINAL ANALGESIA

A spinal block can provide analgesia for several hours after the completion of surgery. Continuous spinal techniques have been shown to provide effective treatment of acute postoperative pain. A combined spinal and epidural technique can provide superior anaesthesia and analgesia during the perioperative period.

EPIDURAL ANALGESIA

Local anaesthetic boluses or infusions can provide profound analgesia. The epidural catheter tip should be near the appropriate spinal cord segments that mediate sensation for the area around the surgical incision.

SPINAL AND EPIDURAL OPIOIDS

Intrathecal opioids are easy to administer either at the time of the spinal analgesic injection for surgical anaesthesia or as an accompanying technique when general anaesthesia is administered. Many patients remain comfortable for 24 h or more after a single injection of intrathecal morphine or diamorphine, and this technique is gaining popularity in the management of caesarean section pain.

Opioids alone produce good analgesia when put into the CSF or epidural space. A combination of low-dose local anaesthetic and opioid work synergistically and can provide excellent analgesia over a prolonged period. Small doses can be effective, and allow early mobilisation because there should be little motor blockade and good analgesia. Patient-controlled epidural analgesia is gaining popularity as this allows the patient to supplement a low background infusion with a small bolus to fine-tune analgesic requirements.

Side-effects of spinal opioids include:

- Sedation
- Respiratory depression
- Nausea and vomiting
- Itching
- Hypotension
- Urinary retention.

Patients with epidurals continuing into the postoperative period require careful monitoring. Routine monitoring should include sedation level, respiratory rate and blood pressure. The extent of sensory and motor blockade should be monitored. Evidence of haematoma or abscess should be excluded. Intravenous access should be maintained. Monitoring should continue for a minimum of 12 h after cessation of the epidural. Patients should be nursed in an easily observable environment. Good staff education, clear guidelines and the support of an acute pain team are imperative.

NON-PHARMACOLOGICAL APPROACHES

Psychological factors are always present, and non-pharmacological therapy can be useful in helping to treat acute pain. It does not necessarily take more time to put some of these forms of therapy to use, but it does take awareness, sensitivity and a willingness to approach pain management from a broad perspective. The techniques that seem to have the broadest application are those that increase the patient's sense of control, provide psychological support and permit relaxation.

BIBLIOGRAPHY

Agency for Health Care Policy and Research. Acute pain management: operative or medical procedures and trauma. Rockville, Maryland: Agency for Health Care Policy and Research; 1992

Allen HH, Ginsberg B, Preble LM. Acute pain mechanisms and management. Mosby, 1992

American Society of Anesthesiologists. Practice guidelines for acute pain management in the perioperative setting. Park Wood: ASA; 1995

Audit Commission. Anaesthesia under examination. London: Audit Commission; 1998

McHugh G, Thoms G. The management of pain following day-case surgery. Anaesthesia 2002; 57:270-275

Macintyre PE. Safety and efficacy of patient-controlled analgesia. British Journal of Anaesthesia 2001; 87:36-46

McQuay H, Moore A. An evidence based resource for pain relief. Oxford: Oxford University Press; 2002

Moiniche S, Kehlet H, Dahl JB. A qualitative and quantitative systematic review of preemptive analgesia for postoperative pain relief. The role of timing of analgesia. Anesthesiology 2002; 96:725-741

Ready BL, Edwards TW. Management of acute pain: a practical guide. Seattle: ASP Publications; 1992

Wheatley RG, Schug SA, Watson D. Safety and efficacy of postoperative epidural analgesia. British Journal of Anaesthesia 2001; 87:47-61

Wilson JA, Colvin LA. Acute neuropathic pain after surgery. Royal College of Anaesthetists Bulletin 2002; 15:739-743

Wulf H, Schug SA, Allvin R, Kehlet H. Postoperative patient management – how can we make progress? Acute Pain 1998; 1:32-44

31

Pseudocholinesterase deficiency

D. Østergaard and J. Viby-Mogenson

Pseudocholinesterase, also known as plasma cholinesterase (acylcholine acylhydrolase E.C.3.1.1.8.), is a soluble enzyme found in the plasma and manufactured in the liver.

IMPORTANCE FOR ANAESTHESIA

Decreased pseudocholinesterase activity may cause a reduction in the rate of hydrolysis and hence a prolonged duration of action of:
• Succinylcholine
• Mivacurium.

DETERMINATION OF PSEUDOCHOLINESTERASE ACTIVITY AND PHENOTYPE

Biochemical analysis involves measuring:
• The rate of hydrolysis of a substrate catalysed by pseudocholinesterase
• The percentage inhibition of the hydrolysis in the presence of different inhibitor substances, often dibucaine.
Structural analysis is at the DNA level.
See Tables 31.13 and 31.14.

GENETICALLY DETERMINED CHANGES

• More than 50 different mutations are known, and about 25% of subjects in a Caucasion population carry at least one pseudocholinesterase variant. Only a few of these have, however, clinical significance.
• The cholinesterase activity of the different phenotypes differ qualitatively as well as quantitatively.
• Because of the above factors, it is not possible to estimate the clinical significance from pseudocholinesterase activity alone. The phenotype (or genotype) must also be identified.
See Table 31.15.

TABLE 31.13

Aetiology of decreased pseudocholinesterase activity

Condition	Change in activity
Physiological variation	
Sex	Males > females
Age	Newborns 50% of adults
Pregnancy	70–80% of pre-pregnancy level until 6–8 weeks after delivery
Disease	
Liver failure	40–70% decrease
Renal failure	10–50% decrease
Malignant tumours	25–50% decrease, depending on localisation
Burned patients	Lowest value 5–6 days after the injury. Depending on the degree of injury, the reduction may exceed 80%

TABLE 31.14

Iatrogenic factors that decrease pseudocholinesterase activity

Factor	Decrease in activity (%)
Glucocorticoids, oestrogen	30–50
Cytotoxic compounds	35–70
Neostigmine	5–100
Echothiophate eye-drops	70–100
Bambuterol	30–90
Organophosphates	100
Plasmapheresis (removes pseudocholinesterase)	60–100

TABLE 31.15

Frequency and biochemical characteristics using benzoylcholine as a substrate of the clinically most important pseudocholinesterase variants in Caucasian populations

Phenotype	Frequency (%)	Pseudo-cholinesterase (units l^{-1})	Dibucaine number
UU	95–97	690–1560	79–87
UA	2–4	320–1150	55–72
AA	0.04	140–730	14–27

CLINICAL IMPLICATIONS OF DECREASED PSEUDOCHOLINESTERASE ACTIVITY IN RELATION TO SUCCINYLCHOLINE

Normally 90% of an injected dose of succinylcholine is hydrolysed in plasma and only a small amount reaches the neuromuscular receptor. If pseudocholinesterase activity is decreased, more succinylcholine reaches the receptor.

LOW ACTIVITY IN PHENOTYPICALLY NORMAL PATIENTS
The duration of action of 1 mg kg^{-1} succinylcholine may be moderately prolonged (20–45 min).

PHENOTYPICALLY ABNORMAL PATIENTS
In patients who are heterozygous for the normal and the atypical genes:
- The duration of action is normal or slightly prolonged (10–15 min)
- More prolonged responses and a phase 2 block may be seen if the pseudocholinesterase activity is further decreased by other reasons (see Tables 31.13 & 31.14).

In patients who are homozygous for two abnormal genes, a very prolonged response (120–180 min) and a phase 2 block are always seen.

MANAGEMENT OF PROLONGED RESPONSE TO SUCCINYLCHOLINE

Management depends on the pseudocholinesterase activity and the phenotype. Often the patient's phenotype is unknown. Therefore:
- Keep the patient ventilated and anaesthetised
- Evaluate the response to peripheral nerve stimulation.

THEORETICAL CONSIDERATIONS CONCERNING RECOVERY

In phenotypically normal patients and in heterozygous abnormal patients, a prolonged response can be antagonised with a cholinesterase inhibitor. In homozygous atypical patients, succinylcholine is not hydrolysed in plasma. The effect of a cholinesterase inhibitor is therefore unpredictable and may eventually potentiate the block. Administration of purified pseudocholinesterase, blood or plasma may antagonise the block. However, because of the risks associated with their use, infusion of banked blood or fresh frozen plasma cannot be recommended.

CLINICAL IMPLICATIONS OF DECREASED PSEUDOCHOLINESTERASE ACTIVITY IN RELATION TO MIVACURIUM

The rate of hydrolysis of mivacurium is 70–80% of that of succinylcholine *in vitro*.

LOW PSEUDOCHOLINESTERASE ACTIVITY IN PHENOTYPICALLY NORMAL PATIENTS:
- May cause a prolonged block
- A prolonged block has been seen in patients with renal and hepatic failure.

PHENOTYPICALLY ABNORMAL PATIENTS
In patients heterozygous for the normal and the atypical genes:
- The duration of action may be moderately prolonged (50%).
- The infusion rate is decreased (33%).
- Reversal with neostigmine is prompt when two responses to train-of-four (TOF) stimulation are present.

In patients homozygous for two abnormal genes:

31

- A normal intubating dose causes a very prolonged duration of action (no signs of recovery for 40–180 min).
- Reversal with neostigmine should not be attempted before two responses to TOF stimulation are present.
- Purified human pseudocholinesterase can be used, but the exact dose and optimal time are not yet known; fresh frozen plasma or blood should not be given.

PATIENT FOLLOW-UP

- The patient should be informed about the prolonged block. Has the patient been awake during the incident? If so, the patient might develop severe psychological problems and require counselling.
- Blood samples should be drawn for determination of pseudocholinesterase activity and phenotype.
- Warning cards should be issued to the patient.

BIBLIOGRAPHY

Belmont MR, Rubin LA, Lien CA, Tjan J, Savarese JJ. Mivacurium. Anaesthetic Pharmacology Review 1995; 3:156–167

Gätke MR, Østergaard D, Bundgaard JR, Varin F, Viby-Mogensen J. Response to mivacurium in a patient compound heterozygous for a novel and a known silent mutation in the butyrylcholinesterase gene. Anesthesiology 2001; 95:600–606

Head-Rapson AG, Devlin JC, Parker CJR, Hunter JM. Pharmacokinetics and pharmacodynamics of the three isomers of mivacurium in health, in end-stage renal failure and in patients with impaired renal function. British Journal of Anaesthesia 1995; 75:31–36

BIBLIOGRAPHY – CONTD.

Jensen FS, Viby-Mogensen J, Østergaard D. Significance of plasma cholinesterase for the anaesthetist. Current Anaesthesia and Critical Care 1991; 2:232–237

Jensen FS, Schwartz M, Viby-Mogensen J. Identification of human plasma cholinesterase variants using molecular biological techniques. Acta Anaesthesiologica Scandinavica 1995; 39:142–149

Jensen FS, Skovgaard LT, Viby-Mogensen J. Identification of human plasma cholinesterase variants in 6688 individuals using biochemical analysis. Acta Anaesthesiologica Scandinavica 1995; 39:157–162

Østergaard D, Jensen FS, Skovgaard LT, Viby-Mogensen L. Dose–response relationship for mivacurium in patients with phenotypically abnormal plasma cholinesterase activity. Acta Anaesthesiologica Scandinavica 1995; 39:1016–1018

Østergaard D, Rasmussen SN, Viby-Mogensen J, Pedersen NA, Boysen R. The influence of drug-induced low plasma cholinesterase activity on the pharmacokinetics and pharmacodynamics of mivacurium. Anesthesiology 2000; 92:1581–1587

Østergaard D, Viby-Mogensen J, Pedersen NA, Holm H, Skovgaard LT. Pharmacokinetics and pharmacodynamics of mivacurium in young adult and elderly patients. Acta Anaesthesiologica Scandinavica 2002; 46:684–691

Østergaard D, Ibsen M, Skovgaard LT, Viby-Mogensen J. Plasma cholinesterase activity and duration of action of mivacurium in phenotypically normal patients. Acta Anaesthesiologica Scandinavica 2002; 46:679–683

Viby-Mogensen J. Cholinesterase and succinylcholine. Danish Medical Bulletin 1983; 30:129–150

Whittaker M. In: Beckman L, ed. Cholinesterase. Exeter; 1986

31

Raised ICP and CBF control

M. Simpson

INTRACRANIAL PRESSURE

The principal constituents within the skull are brain, blood and cerebrospinal fluid (CSF). The Monroe Kellie doctrine describes how an increase in the volume of one component must be accompanied by an equal reduction in another to maintain the same pressure (Fig. 31.9).

Initially, the volume increase is compensated for by extrusion of CSF into the spinal sac. When this mechanism is exhausted, further volume increases result in a sudden large increase in intracranial pressure (ICP).

Further brain swelling causes:
- Herniation of the temporal lobe through the tentorium and of the cerebellar tonsils through the foramen magnum
- Brainstem torsion with reduced cerebral blood flow (CBF) and sudden obstruction of CSF flow with acute hydrocephalus.

CLINICAL SIGNS OF RAISED ICP:
- Nausea and vomiting
- Frontal headaches on waking
- Papilloedema
- Drowsiness
- Hypertension and bradycardia.

CAUSES OF RAISED ICP:
- Severe head injury
- Space-occupying lesions (e.g. tumour, subarachnoid haemorrhage)
- Acute hydrocephalus.

AGGRAVATING FACTORS:
- Venous obstruction (e.g. from poor neck positioning)
- Raised intrathoracic pressure (e.g. from respiratory obstruction).
- Fibreoptic bronchoscopy increases the ICP significantly in brain-injured patients.

AMELIORATING FACTORS:
A head-up tilt of 30° gives maximal benefit from venous drainage, whilst minimising the reduction in cerebral arterial pressure due to the hydrostatic pressure difference between the heart and brain level.

CEREBRAL BLOOD FLOW

Normal CBF is 50–65 ml 100 g^{-1} min^{-1}.

REGULATING FACTORS:
- Cerebral perfusion pressure
- Pao_2
- $Paco_2$
- Other (e.g. adenosine, neuropeptides, ions, neurogenic mechanisms).

CBF doubles as Pao_2 declines from 50 to 30 mmHg.

For every 1-mmHg decrease in $Paco_2$ between 60 and 20 mmHg, the CBF decreases by 1.1 ml 100 g^{-1} min^{-1}. The reduction in CBF is maximal when $Paco_2$ is less than 25 mmHg. If hypocapnia continues for more than 5 h, the CBF returns to control values.

Cerebral perfusion pressure
CPP is defined as the difference between the systemic mean arterial pressure and the ICP.

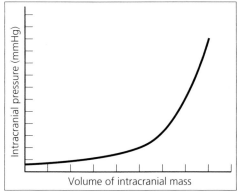

Fig. 31.9 Effect of increasing intracranial mass on ICP. Small changes in ICP, initially, become much greater beyond a critical intracranial mass.

31

Cerebral vascular resistance

This is proportional to the fourth power of the vessel radius.

Autoregulation

This is the coupling of blood flow to metabolic demand in normal brain by the dynamic interplay of vasoconstriction and vasodilatation in the cerebral vascular bed.

LOSS OF AUTOREGULATION

This occurs:

- At CPP < 50 mmHg
- In the traumatised or ischaemic brain
- With vasodilators (e.g. sodium nitroprusside)
- With high doses of volatile agents.

PHARMACOLOGICAL AGENTS THAT AFFECT CBF

Volatile agents

Halothane and enflurane increase CBF by a direct vasodilating effect on cerebral vasculature. Autoregulation is lost at high concentrations. Hypocapnia prevents the CBF rise.

Isoflurane has an indirect vasoconstricting effect secondary to reducing the metabolic rate and a direct vasodilating effect. Isoflurane provides cerebral protection, and ischaemic changes do not develop until the CBF is reduced to 8–10 ml 100 g^{-1} min^{-1} (compared with 18–20 ml 100 g^{-1} min^{-1} for halothane or when awake). At > 1.5 MAC, or in damaged brain, the vasodilating effect predominates.

Sevoflurane has similar effects to isoflurane. It is a cerebral vasodilator increasing CBF and decreasing CVR in a dose-dependent manner. Carbon dioxide reactivity is preserved at 1.5–2.5% inspired sevoflurane concentrations.

Nitrous oxide causes significant global increase in CBF by direct vasodilatation.

Hypnotics

Propofol causes a reduction in ICP and CPP (not less than 70 mmHg). In patients with intracerebral tumours there is less tendency to cerebral swelling after opening the dura than when isoflurane or sevoflurane is used. Propofol without narcotic does not prevent the rise in ICP on intubation.

Barbiturates and midazolam produce a dose-dependent reduction in metabolic rate, CBF and cerebral blood volume.

Narcotics

Unless ventilation is supported, narcotics increase ICP secondary to hypercapnia from respiratory depression. Injudicious use can reduce CPP by reducing systemic blood pressure.

Mannitol

The initial effect of a bolus of mannitol is haemodynamic, augmenting intravascular volume and increasing systolic arterial pressure and CPP. With an intact autoregulation reflex, cerebral vasoconstriction and a decreased metabolic rate reduce ICP. With impaired autoregulation, ICP falls by 5%, but CBF increases by 17%. The osmotic effect occurring 15 min later is less effective in the damaged brain. Mannitol increases flow in the microcirculation improving oxygen delivery and clearance of vasodilating substances.

Other drugs

- Dexamethasone is used to reduce ICP.
- Dimethyl sulfoxide and hypertonic saline have beneficial effects on ICP.
- Suxamethonium raises ICP.
- Calcium channel blockers and magnesium sulfate improve blood flow to ischaemic brain areas.
- In the awake patient dopamine raises ICP whereas adrenaline (epinephrine) and noradrenaline (norepinephrine) have no effect.
- In the anaesthetised patient all three inotropes increase ICP. General anaesthesia may alter blood–brain barrier permeability via a central effect.
- Lidocaine (lignocaine) reduces ICP in a dose of 1.5 mg kg^{-1}.
- In severe craniocerebral trauma, bi-temporal craniotomy has been used to reduce ICP.

BIBLIOGRAPHY

Fessler RD, Diaz FG. The management of cerebral perfusion pressure and intracranial pressure after severe head injury. Annals of Emergency Medicine 1993; 22:998–1003

Peterson KD, Landsfeldt U, Cold GE et al. ICP is lower during propofol anaesthesia compared to isoflurane and sevoflurane. Acta Neurochirurgica. Supplementum 2002; 81:89–91

Ravussin P, Wilder-Smith O. General anaesthesia for supratentorial neurosurgery. CNS Drugs 2001; 15:527–535

Walters FJM. Neuroanaesthesia – a review of the basic principles and current practices. Central African Journal of Medicine 1990; 36:44–51

31

Thrombosis and embolism

B. J. Pollard

A thrombus is a blood clot that forms within a blood vessel. If a piece breaks off and is carried along in the blood to a distant site, it is an embolus. The effect of the embolus depends on where it ultimately lodges. If on the systemic venous side, it will lodge in a pulmonary vessel. If on the systemic arterial side, it will lodge in a peripheral artery. The symptoms and signs will depend on the vessel occluded and the size of the embolus. Thromboembolic disease is a major cause of morbidity and mortality, much of which can be prevented with simple prophylactic measures.

Factors important in the formation of thrombus may still be considered in terms of Virchow's triad:

- Abnormality of the endothelium of the blood vessel (e.g. trauma)
- Slowing or other disturbances of blood flow
- Changes in the composition of the blood, favouring an increase in coagulation potential (e.g. increased platelet aggregation and fibrin formation).

> ### BOX 31.11
>
> Risk factors for venous thromboembolism
>
> **Patient factors**
>
> - Age
> - Obesity
> - Varicose veins
> - Immobility (bed rest > 4 days)
> - Pregnancy and puerperium
> - High-dose oestrogens
> - Previous DVT or pulmonary embolism
> - Thrombophilias
>
> **Factors relating to disease or procedure**
>
> - Surgery or trauma, especially to the pelvis, hip or lower limb
> - Malignancy, especially pelvic, abdominal or metastatic
> - Heart failure
> - Recent myocardial infarction
> - Lower-limb paralysis
> - Infection
> - Inflammatory bowel disease
> - Polycythaemia

DEEP VEIN THROMBOSIS

Deep vein thrombosis (DVT) is a common event in hospital patients. Surgical patients most at risk are listed in Box 31.11 and include especially those with a previous history of DVT or pulmonary embolism, those who are obese and those who have a malignant disease. Surgery involving the pelvis, hip and knee are associated with a significant risk of DVT formation.

DIAGNOSIS OF DVT

Diagnosis based on the clinical features of leg swelling, pain, warmth and positive Homan's sign is unreliable. More accurate diagnostic tests for DVT include:

- Venography – this is the most reliable technique; however, up to 2% of patients may develop a DVT as a result

- Impedance plethysmography – this is sensitive and specific, but not for calf vein thrombi
- Doppler ultrasonography
- Duplex venous scan
- Radiolabelled fibrinogen scan.

TREATMENT OF DVT

Anticoagulation with heparin should be started with a bolus of 100 units kg^{-1} followed by an infusion of approximately 20 000–30 000 units daily, aiming to keep the activated partial thromboplastin time (APTT) between 1.5 and 2.5 times normal. APTT should be monitored daily. Low-molecular-weight heparin may also be used in the treatment of DVT, but the different preparations have different dose schedules and these should be checked in the

31

local formulary before administration. Warfarin is commonly used for longer-term treatment. It may be started on the first day, but heparin should be continued for 5 days while the warfarin becomes effective.

DVT PROPHYLAXIS

Prophylaxis should be related to perceived risk. Low-risk patients may be managed by encouraging them to mobilise early. Intermediate- and high-risk patients should in addition receive prophylaxis. This should include either low-dose subcutaneous heparin (5000 units 8–12 hourly) or a low-molecular-weight heparin of proven efficacy. When heparin is contraindicated, intermittent pneumatic compression or graduated compression stockings should be used. Their effect on prevention of pulmonary embolism is, however, unknown.

PULMONARY EMBOLISM

Pulmonary embolism has been reported to account for up to 10% of hospital deaths. Three of four patients dying from pulmonary embolism have not had recent surgery, emphasising the importance of prophylaxis in medical patients at risk.

DIAGNOSIS AND TREATMENT OF PULMONARY EMBOLISM

Clinical features will depend partly on the degree of obstruction and include tachypnoea, pleuritic or dull central chest pain, tachycardia, cyanosis, raised CVP and gallop rhythm. Massive acute pulmonary embolism usually presents with cardiac arrest. Electrical activity may continue without any cardiac output (electromechanical dissociation or pulseless electrical activity).

Investigations include: ECG (common changes include tachycardia, right bundle branch block, or S1 : Q3 : T3 in 25% of patients); chest radiography, which may show pulmonary oligaemia or a wedge-shaped opacity; and measurement of blood gases, which may show hypoxaemia. Isotope ventilation–perfusion (V/Q) scanning is the most widely used specific investigation. These are reported as representing a low, moderate or high likelihood of pulmonary embolism. When compared with angiography, radionuclide scans underestimate the severity of pulmonary embolism.

The treatment of pulmonary embolism includes the supportive measures of oxygen, fluids and analgesia, depending on the severity of cardiopulmonary disturbance. Obstruction of the pulmonary veins greater than 25% produces raised right ventricular pressure, a fall in left heart filling pressure and displacement of the interventricular septum into the left ventricular cavity. This helps to explain why dyspnoea is eased by manoeuvres to raise left ventricular preload with fluid loading and supine position. Specific treatment options include anticoagulation, thrombolysis and pulmonary embolectomy. The place of pulmonary embolectomy is controversial; surgery can be justified only if the patient is thought to be unlikely to survive without operation.

Acute minor pulmonary embolism with no haemodynamic disturbance can be treated with heparin as described above, followed by warfarin for a period of 3–6 months.

Patients with acute major pulmonary embolism presenting with haemodynamic disturbance will initially require resuscitation with oxygen and fluids and direct haemodynamic monitoring in a HDU. This should be followed by thrombolysis with streptokinase 250 000– 600 000 IU over 20–30 min, with or without 100 mg hydrocortisone, followed by 100 000 IU h^{-1} for up to 72 h. Tissue plasminogen activator produces more rapid resolution of thrombus, but the results are similar after 12–24 h.

Pulmonary embolectomy is occasionally attempted in major centres but the success rate is not good.

ARTERIAL THROMBOEMBOLISM

The source of arterial thromboembolism is often the heart. More than half of all thromboemboli of cardiac origin are the result of atrial fibrillation, particularly when this is associated with mitral stenosis or thyrotoxicosis. Other predisposing conditions include valvular prostheses, recent myocardial infarction with mural thrombus formation and low cardiac output states. Resulting thromboemboli may take the form of peripheral emboli or, more commonly, cerebrovascular events producing a stroke. Studies have demonstrated the benefits of anticoagulation in patients with atrial fibrillation.

31

BIBLIOGRAPHY

Dunn M, Blackburn T. Anticoagulant treatment of atrial fibrillation in the elderly. Postgraduate Medical Journal 1992; 68(Suppl 1):S57–S60

Goldhaber SZ. Pulmonary embolism. New England Journal of Medicine 1998; 339:93–104

Hull RD, Pineo GF. Treatment of venous thromboembolism with low molecular weight heparins. Hematology and Oncology Clinics of North America 1992; 6:1095–1103

Mammen EF. Pathogenesis of venous thrombosis. Chest 1992; 102(Suppl 6):640S–644S

Thromboembolic Risk Factors (THRIFT) Consensus Group. Risk of and prophylaxis for venous thromboembolism in hospital patients. British Medical Journal 1992; 305:567–574

31

Total spinal anaesthesia

M. Y. Aglan

DEFINITION

- Spread of local anaesthetic to block all of the spinal nerves and/or intracranial extension
- Life-threatening extensive block results in severe hypotension which may progress to cardiovascular collapse, respiratory failure, unconsciousness and cardiac arrest
- High spinal anaesthesia includes profound hypotension without respiratory failure.

PHYSIOLOGICAL EFFECTS

See Figure 31.10.

CARDIOVASCULAR COLLAPSE:
- Total preganglionic efferent sympathetic block
- Peripheral sympathetic (T1–L2) block leads to loss of vasoconstrictor tone with profound reduction in systemic vascular resistance and venous return
- Block of cardiac sympathetic fibres (T1–T4) with unopposed vagal nerve supply results in severe bradycardia.

RESPIRATORY FAILURE:
- Progressive intercostal muscles paralysis (T1–T12)
- Diaphragmatic paralysis (C3–C5)
- Inhibition of respiratory centre due to direct effect of local anaesthetic or secondary to cerebral hypoperfusion.

LOSS OF CONSCIOUSNESS:
- Direct action of local anaesthetic on the brain
- Secondary to cerebral hypoperfusion due to severe hypotension.

AETIOLOGY

INTENTIONAL:
Total spinal anaesthesia (TSA), with respiratory and cardiovascular support, has been used for deliberate hypotension:

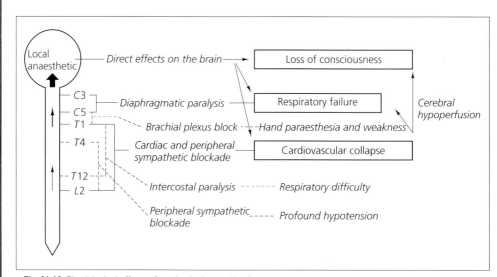

Fig. 31.10 Physiological effects of total spinal anaesthesia.

- To provide a bloodless operative field, for example for ear surgery
- To reduce intraoperative blood loss, for example for surgery in a Jehovah's Witness patient.

In chronic pain management, TSA provides transient relief of intractable pain.

ACCIDENTAL:

As a complication of spinal anaesthesia. Occurs most commonly when larger volumes of local anaesthetic are injected accidentally into the subarachnoid space (SAS):

- Central block:
  —extended epidural – increased risk following dural tap
  —caudal block in children
  —false-negative aspiration (no CSF reflux) and test dose
  —subdural block
  —multicompartment block (epidural, subdural or subarachnoid block with multi-holed catheter or Touhy needle). Delayed collapse can develop after previously normal top-ups. Misplaced catheter – initially incorrect place or subsequently migrates into subdural or SAS
- Peripheral block – local anaesthetic spreads to the SAS along the radicular dural cuff or via the perineural space in case of intraneural injection. Cases have been reported after:
  —retrobulbar block
  —stellate ganglion block
  —brachial plexus (interscalene approach)
  —intercostal block
  —paravertebral block
  —lumbar plexus block for total hip replacement.

DIAGNOSIS

One or more of the following (during a potential risk block):

- Loss of consciousness
- Respiratory collapse
- Cardiovascular collapse or cardiac arrest.

PREVENTION

Pay close attention to details when performing blocks close to the spinal cord.

Factors that may lead to high spinal block are:

- Large-volume local anaesthetic (LA) for spinal anaesthesia in a short patient

- Patient position
- Pregnancy (engorgement of epidural veins)
- Barbotage
- Straining or coughing
- Cephalad direction of a small lateral hole spinal needle combined with rapid injection.

Precautions that should be taken when using an epidural catheter are:

- Aspirate without a filter and aspirate before each injection (top-ups)
- Use a test dose sufficient to produce a reliable subarachnoid block
- Test for S1 motor block 10 min after epidural injection (10 ml bupivacaine is a reliable test to detect accidental intrathecal injection in obstetric patients)
- Wait sufficient time for the block to occur
- Titrate the injected local anaesthetic in incremental doses
- Avoid injection during uterine contractions
- It is essential to assess both sensory and motor blocks frequently.

Precautions to be taken with other blocks are:

- Use the shortest practicable needle
- Careful aspiration.

EARLY RECOGNITION AND TREATMENT OF POTENTIAL TSA

- Resuscitation equipment and anaesthetic help should be available before any regional block.
- Signs and symptoms:
  —respiratory difficulty (weak voice, inability to cough)
  —upper limb paraesthesia and weakness
  —Horner's syndrome (spinal or epidural)
  —Cerebral hypoperfusion (restlessness, nausea, vomiting, headache).
- Management directed at restricting spread of local anaesthetic:
  —hyperbaric solution (spinal), anti-Trendelenburg
  —solutions intended for non-subarachnoid use are likely to be isobaric or hypobaric within CSF; the patient should be kept still; a slight head-down tilt will encourage caudal spread of hypobaric local anaesthetic and help to maintain venous return
  —obstetric patients should be managed in a left lateral tilt to avoid aortocaval compression
  —if a dural puncture is not recognised and a volume of LA is injected into the CSF, an attempt could be made immediately to withdraw a volume of CSF equal to the LA volume through the catheter.

31

Some of the drug will theoretically be aspirated and the remainder will be diluted as the CSF is formed.

TREATMENT

- Support the cardiorespiratory systems until the effects of high block recede.
- Give 100% oxygen to maximise oxygen supply.
- Cardiovascular support:
  —maintain venous return (elevation of legs; left lateral tilt (obstetric patient); intravenous fluids (colloids or crystalloids)
  —give atropine and vasopressor drugs if required (Table 31.16).
- Tracheal intubation and assisted ventilation, which may require general anaesthetic or muscle relaxant.
- Cardiopulmonary resuscitation if cardiac arrest occurs.

TABLE 31.16

Drugs used for the treatment of cardiovascular collapse[a]

Heart rate (beats min⁻¹)	Drug	Comments
Asystole	Adrenaline (epinephrine)	CPR guidelines
< 60	Atropine	Vagolytic
60–90	α and β agonist (e.g. ephedrine)	Increases SVR and cardiac output
> 90	α agonist (e.g. phenylephrine, metaraminol)	Reflex bradycardia

[a]In the obstetric patient, ephedrine is the drug of choice because it does not depress uterine blood flow.

BIBLIOGRAPHY

Aglan MY, Stansby PK. Modification to the spinal Sprotte needle. Anaesthesia 1992; 47:506–507

Bonica JJ. Regional anaesthesia: recent advances and current status. High or total spinal or epidural block. Oxford: Blackwell Scientific; 1971

Daoud Z, Collis RE, Ateleanu B, Mapleson WW. Evaluation of S1 motor block to determine a safe, reliable test dose for epidural analgesia. British Journal of Anaesthesia 2002; 89:442–445

Morgan B. Unexpectedly extensive conduction blocks in obstetric epidural analgesia. Anaesthesia 1990; 45:148–152

Morton CPJ, Wildsmith JAW. Crises in regional anaesthesia. Baillière's Clinical Anaesthesiology 1993; 7:367–375

Russell IF. Total spinal anaesthesia: the effect of spinal infusions. In: Reynolds F, ed. Epidural and spinal blockade in obstetrics. London: Baillière Tindall; 1990:107–120

Yokoyama M, Itano Y, Kusume Y, Oe K, Mizobuchi S, Morita K. Total spinal anesthesia provides transient relief of intractable pain. Canadian Journal of Anaesthesia 2002; 49:432–436

CROSS-REFERENCES

Spinal and epidural anaesthesia
  Anaesthetic Factors 30: 696
Local anaesthetic toxicity
  Anaesthetic Factors 31: 761
Cardiopulmonary resuscitation
  Anaesthetic Factors 31: 731

31

Transport of the critically ill

A. MacKillop

ORGANISATION OF SERVICES

Lack of a functioning ICU bed in the patient's parent hospital is statistically the most common reason for transferring a critically ill patient (Advanced Life Support Group 2002). The second is referral for specialist services.

In the UK, as in most developed countries, the demand for critical care services has constantly outstripped the supply. As the demand increases relentlessly, critically ill patients are increasingly being transferred from one hospital to another. This situation is particularly clear in the UK where there are fewer ICU beds per person compared with many other European countries.

It should also be realised that transfers of the critically ill are not benign. When the Canadian Physician Accompanied Transport System was audited, there was a serious morbidity rate of 7% of transfers and a mortality rate of 1% (Girotti et al 1988).

The public awareness of such problems was heightened by the national media concerning the following case. In 1995 a victim of a road traffic accident in London was unable to be accommodated in an appropriate, local, intensive care unit due to a perceived lack of beds. He was eventually flown to Leeds but died during the transfer. The resulting political outcry led to the development of the following regional bed bureaux in order to coordinate critical care transfers better:

- EBS (Emergency Bed Service) serving the south of England
- ICBIS (Intensive Care Bed Service) serving the north-west of England.
- WYMAS (West Yorkshire Metropolitan Ambulance Service) serving West Yorkshire
- NICBIS (Northumbrian Intensive Care Bed Information Service) serving the north-east of England.

These bed services operate systems that are based on telephone surveys of critical beds.

The Department of Health document *Comprehensive Critical Care* made the local and regional planning for ICU transfers mandatory. This, in part, has led to the development of critical care networks. Critical care networks are responsible for, amongst other things, the development of transfer services within defined groups of neighbouring hospitals.

Each network has a lead clinician and manager who are involved in transfer process mapping, protocols and quality assurance programmes. They are also responsible for the availability of appropriate equipment, training and resources to allow the safe and coordinated transfer of the critically ill.

PRACTICAL CONDUCT OF TRANSFERS

ORGANISATION WITHIN TRUSTS

Transfers for capacity reasons should be kept to a minimum. When a transfer is undertaken it should be to an appropriate local hospital within the designated network.

There must be a consultant in an acute specialty responsible for transfers 24 h a day. This is usually the ICU consultant. Each patient should be accompanied by two people. One should be medically qualified and have relevant experience and competencies in transport medicine. They should be able to reintubate and resuscitate the patient and be comfortable with the transfer equipment used.

Whether regional retrieval services are utilised depends on local arrangements. If a retrieval team is unavoidably delayed and further delays may lead to a worsened patient outcome, a hospital-based transfer team should be used instead.

VEHICLES

Road transport has many advantages. Ambulances with trained paramedical staff are easy and quick to mobilise and are rarely affected by British weather. Dedicated retrieval ambulances have many potential

31

advantages including standardisation of gas and power supplies and installation of permanent equipment. However, a substantial workload has to exist to justify such a resource.

There may be situations when air transport may be preferable. The obvious advantage of speed must be balanced against other considerations. Aeromedical transfers by either helicopter or fixed-wing aircraft have the following disadvantages:

- Organisational delays
- Transfer considerations at either end of the journey
- Staff involved must have previous aeromedical training
- A fall in atmospheric pressure may lead to an increased FiO_2 requirement; any gas-containing cavity will tend to expand (e.g. pneumothorax, pneumoperitoneum, intracranial air)
- Altitude is also accompanied by an increased risk of hypothermia.

MONITORING

Minimal monitoring standards for transfers as defined by the Intensive Care Society (2002) are:

- Continuous ECG
- Non-invasive blood pressure – often unreliable in a moving vehicle and an arterial line should generally be used
- Oxygen saturation (SaO_2)
- End-tidal carbon dioxide in ventilated patients
- Temperature, core or peripheral
- Presence of appropriately trained staff.

PREPARATION:

- Resuscitation of the patient should be complete before the start of the transfer. If it is not, the risk : benefit ratio of the transfer should be re-examined.
- Persistent hypotension after resuscitation should trigger a further search for continuing blood loss and/or systemic inflammatory response syndrome.
- If there is any doubt regarding airway patency, tracheal intubation should be carried out prior to transfer.
- Generally all ventilated patients should be paralysed and stabilised on the transfer ventilator before departure.

- Chest drains should not be clamped. Underwater seals can, if necessary, be replaced by leaflet valves.
- All long-bone fractures should be splinted. This will reduce blood loss, pain and risk of nerve damage.

HANDOVER AND DOCUMENTATION

In many circumstances the transfer personnel have not been involved in the initial treatment of the patient. It is imperative that they make an independent assessment of the patient's condition prior to the transfer. This will include collecting and reviewing relevant radiographs, scans and laboratory results. Formal handovers between medical and nursing staff should occur before departure and on arrival at the receiving hospital. Particular care should be taken to avoid the erroneous administration of blood products during or after the transfer.

Transfer documentation may be standardised within networks or regions. The information recorded should include: patient's diagnosis, reason for transfer, responsible consultants, vital signs, treatment modalities used and drugs given during the transfer.

INSURANCE

In the event of injury or death to transfer personnel the insurance situation is unclear. NHS Trusts would provide employer's liability benefits but it is possible that negligence on the part of the employer may have to be proven first.

However, membership of the Association of Anaesthetists of Great Britain and Ireland or of the Intensive Care Society (UK) provides automatic and fully comprehensive transfer insurance.

BIBLIOGRAPHY

Advanced Life Support Group. Safe transfer and retrieval. London: BMJ Books; 2002

Girotti MJ, Pagliarello G, Todd TR et al. Physician-accompanied transport of surgical intensive care patients. Canadian Journal of Anaesthesia 1988; 35:303–308

Intensive Care Society. Guidelines for transport of the critically ill adult. London: Intensive Care Society; 2002

Trauma

C. Gwinnutt and K. Demaine

In the UK, trauma is the commonest cause of death in people aged between 1 and 35 years. Road traffic accidents alone account for 60 000 admissions annually, and trauma patients occupy more bed-days than cancer and cardiac patients combined. The cost to the nation is around 1% of the Gross National Product.

Most people suffer blunt trauma, with one system sustaining severe injuries and one or two other systems lesser injuries. The incidence of life-threatening injuries to different systems is:
- Head 50%
- Chest 20%
- Abdomen 10%
- Spine 5%.

Approximately 30% of emergency operating workload is trauma related (personal observation). All anaesthetists should have an understanding of the problems they may encounter and how to deal with them.

PREOPERATIVE ASSESSMENT

This is often limited because of the urgency of the situation or because the patient is unconscious. If possible, question paramedics, relatives and the patient's general practitioner about:
- Allergies
- Medications (the elderly in particular)
- Past medical and anaesthetic history
- Last meal
- Time, place and mechanism of injury.

Limit investigations to those influencing management:
- Radiography - chest and pelvis (cervical spine may wait until secondary survey)
- Arterial blood gases
- Urea, electrolytes, blood sugar
- ECG
- Blood group and cross-match
- Pregnancy test in women of child-bearing age.

THEATRE PREPARATION

Having assembled appropriate personnel, check:
- Anaesthetic machine, ventilator
- Intubation equipment, including cricothyroidotomy set
- Equipment for vascular access
- Fluid administration devices (e.g. Level One™ infuser)
- Monitors – check function and correct calibration
- Drugs – anaesthetic, resuscitation
- Patient-warming devices
- Equipment for positioning.

PERIOPERATIVE MANAGEMENT

Establish adequate venous access before surgery. Catheters, drains, etc. already *in situ* must be checked for position, function and security.

ANAESTHETIC TECHNIQUE
The technique used is determined by the physiological status of the patient, surgical plan, availability of equipment and drugs, and experience of the anaesthetist.

General anaesthesia
This is the most commonly used technique:
- Regard all patients as having a full stomach
- Use rapid sequence induction if not contraindicated
- Drugs used for induction and maintenance are dictated by haemodynamic status
- Consider avoiding nitrous oxide if pneumothorax or bowel obstruction is present, or operating time may be prolonged
- Induce unstable patients in theatre to reduce movement, risk of intravenous lines being dislodged, and time to surgery; there is no need to disconnect the patient from the ventilator.

31

Regional anaesthesia:
- Sympathetic block may worsen hypotension
- Difficulty in positioning injured patients for epidural or subarachnoid block
- Delay in achieving adequate block
- Inadequate when surgery in different body areas
- May be appropriate for isolated peripheral surgery.

POINTS TO NOTE

AIRWAY

A tracheal tube may have already been inserted during resuscitation. Check:
- Position – listen, $EtCO_2$, chest radiography
- Cuff integrity
- Security
- Diameter and length.
  Do not forget to protect the cervical spine. Anticipate difficult intubation if there is:
- Trauma to soft tissues of face and neck
- Midface fractures
- Actual or potential injury to the cervical spine
- Upper airway burns
- Obvious pre-existing conditions (receding mandible, 'buck' teeth).
  Consider:
- Inhalation induction and direct laryngoscopy
- Intubating laryngeal mask airway
- Fibreoptic intubation – awake or post-induction
- Surgical airway, cricothyroidotomy or tracheostomy
- Double-lumen tubes if thoracotomy planned.

VENTILATION

IPPV in the presence of multiple rib fractures requires a chest drain to prevent a tension pneumothorax developing. In all ventilated patients:
- Check air entry bilaterally by listening in mid-axillary lines
- Monitor end-tidal carbon dioxide and oxygen saturation
- Measure expired tidal and minute volume, rate and pressure
- Adjust FIO_2, I/E ratio and PEEP to optimise oxygenation
- Consider pressure control ventilation if available.
  Difficult ventilation may be due to:
- Gastric dilatation – pass a nasogastric or orogastric tube

- Pneumothorax or haemothorax – insert chest drain
- Diaphragmatic hernia.

Of patients with chest trauma, more than 50% have a normal chest radiograph initially. Consider CT in these patients if time permits or other body areas are being scanned.

A large air leak (e.g. bronchial tear) may require a double-lumen tube.

The final check of the adequacy of ventilation is by analysis of arterial blood gases.

Aim for normocapnia in order not to confuse interpretation of acid–base status (unless there is a head injury).

CIRCULATION

Maintenance of circulating volume is more important than a normal haemoglobin.
- Intravenous access with short, wide cannulae (Poiseuille's law)
- Secure all intravenous lines
- Whenever possible, avoid intravenous distally to limb fractures
- Check that the cannula is in the vein before administering drugs or fluids
- Central venous access can cause pneumothorax or haemothorax
- Warm all fluids before administration
- Hartman's solution is recommended for crystalloid infusions; excessive use of normal saline can lead to acidosis with an associated worse prognosis
- Use cell-savers or autotransfusion where appropriate
- Aim for a minimum urine output of 50 ml h^{-1} (excluding diuretics).

Measure blood pressure directly in an upper limb. This is more accurate at low pressures, allows repeat sampling of arterial blood, and is less subject to interference (e.g. surgeons).

In patients who present in haemorrhagic shock due to uncontrollable bleeding, do not attempt to resuscitate to normotension; accept a systolic blood pressure of 70–80 mmHg. Administration of large volumes of fluid simply leads to increased blood loss. Delay aggressive fluid administration until there is operative control of haemorrhage.

In persistent hypotension:
- Ensure monitors are correctly calibrated
- Check for occult haemorrhage
- Correct profound acidosis (pH < 7.2)
- Adjust the ventilator to give the lowest mean intrathoracic pressure.
  Then consider:
- *Cardiac tamponade* – low blood pressure, pulsus paradoxus, increased central venous

pressure (CVP). Use fluids and maintain heart rate to preserve cardiac output. Attempt pericardiocentesis if skills available. Maintain spontaneous ventilation as long as possible. Induce anaesthesia using rapid sequence induction with ketamine and suxamethonium.

- *Tension pneumothorax* – low blood pressure, high inflation pressures, hyper-resonant deviated trachea, increased CVP. Emergency decompression by needle thoracocentesis followed by chest drain. Have a high index of suspicion after central line insertion.
- *Neurogenic shock* – low blood pressure, bradycardia, vasodilatation. Use volume expansion initially and institute early measurement of CVP to guide fluid replacement. Atropine and vasopressors may be required when CVP is adequate.
- *Septic shock* – low blood pressure, tachycardia, vasodilatation. Uncommon early after injury and usually associated with abdominal injuries.
- *Myocardial infarction* – low blood pressure, arrhythmias, pulmonary oedema, chest pain (if conscious).

A technique of surgeon-performed ultrasonography to assess patients with blunt abdominal trauma is becoming popular in the USA and Europe. Focused assessment with sonography for trauma (FAST) can identify haemoperitoneum. The examination looks at four areas: perisplenic, perihepatic, pelvic and pericardial. However, small fluid collections can be missed and it is recommended that at least two examinations should take place, with the second occurring no earlier than 6 h after the first. Visceral injuries may be missed in the absence of haemoperitoneum.

DISABILITY

Beware when moving or using fractured or injured limbs. Neurovascular injuries may be worsened or caused, especially around joints. Ensure adequate personnel for safe positioning of patients. A head injury is not a contra-indication to general anaesthesia. Protect peripheral nerves and pressure areas adequately, particularly the eyes, when prone.

EXPOSURE

Around 66% of trauma patients arrive at hospital hypothermic. This will be worsened by the administration of cold fluids and exposure of body cavities (e.g. abdomen, chest), and temperature loss is most severe in the emergency department. Cooling predisposes to arrhy-

thmias, decreases cardiac function, causing an acidosis, adversely affects coagulation, causes left shift of the oxyhaemoglobin curve and enhances anaesthetic drugs. On recovery, shivering increases oxygen consumption dramatically. Therefore:

- Warm all fluids, especially blood
- Monitor core and peripheral temperature
- Warm and humidify all anaesthetic gases
- Cover all exposed parts, including head
- Raise theatre temperature when possible.
- Cover exposed bowel with dry towels or plastic sheet.

Limit initial surgical therapy to life-saving procedures (i.e. 'damage control surgery').

Remember:

- Only blood loss kills early.
- Gastrointestinal injuries cause problems much later.
- Everything takes longer than you think.
- It is easy to miss an injury if you rush.
- Hypothermia, acidosis and coagulopathy only lead to more of the same.
- The best place for a sick patient is the ICU.

The message regarding hypothermia is mixed. It can be protective by reducing metabolic and oxygen demands, especially in patients with brain injuries and following cardiac arrest. However, it is also part of the triad of death – acidosis, hypothermia and coagulopathy, which lead to a worse outcome in trauma.

MONITORING:

- ECG
- Blood pressure (direct)
- SpO_2
- $EtCO_2$
- CVP (or pulmonary artery wedge pressure)
- Temperature (core and peripheral)
- Urine output
- Fluid balance
- Ventilatory parameters
- Coagulation.

In the elderly trauma patient, early invasive haemodynamic monitoring improves outcome as it facilitates the identification and treatment of cardiovascular instability (low-flow cardiac output syndrome). Occasionally this may be due to concurrent acute cardiac ischaemia, unrecognised or unreported by the patient.

POSTOPERATIVE MANAGEMENT

On completion of surgery, ensure the following before extubation:

- Hypovolaemia corrected
- pH normal

31

- Pao_2 acceptable
- Temperature > 34°C
- Reflexes intact
- Adequate analgesia.

Any instability requires transfer to an ITU/HDU until problems are resolved, or if there is a risk of the patient developing adult respiratory distress syndrome (ARDS) (Box 31.12).

Beware of problems of transfer, even over short distances.

Remember the secondary survey if not already completed.

BOX 31.12

Factors predisposing to ARDS

- Aspiration
- Multiple fractures
- Pulmonary contusion
- Blood transfusion > 12 units
- Hypotension > 30 min (< 90 mmHg)
- Sepsis

Risk:
1 factor 18%
2 factors 42%
3 factors 85%

BIBLIOGRAPHY

American College of Surgeons Committee on Trauma. Advanced Trauma Life Support for Doctors. 6th edn. Chicago: American College of Surgeons; 1997

Creteur J, Sibbald W, Vincent JL. Hemoglobin solutions – not just red blood cell substitutes. Critical Care Medicine 2000; 28:3025–3034

Danks RR. Triangle of death. How hypothermia, acidosis and coagulopathy can adversely impact trauma patients. Journal of Emergency Medical Services 2002; 27:668–670.

Dutton RP, Mackenzie CF, Scalea TM. Hypotensive resuscitation during active hemorrhage: impact on in-hospital mortality. Journal of Trauma 2002; 52:1141–1146

Ford P, Nolan JP. Cervical spine injury and airway management. Current Opinion in Anaesthesiology 2002; 15:193–201

Ho MA, Karmaka MK, Contardi LH, Ng SS, Hewson JR. Excessive use of sodium chloride solution in managing traumatised patients in shock: a preventable contributor to acidosis. Journal of Trauma 2001; 51:173–177

Scalea T. What's new in trauma in the past 10 years? International Anesthesiology Clinics 2002; 40:1–17

Shapiro MB, Jenkins DH, Schwab CW, Rotondo MF. Damage control: collective review. Journal of Trauma 2000; 49:969–978

Stern SA. Low volume fluid resuscitation for presumed hemorrhagic shock: helpful or harmful? Current Opinion in Critical Care Medicine 2001; 7:422–430

31

TURP syndrome

D. M. Nolan

The profound alteration in the functioning of the cardiovascular and nervous systems produced by the absorption of large volumes of electrolyte-free irrigation fluid during transurethral resection of the prostate (TURP) is described as the TURP syndrome, although it has also been described in connection with percutaneous ultrasonic lithotripsy, vesical ultrasonic lithotripsy and intrauterine laser endoscopy.

In TURP syndrome, fluid absorption occurs principally through the venous sinuses of the prostatic capsule. Distilled water was the irrigant used originally for TURP, but usage was largely abandoned when it became apparent that the reduction in osmolarity consequent on absorption was responsible for intravascular haemolysis. Water intoxication also occurred and renal failure, due to precipitation of haemoglobin in the renal tubules, was also described. Irrigation by non-electrolyte solutions is necessary in order to reduce dispersion of current through the bladder during electrocautery. Glycine, an amino acid presented as a 1.5% solution, is the most widely used irrigant for TURP and undergoes both renal excretion and metabolism to ammonia by the liver.

PATHOPHYSIOLOGY

As fluid absorption becomes significant, a rise in intravascular pressure results in dilution of both proteins and electrolytes. Reduction of oncotic pressure promotes fluid shifts from the vascular compartment into the interstitial compartments, producing oedema in the tissue beds. The syndrome is particularly likely to occur if uptake of fluid exceeds 50 ml h^{-1} during the first 30 min of surgery.

SODIUM

True water intoxication produces a serum sodium concentration of less than 120 mmol l^{-1}. The low serum sodium level seen in the TURP syndrome is not usually associated with a change in serum osmolality. There is often no observable reduction in osmolality in response to the lower serum sodium concentration because irrigating solutions contain osmotically active solutes. It may be the case that a decrease in osmolality, rather than a reduction in serum sodium level, distinguishes asymptomatic from symptomatic patients. It has been suggested that the reason for the reduction in serum osmolality seen in some patients is a more rapid diffusion of glycine into the cells. A very low serum sodium concentration is, however, associated with more severe symptoms and a poorer prognosis.

POTASSIUM

Transient increases in serum levels of potassium have been observed in the absence of haemolysis, and hyperkalaemia may be implicated in the production of cardiac arrest during uptake of irrigating fluid.

RENAL FUNCTION

In severe TURP syndrome renal function may be impaired due to acute tubular necrosis, which may be the result of the reduction in renal blood flow produced by hypotension or by renal swelling.

SIGNS AND SYMPTOMS

These are related to the volume of irrigant absorbed.

CARDIOVASCULAR SYSTEM:

Chest pain may be observed after 20 min of absorption and initially reflects hypervolaemia.

Blood pressure may rise initially as a result of hypervolaemia. If the plasma sodium level is less than 120 mmol l^{-1}, a reduction in heart rate is usually observed and profound bradycardia may occur. Reduced myocardial contractility produces wide ranging ECG abnormalities including loss of P waves, nodal rhythm, ventricular tachycardia, widened QRS

31

complexes, depression of ST segments and T-wave inversion.

RESPIRATORY SYSTEM:

Oedema in the pulmonary vascular bed may result in dyspnoea, cyanosis and pulmonary oedema.

NERVOUS SYSTEM:

In patients undergoing TURP under spinal or epidural blockade, the first signs of excess absorption have been classically described as mental disorientation and restlessness, often immediately preceded by severe apprehension. Other CNS effects include reduction in level of consciousness and grand mal seizures. Transient blindness has been described and has been attributed to a direct effect of glycine on ocular retinal potentials.

MANAGEMENT

- Early serum sodium measurement should be performed.
- Surgery should be concluded as soon as is feasible, and bladder irrigation with warm normal saline should be commenced.
- Ventilation should be appropriately supported.
- Baseline laboratory investigations should include full blood count, electrolytes, arterial blood gases and clotting screen.
- Administration of an intravenous diuretic, usually furosemide (frusemide) in an initial dosage of 20 mg, and concomitant infusion of normal saline may resolve the problem. As a diuresis commences, fluid balance should be maintained with normal saline. Further administration of diuretic should be based on assessment of initial diuresis.
- In most centres administration of hypertonic saline is restricted to the small group of patients demonstrating severe symptoms (e.g. seizures or severe cardiac dysfunction) as a result of electrolyte imbalance. Infusion of hypertonic saline must be undertaken with caution, via a central line and with appropriate cardiovascular monitoring, and should not exceed a rate of administration of

100 ml h^{-1} in order to avoid further fluid overload. Measurement of pulmonary capillary wedge pressure is desirable in this situation.
- During the diuresis the serum potassium level should be monitored as hypokalaemia frequently occurs during this phase.

PREVENTION OF TURP SYNDROME

- The patient requires appropriate preoperative preparation with monitoring of urea and electrolytes. Adequate hydration should be maintained prior to surgery, particularly if elderly or debilitated.
- The main factor in prevention of development of the syndrome is limitation of the duration of the surgical procedure. Where possible, resection time should be restricted to less than 1 h. If fluid is absorbed at a rate in excess of 50 ml min^{-1}, fluid overload of 3 litres may occur within this time-frame.
- Haemodynamic stability should be maintained. Significant hypotension reduces the venous pressure in the periprostatic bed and permits excess absorption.
- Caution should be exercised with the height of the bag of irrigation fluid which, if placed inappropriately high, may increase the hydrostatic pressure generated within the surgical field thus increasing the risks of absorption.
- Bladder distension should be kept to a minimum; frequent bladder drainage reduces the quantity of irrigant absorbed.
- Techniques now exist for calculation of fluid absorption by addition of trace amounts of ethanol to the irrigation fluid and monitoring of expired ethanol.

BIBLIOGRAPHY

Hahn RG. Ethanol monitoring of irrigating fluid absorption in transurethral prostatic surgery. Anesthesiology 1988; 65:867–873

Hahn RG. The transurethral resection syndrome. Acta Anaesthesiologica Scandinavica 1991; 35:557–567

31

Weaning from mechanical ventilation

J. C. Goldstone

INTRODUCTION

Of all patients receiving mechanical ventilation on the ICU, 20% fail initial trials of spontaneous respiration and further ventilation or re-intubation is required. Those patients in whom weaning is prolonged often present complex respiratory problems. This group, some 2% of all ICU admissions, consists of patients with pre-existing lung disease as well as patients surviving after severe multiorgan failure or neuromuscular disease.

PATHOPHYSIOLOGICAL PRINCIPLES INVOLVED IN WEANING

The ability of the patient to sustain spontaneous ventilation is dependent on the triad of central nervous system drive, the strength of the respiratory muscles and the load that is imposed on them.

CENTRAL DRIVE

Pre-existing intrinsic lung disease is often characterised by a high resting drive. In order that weaning be successful, drive needs to be maintained above that seen in normal subjects. Optimisation of drive may require the patient to be awake and alert and, in some cases, the conscious level needs to be adjusted.

CAPACITY OF THE RESPIRATORY MUSCLES

The respiratory muscles may already be weak before ICU admission or may deteriorate further during critical illness. Acute and chronic causes of weakness are:

- Hypophosphataemia
- Hypomagnesaemia
- Hypocalcaemia
- Hypoxia
- Hypercarbia
- Acidosis
- Infection

- Muscle atrophy
- Malnutrition.

When measured, most studies suggest that the respiratory muscles are severely weak in intubated patients recovering from critical illness.

WORK PERFORMED BY THE RESPIRATORY MUSCLES

Work is performed by the muscles with each breath, and this can be substantially affected by disease. Factors that increase respiratory work include:

- Bronchoconstriction
- Left ventricular failure
- Hyperinflation
- Intrinsic positive-end expiratory pressure
- Artificial airways
- Ventilator circuits.

STRENGTH AND LOAD: A DYNAMIC RELATIONSHIP

Ventilatory failure can occur if the strength of the respiratory muscles is reduced or if the load applied to them is excessive. When patients are weak, small increases in applied load, insufficient to affect ventilation in the fit patient, may precipitate respiratory failure and weaning will not progress.

INITIAL ASSESSMENT PRIOR TO WEANING

The aim of assessment is to prevent patients undergoing trials of weaning that are unlikely to succeed and to set realistic goals to avoid repeated weaning attempts. The ideal patient to assess is an awake, stably oxygenated patient who is comfortable on the ventilator. Often this is not achieved.

A prerequisite of spontaneous breathing is the ability to oxygenate effectively, and this can be assessed by measuring PaO_2 during mechanical ventilation in the light of the inspired oxygen tension. Weaning is generally not attempted until there is:

- A stable inspired oxygen tension
- FiO_2 of 0.40 or less
- PaO_2/FiO_2 ratio of 250 or greater.

31

Occasionally patients are weaned when oxygenation is poor. This would include patients with congenital shunts and some chronic lung conditions.

INITIAL ASSESSMENT OF BREATHING: RAPID SHALLOW BREATHING

Ventilation is best assessed off the ventilator in the majority of patients. Care should be taken to support the patient during spontaneous ventilation, especially when assessment follows many days of intensive treatment. Rapid shallow breathing is frequently found in patients who will not sustain spontaneous breathing, and it occurs during the initial period off the ventilator. Rapid shallow breathing can be quantified as the f/Vt ratio where f is the breathing frequency and Vt the tidal volume measured in litres. In order to assess the patient it is suggested that:

- Use be made of continuous positive airway pressure (CPAP) via high-flow system
- CPAP be set at the level of PEEP required during mechanical ventilation
- The patient be sitting upright.

After 5 min, measure f/Vt by averaging breaths over the previous 30 s, measure Vt with a simple spirometer (e.g. Wright's respirometer) and take an average over five breaths. f/Vt should be 40 in health; when it is greater than 105, spontaneous breathing is unlikely.

Some patients, especially those who have been ventilated for only a few hours, will immediately revert to spontaneous breathing. When f/Vt is a borderline value (80–105) it is sometimes worth continuing with the spontaneous breathing trial for longer than 5 min and reassessing f/Vt at half-hourly intervals.

If the patient responds to spontaneous breathing with hyperventilation and shallow breathing in the first 5 min ($f/Vt > 105$), the likelihood of failure is high and the patient should receive ventilatory support. This should be of a form that allows the patient to continue to breathe spontaneously.

When the patient is back on the ventilator it is important that assessment be systematic to exclude severe disease or an obvious reversible cause.

CONSCIOUS LEVEL

If the patient is not conscious, the respiratory drive may not be adequate for the increased respiratory demands that are common during weaning. The ventilatory parameters set may result in overventilation, and this is especially likely when the patient is not triggering the ventilator. This is seen by the absence of patient-initiated breaths and measured minute ventilation similar to that set. Care should be taken to observe the patient during the assessment as it is often the case that patient efforts are present that are not sensed by the ventilator. Premorbid blood gases may well be abnormal, and this may be reflected by a high bicarbonate concentration in the initial blood gases prior to mechanical ventilation.

CENTRAL DRIVE

Spontaneous breathing is unlikely if:
- The patient is not triggering when $P\mathrm{aco}_2$ is adjusted to likely permission levels
- After a trial of spontaneous breathing, the patient sleeps during IPPV and is apnoeic.

Weaning should not continue in the face of a depressed conscious level; rather he should be fully ventilated until consciousness is lighter.

ASSESSMENT OF RESPIRATORY MUSCLE STRENGTH

Of central importance is to establish whether the patient is weak. If weakness is severe, repeated attempts at weaning are likely to fail, and this effort can be avoided by a simple bedside test. The maximum negative pressure generated at the bedside indicates how strong the inspiratory muscles are:

- Most adults can achieve -100 $\mathrm{cmH_2O}$
- Severely weak patients achieve -20 $\mathrm{cmH_2O}$
- Most patients can breathe spontaneously when $\mathrm{PI_{max}}$ is more than -30 $\mathrm{cmH_2O}$ provided their lungs are compliant.

Inspiratory muscle strength is measured by asking subjects and patients to perform a maximum inspiratory effort through a mouthpiece closed at one end. Marini describes the use of a one-way valve connected to the patient in order that expiration may occur but inspiration is occluded. With verbal encouragement a series of inspiratory gasps can be recorded and the most negative deflection measured. A suitable one-way valve can be found on the ICU by connecting the patient to a CPAP valve via a catheter mount. In order to perform this test:

- The patient should be pre-oxygenated
- The patient should gasp for eight breaths or 20 s
- It is not mandatory for the patient to be awake.

If the patient is weak and has been able to make good efforts (i.e. the maximum strength recorded is likely to be accurate) during respiratory strength assessment, respiratory support should be continued.

If the patient is either strong or has a level of weakness that could be compatible with spontaneous breathing, then the load applied to the muscles is crucial and this should be assessed.

THE LOAD APPLIED TO THE RESPIRATORY MUSCLES

When the respiratory muscles contract, work is performed against the elastic recoil of the lung and chest wall, and against the resistance offered to gas flowing along branching airways. As the load increases, weak patients are likely not to be able to breathe unassisted. Dynamic compliance (Cdyn) measures both elastic and flow-resistive components of load and can be assessed by the bedside during ventilated breaths. For this measurement to be accurate:

- The patient must receive constant-flow ventilation
- The patient must be relaxed or a relaxed breath is selected during ventilated and spontaneous breathing.

Cdyn is calculated from the equation: Cdyn = tidal volume/(peak airway pressure – PEEP).

WEANING MODES

Considerable debate has centred on whether synchronised intermittent mandatory ventilation (SIMV) enhances weaning. Few controlled prospective studies are available, and those that have been reported fail to support the initial hope that SIMV would enable patients to be weaned over a shorter time period. While the form of ventilation itself is unlikely to affect the major determinants of ventilation (drive, respiratory muscle strength and applied load), work performed to initiate a breath can add a considerable load, especially when the respiratory muscles are compromised.

Pressure support ventilation (PSV) has some advantages when partial support of spontaneously breathing patients is required. Unlike SIMV, PSV has no mandatory minute ventilation set by the clinician; rather, each breath is initiated by the patient and the timing and duration of each breath is also set by the patient not the clinician. PSV has many advantages but is dependent on the patient's breathing effort. Furthermore, a preset tidal volume is not ensured and Vt will change if lung compliance alters.

The technique used to wean patients from mechanical support has been the subject of great interest in an attempt to select the best method used to wean. PSV, SIMV or a t-piece have been prospectively compared for weaning in 109 patients according to a defined protocol. The patients were randomly allocated into the three modes of ventilation and studied over a 21-day period. Many of the patients were unlikely to wean (f/Vt > 80), and all the patients adhered to a rigorously controlled protocol-driven assessment. Patients ventilated with PSV were more likely to be weaned. PSV-ventilated patients were also less likely to remain on ventilation, weaning duration was shorter, and the total length of time on ICU was reduced. This contrasts with the findings in patients who were weaned over a shorter period of time (6 days). In this study, daily t-piece breathing was associated with less time spent on mechanical support. On the basis of this current research, patients who are likely to wean within a week would appear to be better breathing on a t-piece circuit, whereas patients who wean over a number of weeks may be more effectively weaned with PSV.

BIBLIOGRAPHY

Brochard L, Rauss A, Benito S et al. Comparison of three methods of gradual withdrawal from ventilatory support during weaning from mechanical ventilation. American Journal of Respiratory and Critical Care Medicine 1994; 150:896–903

Esteban A, Frutos F, Tobin MJ et al. A comparison of four methods of weaning patients from mechanical ventilation. Spanish Lung Failure Collaborative Group. New England Journal of Medicine 1995; 332:345–350

Marini JJ, Smith TC, Lamb V. Estimation of inspiratory muscle strength in mechanically ventilated patients: measurement of maximum inspiratory pressure. Journal of Critical Care 1988; 1:32–38

Yang KL, Tobin MJ. A prospective study of indexes predicting the outcome of trials of weaning from mechanical ventilation. New England Journal of Medicine 1991; 324:1445–1450

31

INDEX